Kamran M. Riaz • G. Vike Vicente • Daniel Wee
Editors

Optics for the New Millennium

An Absolute Review Textbook

Springer

Editors
Kamran M. Riaz
Dean McGee Eye Institute
University of Oklahoma
Oklahoma City, OK, USA

G. Vike Vicente
Clinical Pediatrics and Ophthalmology
Georgetown University Hospital
Washington, DC, USA

Daniel Wee
Center for Sight
Stockton, CA, USA

Eye Doctors of Washington
Chevy Chase, MD, USA

ISBN 978-3-030-95250-1 ISBN 978-3-030-95251-8 (eBook)
https://doi.org/10.1007/978-3-030-95251-8

This Springer imprint is published by the registered company Springer Nature Switzerland AG
The registered company address is: Gewerbestrasse 11, 6330 Cham, Switzerland

Foreword

I have news for optics lovers and opticsphobes (my nomination for the 2022 word of the year): this is a new book on this topic. Some will be excited by this news; (most) others will bemoan it. In fact, all should welcome it, rush to buy it, and keep it handy for easy study and reference.

Nothing is more fundamental to our field than optics. It's everywhere, starting of course with the eye itself, but including glasses, contacts, prisms, lasers, slit lamp, indirect ophthalmoscope, indirect lens, cameras, goniolens, retinoscope, microscope, and, my personal favorite, intraocular lenses. A basic knowledge of optics is essential for caring for patients, and greater knowledge helps us do this even better.

Why a new book on optics? My longtime favorite optics book (if there is such a thing) is Mel Rubin's *Optics for Clinicians,* and Benjamin Milder and Rubin's companion piece *The Fine Art of Prescribing Glasses without Making a Spectacle of Yourself.* Both books make optics understandable for us nonphysicists, and they do so with elegant explanations and a warm sense of humor. However, both are outdated in that there is so much new material that is central to ophthalmic practice.

This three-part volume is elegantly organized as an educational and clinically practical resource. Part I emphasizes the basics: what one needs to study for written board exams. Part II deals with topics for preparing for oral boards. But don't be fooled: each is full of practical information of great value in the clinic. Examples are superb chapters on astigmatism, accommodation and presbyopia, and prisms in Part I, and on refraction pearls, contact lenses, vision testing, and, for those wait-listed for their SpaceX flight, vision in zero gravity.

The third part concerns optics related to surgery, and it is a wonderful compendium of all kinds of practical information: biometry, corneal measurements, IOL calculations, postoperative optical issues, and optics of refractive surgery, and it includes a chapter listing all available IOLs, yes, all in one place.

These parts are long, which is a good thing. Each chapter stands alone as a superb resource on its topic. Each part can serve as a study guide to be read for the task at hand (written or oral boards, surgical optics), or one can peruse an individual chapter to get a detailed but eminently readable discussion on nearly any topic in ophthalmic optics.

Optics for the New Millennium is clearly written, elegantly illustrated, and full of that same warm humor that Mel Rubin employed, updated to 2022. Drs. Riaz, Vicente, and Wee have pulled off the huge challenge of providing a wealth of information with a highly entertaining presentation. Read a chapter, and you will be hooked.

Houston, TX, USA
12/4/2021

Douglas D. Koch
Professor and Allen, Mosbacher
and Law Chair in Ophthalmology
Cullen Eye Institute, Baylor College of Medicine

Preface

Perhaps the best way for me to start this book would be with an anecdote: as a distracted medical student, I often found time (and excuses) to read books outside of medicine. In college, I majored in Middle Eastern History, and I continued to read books related to this subject during medical school. I came across a fascinating work, *The Book of Optics* (*Kitāb al-Manāẓir*), by Ibn al-Haytham (965–1039), an Egyptian polymath referred to as "the father of modern optics." In this text, the author detailed many Optics subjects, including the camera obscura, intromission theory, refraction, and reflection. He described the first real appreciation of the action of a convex lens to produce a magnified image of an object - perhaps a precursor to the dreaded U+D=V equations now studied by ophthalmology trainees. In this seven volume work, he famously contradicted the prevailing theories of Euclid and Ptolemy, which stated that vision occurs because of rays of light emanating from the human eye; instead, he correctly asserted that rays originate from the viewed object and pass into the eye. I was hooked. Reading this medieval Optics textbook was my "a-ha" moment: I knew I wanted to become an ophthalmologist.

Perhaps the best way for me to continue this introduction would be an admission. Despite my initial enthusiasm before residency, I hated Optics as a first-year resident. Like many residents, I found Optics to be abstruse, boring, and unimportant – instead, I thought to myself: *Who cares about this silly incoming light ray and whether it refracts, diffracts, or reflects? How will that help my patient with this dense cataract see again*? And like many trainees, I didn't care to study it much during that first year and instead focused on learning "real" ophthalmology conditions with vision-threatening implications. Unsurprisingly, on my first-year in-service exam, I got a 10th percentile in Optics. Perhaps my score shouldn't have been so surprising…

After I received my score, I thought to myself, *while I am not the most intelligent person in the world, this subject can't be impossible to learn*. I realized that the "joy" of Optics that led me to ophthalmology had been lost somewhere along the way. Unfortunately, there weren't many subject resources written for people like myself: people with limited brain cells who ultimately wanted to know and appreciate *why* they should care about Optics. I took it upon myself as a challenge: I wanted to (painstakingly and patiently) read every Optics resource available and teach myself the subject in a way that made sense to me. In my last year of training, I was fortunate to have my good friend, Daniel Wee, MD, teach our ophthalmology residency program Optics, and I started to finally understand Geometric Optics. Shortly after that, I came across a series of outstanding Optics lectures by my other good friend Vike Vicente, MD, especially regarding Clinical Optics and Refraction. Both of these finally made the subject matter understandable to me.

When I began to teach Optics to my junior colleagues, I wanted to distill what I learned into something beneficial to the next generation of ophthalmologists. Therefore, I adopted a teaching style that maintained the academic integrity of the subject matter, but also heavily incorporated clinical relevance, surgical applicability, and plenty of humor – mainly to keep my students awake! Over the years, numerous residents and course attendees encouraged me to write a text, presented in my teaching style, that combined all the knowledge of Optics needed for certification exams and clinical/surgical practice into a one-stop-shop text. While many excellent Optics resources are available, I could not find a single, comprehensive resource that combined all of this Optics material into a single textbook with sufficient practice questions that could be used during training and in practice, especially one written in a manner and style that could educate and engage readers.

In September 2019, I finally decided to attempt this ambitious (and slightly audacious) plan to create such a work. I also knew that I could not accomplish this on my own, especially not while maintaining a busy cornea and refractive surgery academic practice. I reached out to Vike and Danny to see if they would be interested (and crazy enough) to join me on this challenging (and perhaps Quixotic) project to write such a book – an optics textbook for the new millennium. Amazingly they were crazy enough to agree. Their contributions to this project go beyond simply writing words and drawing images – while many words can be said regarding how thankful I am to both of them for saying yes, I can say with all sincerity that this work would have never been possible without their agreeing to be my partners in crime. Since this book is our group effort, I will now intentionally switch from the first-person singular tense into a first-person plural tense for the rest of these opening comments.

What we present here is a textbook that embodies our teaching philosophy toward Optics: through our irreverence, we hope to show our reverence for the subject matter so that our students will similarly appreciate how Optics permeates every facet of ophthalmology and learn something along the way. We want our readers to learn Optics to pass their certification exams but, more importantly, to deliver excellent care to their patients. Thus, while there are many tongue-in-cheek jokes and humor (liberally) sprinkled throughout the text, we have not sacrificed the scientific accuracy of the material. While it may also seem that this book is meant to entertain (which we freely acknowledge), the primary goal of our work is to educate, especially through its holistic presentation of "exam-based" and "practice-based" Optics.

In this Optics textbook, we have attempted to maintain the content found in other books historically, but we have also intentionally changed the context in which it has traditionally been presented. We want this to be a resource that trainees will use early in their careers, and one that seasoned practitioners will find useful for their day-to-day care of patients. Thus, we have intentionally made this book into a relatively large, singular compendium of Optics information. We hope that readers will find specific chapters of this "one-stop-shop" book of greater interest depending on their training level, upcoming exam preparations, and/or primer for clinical and surgical practice. Whether you are a first-year resident wanting to learn about U+D=V or an experienced practitioner wanting to know about IOL calculation formulas, we think this book is valuable for both kinds of readers – and if you read this book carefully, you will see how both U+D=V and IOL formulas are intimately connected.

We are thankful to a number of people (listed in more detail in the Acknowledgments), but perhaps, strangely enough, we are especially grateful for our health and opportunity during the Great Quarantine of 2020 during the COVID-19 pandemic to be able to dedicate time and effort toward the writing of this book. Since we did not have much to do while bunkered in our homes, we were able to have an opportunity to work on this Optics textbook. This relationship between quarantine and Optics is not a first: fittingly, the social distancing during the Great Quarantine of 1665 allowed Sir Isaac Newton to embark upon a "year of wonders," including exploring Optics and experimenting with prisms and refraction. Similarly, Ibn al-Haytham wrote his Optics magnum opus while under political quarantine (house arrest) for nearly a decade. We do not suppose our work will be nearly as influential as Newton's or Ibn al-Haytham's, but nonetheless, we whimsically observe the historical similarity of our situation 350 years later. We hope that our book is some small measure of good that comes out of this troubling time. On a more solemn note, it is also why we dedicate our work to the memory of every single human life lost during the COVID-19 pandemic worldwide.

We hope that you, dear reader, not only enjoy reading this book but can use this knowledge to better care for your patients. The knowledge that our work may help you improve the vision and lives of our fellow human beings is comforting. We hope we have continued the legacy of Ibn al-Haytham and Newton for this new millennium and a new generation of Optics enthusiasts.

Oklahoma City, OK, USA Kamran M. Riaz

Acknowledgments

Through our work, we also hope to show our admiration for our many teachers and mentors that have taught us Optics through their lectures, papers, and generous mentorship over the years. We would be remiss not to recognize some of them at the very least: David Guyton, MD, David Hunter, MD, Constance West, MD, Surendra Basti, MD, and Douglas Koch, MD. We are also profoundly grateful and thoroughly indebted to the countless students, residents, and colleagues we have met at various conferences, review courses, academic institutions, and even online, who have provided feedback, encouragement, suggestions, and criticism (constructive and otherwise!) over the years to improve our manuscript.

The following residents and trainees deserve special recognition for serving as beta-testers and providing valuable suggestions as we wrote the text. They deserve particular recognition for sacrificing valuable time during training to participate in this work:

1. Karl Becker, MD – Cook County/Stroger Hospital, Chicago, IL
2. Kristen Collister, MD – Dean McGee Eye Institute
3. David A. Murphy, MD – Dean McGee Eye Institute
4. Casey Smith, MD – University of Tennessee
5. Jacob Warmath, MD – Dean McGee Eye Institute
6. Asher Khan, MS4 – University of Oklahoma Medical School

The following colleagues similarly deserve acknowledgment for their critical review and expertise in improving the text:

1. David L. Cooke, MD – Great Lakes Eye Care, St. Joseph, MI
2. Andrew T. Melson, MD – Assistant Professor, Dean McGee Eye Institute
3. Andrew Hou, MD – Cornea Fellow, Dean McGee Eye Institute
4. Rachel M. Caywood, OD, FAAO – Dean McGee Eye Institute
5. M. Edward Wilson, MD – Medical University of South Carolina
6. Thomas Clinch, MD – Eye Doctors of Washington, MD
7. Belinda Weinberg, OD – Washington DC
8. Suleiman Alibhai, OD – Washington DC

We would also like to thank everyone at SpringerNature Publishing, especially Mariah Gumpert, Asja Rehse, and Michelle Tam for their editorial assistance with the production of this work. We also want to acknowledge Jeffrey Taub and Vinodh Thomas (and their respective teams) for proofreading and typesetting. Most publishers would have rejected and balked at the idea of this kind of textbook. Some did. Thank you for taking a chance on this crazy project.

Individually, the editors would like to thank:

I would like to thank my teachers and mentors who shared their love of optics and teaching: Dr. David Hunter, who passed a torch of teaching; Dr. Dave Guyton, who was never tired of answering my questions at conferences and emails; and Dr. Connie West, for great teaching gigs. I would like to thank my wife Wendy for supporting me, and my sons Mark and Peter for allowing me to share the magic of light and physics on the back of many napkins.

– Vike Vicente

I'd like to thank my older brother, Ray (also ophtho), for telling me to get off my butt at the end of medical school and start learning optics. It gave me a huge head start heading into my ophthalmology residency. I'd like to thank the various ophthalmology residents and attendings at the University of South Carolina, Northwestern University, and the University of Arizona for allowing me to teach. I'm extremely grateful to Kamran and Vike for inviting me to be a part of this book. Finally, I'd like to thank my wife, Lydia, and my kids, Nolan and Kyla, for their unconditional love and support.

– Daniel Wee

I am grateful to my family for their support and patience over these past two years, especially my wife, Sanaa, and my three kids, Rabiyah, Nabeel, and Zaynab, for giving me the time, freedom, and encouragement (along with peace and quiet) to embark upon, continue, and finish this laborious project. I am also thankful to the wonderful folks at the Osler Institute for allowing me to teach at the written and oral board review courses. They took a chance on a novice lecturer in 2015 and allowed me to develop my teaching style while helping hundreds of my colleagues pass their certification exams. I suppose I should also be thankful to several people in the world of ophthalmology who doubted my abilities, questioned if I "belonged", and actively sought to hinder my academic career. Thank you for doubting me; I have channeled that into a relentless desire to work harder and have realized that the best revenge is living well. Finally, I dedicate this work to my mother, Fahmeeda Begum, MD, who initially matched into ophthalmology but decided she wanted something more challenging and had a brilliant career as an endocrinologist. You are the reason why I chose my career path so that someday I could be as fractionally good, as a clinician and as a person, as you.

– Kamran Riaz

Contents

Contributors

Shehzad Y. Batliwala, DO Department of Ophthalmology, Dean McGee Eye Institute, Oklahoma City, OK, USA

Kamran M. Riaz, MD Dean McGee Eye Institute, University of Oklahoma, Oklahoma City, OK, USA

J. Scott Samples, NCLE-AC Contact Lens, Dean McGee Eye Institute, Oklahoma City, OK, USA

Dean McGee Eye Institute, University of Oklahoma, Oklahoma City, OK, USA

G. Vike Vicente Clinical Pediatrics and Ophthalmology, Georgetown University Hospital, Washington, DC, USA

Eye Doctors of Washington, Chevy Chase, MD, USA

Daniel Wee, MD Center for Sight, Stockton, CA, USA

Part I

Ophthalmic Optics for Written Exams

Geometric Optics

Kamran M. Riaz

Objectives

- To define and understand terminology used in Geometric Optics regarding:
  - Path of light rays
  - Index of refraction
  - Divergent, parallel, and convergent light rays
- To define, understand, and give clinical examples of:
  - Refraction
    - Distortion and dispersion
  - Reflection (including total internal reflection)
  - Diffraction

Introduction

When we consider Ophthalmic Optics as a universe, we can imagine the various types of optics, such as Geometric Optics, Physical Optics, and Quantum Optics, as different planets within this universe. If you have seen the movie *Interstellar (2014)*, then you may remember how each planet has its unique rules and circumstances. For example, time runs differently on the water planet and gravity functions differently on the ice planet.

When studying Ophthalmic Optics for the purposes of written examinations, we will spend the majority of our time in the world of Geometric Optics. There are several rules we must follow and several assumptions that we will make on this planet, the foremost being that light travels in straight lines (linear rays) (Fig. 1).[1] This is also referred to as a "pencil" of light rays, even though no actual pencil that you can write with exists. The principles we will discuss in this chapter will allow us to later discuss other topics, such as prisms, lenses, and mirrors.

Finally, given the amount of time we will spend on this world, it may also feel like we will age 20 years while doing Geometric Optics.

We will also make several other assumptions that we will point out as we discuss additional topics.

Light Rays in Geometric Optics

A reality on this planet of Geometric Optics is that these linear light rays do not like each other: They are naturally *divergent (mathematically represented as having negative vergence)*, trying to get away from their neighbors as fast as

[1]Chaps. 1-13 "Geometric Optics", "Prisms in Ophthalmic Optics", "Lenses", "Mirrors and Combined Systems", "Power of Lenses in Different Media", "Lens Effectivity", "Schematic Eye", "Magnification and Telescopes", "Accommodation and Presbyopia", "Spherocylindrical Lenses", "Astigmatism", "Glasses for Written Exams", and "Contact Lenses for Written Exams" of this book will primarily discuss principles within Geometric Optics. Chap. 14, "Physical Optics", will discuss light in other forms, such as waves and particles. Quantum electrodynamics, which is the most comprehensive theory of light, unifying macroscopic and microscopic properties of light, is (thankfully) beyond the scope of this book.

K. M. Riaz (✉)
Dean McGee Eye Institute, University of Oklahoma, Oklahoma City, OK, USA

K. M. Riaz et al. (eds.), *Optics for the New Millennium*, https://doi.org/10.1007/978-3-030-95251-8_1

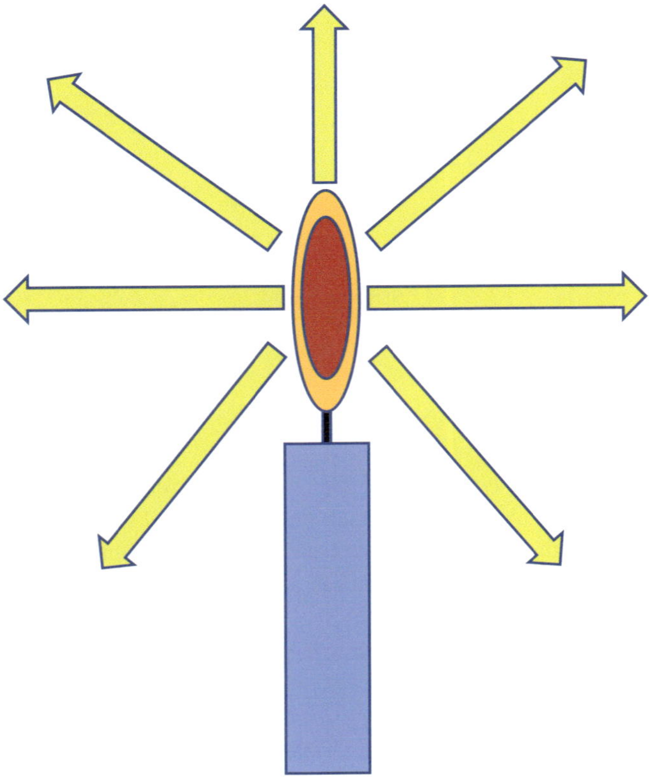

Fig. 1 Light travels in linear rays in all directions in the world of Geometric Optics

they can.[2] However, if we operated with this understanding, then we could not solve any Geometric Optics problems (which you might argue is a wonderful thing), so therefore we have to make another assumption: These divergent light rays are also *parallel* (when originating from an extremely far away distance, which we refer to as "infinity"), which is an assumption we will make when we solve problems, such as object–lens systems and Prentice's Rule type of problems.

Another assumption we will make is that light rays will always travel from "left" to "right" when we draw these problems out. As seen in the candle light figure above, light travels in all directions, but for now, we will draw out most problems with light rays coming in from the left side of the diagram. However, the paths of light rays are reversible, and we will sometimes need to do this to understand why images form in a particular location, for example.

Finally, when linear light rays get affected by an external source (e.g., a plus power lens), then some of these light rays are considered to be *convergent (mathematically represented as having positive vergence)* (Fig. 2). For completeness, external sources may also cause parallel rays to diverge, such as when light rays pass through a minus-powered lens. We can see all three types of light rays when a pencil of light encounters an aperture (Fig. 2).

When light rays are traveling along peacefully in a medium, they may do one of the above three actions. However, when they encounter an object, one or more things may occur:

- Refraction
  - Distortion
  - Dispersion
- Reflection
- Absorption
- Diffraction
- Scattering
- Polarization

For our purposes in this chapter, we will further discuss the first four of the above concepts in the next sections. Discussions pertaining to diffraction, scattering, and polarization can be found in Chap. 14, Physical Optics.

Refractive Index

Light rays will always travel the fastest in a vacuum (approximately 300,000,000 m/s). We can compare this speed to other common materials, such as water, aqueous, and the crystalline lens. The refractive index (n) is simply the ratio of the speed of light in a vacuum compared to the speed of light in a given material. Since light travels faster in a vacuum, n is always >1.

We will discuss how changing the index of refraction can affect the power of lenses in Chap. 5.

Refraction

Refraction simply means that when light rays pass from one medium into another medium, the original path of traveling gets bent in a different direction. Technically, there is also a change in direction in waves as they pass from one medium into another, accompanied by a change in speed and wavelength of the light ray. We are simplifying this phenomenon and rebranding this as "bending of light rays." The quality and quantity of this bending depend on several factors, such as the type of medium (index of refraction) and the surface or barrier that the light ray encounters (e.g., a converging lens vs. a diverging lens).

Snell's Law of Refraction is a valuable tool to quantify how strongly a ray of light is refracted (bent) when passing from one material to another. In other words, this law will give us information about the angle at which an incoming

[2] In other words, light rays are good at practicing social distancing guidelines.

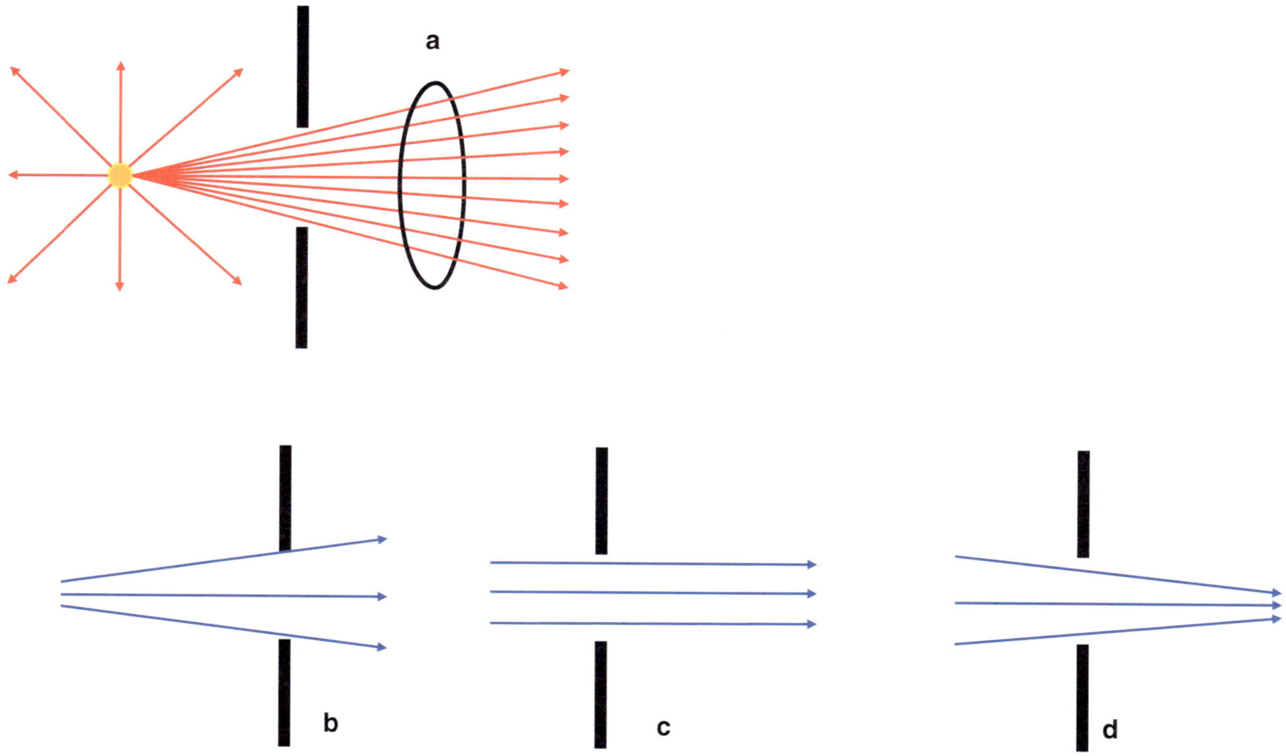

Fig. 2 Panel **a** shows a pencil of light rays as it approaches an opening. At the opening, three different kinds of light rays may be seen: divergent light rays (Panel **b**), parallel light rays (Panel **c**), and convergent light rays (Panel **d**)

light ray, after passing through the medium, exits that particular medium. Snell's Law is defined as follows:

$$n \sin\phi = n' \sin\phi'.$$

The above equation simply states that if we know the 1) index of refraction of the first medium (*n*), 2) the angle at which the light ray strikes the medium (ϕ), and 3) the index of refraction of the second medium (*n*'), then we can determine the angle at which the light ray will exit the medium (ϕ'). Of course, we can also solve any of the four variables used in the above equation if we have information about the other three variables.

At this point, you may be freaking out because the above equation brings back awful memories of high school geometry and scientific calculators! The good news is that you will never be asked to calculate this equation – remember that you will not be given access to a calculator for exams, so no one will ever expect you to do this trigonometry math in your head.

Instead, we can focus on the critical lessons from Snell's Law. One lesson is that light rays that travel from a lower refractive index medium (e.g., air, n = 1.0) into a higher refractive index medium (e.g., water, n = 1.33) will refract (be bent) *toward* the norm. The norm is an artificially constructed line perpendicular to the interface between the two mediums, as seen in Fig. 3. A second lesson is that light rays that travel through a medium of higher refractive index and then encounter a medium of a lower refractive index will be bent *away* from the norm.

The take-home message from Snell's Law is that with an increasing difference between two indices of refraction of two mediums, there will be an increasing amount of refraction when a light ray passes from a medium of lower index of refraction through a medium of higher index of refraction.

Refraction not only occurs throughout Geometric Optics but also has clinical relevance. Spherical eyeglasses and prisms used to quantify strabismus are two examples of refraction used in clinical practice. These topics will be discussed in greater detail in their respective sections.

Two other concepts are related to refraction: *distortion* and *dispersion*.

Distortion refers to the *visual perception of an observer* to refracted light rays. We can see the effects of distortion when a straw is placed in a glass of water (Fig. 4). To an observer, the image of the straw *above* the water appears to be different than the image seen *below* the water. This "distortion" is how the observer has perceived the refraction occurring at the air-water interface.

A classic example often used in many optics textbooks is the "fisherman scenario." The unfortunate fisherman is usually standing at the edge of a pier (or rock) with a spear (why a spear, why not a fishing rod and line or even a net like a normal person?) and sees a fish in the water. Whereas you, dear reader, may need to know optics to pass your examinations, he must rely on his knowledge of optics so that he can catch his dinner (Fig. 5).

The question that is typically asked in this scenario is as follows: *Where must the fisherman throw his spear to hit the fish?* This question also assumes the fisherman is a world-

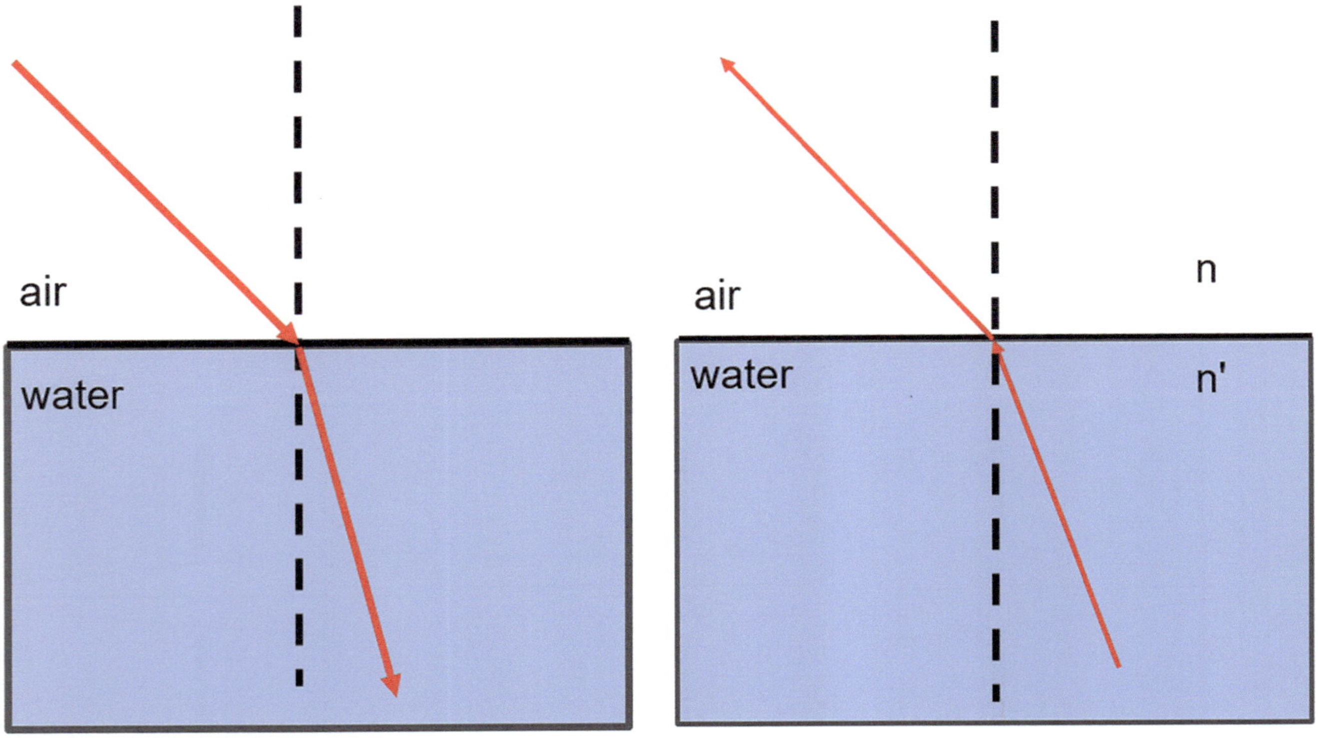

Fig. 3 Light rays entering a material with a higher refractive index will be bent *toward* the norm (left panel). Light rays entering a material with a lower refractive index will be bent *away* from the norm (right panel)

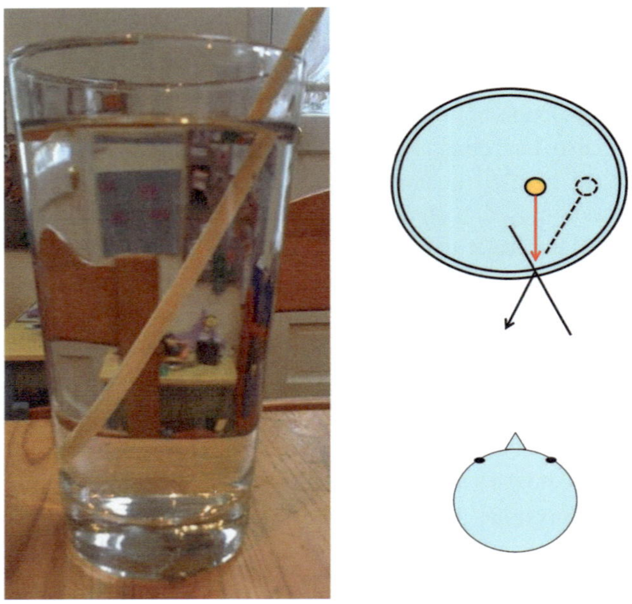

Fig. 4 Principle of distortion. To an observer, the refraction that occurs at the air–water interface will cause the image of the straw above the water to appear different than the image of the straw below the water (left panel). From a bird's eye view (right panel), due to the higher index of refraction, light rays (red arrow) emanating from the object (the straw) will reach the air–water interface and will bend away from the normal. This causes the rays to appear to be coming from further to the right (left panel)

class swimmer and diver because he then has to find his speared fish in the water, but no one ever seems to ask these important details on examinations.

Usually, you will be given several options in regards to where the fisherman should throw his spear (Fig. 5):

- In front of the fish (relative to the fisherman)—i.e., to the left of the fish (the "left" is relative to you as the reader observing the diagram) (Choice A).
- Directly at the fish—i.e., at the exact spot in the water where he sees the fish (Choice B).
- Behind the fish (relative to the fisherman)—i.e., to the right of the fish (the "right" is relative to you as the reader observing the diagram) (Choice C).

The key to solving this problem is to recall your knowledge of the previous discussion. Since light rays emanating from the fish will strike the water–air interface, they are going from a medium of higher refractive index into one with a lower refractive index. Since these light rays will refract (bend) away from the normal, for the fisherman, the actual fish will be "in front" (i.e., to the left to you as the reader looking at the diagram) of where he is "seeing it." Therefore, if he wants to catch his dinner, he must use this knowledge of optics and throw his spear at point A (Fig. 6).

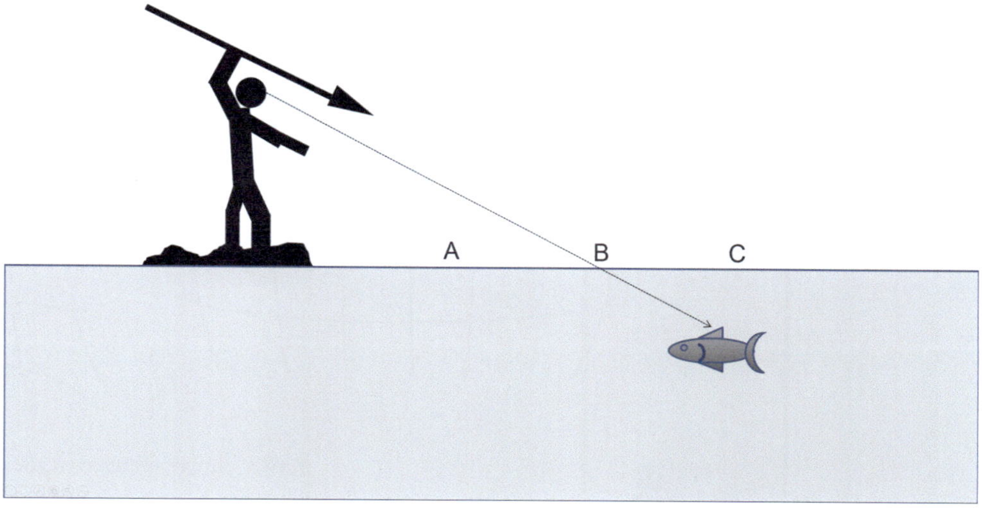

Fig. 5 The fisherman is hungry for his dinner. The image of the fish is what the fisherman sees. Where is the real fish? Should the fisherman aim at A, B, or C?

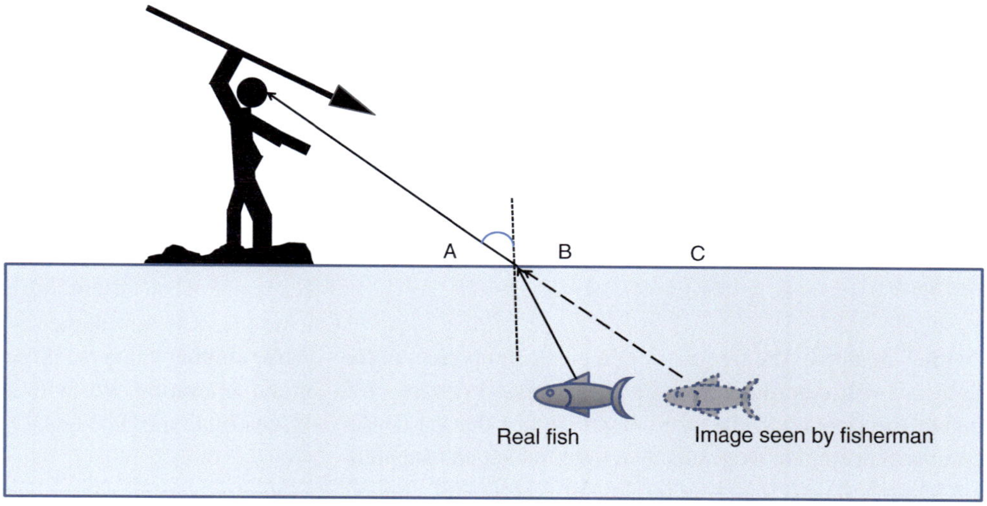

Fig. 6 The fisherman catches his dinner, and you score a few points in optics. The fisherman should aim at A. Light rays coming from the real fish will refract (bend) away from the norm as they enter air (a medium with a lower index of refraction). From the fisherman's point of view, the image will appear to be coming from *behind* the fish

He should also tie a rope to his spear so that it is easily retrievable from the water without diving into the lake.

Technically, distortion is a subset of optical aberrations, which will be discussed later, but it may be helpful to understand some elementary principles of this concept under the discussion of refraction.

One clinically relevant area (also relevant for test purposes) is the concept of *barrel distortion* and *pincushion distortion*, which occur with minus lenses and plus lenses, respectively. You can remember this with the mnemonic *p*lus lens = *p*incushion distortion. We will discuss the differences between plus and minus lenses later, but for now, you should know that the edge of a plus or minus lens is very different from the optical center of the lens. Specifically, a minus lens is much *thicker* at the edges (compared to the center), and a plus lens is much *thinner* at the edges (compared to the center). Therefore, light rays that pass through the edge of each of these lenses will be refracted differently than light rays that pass through the center of the lens.

For minus lenses, because the edge of the lens is thicker than the center, image magnification will decrease further away from the optical center, such that the image at the edge of a minus lens will appear to have been "wrapped" around a sphere or a barrel ("barrel distortion") (Fig. 7). For plus lenses, image magnification will increase further away from the optical center, such that the image of the edge of a plus lens will appear to be stretched out toward the periphery ("pincushion distortion") (Fig. 7). We will discuss this topic in greater detail in the section on troubleshooting glasses in patients (see Chap. 16, "Construction of Glasses: Ophthalmologists as Opticians").

Dispersion occurs whenever light rays undergo refraction. Specifically, dispersion refers to the change in the angle of refraction of the individual colors of light that comprises a

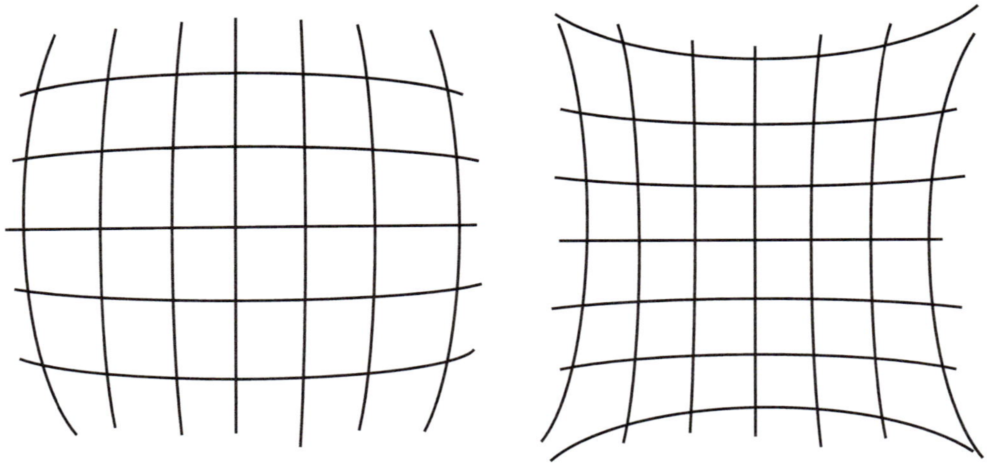

Fig. 7 An observer looking through a high-powered minus lens may report a barrel distortion (left panel), whereas an observer looking through a high-powered plus lens may report a pincushion distortion (right panel). Remember, plus lens = pincushion distortion

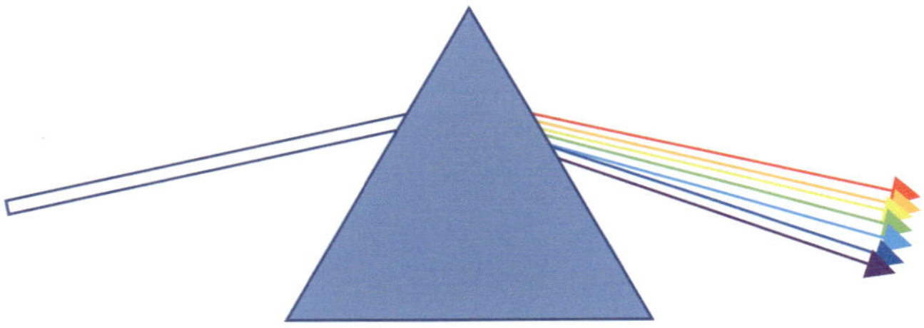

Fig. 8 Dispersion: When a light ray gets refracted, its individual colors will also get refracted according to the frequency of that particular color. Therefore, blue light rays will be dispersed more than red light rays. This concept is a foundation for understanding *chromatic aberration*

"white" light ray. The frequency of a given component of the light ray will determine how much dispersion occurs—the higher the frequency, the more dispersion of that particular color will occur. For example, blue light, which has the highest frequency (and therefore the lowest wavelength), undergoes the most refraction (bending), whereas red light undergoes the least. A useful mnemonic to remember is that **b**lue light rays will get **b**ent the most, whereas **r**ed light rays are **r**arely bent (Fig. 8). This principle is a useful foundation for understanding the more clinically and surgically relevant concept of *chromatic aberration*, which will be discussed in Chap. 14, "Physical Optics".[3]

If blue text and red text are both placed against a dark or black background, then an interesting phenomenon known as *chromostereopsis* occurs. This visual illusion causes the brain to perceive depth when viewing a two-dimensional color image, usually blue-red images. Chromatic aberration effects will cause the brain to view the red portion of the text/image as "closer" to you as the observer than the blue.

Remember that the "red" rays normally land "behind" the retina, and the "blue" rays normally land "in front of" the retina. Since we have to accommodate (generate plus power) in order to see any red text (since usually, those light rays will fall behind the retina), when both red and blue text are placed side by side, the brain will have to accommodate in order to see the red and then relax accommodation to see the blue text. As a result, the brain will falsely think that the red text is closer than the blue text!

Every material has an amount of dispersion known as the *Abbe number (aka the V-number)*. The higher the Abbe number, the lower the chromatic aberration in that particular material and vice versa. Chromatic aberration has clinical relevance when discussing the construction of glasses. For example, it is advantageous to use lens materials with high Abbe number values to minimize the adverse effects of chromatic aberration. We will discuss this further in Chap. 16, "Construction of Glasses: Ophthalmologists as Opticians".

Reflection

We can begin our discussion on reflection by first introducing this concept with a plano (flat, not curved) mirror, such as the one you used this morning while brushing your teeth and preparing yourself to study Geometric Optics.[4] In a plano mirror, every single incoming light ray is "bounced back" away from the mirror's surface; none of the incoming light rays are "refracting" through the mirror (and into the wall). Think of reflection as the term used to describe how some incoming light rays will *bounce back from the optical interface*.

As discussed in the previous section, some light rays will be refracted when they encounter an optical interface. However, some of the light rays will also be reflected, as in the case of the plano mirror. We can be a bit more sophisticated than simply stating reflection is the "bouncing" back

[3]When incoming light encounters water molecules, for example, dispersion *and* scattering help explain why the colors of the rainbow form. We will discuss scattering more in Chap. 14, "Physical Optics".

[4]See Chap. 4 "Mirrors and Combined Systems" for a more detailed discussion of mirrors, including plano and curved mirrors.

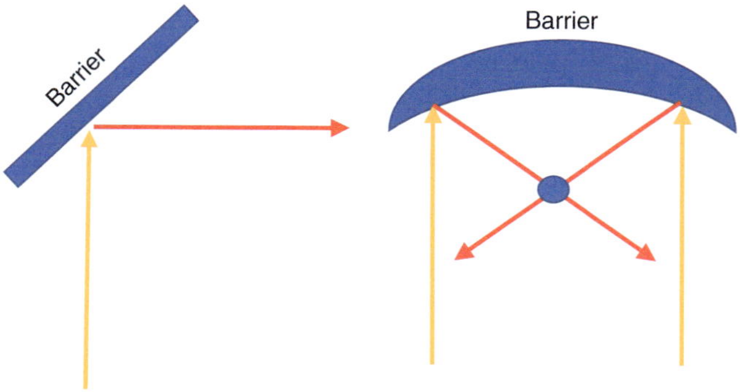

Fig. 9 Reflection. An incident light ray (yellow arrow) will bounce off the barrier (reflection) at an angle equal to the incoming angle (left panel). Reflected light rays (red arrows) from opposite angles may converge at a location known as the *focal point* (blue dot right panel)

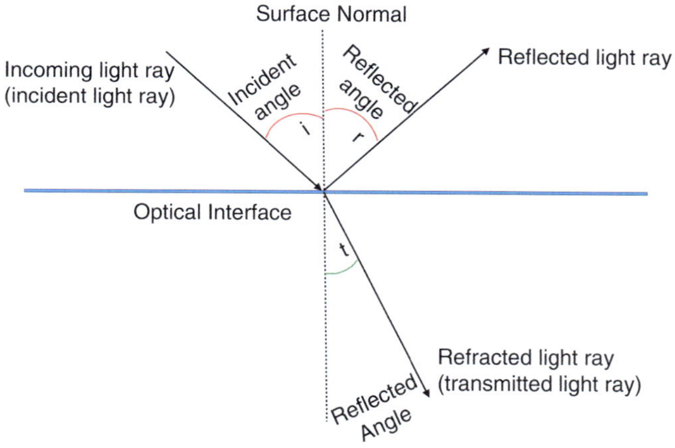

Fig. 10 Whenever reflection occurs at an optical interface (e.g., air–water), light rays that are reflected (θ*r*) will have the same outgoing angle as the incoming angle of the incoming light ray (θ*i*). The refracted (transmitted) light ray (θ*t*) will have an outgoing angle *less* than the incoming angle if the second medium is denser than the first

$$R = \left(\frac{n_2 - n_1}{n_2 + n_1} \right)^2$$

Fig. 11 This scary-looking equation, known as the reflection coefficient, can be used to calculate the amount of light reflected at an optical interface. Believe it or not, it actually has some clinical relevance when understanding topics such as dysphotopsias!

action of incoming light rays: reflection refers to the change in direction of light rays such that the angle at which incident light rays approach a medium will equal the angle at which they reflect away from the medium (Fig. 9). The second medium is essentially a barrier through which light rays cannot penetrate. In other words, when light rays approach a barrier and instead of passing through (refraction), they bounce off the barrier (reflection). Depending on the barrier's geometry reflected light rays from opposite angles will then converge at a single location known as the *focal point* (Fig. 9).

Furthermore, there are two different types of reflection that you may wish to know. *Specular reflection* is when light reflects in a single direction (as seen in clinical practice when using specular reflection as an illumination strategy during slit-lamp examination), and *diffuse reflection*, wherein light reflects in many directions off a given barrier.

The law of reflection states that the incident ray (incoming ray) and the reflected ray (outgoing ray) will lie in the same plane as the surface normal, which means *both rays* will have the *same angle* with respect to the surface normal (Fig. 10). We can compare the angle of reflection to the previously discussed angle of refraction (transmission).

Why do we care about this? The amount of light reflected from a surface is related to the incoming angle and the two media. We can use the *reflection coefficient* to calculate the amount of light transmitted at an optical interface during reflection as follows (Fig. 11)

Do the previous discussions on refraction and reflection have any clinical relevance? Yes.

One area of clinical relevance is the recent interest in the phenomenon of dysphotopsias after cataract surgery. While this will be discussed in further detail in the section on post-cataract surgery (Chap. 29, "Postoperative Optics for Cataract Surgery"), one potential contributing factor toward dysphotopsias may be explained by Snell's Law of Refraction. The index of refraction for most of the popularly used acrylic IOLs ($n = 1.47$–1.55) is significantly higher than the index of refraction of aqueous ($n = 1.33$). Interestingly, dysphotopsias are almost never seen with silicone IOLs ($n = 1.39$), perhaps because there is less refraction of light as it passes from the aqueous through the silicone IOL.[5]

The concept of reflection may additionally play a role in developing dysphotopsias. For example, the reflection coefficient can help us understand one potential contributing factor to the development of dysphotopsia after cataract surgery, especially in the current age of acrylic IOLs (that have a high index of refraction). We can see this with an example comparing the amount of reflection that takes place with a silicone IOL ($n = 1.43$) and an acrylic IOL ($n = 1.55$).[6] Since the IOLs are bathed in aqueous, we will use n_1 for both IOLs as 1.33. Do not worry about solving the math here; instead, focus on the results from these calculations:

[5]Masket S, Fram NR. Pseudophakic Dysphotopsia: Review of Incidence, Cause, and Treatment of Positive and Negative Dysphotopsia. Ophthalmology. 2020 Aug 12:S0161–6420(20)30787–9.

[6]Depending on the acrylic used in popular acrylic IOLs, the index of refraction may range from 1.47 to 1.55, as per manufacturer product inserts.

$$\text{Reflection for silicone } IOL = \left[\frac{(1.43-1.33)}{(1.43+1.33)}\right]^2 = 0.001313 = 0.1313\%$$

$$\text{Reflection for acrylic } IOL = \left[\frac{(1.55-1.33)}{(1.55+1.33)}\right]^2 = 0.005835 = 0.5835\%$$

The preceding fancy math tells us that an acrylic IOL is 0.5835/0.1313 = 4.44 times more reflective than a silicone IOL. This means that up to 4 times the number of light rays that strike an acrylic IOL are reflected (away) from the IOL compared to a silicone IOL, leading to fewer light rays reaching the retina. The increased reflection may be one reason why an acrylic IOL has much higher rates of dysphotopsia (especially negative dysphotopsia) than a silicone IOL.

Critical Angle and Total Internal Reflection

When light rays encounter a barrier, both refraction and reflection will occur, based on the incident angle at which a given light ray approaches the barrier. When considering light rays that pass from a medium with higher index of refraction (e.g., water) into a medium with lower index of refraction (e.g., air), the concept of the *critical angle* states that when incident light rays approach a barrier at any angle *less* than the critical angle, these light rays will get *refracted*—i.e., they will pass through the medium, get bent, and emerge on the other side. When incident light rays approach a barrier at any angle *greater* than the critical angle, these light rays will get *reflected*—i.e., they will not pass through the medium and instead will be bent back into the original medium (Fig. 12). For the sake of completion, an incident light ray that approaches the interface with an angle that equals the critical angle will neither get refracted nor get reflected, but instead will undergo absorption (which is energy lost as heat, which is negligible for the purposes of Ophthalmic Optics and you should not waste brain cells on this any further).

Every material has its respective angle that is unique for that material. You may wish to memorize that ordinary glass has a critical angle of 41 degrees, but do not waste time knowing the values of various critical angles for different media.

Let us use a silly metaphor to drive this home further. Think of light rays as a bunch of senior high school students attempting to have a class ditch day. Those students who can approach the school exits and avoid detection by the hallway monitors at less than the critical angle will be able to escape (i.e., refraction occurs). However, those students who approach at an angle that the hallway monitors can see them will not be able to escape and will be made to stay in the school (i.e., reflection occurs).

Where is this clinically relevant? In clinical examination of the anterior chamber angle for most eyes (i.e., excluding pathologic myopes, megalocorneas, or ectatic corneas), it is impossible to visualize the anterior chamber angle because light rays that emerge from the angle are greater than the critical angle. These light rays are not refracted and instead undergo *total internal reflection* and are reflected into the anterior chamber at the *air–tear film interface*.

Gonioscopy allows us to bypass the tear film–air (1.33–1.00) interface that the emerging light rays from the anterior chamber angle cannot penetrate by creating a "water–water interface" (1.33–1.33; the lens also has an index of refraction, but for our discussion we can ignore it) when the lens is placed on the cornea (Fig. 13). Light rays from the angle are no longer reflected and instead *refracted* at this new interface, thereby reaching the examiner's eye and allowing for examination of the anterior chamber angle structures. For

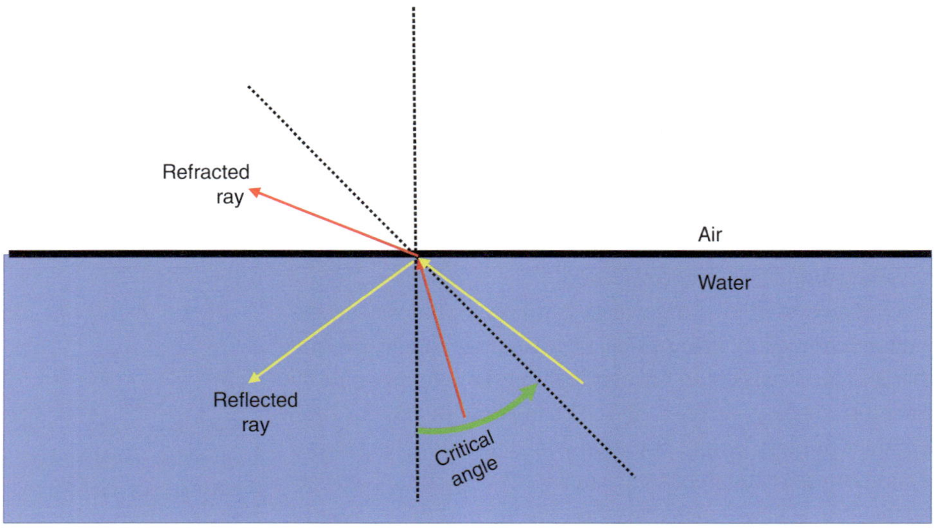

Fig. 12 Incident light rays (red arrow) that approach a barrier at an angle less than the critical angle will undergo *refraction*. Incident light rays (yellow arrow) that approach a barrier at an angle greater than the critical angle will undergo *reflection*

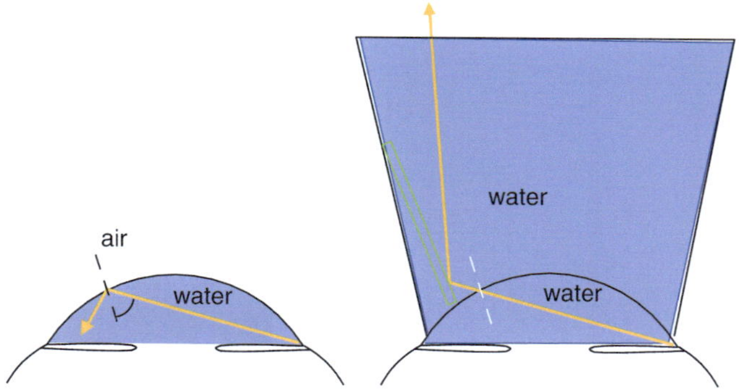

Fig. 13 Gonioscopy allows the examiner to replace the air–water interface with a water–water interface, thereby allowing light from the anterior chamber angle to undergo refraction and reach the examiner's eye

bonus points, you may wish to memorize that the critical angle between air and aqueous is approximately 48.6°.[7]

Total internal reflection is all around us—it is used in fiber-optic cables, binoculars, and even the slit-lamp. You cannot escape optics no matter how much you try.

Diffraction

Technically, diffraction does not occur in the planet of Geometric Optics, but rather in the planet of Physical Optics (Chap. 14) as it deals with light traveling in *waves*, rather than rays. However, since diffraction bears significant relevance in clinical practice, it may be helpful to discuss this concept in light of (pun-intended) the previous discussions on refraction and reflection.

In addition to refraction, reflection, and absorption, light that encounters an opening or barrier in its path will also undergo *diffraction*, which is a change in the direction of light waves to get through the opening or around the barrier (Fig. 14). The figure below shows light waves that encounter water droplets (as in a cloud): some of these waves will refract through (or reflect away from) the water droplet, but other waves will find a path around the droplet through the gaps between the droplets.

Similarly, light waves that encounter a barrier with a small opening will pass through the opening and emerge as waves (Fig. 14). This happens because some peaks of a light wave will be canceled by the trough of another wave (creating a dark spot), and some peaks of a light wave will be amplified by the peak of another light wave (creating a bright spot). As a result of this spacing, the waves that leave the slits will hit the screen at different times (and arrive at different phases).

[7]In case, an enterprising reader wants to check the math on this: sin θ = n2/n1 = 1.00/1.33 = 0.75, giving us the angle calculation of sin-1 (0.75), which is equal to 48.6°.

The amount of diffraction increases with an increasing wavelength of light and decreases with a decreasing wavelength of light. If the wavelength of the waves is smaller than the obstacle, then no noticeable diffraction occurs.

In clinical practice, diffraction occurs at the circular edges of a pupil; in other words, some of the light rays that cannot get "through" the edge of the pupil will find a way to redirect themselves to get through the pupil. When a point source of light travels through the circular pupil, the image formed on the retina is a bright central disk known as the *Airy disc* (Fig. 15).

The Airy disc will have bright and dark rings (Airy pattern). The diameter of the Airy disc can be calculated by a disgusting looking equation:

$$d = (2.44 * \lambda * D)/f$$

(d is the diameter of the disk; λ is the wavelength of light passing through the pupil; "D" is the exit pupil diameter; and "f" is the focal length of the optical system (in this case, the eye)).

If we keep "D" constant, then we can see that longer wavelengths (λ) of light (e.g., red wavelengths) will have more diffraction through the pupil as compared to shorter (e.g., yellow wavelengths) of light. Also, diffraction will limit visual acuity if a patient's pupil size is below 2.5 mm due to the Airy disk principle.

Diffraction is also applicable when discussing the *pinhole test* used in the clinical setting. When a patient looks through the pinhole, we have limited the light rays entering the eye to only those light rays that enter the eye perpendicular to the cornea and lens (i.e., we have eliminated light rays that get refracted (bent)). In theory, a very tiny pinhole would be the most effective optical opening because it would only allow unrefracted light rays to reach the eye. However, diffraction limits the effect of the pinhole because the smaller the pinhole, the greater number of unrefracted rays (proportionally) will hit the edge of the pinhole and undergo diffraction. Basically, there is a "sweet spot" for the pinhole to have the maximum effect of testing a patient's visual potential: 1.2 mm. At this diameter, the beneficial effects of the pinhole (allowing in only the unrefracted rays) will outweigh the negative effects of diffraction. If we use a smaller pinhole, then the negative effects of diffraction will outweigh the potential benefits of the pinhole. The pinhole effect also helps explain why undercorrected patients may squint to increase the number of unrefracted rays that reach their retina. Finally, we should understand that the pinhole test is only practical to assess patients' visual potential in the presence of anterior segment opacities (e.g., corneal scar, cataract) and will not be useful in the presence of retinal pathology (e.g., macular scar). See Chap. 26, "Preoperative Optics for Cataract Surgery" for more information on pinhole testing.

Fig. 14 Diffraction. Light waves may find alternate paths around a barrier (left panel) or may emerge as waves when traveling through a narrow opening within a barrier (right panel)

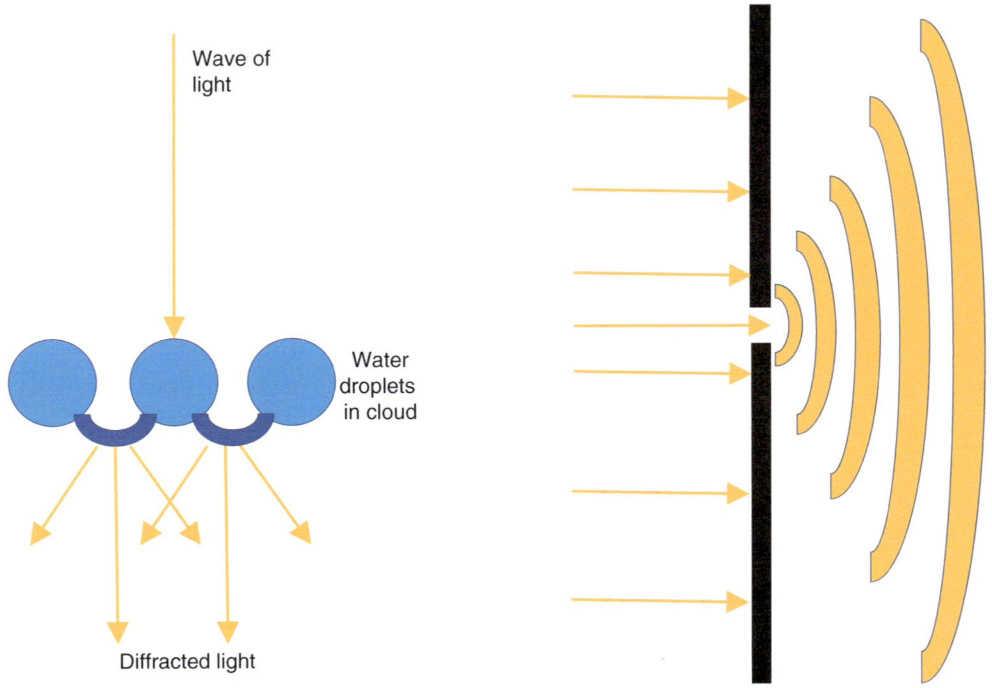

Fig. 15 The Airy disc pattern shows a series of concentric bright and dark rings formed by a point source of light passing through a circular opening (aperture)

In surgical practice, we take advantage of diffraction when we use diffractive multifocal intraocular lenses (MFIOLs). MFIOLs have microscopic steps (diffractive zones, aka "the rings") on the optic (depending on the manufacturer, these steps may be on the anterior or posterior aspect of the optic) that split incoming light toward distant and near focal points based on the height of the microscopic step. If the *step height is one wavelength*, the light that hits that step will be directed toward the *near focal point*. If the step height is a *smaller fraction of the wavelength*, light that hits that step will be directed *toward the distal focal point*. MFIOLs employ a combination of step heights (or a combination of refraction and diffraction) to split and direct incoming light and to distant, intermediate, or near focal points.[8]

Practice Questions

1. What is the critical angle when light travels from air to water?
   A. None
   B. 13.3°
   C. 28°
   D. 42.8°
   E. 56.3°

[8]Optics of MFIOLs are discussed further in Chap. 27, What Is on the Menu: An Overview of Currently Available IOLs and Relevant Optics.

2. If blue text and red text are placed side by side against a black background for an emmetropic patient, which of the following statements is true?
   A. The blue text will appear to be sharper than the red text
   B. The red text will appear to be sharper than the red text
   C. The blue text will appear to be closer to the patient than the red text
   D. The red text will appear to be closer to the patient than the blue text
3. Which of the following statements about light rays is true?
   A. Light rays that emanate from a point source of light are parallel
   B. Light rays that get affected by a lens will always be convergent
   C. Light rays that pass through an aperture will either be parallel or convergent
   D. Light rays must be affected by an external source to become convergent
4. What is the most significant refractive interface when light passes through the eye?
   A. Tear film–anterior cornea interface
   B. Air–tear film interface
   C. Anterior cornea–posterior cornea interface
   D. Posterior cornea–aqueous humor interface
5. Which of the following statements is true?
   A. Refraction describes the process wherein incoming light rays attempt to pass from one medium into another medium but instead are refracted back into the original medium.
   B. Refracted light rays will also be split according to the wavelengths of light that comprise the incoming light ray.
   C. Barrel distortion is experienced by patients who wear high-plus lenses, and pincushion distortion is experienced by patients who wear high minus lenses due to the light rays that strike the edge of the lens undergoing different amounts of refraction compared to light rays that strike the center of a given lens.
   D. The law of reflection states that the angle of the incident ray (incoming ray) is related to the angle of the reflected ray (outgoing ray) based on the index of refraction of the second medium.

Answers

1. Answer: This is somewhat of a trick question (sorry). The critical angle only occurs when light travels from a denser medium (such as water) into a less dense medium (such as air). There is no critical angle when light travels from a less dense medium into a denser one (Answer Choice A). Remember that the critical angle between air and water (aqueous) is approximately 48.6°.
2. Answer: In order to see the red text when placed side by side to blue text on a black background, the patient will have to accommodate. As a result, the patient may falsely think that the red text is actually closer (Answer Choice D). The sharpness of both the blue and red text should be about the same for an emmetropic patient.
3. Answer: Light rays that emanate from a point source of light are always divergent and must be affected by an external source (e.g., a plus lens) to become convergent (Answer Choice D). We artificially consider them parallel in the world of Geometric Optics to gain information about image location, etc. Light rays may be convergent or divergent depending on the type of lens that they pass through (positive or negative lens, respectively). When light rays pass through an aperture, all three types of light rays (divergent, parallel, and convergent) are formed.
4. Answer: The air–tear film interface is the most important refractive interface of the eye (Answer Choice B). This is a very important fact to commit to memory.
5. Answer: Dispersion occurs whenever a light ray undergoes refraction (Answer Choice B). The individual colors that comprise the light ray will also get refracted according to the frequency of that particular color. While both barrel and pincushion distortions occur due to light rays' refractive effects at the edge of a given lens, the former occurs in high-minus lenses, and the latter occurs in high-plus lenses. Remember that blue light rays will be dispersed more than red light rays.

Prisms in Ophthalmic Optics

G. Vike Vicente

Objectives

- To understand how light rays interact with prisms to form images in geometric optics and in clinical practice.
- To define and understand the concept of prism diopters.
- To apply Prentice's rule to clinical practice problems.
- To understand how prisms are used in clinical practice in a variety of settings.

Introduction

This chapter will focus (pun-intended) on prisms used in everyday ophthalmic practice. Prisms have flat transparent surfaces that refract (change the direction of) light rays. They may come in different shapes, but the most commonly encountered are prisms with triangular shapes, which allows us to have "two" refracting surfaces within the same prism. They are usually made of plastic or glass because these materials are transparent to the visible electromagnetic spectrum. Plastic prisms are much more commonly used in modern clinical practice; glass prisms are relics of days gone past.

As a side note, glass prisms are calibrated such that they are held with the frontal plane in the direction of the tropia, whereas plastic prisms are held with the frontal plane of the prism in the direction of the non-tropic eye (Fig. 1).

Prisms are usually made of a material that will have a different index of refraction depending on the wavelength that is going through it. For example, red light will move through the prism faster than blue light and thus will be refracted less. Recall that we previously discussed that the **b**lue component of light rays is **b**ent more when undergoing refraction (mnemonic: **B**lue is **bent** the most).

In 1666, Sir Isaac Newton showed that prisms can be used to disperse light into different wavelengths that can be described as the colors of the rainbow (red, orange, yellow, green, blue, indigo and violet; recall the "ROY G. BIV" mnemonic from middle school!). Previously, before Newton, it was thought that prisms would add color to white light. Using two prisms, Newton first separated the incident light into different colors. Then, he had the red light pass through a second prism showing that no further colors were added and that this second light ray remained red (Fig. 2). Amazingly, Newton is not as famous for this fascinating discovery in the world of optics; instead, he is credited for his work on gravity and modern physics—as if those things ever saved a patient from going blind!

An understanding of this principle will be helpful when discussing the concept of chromatic aberration in chapter, "Glasses in Clinical Practice" and its clinical applications, such as the Duochrome test.

Recall that when incoming light reaches a surface, some of the light rays may undergo reflection, depending on the angle of incidence. In this capacity, prisms may also be used to reflect light using the principle of total internal reflection (see Chap. 1, "Geometric Optics")

Ray Tracing and Prisms

Triangular prisms will refract a real light ray toward its base as seen by ray tracing (Fig. 3).

The light ray is first bent *toward the norm* as it enters the prism, which has a higher refractive index. The ray is then bent *away from the norm* as it exits the prism and enters a medium with a lower refractive index. The net result is that the light ray will be bent toward the base of the prism. Always remember that real light rays love the base of a prism!

G. V. Vicente (✉)
Clinical Pediatrics and Ophthalmology Georgetown University Hospital, Washington, DC, USA

Eye Doctors of Washington, Chevy Chase, MD, USA
e-mail: vvicente@edow.com

K. M. Riaz et al. (eds.), *Optics for the New Millennium*, https://doi.org/10.1007/978-3-030-95251-8_2

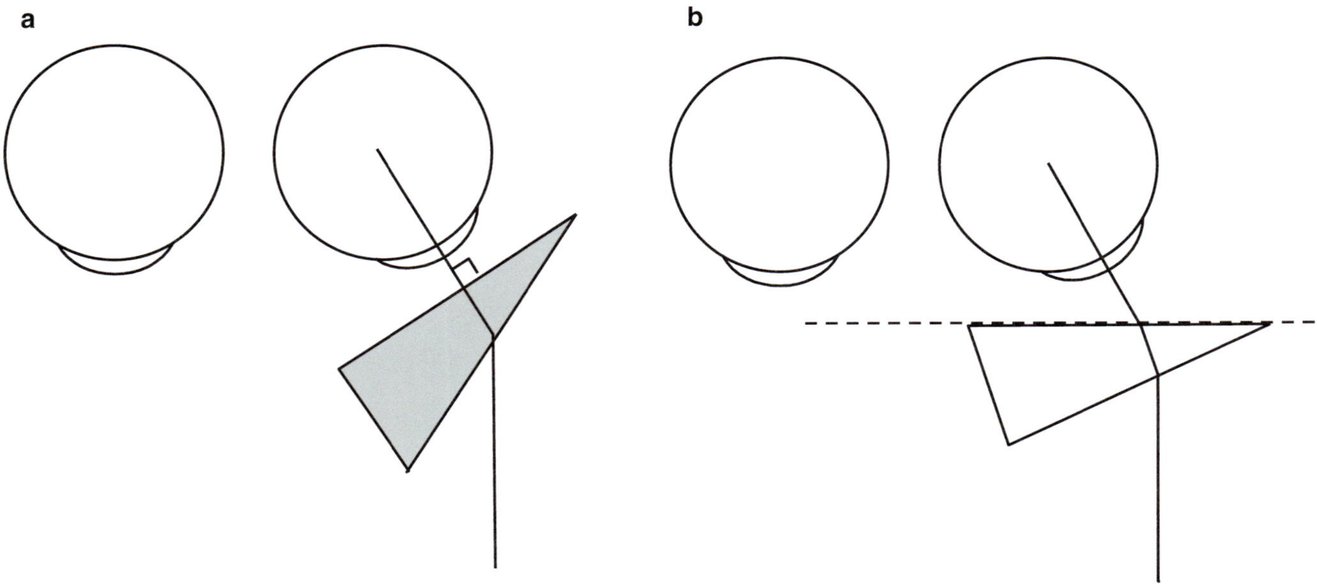

Fig. 1 Calibration of glass (**a**) vs. plastic prisms (**b**). Notice that the glass prism (**a**) is held such that the frontal plane is perpendicular to the tropic eye. The plastic prism (**b**) is held such that the frontal plane is perpendicular to the non-tropic eye

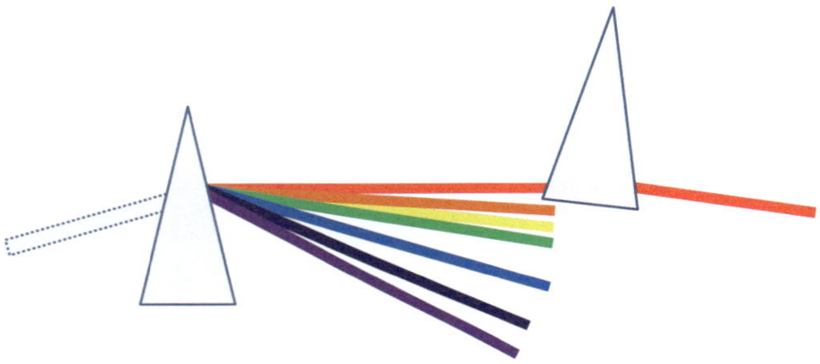

Fig. 2 Newton's experiment of refraction with prisms. Notice that after passing through a prism, a light ray may be separated (dispersed) according to its wavelengths with blue light rays undergoing the most refraction. A second prism can be placed after the first prism to demonstrate that previously refracted light ray will maintain its color because no further significant refraction according to wavelength will occur

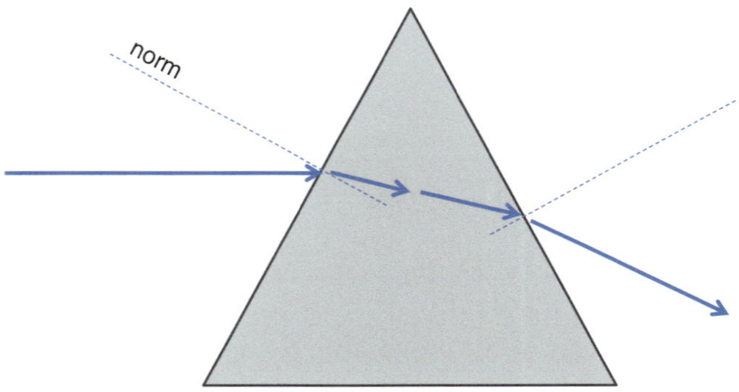

Fig. 3 A real light ray will be refracted (bent) toward the base of a prism

Prism Diopters: Definition and Quantification

The amount of refraction can be quantitated by a unit called a prism diopter (Δ or PD). The technical definition of a prism diopter is a unit describing the refraction of light by a prism equal to 100 times the tangent of the angle of refraction. Since that definition is not very useful; let us rephrase into something a bit more understandable: If a ray of light is refracted 1 cm at a distance of 1 meter from the prism, then that prism is said to have 1 $^{\Delta}$ of effect (Fig. 4). In other words, that prism has a power of 1 PD.

This is one of the few places in geometric optics where centimeters are used instead of meters in the actual definition. A common mistake made here is that many students may erroneously think that the prism causes the light ray to be shifted in millimeters; examinations will often have (wrong) answer choices that will correspond to making this mistake.

For example, a 15 $^{\Delta}$ prism will refract a ray of light 15 cm (toward its base) when measured at a distance of 1 m (Fig. 5).

The amount of refraction can be calculated by the following formula:

$$P = 100 \tan d$$

P is the strength of the prism, and d is the angle of deviation of light.

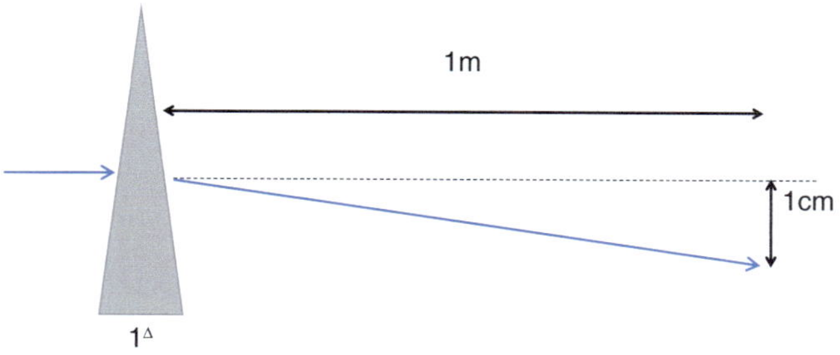

Fig. 4 Prism diopters are defined as the number of *centimeters* a light ray is refracted when measured at a distance of 1 m from a prism. The higher the strength of a prism, the greater amount of refraction will occur at 1 m

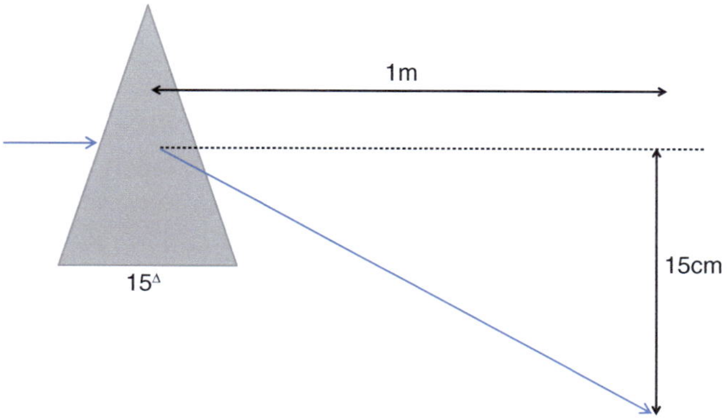

Fig. 5 A 15 Δ prism will refract a real light ray 15 cm (toward its base) when measured at a distance of 1 m to the right of the prism

Again, don't worry about memorizing this formula! We intentionally did not include it in the list of hi-yield formulas that should be committed to memory. Instead, how the relationship between the strength of the prism and amount of refraction is related through this equation is observed.[1]

Prism diopters are nonlinear. For example, a 45-degree angle is equal to 100 prism diopters. However, a 90-degree angle is equal to an infinite number of prism diopters (not 200!) (Fig. 6).

To review, a prism diopter is simply the distance an image is shifted (measured in centimeters) when measured 1 meter away from a prism. Therefore, all prism diopter problems are nothing more than similar triangle problems. Let us see some examples of how this can be tested.

Example #1 A patient with a 6th nerve palsy has an 8 Δ distance esotropia. How far apart do the images of a fixation light at 7 meters appear to the patient?

Answer: 8 Δ means that at 1 meter away from the prism, there is an 8 cm shift in the fixation light due to the prism effect. Therefore, at 7 meters, there is an 8 cm/1 m × 7 m = 56 cm prism effect. So, the images will appear 56 cm apart.

We could also set it up as a comparative triangle problem (Fig. 7).

For these types of problems, we can jump straight to the math or we can visualize it as similar triangles. As there are no "style points" on an examination, it is useful to figure out which approach is easier for you and consistently use that approach, so long as you get the right answer.

Example #2 If you are given a 20 Δ BD prism and shine a light through the prism toward a screen located 2.5 m away, where will the light ray hit the screen (Fig. 8)?

Answer: Since we have been given a 20 Δ BD prism, we know that 1 m away, the light ray will be deflected by 20 cm. Using the laws of similar triangles, we can calculate that the light ray will be deflected by 50 cm at 2.5 meters away. We also are told that this is a BD down prism, and since real light rays will be bent toward the base, the light ray will hit the screen at 50 cm inferiorly (point D). Note that answer choice A is also 50 cm, which would have been correct if the prism was a 20Δ BU prism.

Example #3 If a prism of unknown power deflects a light ray 6 cm at a distance of 50 cm, what is the power of this prism?

Answer: This problem is again testing our knowledge of similar triangles but is asking us to use this in reverse. We can solve this problem by reasoning that since this prism deflects a light ray by 6 cm at 50 cm, then we must determine how much it deflects a light ray at 100 cm (1 m).

$$\frac{6\,\text{cm}}{50\,\text{cm}} = \frac{x}{100\,\text{cm}}$$

$$50x = 600, \text{ so } x = 12\,\text{cm}$$

Therefore, this must be a 12 Δ prism.

In all three of these examples, we have seen how the same concept can be tested via three different methods.

Oblique Prisms: Vector Forces

When combining two prisms of different directions, we must consider vector effects of the prism. For example, if we place an 8 Δ base-out and an 8 Δ base-up over the left eye, and we wish to calculate the net effect of these two prisms, we have to use vector addition. This will allow us to calculate the magnitude of the vector, ignoring the direction for the time being. We cannot simply add the two prisms (8 + 8 = 16) or shortcut the math. In this case, we know that both the BO and BU prism must be accounted for, and in order to calculate the net effect of

[1]A super nerdy way of bringing together Snell's law of refraction and the concept of prism diopters can be considered here. Recall that using Snell's law, if we know the index of refraction of the two surfaces and the incoming angle, we can calculate the outgoing angle: n1 sin θ1 = n2 sin θ2. Suppose we are asked to calculate the outgoing angle (θ2), we can then calculate the strength of the prism by first calculating the difference between the incoming angle and outgoing angle (θ2 – θ1) and then taking the tan of this difference. Hopefully, this type of calculation will never appear on an examination.

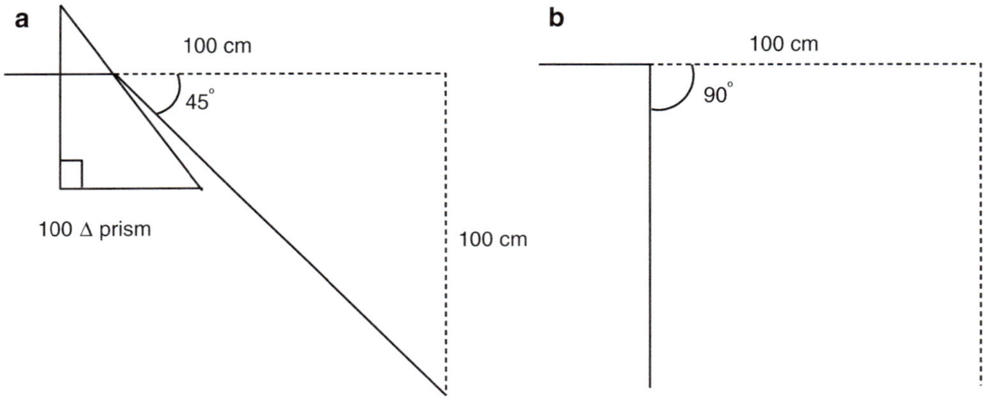

Fig. 6 Prism diopters are nonlinear: a 45-degree angle is equal to 100 prism diopters, but a 90-degree angle is equal to an infinite number of prism diopters (not 200)

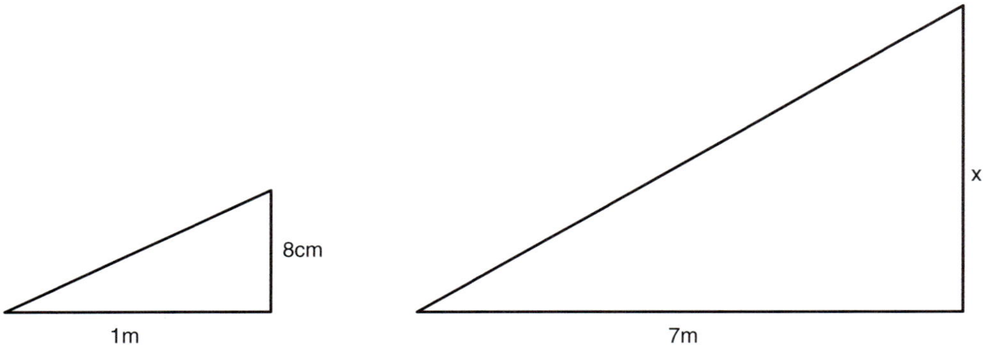

Fig. 7 Similar triangles can be used to solve for *x*

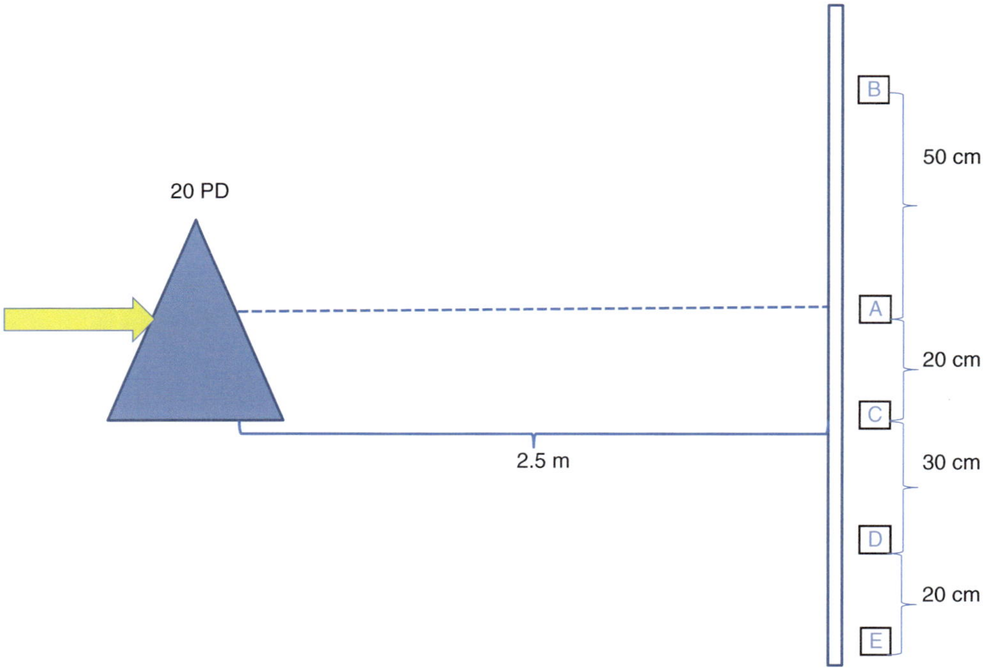

Fig. 8 Where will the light ray hit the screen?

these two prisms, we have to think back to high school geometry and recall the good ole Pythagorean theorem (Fig. 9):

$$a^2 + b^2 = c^2$$

Admittedly, the math on this problem is a bit difficult and may require a calculator:

$$a^2 + b^2 = c^2 \qquad 64 + 64 = \sqrt{128} = 11.31 \text{ prism diopters base-up and base-out effect.}$$

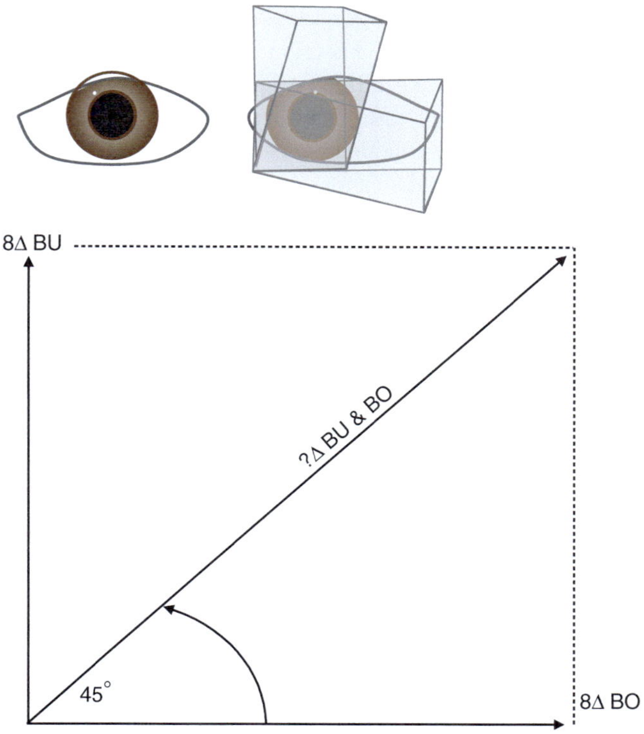

Fig. 9 When considering the vector effects of prisms of different directions and magnitude, we can use the Pythagorean theorem to calculate the value of the hypotenuse, which will be our vector force

Notice that the answer cannot be obtained by simple addition or subtraction—we can be certain that this "wrong math" will be a distractor answer choice on an examination.

We can do an example that is more likely to appear on examinations as the math involved does not require a calculator.

Example #1 If we measure a 3 PD BU and a 4 PD BO for a patient's right eye, what oblique prism would we need to prescribe for this patient? Assume we cannot prescribe anything for the left eye (Fig. 10).

Answer: We must calculate the vector forces by using the Pythagorean theorem.

$a^2 + b^2 = c^2$ $9 + 16 = \sqrt{25} = 5$ prism diopters base-up and base-out. Of course, you may have remembered that this is one of those "golden triangles" as well. Look at you, you overachiever, remembering things from high school geometry that the rest of us have forgotten!

Example #2 If we measure a 5 PD BU and 12 PD BO for the left eye, what oblique prism would we prescribe to this patient? Assume we cannot prescribe anything for the right eye.

For the sake of brevity, we will not draw out the diagram for this problem. But if you are just starting out, you can go

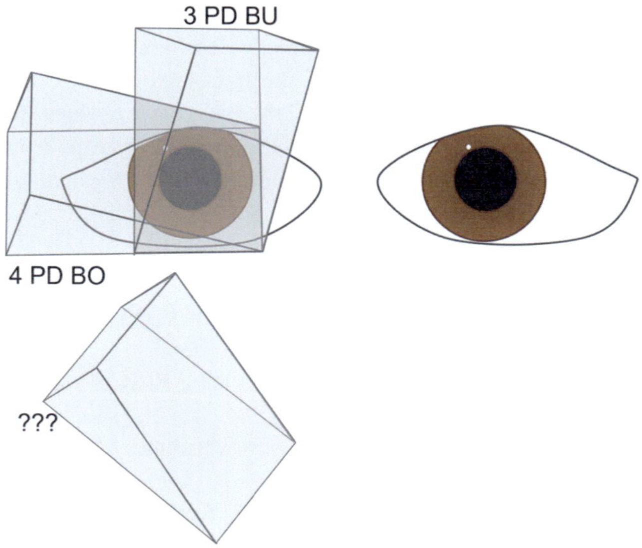

Fig. 10 An oblique prism can be used to correct this patient's double vision instead of a combination of base-up/base-down prisms

ahead and draw out the diagram of the vector forces if it helps you to visualize the problem.

$a^2 + b^2 = c^2$ $25 + 144 = \sqrt{169} = 13$ prism diopters base-up and base-out effect. Of course, you may have remembered that this also is one of those "golden triangles" as well. #Pro tip: You may want to brush up on your Pythagorean triples since test problems have a strong possibility of using golden triangle numbers since it makes for easy mental math.[2]

Effect on Real and Virtual Images

At this point, we should clarify some confusing terminology, depending on whether we are talking about prisms in optics vs prisms used in the clinical setting. This is a concept that can be very confusing if we are not careful about whether we are discussing **REAL** light rays ("Optics") or ***VIRTUAL*** light rays ("Clinical Setting").

For example, we may hear in clinical practice when using prisms that the "image goes to the apex" and the "eye goes to the base." The mnemonic "AIBE" may be helpful here to remind us that *a*pex—*i*mage, *b*ase—*e*ye. For example, for a patient with an RXT, we would place a base-in prism over the right eye to correct this deviation; as examiners, we will see the right eye appear to move "nasally" toward the base of the prism.

For ophthalmic optics, the nuance is you have to ask yourself if we are dealing with real or virtual light rays. When

[2] A few useful "Pythagorean Triples" values you may wish to memorize are the following (including multiples of these numbers): 3,4,5; 5,12,13; 8,15,17; 7,24,25; and 20,21,29.

solving optics problems, we are dealing with real light rays. When treating patients in the clinic, we are dealing with virtual light rays—this is because the light rays coming from the patient's eye are not "real," the patient's eye does not produce the light rays (unless your patient is Cyclops from the *X-Men*, in which case you should start running because his laser beams are deadly…).

Here is how we can keep them separated:

- **Real light rays** are displaced toward the **BASE** of a prism ("optics")
- **Real images** are displaced toward the **APEX** of a prism ("optics")
- **Virtual light rays** are displaced toward the **APEX** of a prism ("clinic")
- **Virtual images** are displaced toward the **BASE** of a prism ("clinic")
- The light ray that goes INTO the eye is REAL, so it is bent toward the base. For the patient, it appears that the image is coming from the apex side. The light ray coming FROM the eye (i.e., what you as the examiner see through the prism) is VIRTUAL, so those virtual light rays move toward the apex, but the image of the eye (as you as the examiner see it) moves toward the base as well.

Therefore, the "AIBE" mnemonic is a combination of the following: *Apex* is where real *images* go toward, and *base* is where the *eye (virtual image)* will go toward.

Prentice's Rule

Charles F. Prentice (an optician!) developed a formula to determine the amount of induced prism in a lens. Your one job is to know Prentice's rule equation well!

Prentice's rule determines how much deviation is present when one looks away from the optical center of a given lens. There is no prismatic power at the optical center of the lens. If everyone would only look through the optical center of their glasses, then we would never have to worry about the good Mr. Prentice's rule!

The formula for Prentice's rule, which you must commit to memory, is as follows:

$$P = \Delta = h \mathrm{X} D.$$

where P or Δ is the amount of prismatic effect in prism diopters, h is the distance in *centimeters* from the optical center, and D is the power of the lens. A mnemonic you can use to help you remember this rule is "PhD":

$$P = hD$$

#Protip1: *Make sure you convert h from mm to cm!!! This is where they mess with you.* The question stem will often have a scenario where a patient looks "x" mm away from the optical center of the lens. It is important to remember to convert the "x mm'' into centimeters before plugging it into the above equation. You can be certain that one of the wrong answer choices on examinations will include a numerical value obtained by using "x mm'' instead of changing it to "x cm."

#Protip2: Even though it may seem unnecessary, draw out the lens, especially if you are still getting the hang of prisms. This will help you keep the BO/BI or BU/BD effect organized visually.

When drawing out lenses, use the following figure to help you remember how to draw out the lens. Think of lenses as basically a combination of two prisms (Fig. 11).

If we place the same type of prism (with equal quantitative magnitude) in front of both eyes, there may or may not be a resulting diplopia (Fig. 12). For example, placing BU or BD prisms in front of both eyes will move the eyes in the same direction. However, placing BI or BO prism in front of both eyes may move the eyes in the same or opposite directions (depending on what part of the lens/prism the patient is looking through). For example, if a patient looks nasal to the optical center of +3D lenses placed in front of both eyes,

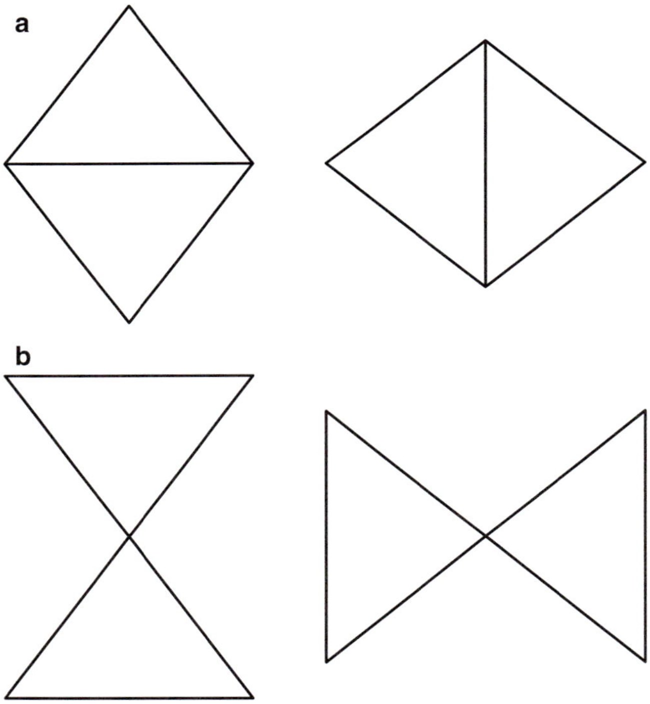

Fig. 11 Think of lenses as a combination of two prisms. Depending on the direction of gaze, drawing out the lens in this manner will make it easier to determine the prismatic effect caused by looking away from the optical center. Panel A shows how a plus lens should be drawn in vertical gaze (top left) and horizontal gaze (top right). Panel B shows how a minus lens should be drawn in vertical gaze (bottom left) and horizontal gaze (bottom right)

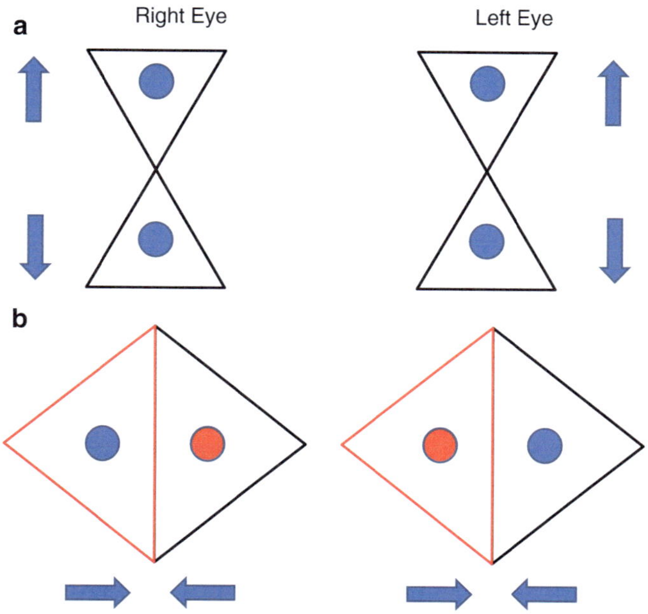

Fig. 12 Summary of prismatic effects when a patient looks away from the optical center of lenses with both eyes. The blue or red dot represents where the patient's eye is looking through (instead of the optical center). Assuming equal magnitude, base-up/base-down over both eyes will move the eyes in the same direction (**a**). Base-in/base-out over both eyes (**b**) will move the eyes in the same or opposite directions (depending on what part of the lens/prism the patient is looking through). For example, if the patient looks nasal to the optical center (red dots), then the eyes will move in different directions due to the base-out effects encountered when looking at this position. However, if a patient looks to the *right* of the optical center in both eyes (red triangles), then the eyes will move in the same direction (toward the patient's left ear)

there will be a BO prism induced, and therefore, a diplopia will result. However, if the patient is looking to the "right" of the optical center of +3D lenses, then for the right eye, there will be a BI effect, and for the left eye, there will be a BO effect; since both eyes are shifted in the same direction (i.e., toward the patient's left), there will be no diplopia.

Example #1 If you look 6 mm below the optical center of a + 3D lens with your right eye, what is the induced prismatic effect?

Answer: Even though this seems like a relatively simple question, start off by drawing out the lens so that we can visualize the qualitative deviation (BU or BD) (Fig. 13).

We can see that when we look inferior to the optical center of this +3D lens, there will be a BU prismatic effect induced. Now, we can use Prentice's rule to solve for the numerical deviation, remembering to convert to cm:

$$P = hD = (0.6)(3) = 1.8 \text{ prism diopters base} - \text{up effect.}$$

Note that one benefit of drawing the prism out is that it helps with visualizing the BU/BD effect in this eye. For example, a common mistake is to read the phrase "the patient looks down" or "the patient looks below" and to simply assume that this will imply a base-*down* effect. Drawing out the lens as a combination of two prisms helps to avoid this error.

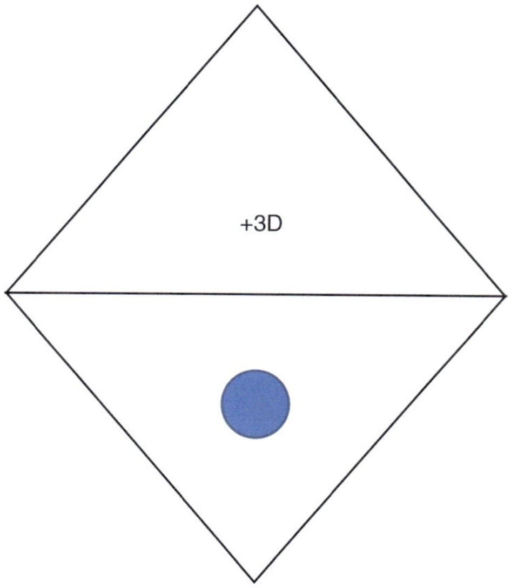

Fig. 13 The blue dot represents the line of sight 6 mm below the optical center of a + 3D lens

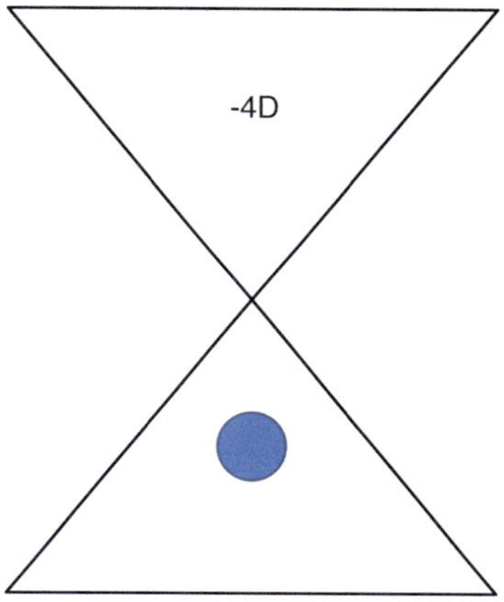

Fig. 14 The blue dot represents the line of sight 8 mm below the optical center of this -4D lens

Example #2 If you look 8 mm below the optical center of a -4D lens with your left eye, what is the induced prismatic effect?

Answer: Again, we can start off by drawing out the lens (Fig. 14).

We can see that when we look inferior to the optical center of this -4D lens, there will be a BD prismatic effect induced. Notice how this is different from the previous problem we just did. In both cases, we looked inferior to the optical center. However, for this problem, we will have to deal with a BD effect.

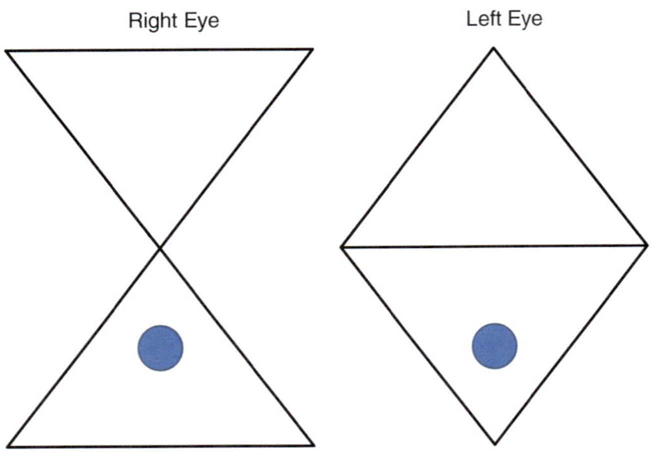

Fig. 15 The blue dot represents the line of sight of the right and left eye, respectively, when looking 4 mm inferior to the optical center of a – 5.00D lens and a + 2.50D lens

Now, we can use Prentice's rule to solve for the numerical deviation, taking care to convert to cm:

$$P = hD\ (0.8)(4) = 3.2\,\text{prism diopters base} - \text{down effect.}$$

Now we can do some more challenging examples (yippee!).

Example #3 If you look 4 mm below the optical center of glasses with the following prescription: OD: -5.00D, OS: +2.50D, what is the net induced prismatic effect?

First, find the resident that did such an awful refraction and administer ophthalmic justice: making the resident refract every VA patient for the rest of the week. Second, solve the problem. Again, start off by drawing out the two lenses (Fig. 15).

Now, we have to calculate each eye separately:

$$\text{OD}: P = hD\ (0.4)(5) = 2\,\text{PD BD.}$$

$$\text{OS}: P = hD\ (0.4)(2.50) = 1\text{PD BU.}$$

Net (total) effect: 3 PD deviation between the two eyes.

Bonus points: How could you correct this deviation?

Answer: Since the right eye is 3 PD "inferior" compared to the left eye, we could either give 3 PD BU prism to the right eye (to shift it superiorly) or 3 PD BD to the left eye (to shift it inferiorly). And yes, it is quite possible that if the patient had normal vertical fusion amplitudes, he/she could probably fuse this small induced tropia and we could skip the bonus question(!).

Example #4 If you look 8 mm to the right while wearing a pair of glasses with the following prescription: OD: –6.00 sphere, OS: +6.00 sphere, what is the net induced prismatic effect.

Answer: Note the (tricky) wording in the stem of this question. It states that you are *looking to the right* with both eyes, meaning you are looking to the right of the optical center in both eyes. This means that the right eye will be looking temporally and the left eye will be looking nasally (both eyes will be directed toward the right ear). Also, this pair of glasses would be awful to wear even if we were looking through the optical centers due to the likely anisometropia/aniseikonia![3] Nevertheless, we can play this game: drawing out the lenses will make the direction of the deviation relatively simple to figure out (Fig. 16).

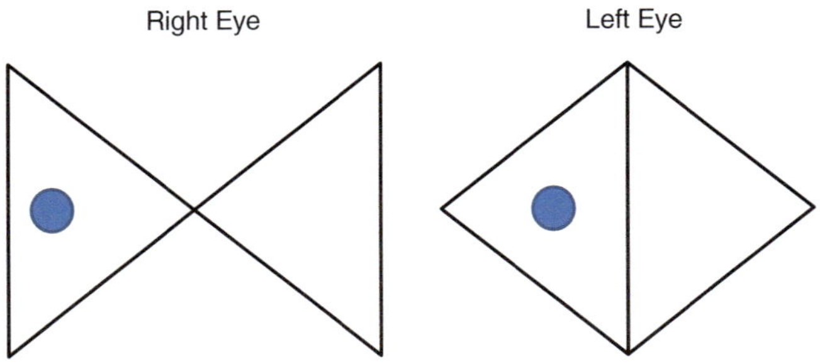

Fig. 16 The blue dot represents the line of sight of the right and left eye, respectively, when looking 8 mm to the right of the optical center of a – 6.0D lens and + 6.0D lens

We can see that there will be a BO prism effect for the right eye, and a BO prism effect for the left eye—i.e., there will be diplopia. We can now calculate how much prismatic effect will be present:

$$\text{OD}: P = hD\ (0.8)(6) = 4.8\,\text{prism diopters base} - \text{out.}$$

$$\text{OS}: P = hD\ (0.8)(6) = 4.8\,\text{prism diopters base} - \text{out.}$$

Since the eyes will be moving in opposite directions, we have to add the two deviations. The net deviation will be 4.8 + 4.8 = 9.6 prism diopters (between the two eyes) (XT induced).

Bonus points: how could you correct this deviation?

Answer: We can either give 9.6 PD BI to the right eye or 9.6 PD BI to the left eye.

Even more bonus points: What is the problem with the above answer?

Answer: Prisms are only made in whole number values. So, we could either give a 9 PD or a 10 PD prism since a 9.6 PD is not available. C'est la vie.

Finally, notice that in the above examples, we were only asked to calculate the deviation when looking away from the optical center of *spherical lenses*. When dealing with *spherocylindrical lenses*, the calculations are a bit trickier, depending on where the cylinder will have an effect (or not have an effect). We will therefore revisit this advanced topic under "Prentice's Rule," in Chap. 10, Spherocylindrical Lenses. Note: Problem #10 in the end-of-chapter questions involves a spherocylindrical lens.

[3] See Chap. 8, "Magnification and Telescopes" for a detailed discussion of anisometropia and aniseikonia.

Prisms in Clinical Practice

Prisms and Strabismus

In clinical practice, prisms are used to measure a patient's strabismus. This will allow a surgeon to know how much strabismus surgery to perform or how many prism diopters to prescribe. Using the alternate cover technique, a prism is held with its *apex toward the eye deviation.*

For example, suppose that we have a patient with a LXT (Fig. 17, left panel). Without prism correction, when the patient is looking at an object, an inverted real image is projected onto the retina (by real light rays); for the right eye, the light rays strike the fovea, but for the left eye, the light rays fall temporal to the fovea. In order to correct this LXT, we would place a BI prism over the patient's left eye with the apex directed toward the patient's ear (Fig. 17, right panel). Since real light rays are bent toward the base of the prism, this will "bend" the light rays to hit the fovea of the left eye, thereby resolving the diplopia. In the alternative cover test, prisms of increasing strength are used until the patient's eyes no longer need to re-fixate on the target. This amount of prism will be the amount of strabismus present.

Before dispensing the measured prism, a prism adaptation test (PAT) may be performed in the clinic (for a few minutes to few hours) or with trial Fresnel prisms (for several days to several weeks) to allow the patient to get used to the prism and bring about any latent strabismus not initially observed. Some patients may require repeat measurements after a PAT in order to titrate the final amount of prism needed, especially if they have a deviation with both vertical and horizontal components.

We can review some hi-yield facts regarding dispensing prisms:

- If a patient is suffering from binocular diplopia, and the amount of strabismus measured is less than 18 prism diopters (PD), then a prism may be prescribed. This may serve as a palliative "crutch" and may help avoid surgery.
- When the prisms are greater than 3 PD, then the optician will typically split the prism and provide half the strength over each eye. For example, for an 8 PD LXT, the optician may give 4 PD BI for the left eye and 4 PD BI for the right eye.
- Typically, about 70–75% of the full deviation measured will be prescribed. This will avoid exacerbating a patient's dependence on prisms. For example, if a patient has 16 PD of exotropia, a clinician may offer 12 PD base-in for one eye, or 6 PD base-in each lens over each eye.
- With the prescribed prism(s), the patient should experience relief of diplopia for most of the day. However, even with the prismatic correction glasses on, double vision is expected at the end of the day when the patient is tired and the strabismus is harder to control.
- Prescribing partial strength prisms (e.g., giving 8 PD BI for the right eye for a patient with 14 PD RXT) will compassionately provide some relief to the patient while still promoting fusion and encouraging them to develop some fusional amplitude by fighting their strabismus. Think of this as sending the patient to the gym to work out and get stronger for building up the ability to compensate for the remaining needed prism. This will also hopefully avoid the patient becoming "lazy" and "eating

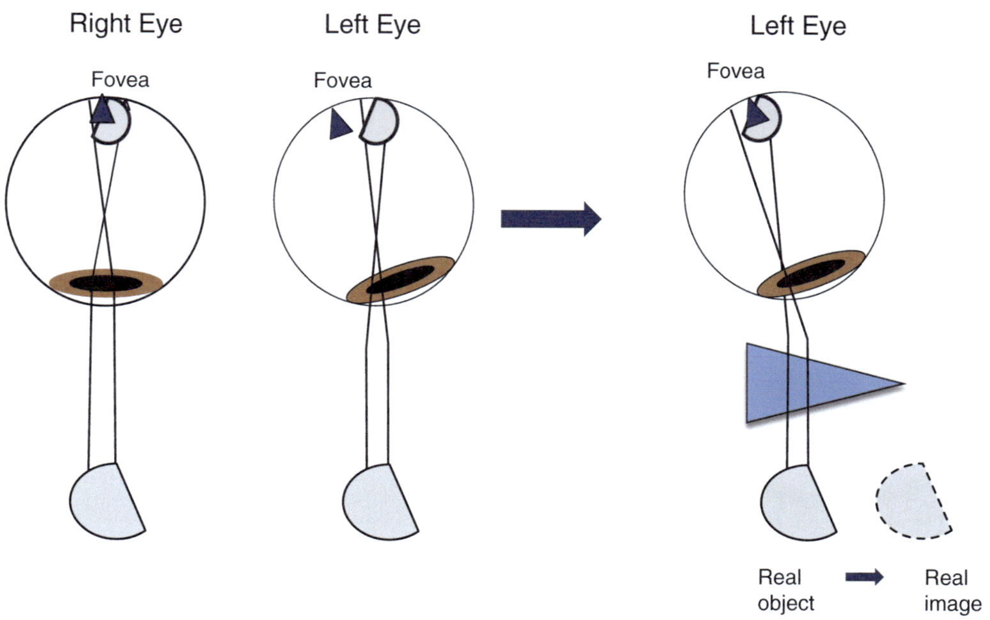

Fig. 17 Without prism correction, real light rays will fall temporally to the fovea of the left eye for a patient with LXT (left panel). When a BI prism is placed over the left eye (right panel), real light rays are bent toward the base (nasally) such that they will now fall on the fovea of the left eye, thereby resolving the diplopia

up" their prescribed prism, therefore requiring stronger prisms in the future.

- If necessary, a second pair of glasses with full-strength prisms may be provided to use only at night if the patient really needs it to drive safely or has high demands for excellent vision at night time. The patient could wear her partial strength prisms during the day and switch to the full-strength prisms in the evening.

Clinical Examples of Prism Dispensation.

Example #1 For a patient named Lefty N. Wards with LET of 20 PD (measured in clinic), 7 PD BO can be given for both eyes (Fig. 18).

Example #2 For a patient named Lefty Ootward with LXT of 20 PD (measured in clinic), 7 PD BI can be given for both eyes (Fig. 19).

Example #3 For a patient named Wright I. Down with LHT of 20 PD (measured in clinic), 7 BU can be given for the right eye, and 7 PD BD can be given for the left eye (Fig. 20).

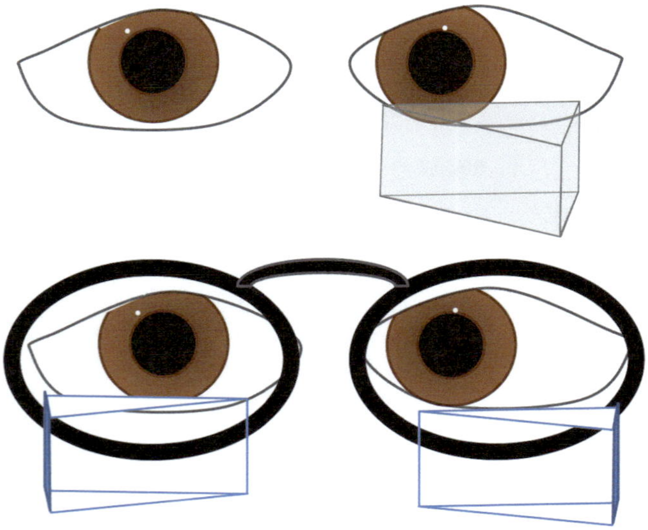

Fig. 18 A partial strength split prism: 7 PD base-out over both eyes can be issued for this patient with 20 PD base-out esotropia

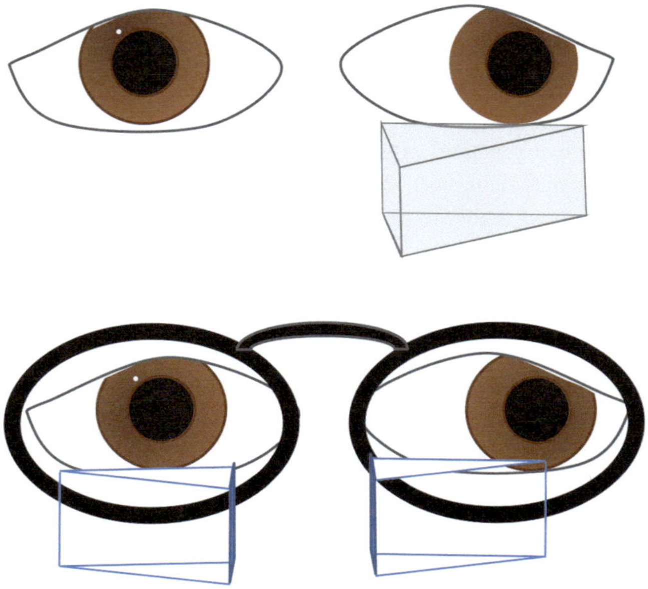

Fig. 19 A partial strength split prism: 7PD base-in over both eyes can be issued for this patient with 20 PD base-out exotropia

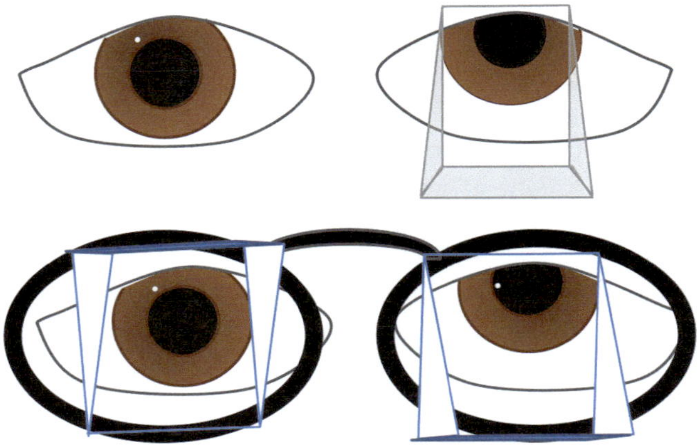

Fig. 20 A partial strength split prism: 7PD base-up over the right eye and 7PD base-down over the left eye can be issued for this patient with 20 PD base-down LHT

Fresnel (Temporary) Prisms

In addition to a ground-in prism in the patient's glasses, the clinician may choose instead to give a temporary, inexpensive, plastic Fresnel prism, or a "press-on" prism (Fig. 21). Fresnel prisms (pronounced as "Freh-NELL"; don't be a noob and pronounce it as "FREZ-nel"…) can be easily attached to the patient's glasses and can be moved, rotated, and exchanged (Fig. 22). Basically, a Fresnel prism is a series of parallel smaller prism surfaces at the same angle. In patients with diagonal diplopia, Fresnel prisms may also be rotated to an oblique angle.

Advantages of Fresnel prisms include the following:

1. Useful for the temporary control of diplopia, such as:
   - Ischemic diabetic sixth nerve palsy,
   - Postoperative diplopia in patients with consecutive strabismus.
2. Ability to function as experiment ("Trial Prisms") prisms when clinical measurements of the deviation are inconsistent, and a clinician may therefore use a Fresnel prism to help titrate the final required prism power, or perform a prism adaptation test to confirm how much strabismus surgery should be performed.
3. Relatively inexpensive (compared to ground-in prism).

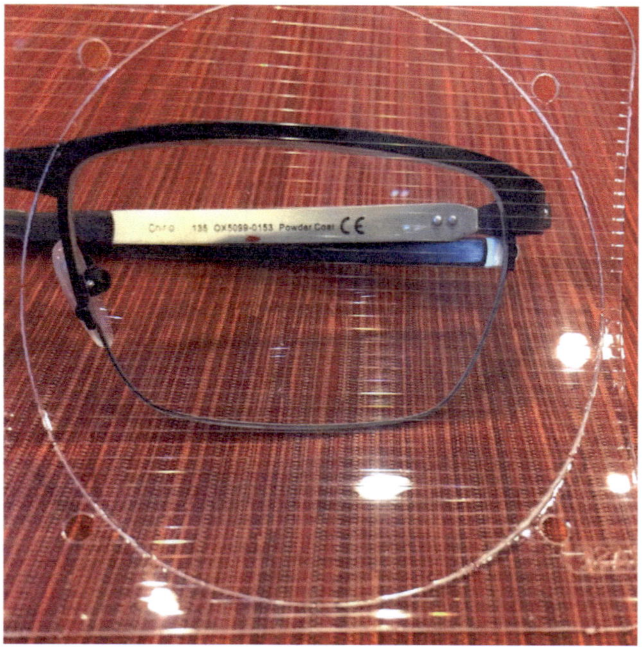

Fig. 21 8 PD base-down Fresnel prism prior to trimming the size

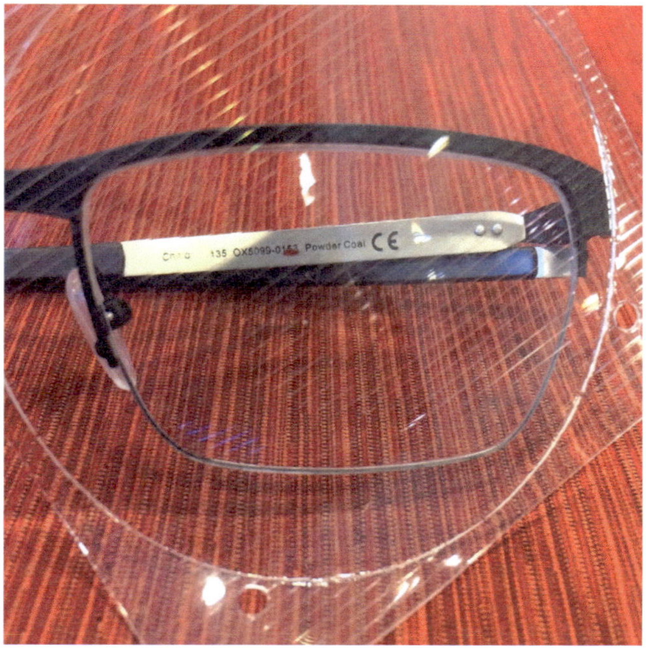

Fig. 22 Rotated Fresnel prisms 8 base-down and base-out, before and after trimming

Disadvantages of Fresnel prisms include:

1. Fresnel prisms may easily smudge or get dislodged from the spectacle lens.
2. The Fresnel prism, due to its "press-on" nature, may have a level of opacity/blurriness of the material, and thus are less transparent (and more easily noticeable, especially to observers), than ground-in prism.
3. Higher prism powers will require thicker material, which may lead to further blurriness of vision.
4. Some level of visual acuity is compromised, mainly due to negative effects of chromatic aberration.

Convergence Insufficiency

See Chap. 22, "Optics for Clinical and Surgical Management of Strabismus" for a more detailed explanation of this topic.

Patients with convergence insufficiency (CI) will suffer from diplopia with near activities. Orthoptic exercises to increase convergence will often improve convergence insufficiency, especially in younger patients; however, these may not work well in older patients, especially in patients with brainstem pathology or Parkinson's disease.

Several options exist to help patients with CI. If the patient is myopic, one option is to simply prescribe them their full myopic prescription since myopic glasses will have a BI prismatic effect when looking at near. For younger patients, and this may seem somewhat counterintuitive, another option may be to do the opposite: *intentionally under correct the needed myopic prescription*. This intentional under correction may stimulate the patient to build up their convergence abilities. A second option is to prescribe monofocal reading glasses with a (plus) +2.0 D add. The lower add will increase the working distance (out to 50 cm) and alleviate some convergence symptoms by forcing the patient to read further away. If the patient is still diplopic, a third option is to add up to 7 PD base-in prism to each lens. Remember, BI prism will cause the eyes to "shift towards the base," so giving extra BI prism can "help" these patients who are not otherwise able to generate the convergence amplitudes needed. A fourth option involves taping one lens as the last resort to alleviate the symptoms. A fifth option may be a situation that may require full correction with base-in prism may be for a patient who has a time-sensitive need for improved convergence, such as a young patient with an upcoming prolonged standardized examination, and thus cannot wait for the convergence exercises to take effect.

In general, younger patients with CI should not be given the full prismatic correction as they can work to improve their convergence abilities. For older patients, however, we should be a bit more lenient and merciful; these patients should be given the full prismatic correction to help alleviate CI as described above.

Combined Vertical and Horizontal Diplopia

Say a patient, Wright I. Diagonal (who is right eye dominant) has diagonal diplopia, with an esotropia and a right hypertro-

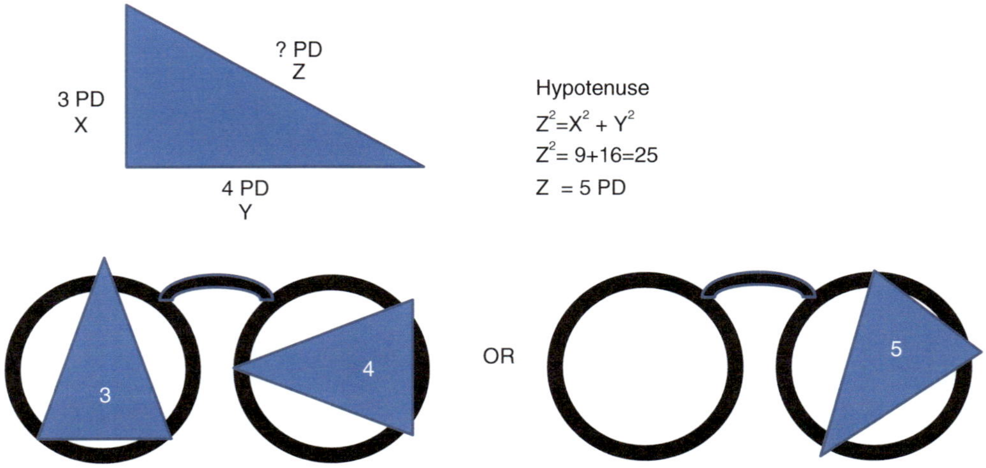

Fig. 23 A 5 base-up and base-out Fresnel prism over the left eye would compensate for this patient with vertical and horizontal strabismus

pia, and he requires a 4 PD base-out and a 3 PD base-down on the RIGHT side. The clinician can prescribe this combination as ground-in lenses: 4 PD base-out OS, and 3 PD base-down OD or place a Fresnel prism over the non-dominant LEFT eye base-up and base-out (Fig. 23). The amount of a diagonal prism is estimated by calculating the hypotenuse of the triangle formed (as we discussed in Section D).

We can now do a few more examples of combined vertical and horizontal strabismus that may require us to prescribe prismatic correction.

Example #1 Suppose a patient named I.C. Good presents with complaints of double vision. You measure a 4 PD RHT and a 5 PD LET. We can prescribe prisms for both eyes separately, using our rule of thumb to give ~75% of the measured deviation. One option is to give 3 PD BD for the right eye and 4 PD BO for the left eye (Fig. 24). A second option is to give a Fresnel prism placed over the left eye of 5 PD placed base-up and base-out as a trial prism.

Finally, one more advanced point: Patients with cranial nerve IV palsies will often have a torsional diplopia in addition to a vertical and a horizontal one. The torsional diplopia unfortunately cannot be ameliorated with prisms; however, if the horizontal and vertical diplopia can be neutralized with prisms, then the patient may find it easier to tolerate and fuse the tilted images.

Prisms for High Reading Add Powers

In the clinical management of patients with low vision, single-vision reading glasses with high-plus power in both eyes may be necessary to improve functional near vision.[4] The high plus lenses will decrease the working distance, but will also increase the convergence demands due to the

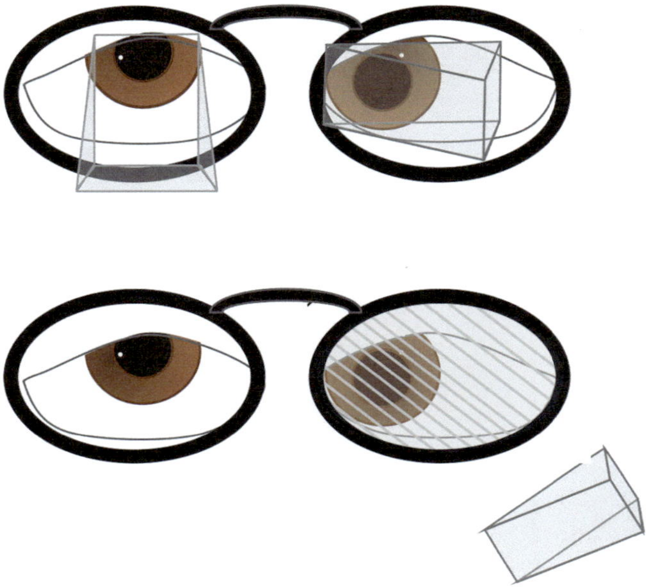

Fig. 24 Ground-in and Fresnel prism options

induced BO effect when patients look nasal to the optical center of these lenses (Fig. 25).

To decrease the additional convergence demands in this situation, additional BI prism may be needed in the glasses. As a rule of thumb, you should prescribe 2 PD BI greater than the power of the plus lens. For example, if we prescribed +8.00D glasses, then we would need to give 10 PD BI for each eye. (Depending on the frame and the prescription, most opticians can make ground-in prisms up to 8–9 PD.)

Prisms and Nystagmus

Patients with nystagmus will often have a null point in which they can dampen their nystagmus and improve their best corrected vision. If the null point is not in primary gaze, they will develop a compensatory head posture to basically arrive

[4]See Chap. 19, "Low Vision and Vision Rehabilitation" for more information.

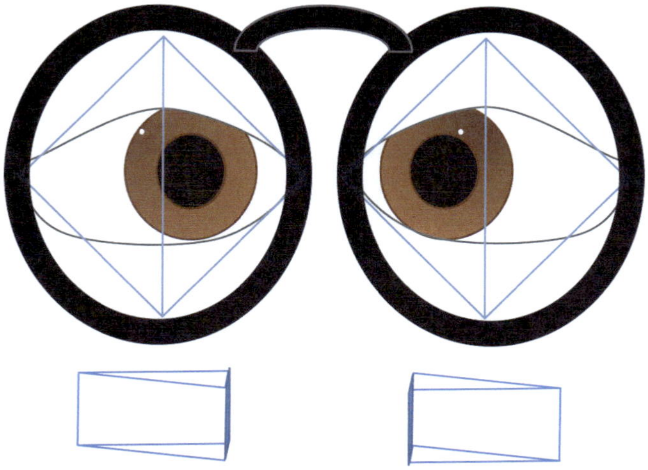

Fig. 25 High plus lenses will increase convergence demands when a patient attempts to focus at near due to the induced base-out prismatic effects when looking nasal to the optical center. These patients may fatigue easily if they are not given additional base-in prism to alleviate the base-out prism due to the high plus lenses

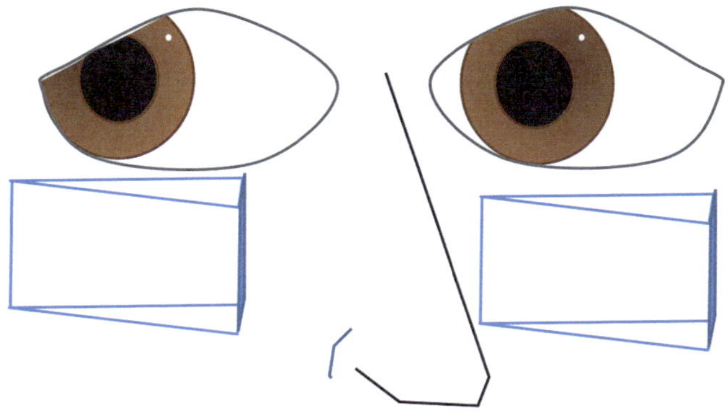

Fig. 26 Prisms and nystagmus with null point in right gaze

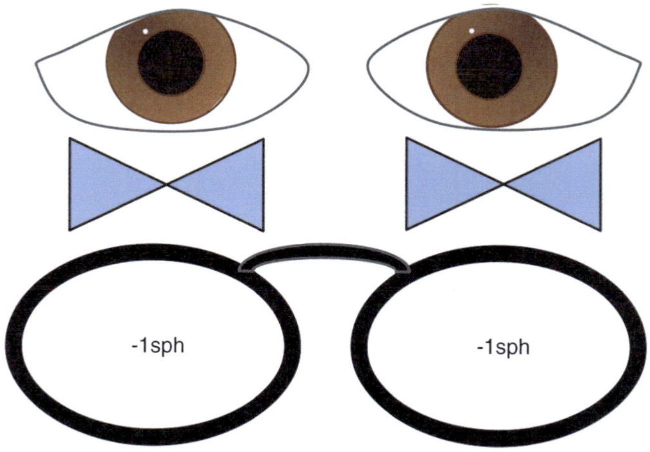

Fig. 27 Prisms and nystagmus with null point in primary gaze and dampening with convergence. Adding extra minus power allows a patient to use the base-in effect of the minus lens to decrease the demands for convergence

at the null point through the head turn. If the head turn is small, prisms can be used to "shift the eyes" toward the null point, thereby reducing the need to turn the head as much. However, most symptomatic head turns are too large to ameliorate with prism. These patients may require surgical intervention, such as a Kestenbaum procedure.

Patients with mild–moderate nystagmus patients may try prisms in the office in the following way:

- Point the apex of the correcting prism in the direction of the null zone: For example, if a patient presents with a left head turn and clinical examination reveals a *null point in right gaze*, this means we need to figure out a way to "move" the incoming image to the patient's right visual field (Fig. 26). This will motivate the patient to move the eyes into the null point (since this is where the image will now appear) so that he/she does not have to do a constant head turn anymore. Several options include the following:
  - 7 PD BI given to the right eye, with apex of prism toward the right ear.
  - 7 PD BO given to the left eye, with apex of prism toward the right ear.
  - A combination of the above two options.

Note that all of these options aim to shift the incoming images to the right (i.e., toward the patient's right ear) and the patient will move his/her eyes towards the null point.

- If the patient has a chin down posture, this means that both eyes are hypertropic. A base-down prism may be given to both eyes to move the eyes "down."
- Patients with infantile idiopathic nystagmus will have better vision at near because they are able to dampen their nystagmus with convergence. Therefore, prescribing 5 PD *BO prisms* for both eyes *can be used to induce convergence* at distance and possibly improve their best corrected distance vision.[5]
- It is important to remember that when young patients converge, they will also accommodate and thus fog themselves. By giving patients extra myopic correction (i.e., additional −1 to −1.5D myopic correction), when the patient converges, he/she will look through the "base-in" portion of the myopic lens (Fig. 27). This base-in prismatic effect will decrease the amount of convergence (and subsequent accommodation) needed, thereby alleviating fogging and asthenopia symptoms.

[5]This may initially seem counterintuitive: If the patient can dampen the symptoms with convergence, why are we giving base-out prism, should not we give base-in prism (to facilitate convergence)? This can be explained by the idea that giving base-out prism is *forcing* the patient to converge (rather than passively converge), similar to the "stick" method in a "carrot and stick" approach.

Miscellaneous Pearls for Prism Dispensation

- The patient should be warned that different prism strengths may be necessary over time and that their strabismus may change over time independent of whether prisms were worn.
- Strabismus surgery may still be necessary despite prisms. Remember that prisms do not halt or reverse the disease process. They are simply a workaround for the pathology that is present.
- If the patient has an incomitant strabismus, he/she should understand that they may still have diplopia in non-primary gazes.
- Patients should be warned about the optical quality of eyeglasses with prisms. Specifically, they should be aware of seeing rainbows around light sources and heavier weight of the frames.
- The patient should be told that it is very difficult to make prisms. They should not be surprised if it takes most optical shops a few weeks and a couple of tries to get the prism lenses just right.
- Patients should also be told about the higher cost of making glasses with ground-in prisms. This is why a Fresnel prism may be a good option as a "test-drive" prism until the patient is happy with a certain prism power that can then be made permanent.
- On that note, it is very difficult, but not impossible to make the following prisms; they will have a high error rate at the optical shop and thus should be avoided:
  A. Progressive lenses and ground-in prisms.
  B. Diagonal ground-in prisms.
  C. Ground-in prisms stronger than 8–9 PD (they are too thick).
  D. Ground-in prisms in only one segment of a bifocal prescription.
  E. Fresnel prisms stronger than 15 PD (they are too blurry).
- Prisms may also be given to patients with hemispheric visual field defects (such as those that would occur with a stroke, for example). By shifting the "missing" visual field into the "visible area of vision," the patient's symptoms may be partially alleviated. For example, if a patient presents with a *left homonymous hemianopia*, one way to alleviate this patient's symptoms may involve *shifting the "missing" visual field toward the right side* (i.e., the visible) visual field. One way to do this would be to place BI prism over the right eye and BO prism over the left eye. Recall that since real light rays will bend toward the base of the prism, incoming light rays would be shifted to the nasal retina in the right eye and temporal retina in the left eye. Remembering our neuroanatomy, we can then deduce that these light rays will project into the right visual field.

  As a rule of thumb, when prescribing prisms to correct hemispheric defects, place the prism such that the BASE of the prism is directed TOWARDS the hemianopic visual field defect:
  – For a LEFT homonymous hemianopia, orient the bases of the prisms placed over each eye in the direction of the patient's LEFT ear.
  – For a RIGHT homonymous hemianopia, orient the bases of the prisms placed over each eye in the direction of the patient's RIGHT ear.

Practice Questions

1. A prism of unknown power bends a light ray 50 mm when measured 100 cm away. What is the power of the prism?
   A. 5 PD
   B. 20 PD
   C. 25 PD
   D. 50 PD
2. A prism deflects a light ray 20 cm at a distance of 80 cm. What is the power of the prism?
3. A prism deflects a light ray 40 cm at a distance of 250 cm. What is the power of the prism?
4. A patient looks 11 mm below the optical center of the following prescription:
   OD: plano OS: -3.00 sphere
   What is the induced prism?
5. A 52 year old patient named I.C. Googly presents to your office with complaints of double vision when he looks down to read. He wears glasses with the following prescription:

$$\text{OD}: -6.00\text{D sphere}$$

$$\text{OS}: -4.00\text{D sphere}$$

$$+2.00\,\text{add OU}\left(\text{Executive style}\right)$$

What is the induced prism? Assume that the reading position is 8 mm downwards and 2 mm inwards to the optical center.

6. A patient presents complaining of vertical diplopia, most prominent when he wants to read. You note that he has a -12D sph prescription for both eyes. In addition, you measure a 6 PD RHT. How can you correct his vertical diplopia?
   A. Move the optical center down by 2.5 mm for both lenses
   B. Move the optical center down by 2.5 mm for the right lens only

C. Move the optical center up by 2.5 mm for the right lens and down by 2.5 mm for the left lens
D. Move the optical center down by 2.5 mm for the right lens and up by 2.5 mm for the left lens

7. A patient presents complaining of vertical diplopia, most prominent when he wants to read (which is 12 mm below the optical center of the glasses). You note that the patient has +8.75D sphere for the right eye and + 6.25D sphere for the left eye. You also measure a 4 PD RHT. How can you correct this vertical diplopia?
   A. Prescribe 4 PD BU to the right eye, 3 PD BD to the left eye
   B. Prescribe 4 PD BD to the right eye, 3 PD BU to the left eye
   C. Prescribe 4 PD BU to the right eye, 3 PD BU to the left eye
   D. Prescribe 4 PD BD to the right eye, 3 PD BD to the left eye
8. A patient presents with a history of a left occipital lobe stroke. Which of the following combinations of prisms will help alleviate his symptoms?
   A. BI prism for the right eye; BI prism for the left eyes
   B. BI prism for the right eye; BO prism for the left eye
   C. BO prism for the right eye; BO prism for the left eye
   D. BO prism for the right eye; BI prism for the left eye
9. If a low-vision patient requires +9.00D add for reading, how much total prism power should be given to decrease this patient's convergence demands?
   A. 9 PD BO prism for each eye
   B. 9 PD BI for each eye
   C. 11 PD BO prism for each eye
   D. 11 PD BI prism for each eye
10. Suppose a patient has the following prescription:

$$\text{OD}: -4.00\,\text{D sph}$$

$$\text{OS}: +1.00 + 4.00 \times 90$$

The patient presents to your office complaining about vertical diplopia whenever they wear their glasses. Suppose that a repeat EOM examination reveals a 5 PD LHT in downgaze (when looking through the glasses 1 cm below the optical center). Why is this patient unhappy? How can we correct her symptoms?

Answers

1. Answer: This is a seemingly simple question regarding prism diopters. The nuance here is that in the in-text problems, we were given the deflection in cm. Here, we are given the deflection in mm, requiring us to make an additional adjustment.

   At 100 cm (1 m), the light ray was bent 50 mm (5 cm). Therefore, the unknown prism's power is 5 PD (**Answer Choice A**).
2. Answer: We can solve this using the law of similar triangles:

$$\frac{20\,\text{cm}}{80\,\text{cm}} = \frac{\times}{100\,\text{cm}} 80\times = (100)(20) \times = 25\,\text{cm, so } \mathbf{25\ PD}$$

3. Answer: We can solve this using the law of similar triangles:

$$\frac{40\,\text{cm}}{250\,\text{cm}} = \frac{\times}{100\,\text{cm}} 250\times = (100)(40) \times = 16\,\text{cm, so } \mathbf{16\ PD}$$

4. Answer: It may help to draw out the −3.00D lens of the left eye as an hourglass shape as done in the in-text problems. Doing this will make it clear there will be a BD effect when the patient looks inferior to the optical center. We can quantify this deviation using Prentice's rule (again, take care to convert 11 mm to 1.1 cm!)

$$P = hD = (1.1)(3) = \mathbf{3.3\,PD\ base\ down\ effect}$$

5. Answer: This is a problem that builds upon some of the concepts we have already done. In essence, it requires us to solve for Prentice's rule twice (even though we are only getting one point on an exam!)

   First, we need to calculate the effective power of the glasses when the patient is reading. Since he is wearing an executive style bifocal, we can simply add the power of the distance glasses with the added power to give us the "effective" power of the glasses when the patient is reading. So for the right eye, he is basically reading with a -4D lens (−6 + 2 = -4D), and for the left eye, he is basically reading with a -2D lens (−4 + 2 = -2D).

   Since these are myopic glasses, there will be a base-down effect when looking inferiorly and a base-in effect when looking nasally.

   Now, we can use Prentice's rule to determine the deviations:

   Inferior gaze

$$\text{OD}: P = hD\ (0.8)(4) = 3.2\,\text{PD BD}$$

$$\text{OS}: P = hD(0.8)(2) = 1.6\,\text{PD BD}$$

   The net deviation in inferior gaze is 3.2–1.6 = 1.6 PD, with the right eye inferior to the left eye (you can think of this as a small LHT). Since both eyes are shifted inferiorly, we can subtract the deviation between the two eyes.

   Nasal gaze

$$\text{OD}: P = hD\ (0.2)(4) = 0.8\,\text{PD BI}$$

$$\text{OS}: P = hD\ (0.2)(2) = 0.4\,\text{PD BI}$$

The net deviation in nasal gaze is 0.8 + 0.4 = 1.2 PD BI (additive effect since both eyes are looking in opposite directions).

The *total deviation* would be *1.6 PD BD effect and 1.2 PD BI effect OU.*

6. Answer: Since the patient has a 6 PD RHT, we need to "move" the right eye down by either moving the right eye down (by giving this eye a BD prism) and/or moving the left eye up (by giving this eye a BU prism) for a net shift of 6 PD.

   Using Prentice's rule: *P* = hD (0.25)(12) = 3. We can get a 3 PD BD in the right eye by moving the optical center down by 2.5 mm and 3 PD BU in the left eye by moving the optical center up by 2.5 mm (**Answer Choice D**).
7. Answer: Since the patient has a 4 PD RHT, we need to "move" the right eye down by either moving the right eye down (by giving this eye a BD prism) and/or moving the left eye up (by giving this eye a BU prism) for a net shift of 4 PD.

   Currently, the prismatic effect can be calculated using Prentice's rule for each eye. Note that since the patient is looking inferior to the center of a plus lens, there will be a BU effect in each eye:

$$\text{OD}: P = hD\ (1.2)(8.75) = \ 10.5\,\text{PD BU.}$$

$$\text{OS}: P = hD\ (1.2)(6.25) = 7.5\text{D BU.}$$

   The net result is a 3 PD difference between the two eyes, with the right eye shifted 3 PD BU more than the left eye.

   On top of this, there is also an existing 4 PD RHT. So the total difference between the two eyes is 7 PD. In essence, when the patient looks downwards to read, the 4 PD RHT will become a 7 PD RHT. The only answer choice that allows us to correct this 7 PD RHT is to prescribe 4 PD BD to the right eye, 3 PD BU to the left eye (**Answer Choice B**).
8. Answer: As mentioned in the text, when prescribing prisms to alleviate hemispheric visual field defects, we should place the prisms such that the **BASE** of the prism is directed toward the hemispheric visual field defect. In this case, we have a left occipital lobe stroke, which will cause a RIGHT HOMONYMOUS HEMIANOPIA. Therefore, we want to place the bases of each prism to be pointing in the direction of the patient's right ear. For the right eye, this will involve giving a BO prism; for the left eye, this will involve giving a BI prism (**Answer Choice D**).
9. Answer: Patients with high add in their low-vision glasses will have increased convergence demands. We can help decrease these demands by giving additional BASE-IN power to each eye. As a rule of thumb, we should give 2 PD extra base-in compared to the total add. Since we have already given +9.00 add for reading, the total prism necessary is (9 + 2 = 11): 11 PD BI prism for each eye (**Answer Choice D**).
10. Answer: First of all, we messed up by giving the patient glasses that will cause anisometropia and aniseikonia, so there is that issue, but since we are in the chapter of prisms, let us apply some of the concepts we have previously discussed.

    Second, you may be intimidated by the spherocylindrical lens in the left eye. We will deal with spherocylindrical lenses and their bearing on Prentice's Rule in chapter "Spherocylindrical Lenses",: Power Crosses and Spherocylindrical Notation. But for now, suffice to say that +1.00 + 4.00 × 90 means that 4D of cylinder has been placed IN the 90-degree (axis) meridian and will exert an effect at the 180-degree (power) meridian; in other words, when the patient looks down to read, the +4.00 will not have any role in the power of the glasses. We can basically treat the left eye lens as a simple +1.00 D lens.

    Applying Prentice's rule, we can get a better understanding of what is happening (Fig. 28).

    Basically, when the patient is reading, she is looking through a base-down prism in the right eye and a base-up prism in the left eye (Fig. 29).

    Using Prentice's rule, we can calculate the prismatic effect at 1 cm below the optical center as follows:

$$\text{OD}: P = hD\ \ (1)(4) = 4\,\text{PD BD}$$

$$\text{OS}: P = hD\ \ (1)(1) = 1\,\text{PD BU.}$$

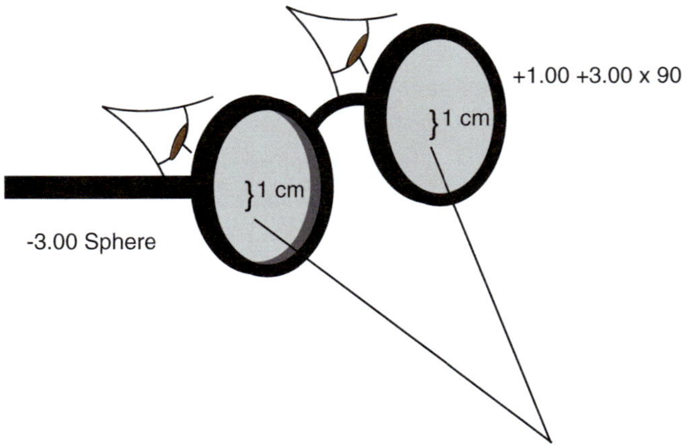

Fig. 28 Prentice's rule can help quantify the prismatic effects in the reading position

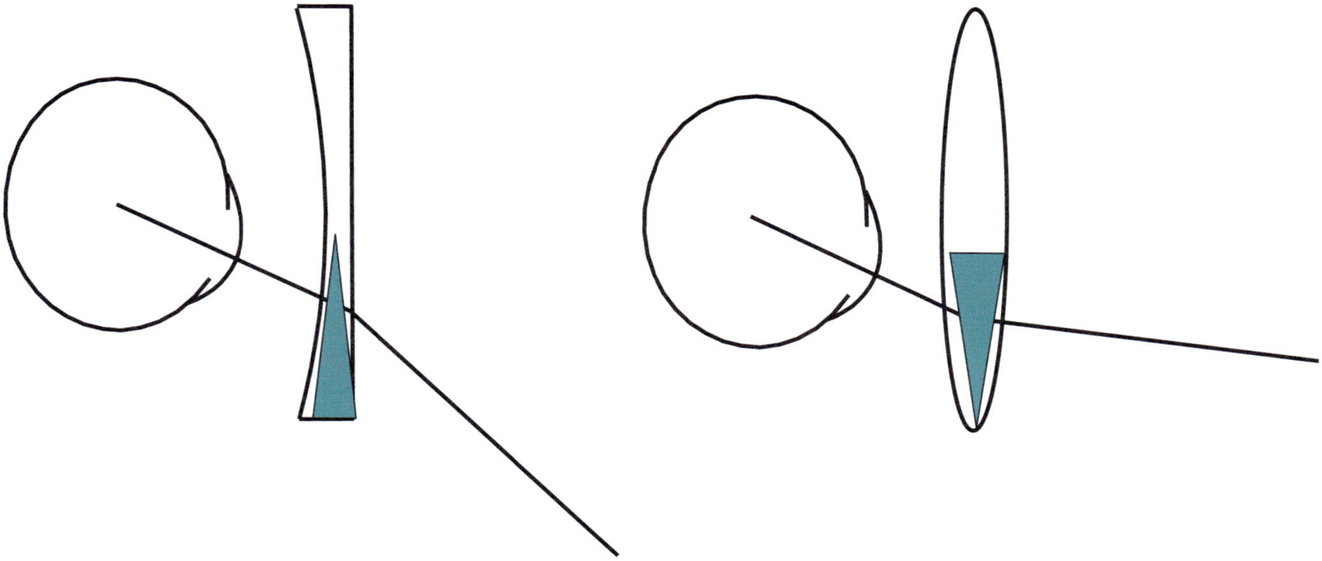

Fig. 29 Prismatic effect of reading position (lenses viewed from the side). Because the right lens is a minus lens and the left lens is a plus lens, there will be a 4 PD base-down in the RT lens and 1 PD base-up in the left lens, respectively

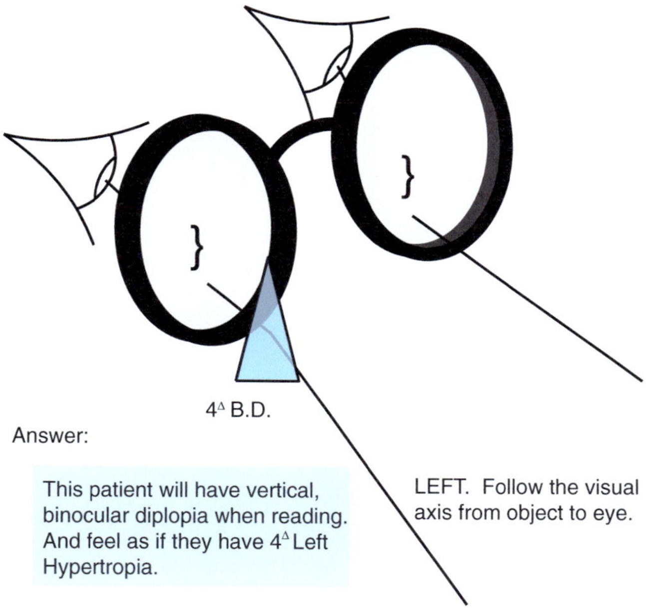

Fig. 30 Total prismatic effect = 5 PD base-down OD. This prescription will induce an annoying vertical, binocular diplopia due to a right hypodeviation. This would be observed in alternate cover only when the glasses are on

Therefore, the total prismatic effect will be 5 PD BD in the right eye. This will induce a right hypodeviation (or left hyper deviation, depending on your preferred frame of reference), which would be observed on alternate cover testing (Fig. 30).

In order to alleviate the problem in downgaze, we have a few options at our disposal:

1. Lower the optical center, if "h" is smaller, then the prismatic effect will be smaller.
2. Decrease the anisometropia, prescribe values closer to one another.
3. Consider contact lenses, or refractive surgery to decrease the anisometropia.
4. Be patient as young patients can develop larger fusional amplitudes over time and adjust to the induced tropia from the glasses.

   And the last and favorite concept to quiz on the oral boards is…
5. Write "slab off 5 $^{\Delta}$ base down OD" on the prescription. To determine the amount of slab off you can follow the above rule or simply do an alternate cover test to see how much strabismus is being induced in the reading position. In general, "SLAB OFF" prism is always placed on the *more minus* lens (Figure 31). "Reverse slab-off" is always done to the *more plus lens*. We will discuss more about slab-off in relation to the construction of glasses in chapter, "Construction of Glasses: Ophthalmologists as Opticians"

Bonus points (extra question): Again, we will discuss this concept more broadly in later chapters, but suppose the patient was looking 1 cm to the left of the optical center in both lenses. What would be the new deviation? Horizontal gaze for reading is not as clinically relevant as the vertical gaze, but in case you were curious5.

Answer: If our patient was now looking 1 cm to the left of the optical center in both lenses, then using $P = hD$, the right eye would have a 4 PD BI effect. The left eye is a bit

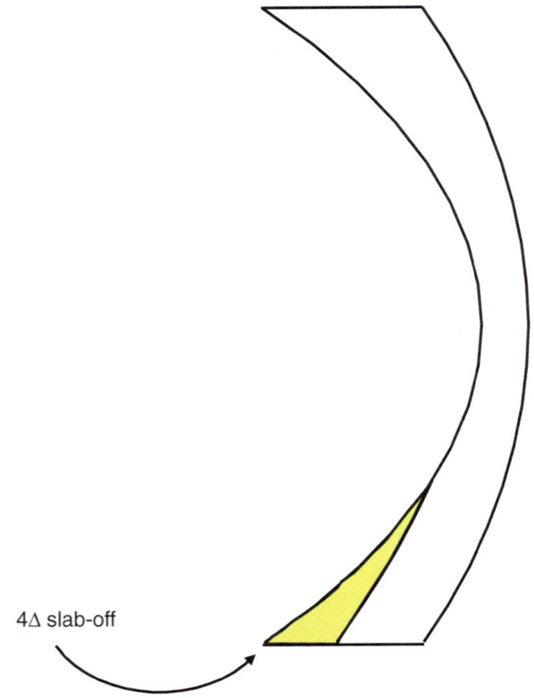

Fig. 31 Slab-off prism to be removed, side view of right lens. "Slab-off" is always done to the more minus lens. "Reverse slab-off" is always done to the more plus lens

trickier as we have to account for the full +1.00 + 4.00 × 90.[6] Since the +4.00 D cylinder has been placed in the 90-degree (axis) meridian, it will have an effect at the

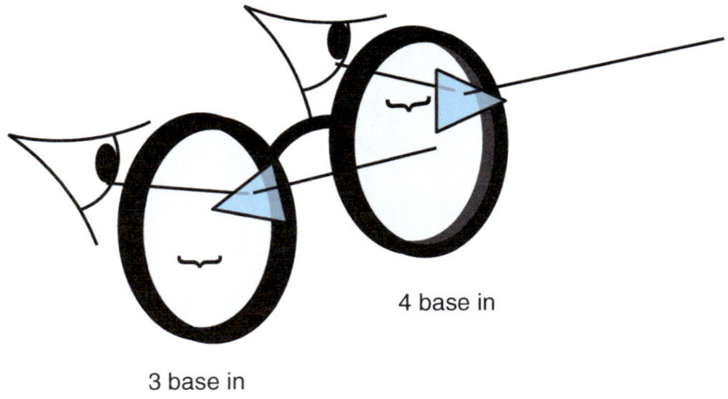

Fig. 32 Total prismatic effect if looking to the left will be 9 PD BI for the right eye for this patient with OD lens −4.0 sphere and OS lens +1.00 + 4.00 x 90

180-degree (power) meridian, when looking horizontally, the left eye lens will now function like a + 5.00D lens. Since the patient will look to the left of the optical center of this lens, again using $P = hD$, we can determine that there will be a 5 PD BI effect. Since both eyes are moving in opposite directions, there will be additive prismatic effect, so the total deviation will be 4 BI +5I = 9 BI OD (Fig. 32).

[6]See Chap. 10, Spherocylindrical Lenses, specifically the section "Prentice's Rule, Part I" for more information on how to deal with spherocylindrical lenses.

Lenses

Daniel Wee

Objectives

- To define and understand the concept of positive and negative vergence.
- To discuss the concept of objects and images in lens and mirror systems problems.
- To understand object and image properties (real vs virtual, upright vs inverted, magnified vs minified).
- To understand the common types of lenses (convex and concave), primary and secondary focal points, and how they function to create images.
- To introduce the concept of ray tracing and its usage in lens system problems.
- To be able to apply the simple lens formula (and central ray tracing) to determine image positions; image orientation; type of image; and transverse (linear) magnification of images formed by both lenses and mirrors.
- To discuss how lens systems can be affected by different media.
- To apply concepts of calculating vergence along a lens system.
- To briefly discuss the concept of thick lenses, including the thick lens formula.

Introduction

This chapter is the first of two chapters that will cover lenses and mirrors in preparation for the purposes of written examinations. Object–lens and object–mirror system problems are the quintessential tested concepts in geometric optics and are often very confusing or boring to trainees. When vague terms such as "vergence" are mentioned, the initial reaction for many people is to have glazed eyes in confusion and existential angst as to why is this important and necessary to take care of patients? This does not have to be the case! While this may *seem* to be a complex and confusing topic, one solace is that all the questions on this topic that may appear on written examinations will follow the same general format. There is no groundbreaking research or developments taking place on this topic. Pharmaceutical companies are not spending millions of dollars to develop a new or more efficient way of calculating where an image will end up after a light ray passes through a convex lens![1]

Given that these concepts are unlikely to ever change in the foreseeable future, this chapter (and the following chapter) will prepare you to answer questions based on lens and mirror systems. While mainly relevant for examinations, we will also briefly discuss how this may have relevance to clinical practice (such as IOL calculation formulas). This chapter (chapter "Lenses") will focus on introductory concepts to object–lens and object–mirror systems and primarily focus on lenses, including some advanced concepts for lens systems, such as thick lenses. The next chapter (Chap. 4, "Mirrors and Combined Systems") will introduce mirrors, as well as combined object–lens–mirror system problems. The usual end-of-chapter questions will therefore appear at the end of chapter "Mirrors and Combined Systems", but will include concepts in both chapters "Lenses" and "Mirrors and Combined Systems".

One assumption that we will be making for most of this chapter is that we will only deal with thin lenses ("thin lens approximation"). This means that we will ignore the "thickness" of a given lens (until we reach the thick lens section at the end of this chapter) and its associated aberrations and dispersion that will take place as the light ray passes through the lens.

For thick lenses, due to the "substance" (thickness) of the lens, we will have to account for these additional aberrations and dispersions. Aberration means that light rays that originate from the same point will converge to slightly different focal points because of the lens thickness and curvature of

[1] A second solace is that much of this information has relevance to fun things in ophthalmology, such as IOL calculation formulas.

D. Wee (✉)
Center for Sight, Stockton, CA, USA

K. M. Riaz et al. (eds.), *Optics for the New Millennium*, https://doi.org/10.1007/978-3-030-95251-8_3

the front and back surface; dispersion means light rays will get slightly shifted (displaced) as they pass through the lens. Basically, for thick lenses, "three refractions" will actually occur (i.e., the light rays will bend once at the front surface, once at the "middle" surface and once at the back surface). If all of that seems needlessly complicated, we agree! That is why we will stick with thin lenses for the majority of this chapter—these are much more likely to be tested.

Finally, the best way to prepare for these types of questions is to practice them over and over, so we will present multiple examples in the text and at the end of the next chapter. We will share some shortcuts and pearls that may help you avoid making common mistakes made by trainees while solving these problems. You may also wish to consult other resources and question databases for more practice problems.

Objects and Images in Lens and Mirror Systems Problems

Conventions and Assumptions

Most of these problems involve the three musketeers: an object, a lens (or mirror), and the image. Usually, we will be given information about two of these musketeers and asked to calculate the third musketeer.

When setting up and solving object–lens and object–mirror system problems, we will make several assumptions as follows:

- Light rays (originating from either an object or an unknown "great beyond" distance) travel from left to right in a formation of parallel rays.
- When light rays encounter a lens, the lens is assumed to be a thin lens unless explicitly stated otherwise. This allows us to ignore more complex calculations that are needed for thick lens problems (which are briefly discussed in the next chapter).
- When light rays encounter a lens, they will either converge or diverge based on the type of lens.
- Unless explicitly stated, otherwise, all of these fascinating object–lens system problems are happening in an air medium. This will allow us to ignore more complex calculations for index of refraction adjustments until the end of the chapter.

Definitions

Vergence

Vergence is probably the most confusing thing about this chapter. The official definition of vergence is listed as "the curvature of optical wavefronts." Don't panic if that doesn't make sense! We can come up with another way of understanding this concept: Vergence is a term used as a description given to light rays that are coming together (converging) or spreading apart (diverging). For objects, light rays emanating from the object are almost always diverging (going away from the object), meaning that light rays emanating from an object have *negative vergence*. For images, light rays that form the image have passed through a lens (or mirror) and may be converging or diverging—this means that images may have a positive or negative vergence, respectively (Fig. 1).

In other words, if light rays pass through a lens and come together in love and harmony, then they will be converging (positive vergence). If these light rays are going away from each other after passing through a lens because they hate each other, then they will be diverging (negative vergence).[2]

For examination purposes, vergence is simply a number that we need to calculate the answers. We will later see how we use vergence as object vergence (U) and image vergence (V) in the equations to follow, especially the "Reduced Vergence Formula (RVF)." Note that when we refer to object or image vergence, we will use the capital letters "U" and "V," respectively. This is important because we will later on use small "u" and "v" to refer to object distance and image distance, respectively. Note that "U/V" and "u/v" are not exactly interchangeable, especially when it comes to calculating magnification! When solving these problems, it is crucial that we make sure to keep these letters (capitalized vs. lower-case) separate.

The next two definitions are primarily relevant to objects and images—we will discuss lenses in greater detail in the next section.

Real vs Virtual

In *The Matrix* (1999), Morpheus famously says: "What is real? How do you define 'real'? If you're talking about what you can feel, what you can smell, what you can taste and see, then 'real' is simply electrical signals interpreted by your brain."

For ophthalmic optics, we are going to define "real" slightly differently. A *real object* is an object that is not formed by any other lens system and gives off its own light rays (diverging light rays). Looking back at Fig. 1, we can see that both objects are "real" objects.

A *real image* is formed when light rays converge. A *virtual image* is an image where light rays actually diverge and we have to draw imaginary extensions to make them appear to converge. Again, looking back at Fig. 1, the top panel

[2]Alternatively, we can think that light rays that have negative vergence are practicing good social distancing. Remember, we wrote this book during the Great Quarantine of 2020.

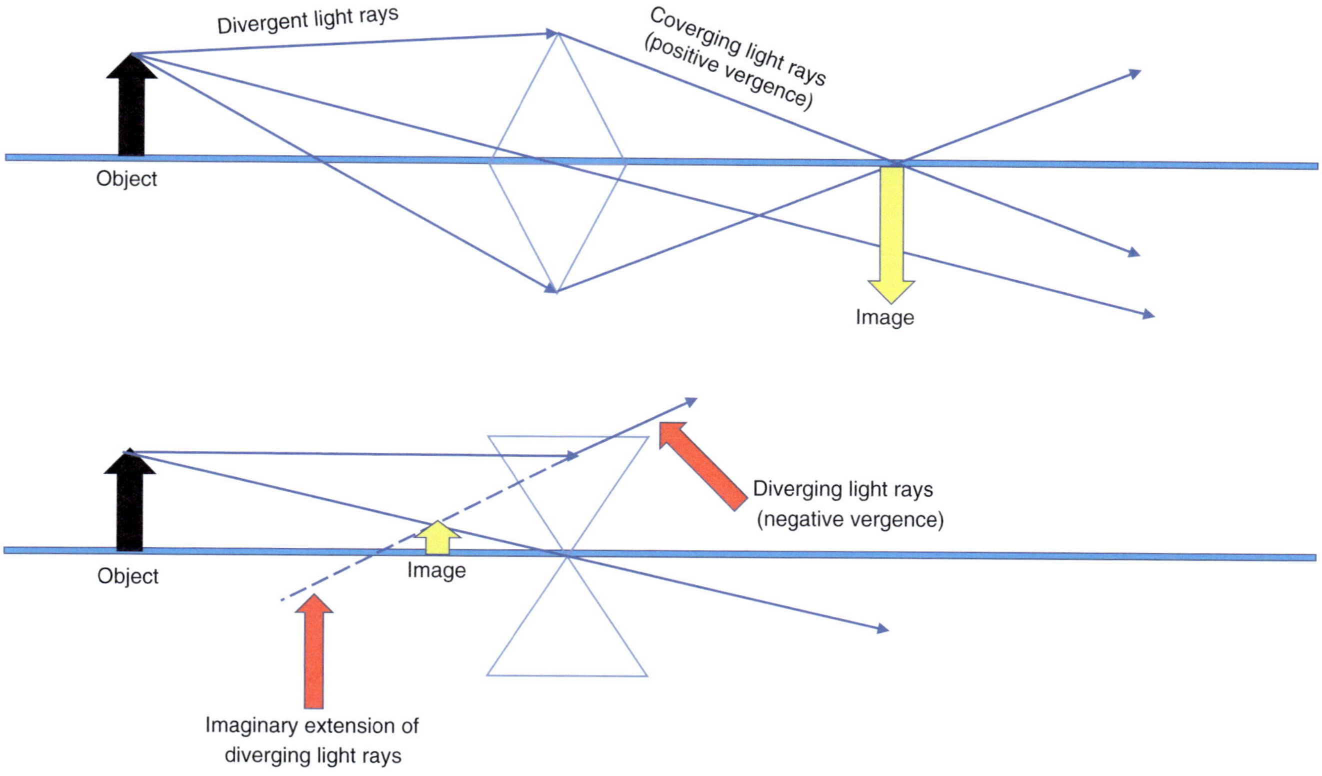

Fig. 1 Light rays that emanate from an object will always have a negative vergence. Light rays that form an image may have a positive or negative vergence, depending on the type of lens that affects these light rays

shows a real image (formed by converging light rays) and the bottom panel shows a virtual image (formed by imaginary extensions of diverging light rays). Did we lose any of you in this matrix? Find a phone booth and call us for help—we'll get you out of there!

For problem-solving, a real image is when the image distance (v) is a positive number and a virtual image is when the image distance (v) is a negative number. Note that we are using lower case "v" to when referring to the image distance. We will discuss this in greater detail when we introduce the RVF later in the chapter.

Upright vs Inverted

We previously introduced "real" and "virtual" to describe one feature of objects and images. Another important feature is the orientation of objects and images. Objects and images can be upright (erect) or inverted. In general, objects will always be upright so long as they are real objects. But for images, they may be upright or inverted, depending on how the image is formed. Later in this chapter, we will discuss how both ray tracing and RVF allow us to determine if the image is upright or inverted. In Fig. 1, the top panel shows an inverted (and real) image; the bottom panel shows an upright (and virtual) image.

Magnified vs Minified Images

A third feature of object–lens (and object–mirror) systems is exclusive to images. Images that are formed by lenses (or mirrors) may be either magnified or minified. While ray tracing can give us information about image orientation, it may not be accurate enough to determine magnification or minification of the final image(s). The best way to determine magnification or minification is to use the RVF. Again, we will save the math for this concept until the end of the chapter.[3]

Lenses

In the previous section, we discussed certain features of objects and images. In this section, we will focus on lenses. Note that these concepts are important not only to better understand lenses, but also to appreciate how these concepts are *similar* and *different* when dealing with mirrors (Chap. 4, "Mirrors and Combined Systems").

[3] Note that this refers to linear (transverse) magnification. We will discuss other types of magnification in Chap. 8, "Telescopes and Magnification".

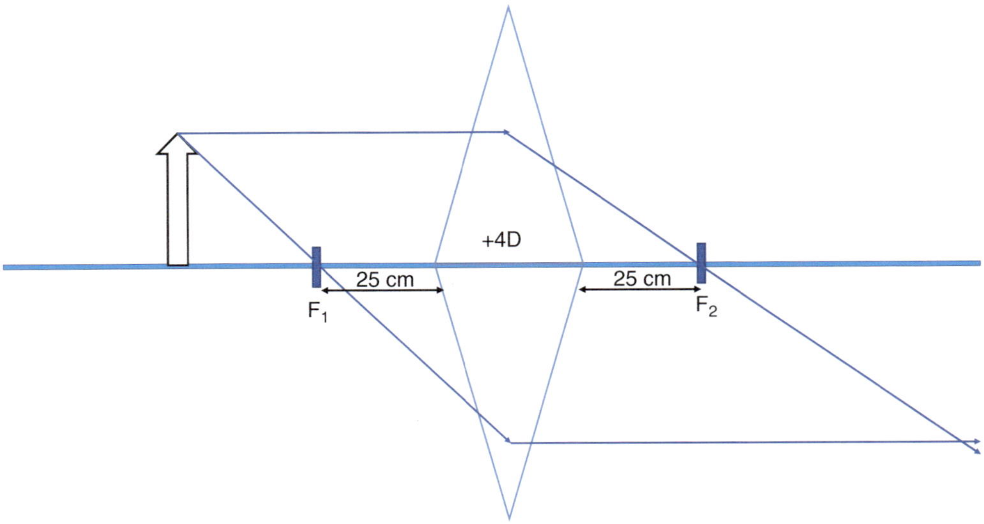

Fig. 2 Primary (F1) and secondary (F2) focal points for a plus lens. Light rays that undergo refraction by the lens will be focused at the secondary focal point. The primary and secondary focal points can be calculated by taking the reciprocal of the lens power

Positive Lenses

A positive (plus) lens is also known as a *converging lens*. We can represent a positive lens by stacking two prisms together such that the bases of each prism are touching each other.[4] When we draw them out, it is helpful to maintain this "diamond" shape as it will help us to do ray tracings. Recall from Chap. 2, "Prisms in Ophthalmic Optics" that real light rays will bend toward the base of a prism. Therefore, light rays that travel through a plus lens at either end will be bent toward the base. This will give us an idea of where these light rays will converge (Fig. 1). This will also help us to perform ray tracings.

Note that we can also draw positive lenses as horizontal diamonds. This will be helpful in later sections to understand concepts such as convergence and strabismus. For lens and mirror problems, however, we will only need to use the "vertical diamond" configuration for positive lenses.

Primary and Secondary Focal Points

Both plus and minus lenses have a primary and secondary focal point. Let us first define these terms and then discuss why they are important.

For a plus lens, the *primary focal point* is located to the *left of the lens*. This is the location for which a light ray emanating from the object passes through until it strikes the lens, undergoes refraction, and then exits the lens in a path parallel to the optical axis (i.e., with zero vergence).

The primary focal point can be calculated by taking the inverse of the lens power. For example, if we are given a + 4D lens, we can calculate the primary focal point as 1/4 = 0.25 m (25 cm), located to the left of the lens (Fig. 2).

[4]See Fig. 11, in chapter "Prisms in Ophthalmic Optics", Prisms, for a review of this concept.

Note in Fig. 2 that the inferior light ray from F1 strikes the bottom portion of the lens, undergoes refraction, and exits with zero vergence.

The *secondary focal point* is the location at which light rays parallel to the optical axis (which have zero vergence), strike the lens, undergo refraction, and come together (converge) *to the right of the lens* (Fig. 2). The secondary focal point is extremely important for solving object–lens system problems because it gives the location of light rays that undergo refraction by the plus lens. Just as we calculated the location of the primary focal point for our given +4D lens, we can use the same reciprocal to calculate the secondary focal point as 0.25 m (25 cm) located to the right of the lens.

Negative Lenses

We will always draw negative lenses as two prisms stacked on top of each other such that the apices of each prism are touching ("hourglass shape") (Fig. 1, lower panel).

Note that we can also draw negative lenses horizontally in a "bowtie" configuration. This will be helpful in later sections to understand concepts such as convergence and strabismus. For lens and mirror problems, however, we will only need to use the "hourglass" configuration for negative lenses.

For a minus lens, the *primary focal point* is still defined as the location at which light rays that emanate from the object will strike the lens and exit the lens with zero vergence (i.e., they remain parallel) (Fig. 3). The key difference for a minus lens is that the primary focal point is located to the *right of the lens*. This would mean that the object would have to be placed to the right of the lens in order to have light rays that converge. Thus, light rays that are located to the left of a minus lens will always *diverge* away from the minus lens.

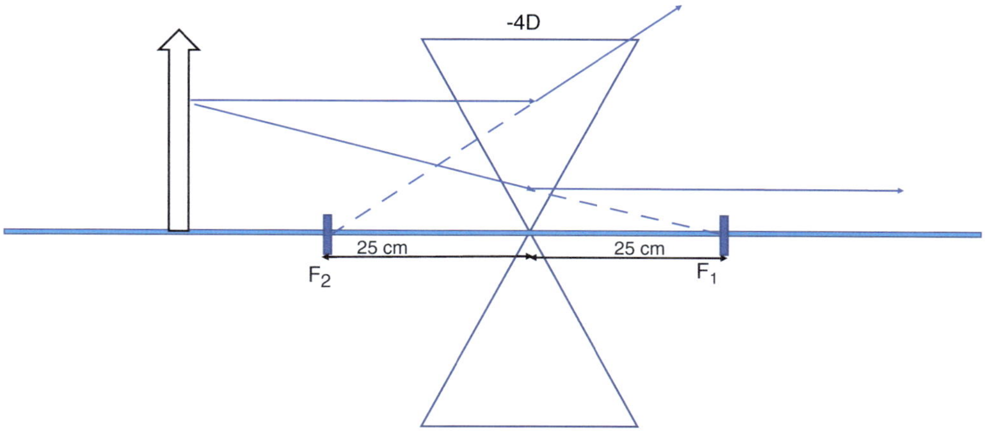

Fig. 3 Primary (F1) and secondary (F2) focal points for a minus lens. Light rays that undergo refraction by the lens will be focused (via imaginary extension) at the secondary focal point. Note that for a minus lens, the secondary focal point is located to the left of the lens. The primary and secondary focal points can be calculated by taking the reciprocal of the lens power

Therefore, for minus lenses, the *secondary focal point* is still defined as the location at which light rays parallel to the optical axis (which have zero vergence) come together (*to the left of the lens*) after undergoing refraction. The key difference is that for minus lenses, we have to create imaginary extensions of the refracted rays (note the dotted line in Fig. 3) onto the secondary focal point. The secondary focal point is extremely important for solving object–lens system problems because it gives the location of light rays that undergo refraction by the minus lens.

The calculation of the primary and secondary focal point location for minus lenses is still the same: We can use the same reciprocal calculation for a given -4D lens to calculate a primary focal point of 0.25 m (25 cm) located to the right of the lens and a secondary focal point of 0.25 m (25 cm) located to the left of the lens.

Ray Tracing

Before we get into the mathematical problem-solving of object–lens systems, we will first discuss the concept of ray tracing as a useful foundation to understand later problems. In the previous discussion of primary and secondary focal points, we used some elementary concepts of ray tracing. Ray tracing is helpful because it gives us a visual idea of where light rays will end up after undergoing refraction by a lens (or undergoing reflection by a mirror).

Note that ray tracing is not crucial to solving object–lens system problems! We can instead use the equations presented in the next section to calculate information such as image location, size, and orientation. If this section seems to be confusing on a first-time read, you may wish to skip ahead to the next section and come back to this section on a future reading.

Definitions

Optical Axis

The "optical axis" used in geometric optics is different than the optical axis used for cataract and refractive surgery, which is discussed in Chap. 26, "Preoperative Optics for Cataract Surgery". For our discussions in this chapter, the optical axis refers to an imaginary perpendicular line that passes through the center of a lens. For example, the optical axis is the "thick" blue line in Figs. 1, 2, and 3 presented earlier. The optical axis is useful when drawing ray tracing diagrams for object–lens systems because it primarily serves as a frame of reference. Note: Some texts may refer to this as the "optic axis" as well.

Cardinal Rays

While there are an infinite number of light rays that emanate from an object, we do not have time to deal with every whiny little light ray. Starting with a given object–lens system using a *plus lens*, we can focus our attention instead on the cardinal rays, which are the three most important light rays that help determine the location of the image (Fig. 4), if we know the focal point(s) of the lens. Remember that we can calculate the primary and secondary focal points by taking the reciprocal of the lens power.

- Cardinal Ray #1: Light ray from the object that starts on a course parallel to the optical axis until it reaches the lens, then undergoes refraction (positive vergence) and continues in a straight line through the *secondary focal point*
- Cardinal Ray #2: Light ray from the object that passes through the *center of the lens* and ignores the primary and secondary focal points altogether. This is also known as the *central ray*

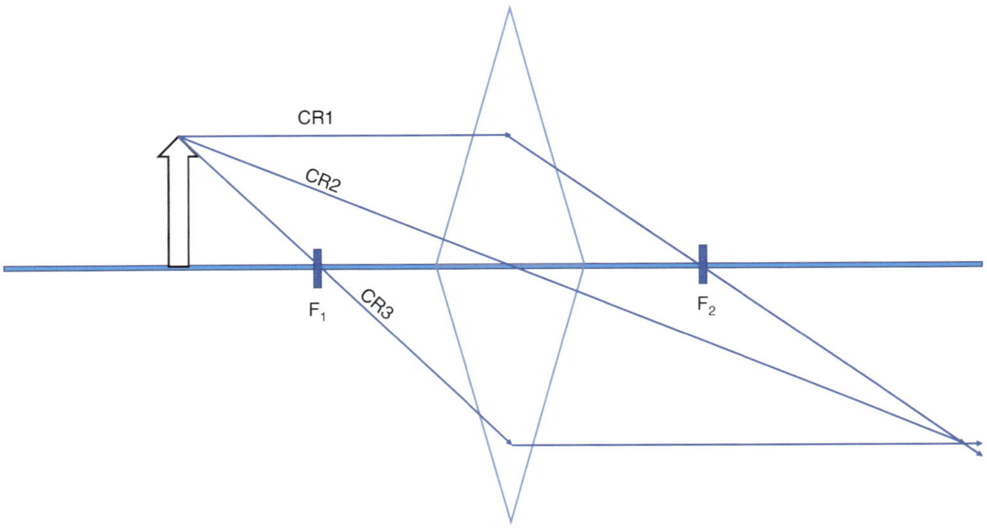

Fig. 4 The three cardinal rays (CR1, CR2, and CR3) can be used with a plus lens to help determine the image location. CR1 will undergo refraction and will be focused at the secondary focal point (F2). CR2 will pass through the center of the lens without undergoing any refraction. CR3 will pass through the primary focal point (F1) until it reaches the lens, then exit the lens with zero vergence (parallel to the optical axis)

- Cardinal Ray #3: Light ray from the object that passes through the *primary focal point* until it reaches the lens, then continues on a course parallel to the optical axis (zero vergence)

Note that the image can usually be determined by the meeting point of *two out of the three cardinal rays* as well. For the sake of sophistication and showing people we know geometric optics, we can draw all three rays whenever possible.

Concepts and Methods of Ray Tracing

If we have an object located to the left of a given lens, we can use the optical axis and the cardinal rays to set up ray tracing and determine the location of the image in a given object–lens system. In the previous example, we showed the ray tracing for a plus lens.

As an additional note regarding plus lenses, we can use ray tracing to determine where the image will form based on 4 potential object locations. You can practice this on your own, but we can summarize this as follows:

- Object very far away from the lens (*extremely* left of the focal point): the image will be real, inverted, and minified
- Object close to the lens (*minimally* left of the focal point): the image will be real, inverted, and magnified
- Object placed at the focal point: trick question—no image is formed! Mathematically, the image is located at "infinity"
- Object placed to the right of the focal point: image will form to the left of the object (virtual image) and will be upright and magnified.

We can similarly draw the three cardinal rays for a *minus lens* using the same strategy we used with a plus lens (Fig. 5). The first cardinal ray undergoes refraction *away* from the minus lens (negative vergence)[5]; therefore, we can draw an imaginary extension toward the *secondary* focal point to the left of the lens. The second cardinal ray passes through the center of the lens, similar to the second cardinal ray for a plus lens. Finally, the third cardinal ray passes through the secondary focal point until it strikes the lens and continues on a path parallel to the optical axis (zero vergence). Note that the image can be determined simply by the intersection of the first and second cardinal ray (red arrow).

Finally, the concept of ray tracing is clinically helpful for understanding concepts used in cataract surgery. For example, the Olsen formula uses ray tracing (and a thick lens model) to help calculate the IOL power. In addition, ray tracing is helpful to understand postoperative problems such as Holladay's model of negative dysphotopsia.[6]

Important Equations for Lens and Mirror System Problems

While ray tracing is helpful to visualize the path of light rays in an object–lens system, it is more likely that one will encounter examination problems wherein one will be asked to calculate the exact location of the image, its size (magnified/minified), its orientation (upright/inverted), and its nature (real/virtual).

[5]This is a good time to review a lesson from Chap. 2, "Prisms in Ophthalmic Optics". Notice that this CR1 is hitting the base-up prism component of this lens; since it is a real light ray, it will be bent toward the base.

[6]Holladay JT, Zhao H, Reisin CR. Negative dysphotopsia: the enigmatic penumbra. J Cataract Refract Surg. 2012 Jul;38(7):1251–65.

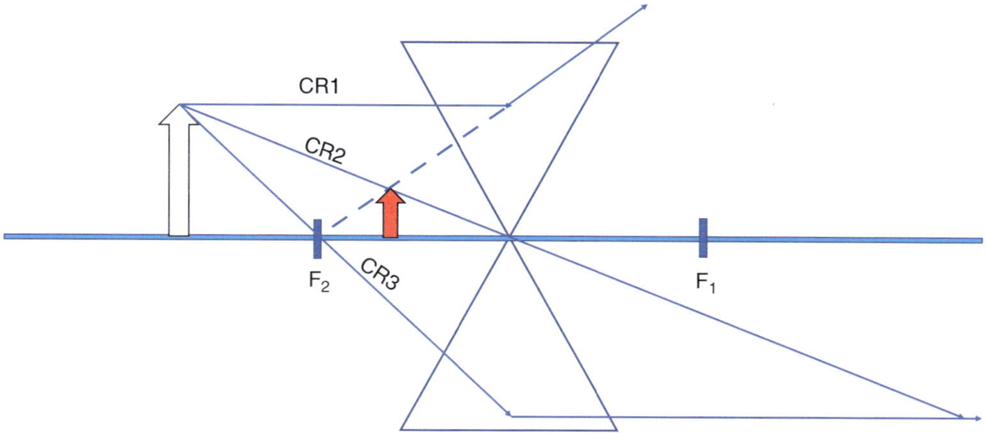

Fig. 5 The three cardinal rays (CR1, CR2, and CR3) can be used with a minus lens to help determine the image location (red arrow). CR1 and CR2 can be used to determine that the image will form to the left of the lens. Ray tracing can also help determine that the image will likely be upright and minified (relative to the original object)

There are only two key equations we need to know in order to solve these object–lens (and object–mirror) problems. Neither will be provided on examinations so you must memorize them!

The reduced vergence formula (RVF) is the bread-and-butter equation for object–lens system problems.[7] It is based on the principle that the sum of the object vergence (U) and the power of the lens (D) equal the image vergence (V). The other equation is the magnification formula; in addition, to giving information about magnification, it can also give information about image orientation and nature (real/virtual).

Let us explore each of these formulas in greater detail.

Reduced Vergence Formula (Simple Lens Formula)

$$\boxed{U + D = V}$$

- (big)U = object vergence (almost always negative!): calculated as $1/u$ (in meters) or $100/u$ (in cm).[8]
- (little) u = object distance (almost always negative!)
- D = lens or mirror power (may sometimes be written as P in other texts). We will use D to represent diopters, since the power of the lens is measured in diopters.
- (big) V = image vergence: calculated as $1/v$ (in meters) or $100/v$ (in cm)[9]
- (little) v = image distance

A few helpful comments regarding this equation[10]:

- It may help to convert calculations into "100/x" and work with cm instead of working with decimals. You can choose to work with 1/x or 100/x depending on which kind of math is easier for you to do in your head (or with pen and paper).
- For all of these problems, we will assume that light travels from left to right, unless explicitly stated otherwise.
- If the problem does not state where the light rays are originating from or use terminology ("light rays from infinity," "parallel light rays strike a lens," etc.), then we can assume that $U = 0$. Mathematically, if the light rays are originating from a (galaxy) far, far away, then the 1/u will be such a small number that we can make it zero in order to calculate the rest of the problem.
- Finally, remember that the math for these problems should be relatively easy because they would not allow you to use calculators on the actual examination. If you suddenly find yourself calculating some very ugly numbers, stop and re-assess: You may have flipped the numerator/denominator somewhere, or plugged in the wrong number for the wrong variable.

---

[7]We will skip how this formula is derived for the sake of keeping your sanity. For those who wish to understand how this formula is derived, consult other texts or Google it if you are extremely bored. This formula also has several other names, such as simple lens formula and vergence formula.

[8]We use $1/u$ (or $100/u$) for the majority of these calculations because we assume that we are working in air (index of refraction = 1.00). If an object–lens system were immersed into a different medium, such as water (index of refraction = 1.33), then we would have to accordingly calculate $U = 1.33/u$ (or $133/u$).

[9]We use $1/v$ (or $100/v$) for the majority of these calculations because we assume that we are working in air (index of refraction = 1.00). If an object–lens system were immersed into a different medium, such as water (index of refraction = 1.33), then we would have to accordingly calculate $V = 1.33/v$ (or $133/v$).

[10]The RVF is a modification of Snell's law of refraction. The full mathematics for this has been nicely described in other texts and is beyond the scope of our discussion. Another confusing aspect of this terminology is that some textbooks refer to this formula as the lens maker's equation. We will discuss the lens maker's equation (i.e., a different equation) in Chap. 5, "Power of Lenses in Different Media".

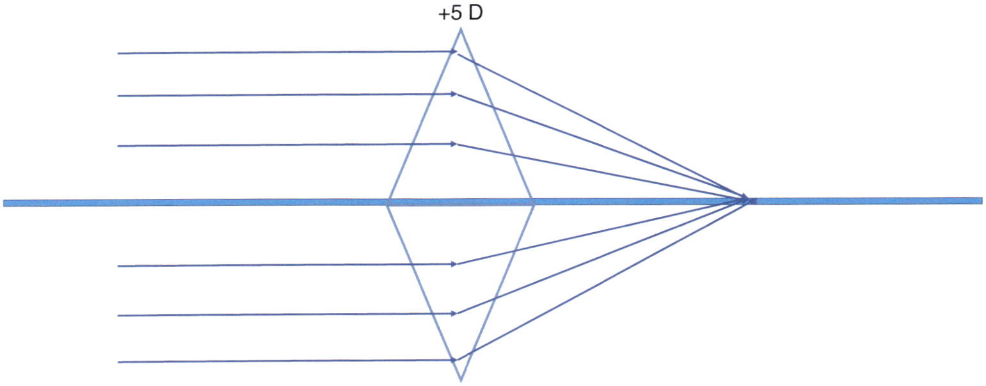

Fig. 6 If parallel rays approach a + 5D lens, where will the image form?

While many of these reciprocals (diopters and distances) can be easily calculated, the following table may help serve as a refresher for commonly encountered powers and distances[11]:

Diopter values (D)	Distance (in cm)
0.25	400 cm
0.33	300 cm
0.50	200 cm
1.00	100 cm
1.33	75 cm
1.50	67 cm
2.00	50 cm
2.50	40 cm
3.00	33 cm
4.00	25 cm
5.00	20 cm
6.00	16.6 cm
7.00	14 cm
8.00	12.5 cm
9.00	11 cm
10.00	10 cm

We can see how the RVF can help us solve commonly asked questions about object–lens system problems in the following examples.

Example #1 If parallel light rays approach a + 5D lens, where will the image form (Fig. 6)?

Answer: Since the question stem gives us no information about the origin of the light rays, we can assume that the light rays are originating from an extremely far-off distance. Therefore, if u is an incredibly far away distance, then $1/u = 0$, for the purposes of this problem.

So, our $U + D = V$ will become $D = V$.

$V = D = 1/0.05$ (or 100/5) = 20; the image will form 20 cm to the right of the lens.

[11]We have included this table based on years of feedback from trainees expressing frustration how they had set up the equation correctly but goofed the reciprocal calculation and ended up with the wrong answer.

Example #2 If an object is located to the left of a + 7D lens and forms an image 25 cm to the right of the lens, where is the object?

Answer: We can draw this problem out if we would like, but we can skip to the chase and use our RVF equation. The question is asking us to calculate "*u*," which is the reciprocal of *U*. If we can calculate *U*, we can easily calculate *u*. We are given v as 25 cm, so we can calculate *V* as 100/25 = +4.

Therefore: $U + D = V$, which can be re-arranged so that $U = V - D$.

$U = 4–7 \rightarrow U = -3$. Therefore, $u = 100/-3 = -33$ cm, or 33 cm to the left of the lens.

At this point, you may wonder: "Who cares about U+D=V? I just want to do cataract surgery and help people see well!" Well, most IOL calculation formulas, including some current multi-variable generation formulas, are essentially modifications of RVF from the nineteenth century adapted to modern technology. In order to calculate the IOL power needed, modern formulas use various biometric measurements of the eye to approximate "*U*" and "*V*" in order to calculate "*D*" (the IOL power). An example of a modern IOL formula is shown in Fig. 7. If you do cataract surgery, you have to care about $U + D = V$!

Magnification Formula

$$\boxed{m = U / V \text{ or } v / u}$$

The magnification formula does not simply give us information about the linear (transverse) magnification of an object–lens system. It can also be used to determine (1) orientation of the image (upright/inverted) and (2) nature of the image (real/virtual).

In this equation, the following terms are defined as follows:

- *m* is linear (transverse) magnification.[12]

[12]We will discuss other types of magnification in greater detail in Chap. 8, "Magnification and Telescopes".

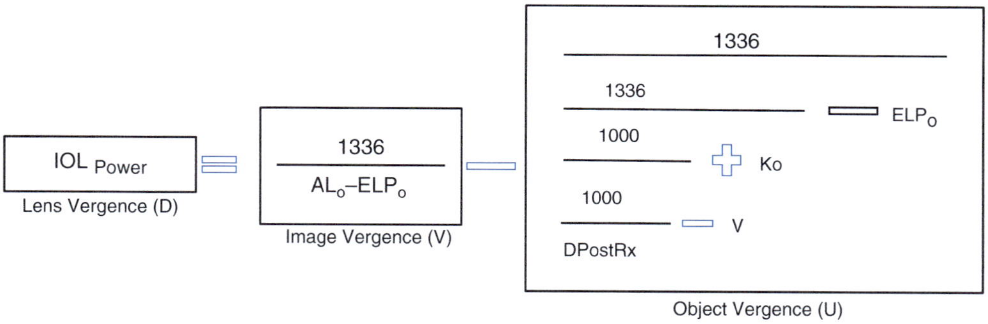

Fig. 7 Modern IOL calculation formulas are modifications of the simple lens formula. Different variables (e.g., axial length, keratometry, central corneal thickness, white-to-white ratio, refraction, and anterior chamber depth) are used to enhance the accuracy of "*U*" or "*V*" in order to calculate the IOL power ("*D*")

- *U* is the object vergence.
- *V* is the image vergence.
- *u* is the object distance (from the lens or mirror).
- *v* is the image distance (from the lens or mirror).

A few helpful comments regarding this equation:

- Magnification can be determined by both $m = U/V$ or v/u → a helpful mnemonic is as follows: "big MOVIE, little VIEW." "MOVIE" may help you to remember that the "big *U*" goes over the "big *V*," and "VIEW" may help you to remember that "little v" goes over the "little *u*" when you want to calculate magnification. Depending on the question, you may only be given "*U*/*V*" or "*v*/*u*," so it is important to know how to use this equation using both terms. Of course, if given "*U*," you can always calculate "*u*" by $u = 1/U$, etc.
- Positive m is upright; negative m is inverted. You can always use this to mathematically make sure that you have correctly determined the orientation of the image. Note that *negative m does not mean that the image is minified, it simply means that the image is inverted.* This is a common mistake that many trainees make when first doing these problems.
- For magnification, we will use the absolute value of m. Therefore, $|m| > 1$ is magnified and $|m| < 1$ is minified. The value of m can be used to determine how large the image will be relative to the original object.
- Remember that positive *V* is a real image, and negative *V* is a virtual image.

For example, suppose we solve an object–lens system using the RVF, and then using the magnification formula, we get $m = 2$. This means we have an upright, magnified image with 2x magnification. If our original object is 2 m tall, then our image is 4 m tall and upright.

As another example, suppose we use the magnification formula for another object–lens system and we get $m = -0.5$. This means we have an inverted, minified image with 1/2× magnification (i.e., the image is 50% the size of the original object). If our original object is 2m tall, then our image is 1m tall and upside down. As a final point, suppose $m = -5$. This means we have an inverted, *magnified* image with 5× magnification. Remember that the minus sign denotes *inversion, not minification.*

We can now use a few examples to reinforce some of the concepts we have discussed so far with both the RVF and magnification equations. These should be fairly easy to understand at this point. If you are having any difficulty with these examples, re-read the above sections until they make (some) sense.

Convex (Positive) Lens Example #1

An object is 20 cm to the left of a + 7 D converging lens. Where is the image? Is it real or virtual? Is it upright or inverted? Is it magnified or minified?

We can walk through this one together step by step. It is always helpful for these problems to start off by drawing out a rough sketch of the object–lens system (Fig. 8).

The object is 20 cm or 0.20 m to the left of a lens. That tells us $u = -0.2$ m.

Remember that U and u are almost always negative. The exception to U being negative is when we are dealing with multiple lenses or mirrors wherein the intermediate image (aka secondary object) appears to the right of the lens—we will do this example in the end-of-chapter problems.

In order to reinforce some of the concepts we have discussed thus far, we can draw out the ray tracings for this problem. While not necessary for every problem, drawing a ray tracing may be helpful because it will give us some information about the image.[13]

In the previous section, we discussed how to use three cardinal rays for ray tracing. We can take a shortcut by simply using the first two cardinal rays (CR1 and CR2): start by drawing a ray from the top of the object that strikes the top part of the lens—this ray will bend toward the base and pass through the secondary focal point. Do not worry if you do not know the exact location of the secondary focal point, just draw a line that gets refracted by the lens, emerges to the right of the lens, and bends toward (and through) the optical axis and the assumed secondary focal point location. Then draw a ray from

[13] Refer to the previous section for a detailed discussion on ray tracing.

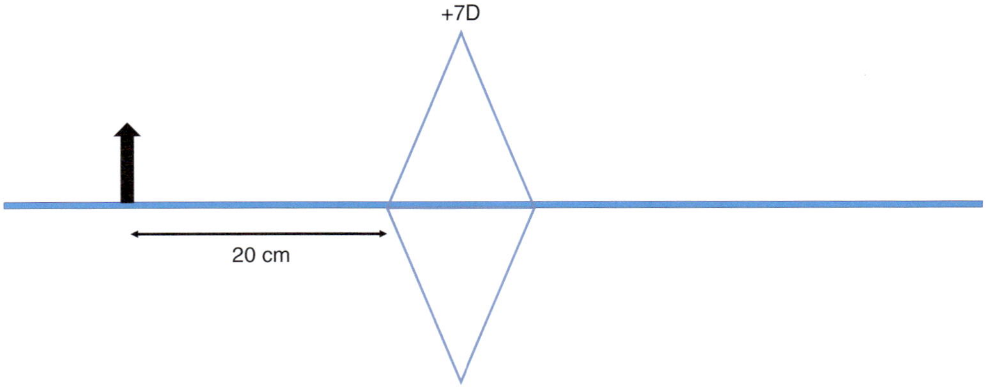

Fig. 8 Object–lens system for an object located 20 cm to the left of a + 7D converging lens. Where will the image form?

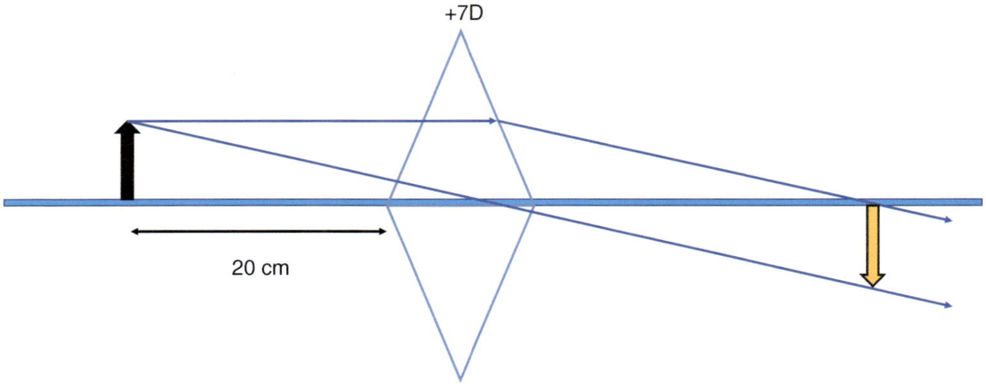

Fig. 9 The first two cardinal rays can be used to give information about the location, orientation, size, and nature of the image located to the right of the lens

the top part of the object that passes through the central part of the lens (the central ray) that does not get refracted. This will give you a rough idea of where the image will form. It may also give you information about the orientation and size of the image if you have drawn it correctly (Fig. 9).

From the ray tracing, we can see that the image will be located to the right of the lens (real image) and it will be inverted. It may also be magnified but we cannot be certain of this, so we will have to do put on our hard hats and do some real work now using the RVF:

$$u = -0.2\text{m} \left(\text{this is the object distance}\right) \text{ or } -20\,\text{cm}$$

$$U = 1/u = 1/-0.2\text{m} = -5 \left(\text{this is the object vergence}\right) \text{ or } 100/-20 = -5$$

$$U + D = V$$

$$-5 + 7 = V = 2 \left(\text{this is the image vergence}\right)$$

$$v = 1/V = 1/2 = 0.5\text{m} \left(\text{this is the image distance}\right) \text{ or } 100/2 = 50\,\text{cm}$$

Now we know the image is 0.5 m or 50 cm to the right of the lens. We know it is a real image because v is a positive number.

$$m = U/V = -5/2 = -2.5 \text{ or } m = v/u = 50/-20 = -2.5$$

(Note that we can calculate magnification using either *U*/*V* or *v*/*u*; we should get the same number either way).

Wonderful! We have a magnified image (2.5×), an inverted image (since *m* is negative), and a real image because v is positive.

Convex (Positive) Lens Example #2

An object is 10 cm to the left of a + 8D converging lens. Where is the image? Is it real or virtual? Is it upright or inverted? Is it magnified or minified?

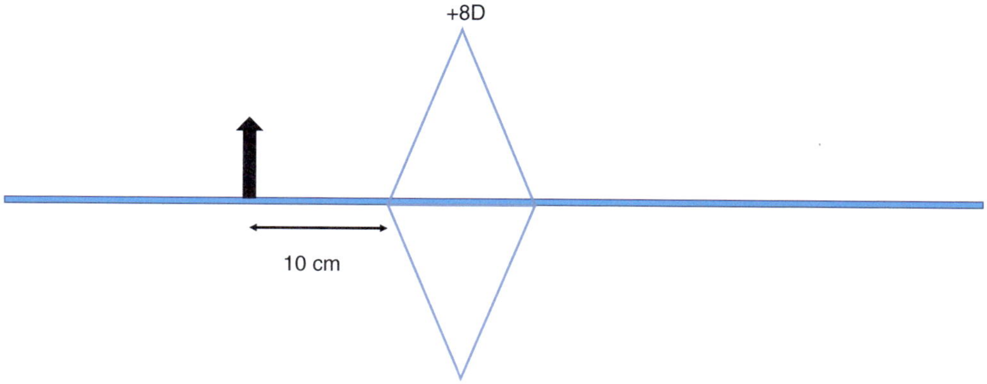

Fig. 10 Where will the image form if the object is 10 cm away from this +8D converging lens?

Answer: Again, start off by drawing out the lens system as presented in the question stem to get your bearings (Fig. 10).

We will skip drawing the ray tracing for this problem and get to the chase:

$$u = -10\,\text{cm or } -0.10\,\text{m} \left(\text{make sure that "}u\text{" is negative!}\right)$$

$$U = 1/u = 1/-0.1 = -10 \left(\text{this is the object vergence}\right) \text{ OR } 100/-10 = -10$$

$$U + D = V$$

$$-10 + 8 = V = -2 \left(\text{this is the image vergence}\right)$$

$$v = 1/V = 1/-2 = -0.5\,\text{m} \left(\text{this is the image distance}\right) \text{ OR } 100/-2 = -50\,\text{cm}$$

$v = -0.5$ m means the image is virtual (since it is negative) and 50 cm to the left of the lens. Remember, positive v means there is a real image to the right of the lens and a negative v means there is a virtual image to the left of the lens.

$$m = U/V = -10/-2 = 5 \text{ OR } v/u = -50/-10 = 5$$

So, we have a magnified, upright image that is 50 cm to the left of the lens.

Suppose the question stated that the original object was 8 cm in height. The final image size will be 8 cm × 5 = 40 cm in height.

In the previous two examples, we have shown how a positive lens can give an image to both the right and the left of the lens. As we do more problems, we will see how (a) the location of the object and (b) the power of the lens can affect where the image will be located. Do not always assume that a convex (plus) lens will always lead to an image on the right!

We can solve a few additional examples with minus lenses to reinforce some of the concepts, we have discussed so far.

Concave (Minus) Lens Example #1

A 10-meter-tall object is 50 cm to the left of a – 3 D lens. How tall is the image and is it upright or inverted?

Answer:

Start off this problem by drawing out a rough sketch of the object–lens system and doing the ray tracing. We will draw one ray from the top of the object that strikes the top part of the lens and gets bent toward the base—this line will have to then have an imaginary extension "backward" to the left of the lens. Then, we will draw a ray from the top part of the object that passes through the central part of the lens (central ray) that does not get refracted (Fig. 11).

The point at which the first two light rays will intersect with the optical axis will give you a rough idea of where the image will form. It may also give you information about the orientation and size of the image if you have drawn it correctly. From the figure above, it would seem that our image will be upright, virtual, and minified. But we should do the actual work here and make sure that our initial conclusions are correct.

$$u = -0.50\text{m} \left(\text{make sure } U \text{ and } u \text{ are negative!}\right) \text{ or } -50\,\text{cm}$$

$$U = 1/u = 1/-0.5 = -2 \left(\text{this is the object vergence}\right) \text{ OR } 100/-50 = -2$$

$$\text{U} + \text{D} = \text{V}$$

$$-2 + (-3) = V = -5 \left(\text{this is the image vergence}\right)$$

$$v = 1/V = 1/-5 = -0.2\text{m} \left(\text{this is the image distance}\right) \text{ OR } 100/-5 = -20\,\text{cm to the LEFT of the lens}$$

$$m = U/V = -2/-5 = 0.4 \left(\text{this is the magnification}\right) \text{ OR } v/u = -20/-50 = 0.4$$

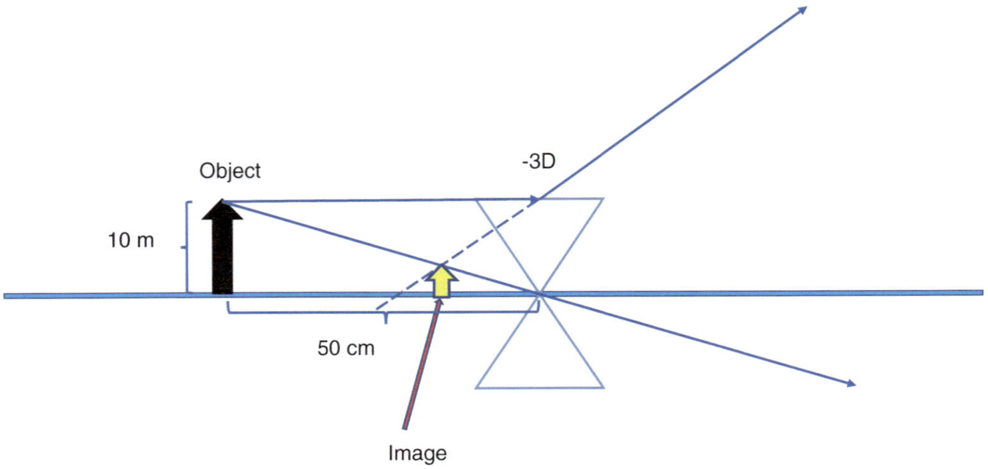

Fig. 11 Ray tracing for an object (10 meters height) located 50 cm to the left of a –3D lens. Note: The object–lens system is not drawn to scale

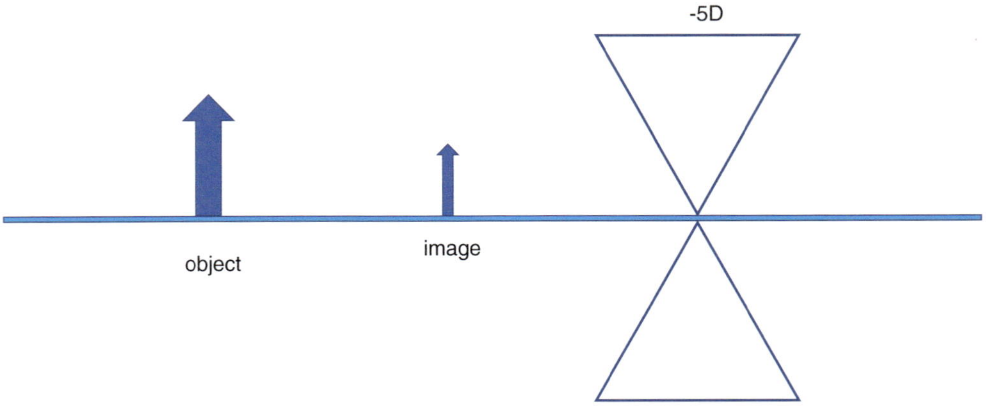

Fig. 12 An object is placed in front of a −5D lens. The image is formed at the midpoint between the object and the lens. At what distance from the lens was the object?

Based on these calculations, our image is upright (since m is positive), virtual (since v is negative), and minified (since $|m| < 1$). The image is 20 cm to the left of the lens.

As for the size of the image: 10 m × 0.4 = 4 m image size.

Concave (Minus) Lens Example #2

An object is to the left of a diverging lens. Is the image upright or inverted? Real or virtual? Magnified or minified?

Answer: Do we have enough information to solve this? We did not get any numbers! Was this a typo? An experimental question? No problem! If the examination gives you a question with no numbers, make them up!

We can make our lives easier by making the numbers easy. Let us make $u - 1$ and the power of the lens −1D.

$$u = -1$$

$$U = 1/u = -1$$

$$U + D = V$$

$$-1 + (-1) = V = -2$$

$$v = 1/V = 1/-2 = -0.5\text{m} \ (\text{our image is 50cm to the left of the lens})$$

$$m = U/V = -1/-2 = 0.5$$

Therefore, our image will be upright (m is positive), virtual (v is negative), and minified ($|m| < 1$). If this was an experimental question, they better give us extra points for doing this extra work!

The takeaway from this example is that if a problem has no numbers, you can make them up in order to determine the piece(s) of information being asked. Remember, the basic information for this topic is never going to change—how this concept may be tested, however, may change over time.

Concave (Minus) Lens Example #3

An object is placed in front of a −5D lens. The image is formed at the midpoint between the object and the lens. Where is the object?

Answer: This is a bit of a trickier question. Let us start off by drawing out what the problem stem is describing (Fig. 12).

We know that the image is between the object and the lens; we also know that this is a diverging lens, so it must be a virtual image. Since the image distance is half of the object distance, this means that $v = ½\,u$.

$$\text{We can now solve for } U \text{ and } V: V = 1/v = 1/\left(1/2u\right). \text{ So } 2U = V$$

Now we can use our trusty equation:

$$U + D = V \rightarrow U + D = 2U$$
$$U + \left(-5\right) = 2U$$
$$\text{So}, U = -5, V = 2 \times \left(-5\right) = -10.$$

Therefore, the object distance (u) from the lens is 100/−5 = −20 cm to the left of the lens.

The image distance (v) from the lens is 100/−10 = −10 cm to the left of the lens.

Lens System with Different Media

In the previous examples, we assumed that the object–lens system was occurring in air. For example, we were able to use $1/u$ (or $100/u$) to calculate U and $1/v$ (or $100/v$) to calculate V. However, not all object–lens systems occur in air as sometimes the image will form in a different medium. The best example for this is the eye itself: We view objects (in air), but the image forms in a water (vitreous) medium. Therefore, we have to account for the *different indexes of refraction* when calculating the location of an image. The clinical relevance for this concept occurs all throughout ophthalmology; IOL calculation formulas are one example of why it is important to account for a different indexes of refraction in regards to image location.

Consider the following example: Suppose we had an object that is located 1 m to the left of a + 3D lens that has been placed in a water medium. To make the math easier, assume that the front surface of the lens is in air and the back surface of the lens is in water.

We can use our familiar $U + D = V$ equation:

$$U + D = V \rightarrow U = -100/100 = -1$$
$$-1 + 3 = V = +2$$

At this point, if the system was in air, we can simply use 100/2 = 50 cm to state that the image would form 50 cm to the right of the lens. However, we have to account for the water medium (n = 1.33).

Therefore: $V = 1.33/v$, $v = 1.33/V = 1.33/2 = 67$ cm. The image will form 67 cm to the right of the lens (in water).

As should be evident, this has implications because the image is significantly shifted to the right in a water medium as compared to an air medium. Suppose we wanted a lens (imagine this is an IOL) such that the image formed at 50 cm.[14] If we simply used "in-air" calculations, the image would be shifted to the right considerably, causing a hyperopic shift. Therefore, the power of the lens needs to be adjusted (increased) in order to form an image at the desired location when considering a medium with stronger index of refraction.

[14]Obviously, this would be a giant eye, but just use this example to understand the concept.

Calculating Vergence Along a Lens System

Another way these concepts can be tested is to ask questions about vergence along a lens system. We have previously discussed how vergence can be positive (convergence) or negative (divergence).

For this subtopic, suppose that we are using a positive lens: We can remember that the vergence of light rays immediately as they leave the lens is equal to the power of the lens. As these light rays approach the focal point (where the image will form), they will converge until the focal point. Mathematically, this means that their vergence will *quantitatively increase* until the focal point—at this point, they will have joined together in love and harmony and the vergence will be infinity.

In order to calculate the numerical vergence along a lens system, follow these simple rules:

1. Solve the lens system using $U + D = V$.
2. Calculate the distance from the given point from the image by subtracting the distance between the point and the location of the final image.
3. Divide this distance by 100. This will be the vergence of the light rays at that given point.
4. Again, as you move closer to the focal point, the vergence should continue to increase.

Let us do an example (Fig. 13). In the lens system below, what is the vergence at points A, B, C, D, E, and F?

Let us set up our equation:

$$U + D = V \rightarrow 100/-11 = -9$$
$$-9 + 14 = 5\left(V\right)$$

Therefore, v = 100/5 = 20 cm to the right of the lens.

At point A: The vergence here should equal V = +5D.

At point B: Point 5 is 5 cm to the right of the lens, but more importantly, it is 15 cm from the location of the image. So, vergence at this point will be 100/15 = +6.67 D vergence.

At point C: Point C is 12.5 cm from the location of the image. Vergence at this point will be 100/12.5 = +8D vergence. Notice how our numbers are increasing at each point as we are approaching the image.

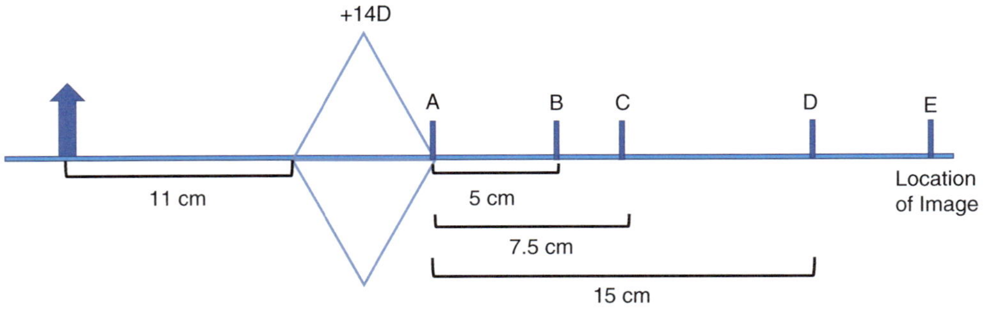

Fig. 13 Calculating vergence along a system: What is the vergence of light at each of these locations?

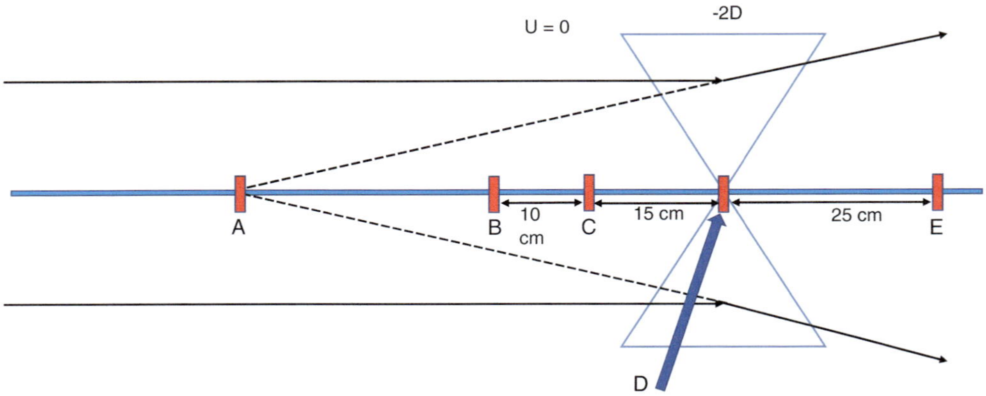

Fig. 14 What is the vergence of light at each of these locations?

At point D: Point D is 5 cm from the location of the image. Vergence at this point will be 100/5 = +20D vergence. Again, our numbers are continuing to increase, so we must be doing something right!

At point E: Point E is 0 cm from the location of the image (because it's right at the image, duh!). Therefore, 100/0 = ∞. This makes sense because at this point all the light rays have finished converging.

For minus lenses, the vergence of all real light rays after they have passed through the lens will be zero (because they will diverge). We will have to calculate the "vergence" of the imaginary light rays in a similar fashion to the problem above. Mathematically, we will use "negative vergence" to describe these imaginary light rays, as technically they are not converging in the same manner as real light rays. Do not think about this topic for too long lest you get lost in the abyss of vergence… just understand the concept as described above and the associated calculations.

We can do one more example (Fig. 14). In the lens system below, what is the vergence at points A, B, C, D, and E? We will assume the incoming pencil of light rays are originating from infinity ($U = 0$).

Answer: We can again start by using our $U + D = V$ equation. We are told that $U = 0$, so $D = V$, so $V = -2$. Solving for v (100/V), we can determine that the image will form 50 cm to the left of the lens at point A.

At point A: Point A is 0 cm from the location of the image, so 100/0 = ∞. Infinite vergence (of the imaginary, extended rays).

At point B: Point B is 25 cm from the location of the image. Vergence at this point will be 100/−25 = −4.0D (because we are dealing with divergent light).

At point C: Point C is 35 cm from the location of the image. Vergence at this point will be 100/−35 = −2.86D (admittedly a yucky number).

At point D: This is the vergence of light rays leaving the lens, aka the "V" in $U + D = V$. Vergence at this point will be −2D.

At point E: Point E is 75 cm from the location of the image. Vergence at this point will be 100/−75 = −1.33D.

In summary, calculating vergence along a lens system is simply a wrinkle to the previously discussed concepts. If we first solve the RVF, we can then use this information to calculate vergence at a given point in the object–lens system.

Thick Lenses

A word of caution: We hope this section is low yield. We hope that examination makers will not be mean enough to put these problems on the examination because the math is often quite difficult and requires calculators. However, there may be several ways to test this concept.

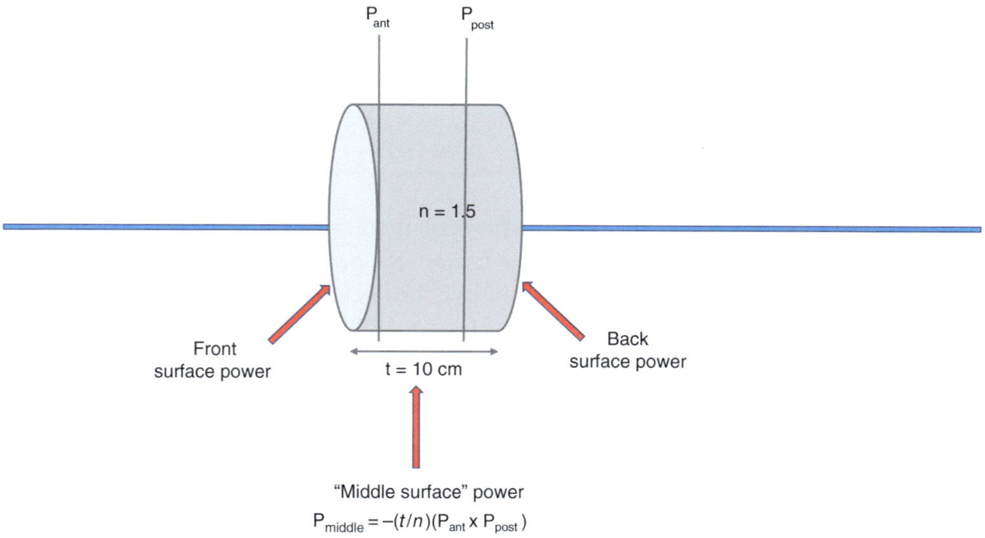

Fig. 15 The power of a thick lens is a sum of the powers of the anterior surface, posterior surface, and the "middle surface." The middle surface power is determined by the lens thickness, index of refraction, and power of the anterior and posterior surface: ($P_{middle} = -(t/n)(P_{ant} \times P_{post})$. In this example, the thickness of the lens is 10 cm ($t = 0.1$) and the index of refraction is 1.5

We should pause for a moment here and understand why this has clinical and practical significance. Recall that we earlier said we will make a "thin lens approximation" when doing $U + D = V$ problems. In reality, all lenses (e.g., the cornea, crystalline lens, and spectacle lenses) have both a front surface and back surface that contributes to the refractive power of the lens.[15] In addition, the thickness of that lens (and index of refraction) will also contribute to the refractive power of the lens. This means that there are 3 places of refraction when light rays pass through a thick lens (Fig. 15).

In order to calculate the power of a thick lens, we have to account for all three places of refraction: the front surface (and its power), the back surface (and its power), and the "middle surface" (the adjustment for the thickness of the lens). The "middle surface" power relies on the thickness (t) of the lens (in meters!), the index of refraction (n), and the power of the anterior surface and posterior surface (P_{ant} and P_{post}). When given a thick lens, usually the front surface will be a convex lens (plus power) and the back surface will be a concave lens (negative power).[16] When we look at Fig. 15, we can see how the shape of the front surface of the cylinder resembles a convex lens, and how the shape of the back surface of the cylinder resembles a concave lens.

The power of the "middle surface" is as follows: $P_{middle} = -(t/n)*(P_{ant} \times P_{post})$.

[15] This is one (of many) reason(s) that older generation IOL formulas are often inaccurate as they rely on the thin lens approximation. For example, the cornea is reduced to a single refractive surface. While this may work (relatively) accurately for very normal eyes, these formulas' accuracy drops off significantly in eyes with unique biometric data. See Chap. 26, "Preoperative Optics for Cataract Surgery" for more information.

[16] The cornea is a great example of a thick lens with a convex front surface and concave back surface.

Therefore, the power of a thick lens is as follows: $P_{ant} + P_{post} - (t/n)*(P_{ant} \times P_{post})$.

Note that we did not include this in the hi-yield list of formulas to know!

Let us do some thick lens examples:

Example #1

If a lens has a front surface power of +8.00D, back surface power of −3.00D, thickness of 5 cm, and index of refraction of 1.5, what is the total (net) power of the lens?

Answer:

We can simply plug in the values into our thick lens equation:

$$\begin{aligned}\text{Power of Thick Lens} &= P_{ant} + P_{post} - (t/n)*(P_{ant} \times P_{post})\\ &= +8 + (-3) - (0.05/1.5)*(8 \times -3)\\ &= 5 - (0.033)*(-24)\\ &= 5 - (-0.8)\\ &= +5.8\text{D}\end{aligned}$$

Two other points we can note at this time:

1. The thicker the lens, the more "power" that the "middle surface" will have. This is subtracted from the other two surfaces, leading to an overall decreased power of the lens.
2. The higher the index of refraction, the less "power" that the "middle surface" will have. This is subtracted from the other two surfaces, leading to an overall increased power of the lens.

Example #2 (Clinical Relevance)

If a cornea has a front surface power of +48D, back surface power of −6.00D, thickness of 550 microns, and index of refraction of 1.376, what is the total (net) power of the cornea?

Answer: We can again use our thick lens equation:

$$\text{Power of Thick Lens} = P_{\text{ant}} + P_{\text{post}} - (t/n) * (P_{\text{ant}} \times P_{\text{post}})$$
$$= +48 + (-6) - (0.00055/1.376) * (48 \times -6) \rightarrow (\text{ugly math follows})$$
$$= 42.12\text{D}$$

No one would expect you to be able to do the math for this example. The main learning point is to appreciate how the "middle surface" of a thick lens has to be accounted for when calculating the total power of the lens. Hence, some of the newer IOL calculation formulas use the central corneal thickness measurement as an additional factor to potentially increase accuracy. We can also see how corneal edema (e.g., Fuchs' endothelial dystrophy) can skew the corneal power measurements if considering combined cataract surgery with endothelial keratoplasty. The second learning point is we should appreciate how the back surface of the cornea contributes negative power to the total net power of the cornea. The third learning point is we should be thankful we have calculators to solve these problems for real-life, clinical purposes.

Mirrors and Combined Systems

Daniel Wee

Objectives

- To understand common types of mirrors (plano, convex, and concave) and how they function to create images
- To understand how mirror systems will share similar features as lens systems and also have their own unique image characteristics
- To solve problems with multiple lenses and lens–mirror combinations
- To review common mistakes made when solving lens and mirror system problems

Introduction

In the previous chapter, we primarily focused on (no pun-intended) lenses. In this chapter, we will direct our attention toward mirrors.

It is important to be comfortable with certain principles and concepts discussed in the previous chapter, such as using the reduced vergence equation/simple lens formula (RVF/SLF), calculating the orientation and magnification of images, etc. In general, object–mirror system problems are set up in a similar fashion, and many of the equations and concepts we previously discussed have relevance for the discussion of mirrors. However, some of the rules we introduced (and emphasized) in the previous chapter are no longer valid.

Before you get mad, imagine that the world of mirrors is a parallel universe wherein some of the rules of our universe are still valid, but others are not.

Why is this? With lenses, we previously dealt with <u>refracted</u> light rays. With mirrors, we are primarily dealing with <u>reflected</u> light rays. This is why we are in the parallel universe of mirrors.

D. Wee (✉)
Center for Sight, Stockton, CA, USA

Mirrors

In order for a smooth surface to function as a mirror, it must reflect as many light rays as possible, while minimizing refraction and absorption. For ophthalmic optics, we will focus our discussion on three kinds of mirrors: plano mirrors; positive (concave) mirrors; and negative (convex) mirrors.

Plano Mirrors

Think of plano mirrors as objects that contain a portal to an entire parallel universe that exists in the mirror. This parallel universe is basically a "mirror image" of the world on the other side of the mirror (see what we did there?). Basically, this means that any object located at a certain distance to the left of the mirror (by convention) will have the same distance to the "right" of the mirror. This is somewhat confusing because if you have a mirror on the wall, then there obviously is no image that is forming to the "right" of the wall. However, since mirrors reverse the image space, there is the same "space" inside the mirror as there is outside the mirror—if you think about this for too long, your head will hurt.

We can understand this by falling back on our good old $U + D = V$ equation. Basically, plano mirrors will have zero power, so $D = 0$. Therefore, $U = V$ (and by extension, $u = v$ as well). So, if we have an object 50 cm to the left of a plano mirror, then its image will form 50 cm to the "right" of the mirror (in the mirror).

Images formed by plano mirrors are always a follows:

- upright
- virtual
- same size
- left–right reversed

We can do some examples to reinforce these properties of plano mirrors.

K. M. Riaz et al. (eds.), *Optics for the New Millennium*, https://doi.org/10.1007/978-3-030-95251-8_4

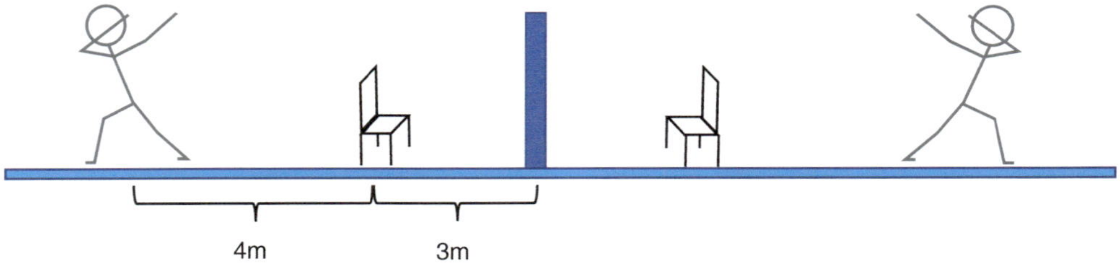

Fig. 1 Plano mirrors. How far away will the images formed on the right be located in relation to the person and the chair?

Example #1

If you are standing (and dabbing) 4 meters behind a chair that is located 3 meters to the left of a mirror, how far away is:

(a) the image of the chair from its object (i.e., the chair)
(b) the image of the chair from you

Answer: Start off as always by drawing out the problem. This eventually will become easy enough to solve without a diagram, but it may help initially to draw these diagrams to get your bearings (Fig. 1). Notice the left–right reversal of the images compared to the objects, in addition to being upright, virtual, and same size.

Since the "world" inside the mirror (to the right) is basically the same as the world to the left of the mirror, then the image of the chair will be located 3 m to the right of the mirror, and your image will be 4 m to the right of the image of the chair (and 7 m to the right of the mirror).

The image of the chair will therefore be 6 m from the chair. The total distance between you (in the real world) and the image of the chair will be as follows: 4 m + 3 m + 3 m = 10 meters.

Recall our previous discussions on reflected light rays (Chap. 1, "Geometric Optics"). We learned that incoming light rays that strike an optical surface will get reflected at an angle equal to the angle of incidence. However, when we have a plano mirror, the brain will think that the light is originating in a straight line from the "image" in the mirror.

Why is this useful? One advantage of knowing this rule is that we can determine the "height" needed of a mirror in order to fully visualize the object. This leads us to a second classically presented example.

Example #2

Suppose a 6-foot-tall male ophthalmology resident wished to see himself (head to toe) in a mirror, but he is on a bit of a budget (residents' income being what it is these days…). He goes to a mirror store that sells mirrors by foot length. He wants to buy the absolute minimum length of mirror in order for him to be able to see himself head to toe. However, he has not been paying attention during his optics lectures and is confused now at the store. What is the minimum length of the mirror that he will need to buy? How far away from the mirror must he stand in order to visualize himself head to toe completely? (Fig. 2).

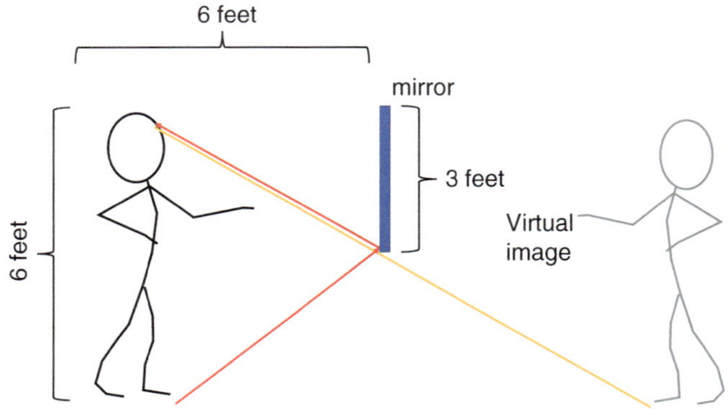

Fig. 2 Six-foot ophthalmology resident is on a bit of a budget, so he wants to buy the bare minimum length of mirror in order to see himself completely. A 3-foot mirror will allow him to be able to do this if he stands six feet away from the mirror

Since incoming (incident) light rays that hit the mirror at a given angle will leave the mirror at the same angle, he basically needs a mirror length that is *half his height*. This will allow the light rays that originate from his toe to be reflected toward him if he stands six feet away. Light rays that originate from the top half of his body will be reflected back toward him in a straight line. Therefore, he will only need a 3-foot mirror in order to see his entire body.

Note that he must be standing (at least) six feet away from the mirror in order to visualize himself completely. If he stands any closer to the mirror, for example, five feet away, he will only be able to see five feet of himself (from eye level to approximately knee level).

As an aside, a 5-foot ophthalmology resident will only need a 2.5 foot length mirror; a 7-foot ophthalmology resident[1] will need a 3.5 foot length mirror.

Example #3

Suppose you are standing 10 meters away from a mirror and begin walking toward the mirror at a rate of 0.6 meters/second, how fast is your image moving? How close are you and your image coming together in one second?

[1]This fellow loves ophthalmology so much that he chose it over becoming a professional basketball player.

Consider this example, the optics equivalent of the age old "two trains leave separate stations traveling toward each other at *x* speed at *y* time" problem. Thankfully, our math is much simpler. If an object is moving toward the mirror at a certain speed, then the image is also moving toward the mirror at the same speed. For example, if you walk toward a mirror at a rate of 0.6 meters/second, then your image will also "walk" toward the mirror at that same speed. Therefore, in one second, it will seem that you and your image have moved a net distance of 1.2 meters closer together.

Important Definitions and Equations

Before we define our two curved mirrors, positive (concave) and negative (convex) mirrors, we have to pay our dues and understand a few definitions. Notice the similarities and differences of these terms compared to how we used them with lenses (Fig. 3). Note that we have used a positive (concave) mirror in the diagram below.

Therefore, some important definitions and rules regarding mirrors are as follows:

- Focal length (*f*): It is the point at which incident parallel reflected light rays intersect (just like lenses). Mnemonic: Light rays that hit the mirror will be de<u>F</u>lected and **<u>FOCUSED</u>** onto *f*.
- Radius of curvature (*r*): The central ray for mirrors passes through this point. This is always <u>twice the focal length</u> and is located OUTSIDE the "center" of the mirror. No light ray will pass through the "center" of the mirror. Think of this as the "center" of the mirror that is "outside" the mirror.
- The power of the mirror can be calculated either by $D = 1/f$ or $2/r$ (more on this in a minute). Do not confuse "*r*" and "f" and erroneously calculate $1/r$ or $2/f$. Just remember that "*r*" is "later" in the alphabet, so it is the denominator of the "later" number in the numeral system: $1/f$ or $2/r$ (mnemonic).
- Optically, *r* and *f* are useful because they give us information about where non-reflected and reflected light rays, respectively, will pass through.
- When doing ray tracings with mirrors, draw a reflected ray that passes through *f*. Then draw an unreflected ray from the top of the object that passes through *r*. The intersection of these two rays (Fig. 3) will give you an idea of where the image will form, in addition to its orientation and size.

Calculating the Power of Mirrors

With lenses, the only way to calculate their power was to take the reciprocal of the focal length: $D = 1/F$ (or $100/F$ for cm). With mirrors, we can calculate the power either with the <u>focal length</u> (like we did with lenses) or the <u>radius of curvature</u> (both in meters), using the formula as follows:

$$D_{\text{mirror}} = 1/f \text{ OR } 2/r$$

- Of course, you can use $100/f$ and $200/r$ to work in centimeters.

Let us do some warm-up sample problems.

Example #1 What is the power of a mirror with a radius of curvature of 4 cm?

Answer: $D = 2/r = 2/0.04$ (or $200/4$) = + 50 D.

Note: A distractor answer choice may appear as +25D (which would be erroneously obtained by calculating 1/0.04 (or 100/4). Since we are given the radius of curvature, we must use $D = 2/r$.

Example #2 What is the power of a mirror with a focal length of 10 cm?

Answer: $D = 1/f = 1/0.1$ (or $100/10$) = + 10 D.

Note: Again, a distractor answer choice may appear as +20D (which would be erroneously obtained by calculating

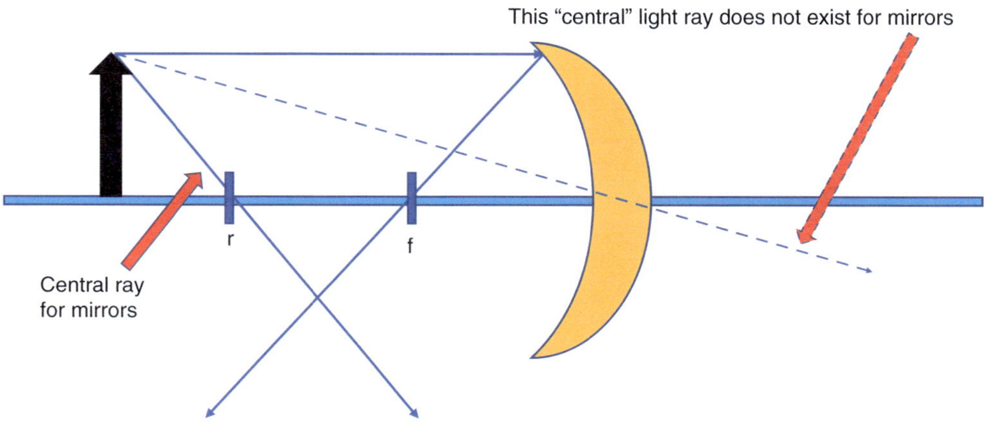

Fig. 3 Focal length (*f*) of a mirror is similar to the length of lenses: Light rays that get reflected off the mirror will pass through this point. The radius of curvature (*r*) is located outside the mirror and is the location through which the central ray passes. Note that no light ray passes through the "center" of the mirror (unlike the central ray for lenses)

2/0.01 (or 200/10). Since we are given the focal length, we must use $D = 1/f$.

Finally, the key to understanding mirrors is to know how they are similar to lenses and how they are completely different. In some aspects, including terminology, everything we learned with lenses must be (temporarily) unlearned as we will seemingly tell you the exact opposite. Remember, when dealing with mirrors, imagine that we are in an upside-down universe wherein some of the rules are totally reversed.

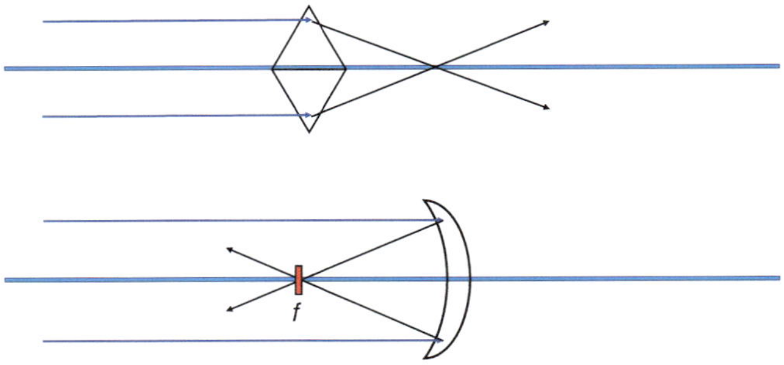

Fig. 4 Real images form at the RIGHT of the positive (convex) lens (where real light rays converge) and at the LEFT of a positive (concave) mirror (where real light rays converge)

Positive (Concave) Mirrors

Positive (plus power) mirrors are known as concave mirrors. This is different from the terminology we used for positive lenses (aka convex lenses). Remember how we said that we are in an upside-down universe?

One mnemonic to remember what a concave mirror looks like is to imagine that if you are standing to the left of a concave mirror (shown in Fig. 3), it will seem like you are "looking into a (con)cave."

Like people, images formed by concave mirrors come in all shapes in sizes. They may be as follows:

- upright or inverted
- real or virtual
- magnified, same size, or minified.

The location of the object (i.e., its distance from the mirror) will determine which characteristics the image will demonstrate.

For concave mirrors, the radius of curvature point (r) is to the LEFT of the mirror (Fig. 3). Because these mirrors can give a variety of image sizes and orientations, they are the most commonly tested type of mirrors. One example of a concave mirror is a vanity/shaving mirror. If you have one handy, notice how your image will change in size and orientation depending on how far away you are from the mirror. There is even a point wherein your image will disappear—rest assured; it is highly unlikely you have also disappeared! We will see this in more detail in the examples below.

When dealing with object–mirror systems, the equations are exactly the same as object–lens systems (our friend $U + D = V$!). Recall that for object–lens systems, a real image (positive v) is to the RIGHT of a lens and a virtual image is to the LEFT of a lens.

However, for mirrors, it is the **TOTAL OPPOSITE!** For mirrors, a real image is to the LEFT of the mirror and a virtual image is to the RIGHT of the mirror (Fig. 4).

What sorcery is this? Remember that real images form as a result of real light rays converging: If you can determine where the real light rays will converge (whether dealing with lenses or mirrors), you can determine whether the image is real or virtual. With mirrors, remember that the light rays are not refracting through the mirror, and they are reflecting away from the mirror, so we are still dealing with real light rays in the above example.

Here is another spot where people get confused. You may think, "Wait, I thought that if u (or U) is negative because it is to the left of the lens, then anything left of the mirror should also be negative!" Well friends, this is again where the upside-down world of mirrors has to be acknowledged: The object is still negative to the left of the mirror, but the image is positive even though it forms to the left of the mirror (because it is formed by real light rays).

"LOST" Method for Concave Mirrors and Image Characteristics

Since concave mirrors can create a variety of images, the "LOST" nomenclature system helps us to remember 4 key characteristics of the image as follows:

- L = location of the image
- O = orientation (upright or inverted)
- S = size (magnification or minification)
- T = type (real or virtual).

For a single concave object–mirror system, the object can be located in 5 potential locations as follows:

- Case 1: beyond (to the left of) the radius of curvature (r)
- Case 2: at the radius of curvature (r)
- Case 3: between the radius of curvature (r) and the focal point (f)
- Case 4: at the focal point (f)
- Case 5: to the right of the focal point (f) (between the focal point and the mirror).

Figure 5 summarizes these 5 possible cases based on the location of the object.

We can discuss each of these 5 cases in greater detail.

Case #1 Object located beyond (to the left of) the radius of curvature (*r*)

We can use ray tracing for the two chief rays: one ray that is drawn from the top of the object to the mirror that gets reflected through the focal point (*f*). The second ray (unreflected) will pass through the radius of curvature. The intersection of these two rays will form an image that is between *r* and *f* (location); inverted (orientation); minified (size); and real (type) (Fig. 6).

Case #2 Object located at the radius of curvature distance (*r*)

We can again use ray tracing: The first ray will similarly be reflected off the mirror and pass through the focal point (*f*). The second ray basically passes "through itself" since the object is already located at *r*. So, the image will form at *r* (location); it will be inverted (orientation); same size (size); and real (type) (Fig. 7).

Case #3 Object located between the radius of curvature (*r*) and the focal point (*f*)

We can again use ray tracing to draw our two rays: one ray that reflects off the mirror and through the focal point (*f*) and a central ray (extended backward) through *r* (Fig. 8). Note that the image is not drawn to scale and some liberties were taken with the object light rays. The image will always form to the left of *r* (location); it will be inverted (orientation); magnified (size); and real (type).

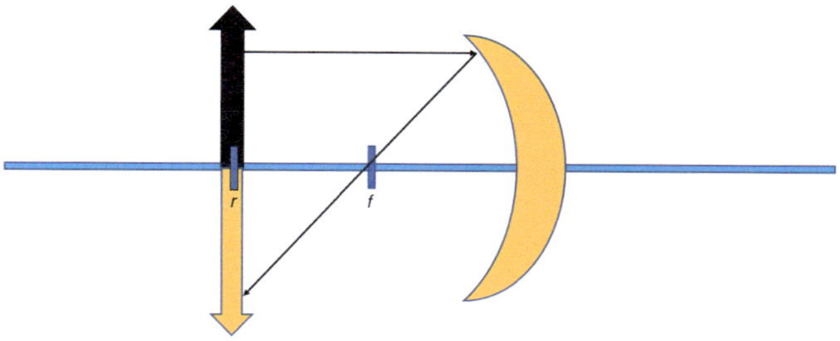

Fig. 7 "LOST" characteristics for an object located at the radius of curvature (*r*). The image will form at *r* (location); it will be inverted (orientation); same size (size); and real (type)

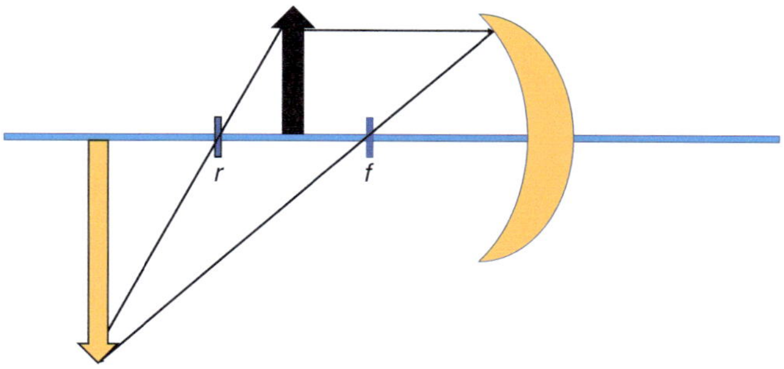

Fig. 8 "LOST" characteristics for an object located between the radius of curvature (*r*) and the focal point (*f*). The image will always form to the left of *r* (location); it will be inverted (orientation); magnified (size); and real (type)

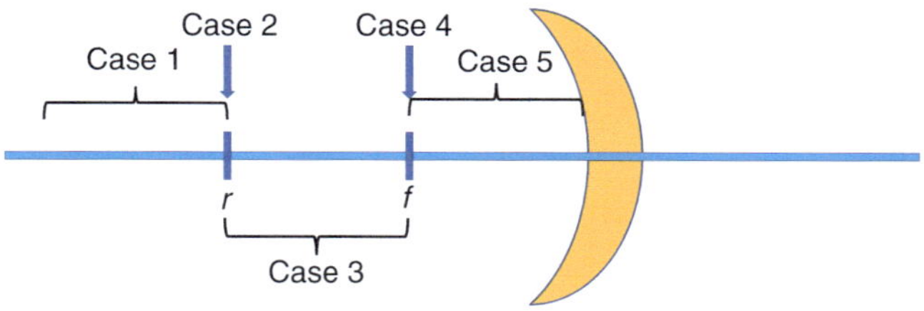

Fig. 5 Five potential locations for an object when placed to the left of a concave mirror. The "LOST" characteristics of the image formed will vary based on these five locations

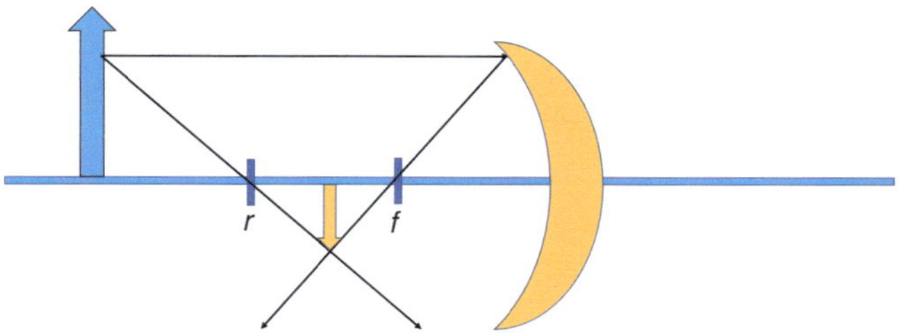

Fig. 6 "LOST" characteristics for an object located to the left of the radius of curvature (*r*). The image will form between *r* and *f* (location), and it will be inverted (orientation), minified (size), and real (type)

Case #4 Object located at the focal point (*f*)

Using ray tracing, we can see that our two familiar rays will both pass through *f* and *r*, but they will remain parallel. As a result, they will never intersect and *no image is formed*. You can try this with a shaving mirror: If you approach the mirror slowly, you will see that your image will be inverted, and then as you draw closer, it will disappear before it becomes upright. The point where it disappears is because you are standing at the focal point (not that you have suddenly become invisible!) (Fig. 9).

Case #5 Object located between the focal point (to the right of the focal point) and the mirror

Using ray tracing, we can see that our two familiar rays (with some liberties taken for the sake of scale and convenience) will form an image that is to the RIGHT of the mirror (location); upright (orientation); magnified (size); and virtual (type) (Fig. 10). Remember, it is virtual because it is forming to the right of a mirror. The previous images were all real images because they were formed by real light rays that converge to the left of a mirror. In this case, we are using the

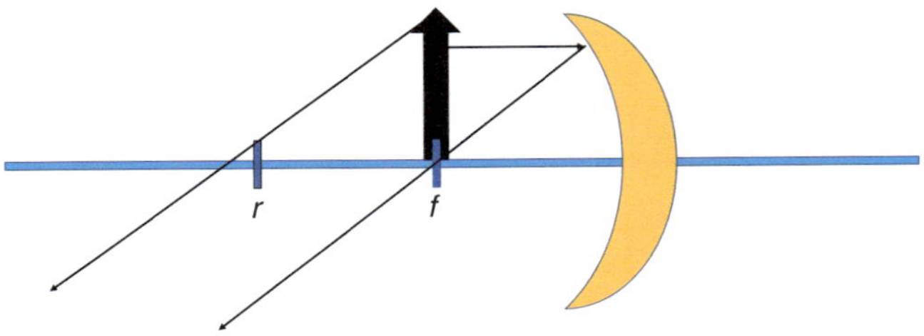

Fig. 9 If an object is located at the focal point (*f*), no image will form because the deflected ray and the central ray will travel parallel to each other and never converge

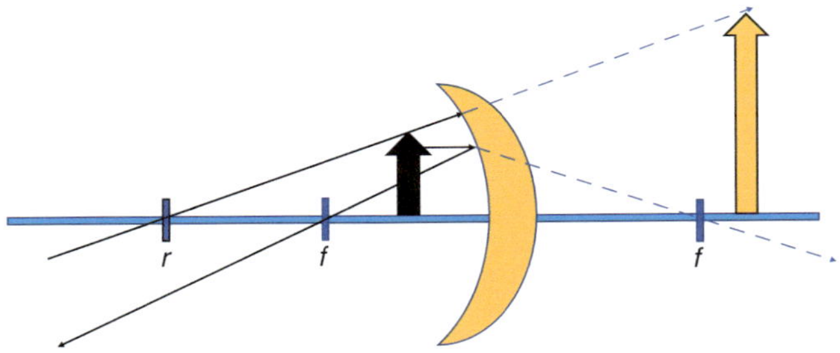

Fig. 10 When an object is located to the right of the focal point, the image is to the RIGHT of the mirror (location); upright (orientation); magnified (size); and virtual (type)

extension of our two light rays (imaginary [dashed] lines). For relevance, this is when the vanity/shaving mirror actually becomes useful and generates an upright and magnified image. In other words, when you use a vanity mirror, you are standing to the right of that mirror's focal point; this is why you are able to have a "useful" image of yourself to make yourself look dapper.

One other point about Case #5: The object will yield the largest image when it is immediately to the right of the focal point (*f*). As the object is brought closer to the mirror, the image size will get smaller (but never smaller than the size of the original object). Ultimately, as the object distance approaches zero (to the mirror), the image distance will also approach zero, and the image height will ultimately become equal to the object height (Fig. 11). You may have noticed this with the vanity/shaving mirror example. If you stand too close to the mirror, your image will become slightly smaller until it basically will have the size as yourself. In other words, if you stand extremely closer to a vanity mirror, it will function like a plano mirror! So, if you want to maximize the use of your vanity mirror, stand immediately to the right of the focal point; otherwise, if you forget your optics and stand too close, you are a NooB and you might as well use a plano mirror.

Table 1 provides a hi-yield summary of the previous 5 cases combined into a single table for review and comparison purposes

Object–Mirror System Examples with Concave Mirrors

Example #1

An object is 25cm to the left of a + 1D mirror. Where is the image? Is it real or virtual? Is it upright or inverted? Is it magnified or minified?

Answer:

$$u = -25\,\text{cm}\ (\text{make sure } U \text{ and } u \text{ are negative!})$$

$$U = 100/u = 100/-25 = -4\ (\text{this is the object vergence})$$

$$U + D = V$$

$$-4 + 1 = V = -3\ (\text{this is the image vergence})$$

$$v = 100/V = 100/-3 = -33\ \text{cm}\ (\text{this is the image distance})$$

$$m = U/V = -4/-3 = 1.33.$$

The final image is 33 cm to the RIGHT of the mirror. It is virtual (v is negative), upright (m is positive), and magnified ($|m| > 1$). We can also see that since the focal length of this mirror is 100 cm, the object is located to the right of the focal length (Case #5 as discussed above). Our math confirms the previous discussion.

Notice that the equations are exactly the same for lenses and mirrors. The only thing that differs is whether the image is to the right or the left of the mirror. If this were a lens, $v = -33$ cm means the image would have been to the left of the lens. Since this is a mirror, $v = -33$ cm means the image is 33 cm to the **right** of the mirror.

Example #2

An object is 50 cm to the left of a + 8D mirror. Where is the image? Is it real or virtual? Is it upright or inverted? Is it magnified or minified?

Answer: $u = -50$ cm (make sure U and u are negative! We keep saying this because it is such a common mistake!)

$$U = 1/u = 100/-50 = -2\ (\text{this is the object vergence})$$

$$U + D = V$$

$$-2 + 8 = V = +6\ (\text{this is the image vergence})$$

$$v = 100/V = 100/6 = 16.7\,\text{cm}\ (\text{this is the image distance})$$

$$m = U/V = -2/6 = -0.33\ (\text{this is the magnification})$$

The final image is 16.7 cm to the LEFT of the mirror. It is real (v is positive), inverted (m is negative), and minified

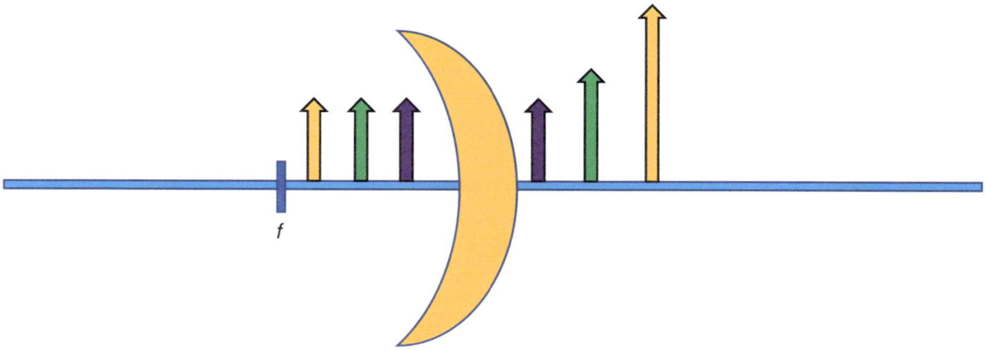

Fig. 11 An object will have the largest image size if it is located immediately to the right of the focal point (*f*). As the object draws closer to the mirror, the image size will also decrease. As the object distance to the mirror approaches zero, the image height will ultimately become equal to the object height. Notice the size and location of the yellow, green, and purple images in relation to the location of their respective objects. The yellow image is the largest because the yellow object is immediately to the right of the focal point

Table 1 Summary of object locations and image characteristics with concave mirrors

Case	Object location	Image characteristics
1	Left of *r*	Image forms between *r* and *f*. It will be inverted, minified, and real.
2	At *r*	Image forms at *r*. It will be inverted, same size, and real.
3	Between *r* and *f*	Image forms to the left of *r*. It will be inverted, magnified, and real.
4	At *f*	No image.
5	Right of *f*	Images will be upright and virtual. Image size will be greatest when the object is located immediately to the right of *f* and will continue to decrease in size. When the object is immediately to the left of the mirror, the image will have the same size as the object.

($|m| < 1$). Note that for this mirror, the focal point (*f*) is 12.5 cm to the left of the mirror and the radius of curvature (*r*) is 25 cm to the left of the mirror. Since the object is located 50 cm to the left of the mirror, this is an example of Case #1 as discussed above. Once again, our math confirms the previous discussion.

Negative Mirrors (Convex Mirrors)

Negative mirrors are known as convex mirrors (Fig. 12). Think of them as "vexing" mirrors to look at because they give weird images, such as a funhouse mirror, surveillance mirror (such as used in a convenience store or hospital hallway), rear-view mirror (objects in the mirror are closer than they appear), or the back of a spoon. The radius of curvature point for these mirrors is located to the RIGHT of the mirror. When a light ray from an object hits a convex mirror, the

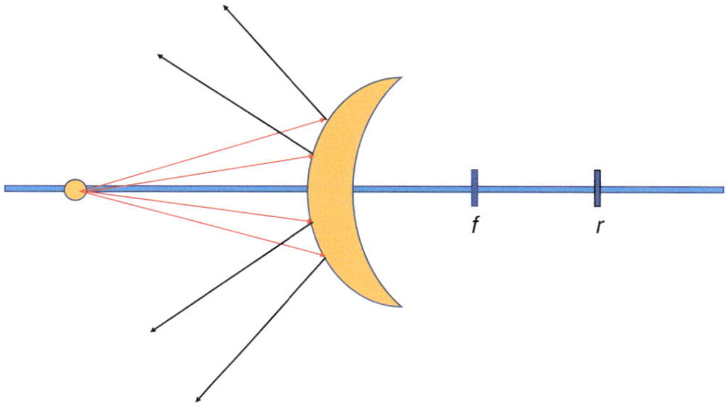

Fig. 12 Convex mirrors. All light rays that strike a convex mirror will be deflected away from the mirror

light rays diverge (spread out) since the normal to the surface differs with each spot on the mirror.

Two Rules for Convex Mirrors

Even though these vexing convex mirrors are vexing us more than anti-vaxxers (drum shot here), in some ways, they are a bit easier than concave mirrors. Why? Because there are only two rules that you need to know for convex mirrors (Fig. 13) as follows:

- Rule #1: A reflected ray from the anterior surface of the convex mirror will have its imaginary extension pass through the focal point (*f*) (to the right of the mirror).
- Rule #2: An undeviated ray from the object will pass through the radius of curvature (*r*), which is also located to the right of the mirror.

As a result, concave mirrors will ALWAYS give images with certain characteristics, no matter how close or far away

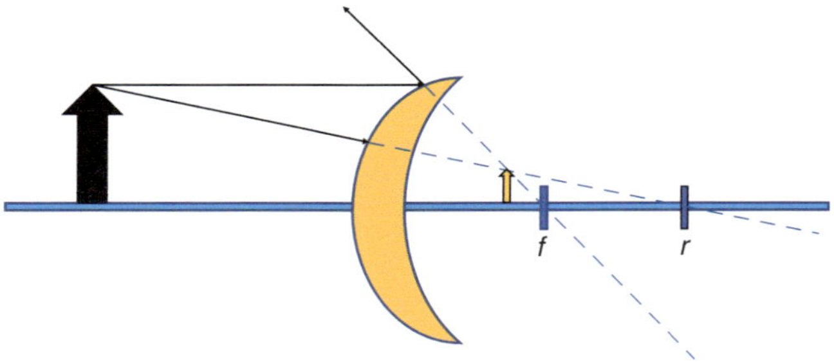

Fig. 13 Convex mirrors. Note that the r and f are located to the right of the mirror. Convex mirrors will always produce images that are Virtual, ERect (upright), and MINified

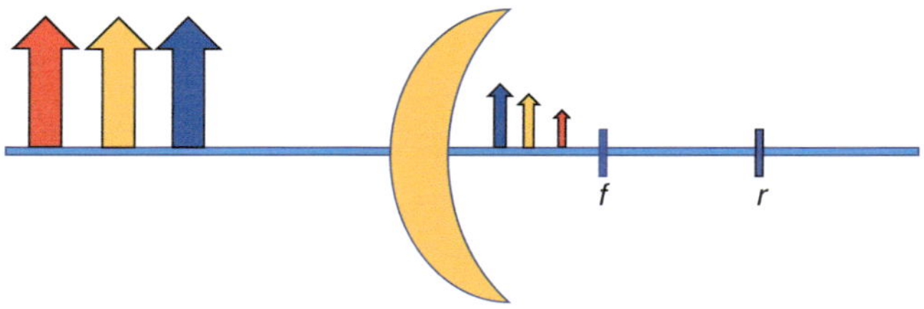

Fig. 14 As an object approaches a convex mirror, its virtual image will also shift closer (shift left) to the mirror and increase in size. However, all images will still remain minified relative to the size of the original object

the object is from the mirror. The images formed by convex mirrors can be remembered by the mnemonic "VERMIN." Convex mirror images are always as follows:

- Virtual
- ERect (upright)
- MINified

One other point about convex mirrors is as follows: As an object approaches closer to the convex mirror, its virtual image (located to the right of the mirror) will also approach closer to the mirror and will become larger, though it will always be smaller than the object (Fig. 14). This is different than concave mirrors (see Case #5 discussion).

As for the math, convex mirrors will use the same equations and principles we discussed with concave mirrors, but it is important to remember the image characteristics that we can (hopefully) confirm mathematically.

Object–Mirror System Examples with Convex Mirrors

Example #1

An object is 33 cm to the left of a −2D diverging mirror. Where is the image? Is it real or virtual? Is it upright or inverted? Is it magnified or minified?

$$u = --33\,\text{cm}\ (\text{this is the object distance and once again negative})$$

$$U = 100/u = 100/-33 = -3\ (\text{this is the object vergence})$$

$$U + D = V$$

$$-3 + (-2) = V = -5\ (\text{this is the image vergence})$$

$$v = 100/V = 100/-5 = -20\,\text{cm}\ (\text{this is the image distance})$$

$$m = U/V = -3/-5 = 0.6\ (\text{this is the magnification})$$

The final image is 20 cm to the RIGHT of the mirror. It is virtual (m to the RIGHT of the mirror. It is viis negative), upright (m is positive), and minified (|m| < 1). Note that it follows our "VERMIN" mnemonic.

Suppose we placed both the object and the mirror underwater. Will this change our answer.

We should do the math, now taking into account the index of refraction (1.33) as follows:

$$u = -33\,\text{cm}$$

$$U = 133/u = 133/-33 = -4\ (\text{this is object vergence})$$

$$U + D = V$$

$$-4 + -2 = V = -6\ (\text{this is the image vergence})$$

$$v = 133/V = 133/-6 = -22\,\text{cm}\ (\text{this is the image distance})$$

$$m = U/V = -4/-6 = 0.67\ (\text{this is the magnification})$$

The final image is therefore 22 cm to the RIGHT of the mirror. It is virtual (v is negative), upright (m is positive), and minified ($|m| < 1$). Note that it follows our VERMIN mnemonic.

We can observe a few things at this point as follows:

- Notice that the change in index of refraction slightly changed the location of the image (by 2 cm further to the right).
- Notice that the image magnification slightly increased underwater, relative to the magnification in air. However, both images are still minified compared to the size of the original object.

Optical Systems with Multiple Lenses and Mirrors

So far, we have given examples of optical systems with a single lens or mirror. If only lenses or mirrors would just stay single—but they sometimes enjoy each other's company, and they get together to form a complex lens or complex mirror system. While they may enjoy each other's company, it makes our lives more difficult because we have to figure out commonly tested concepts of complex optical systems, such as the following:

- Location of the intermediate and final image
- Orientation of the intermediate and final image
- Total magnification of the lens (mirror) system.

These problems are made much easier if we simply tackle one lens (or mirror) at a time: First, ignore the second (or third, fourth, etc.) lens and then use $U + D = V$ for the first lens/mirror to find where the first image will form. Hopefully, it will be to the left of the second (or next) lens (or mirror).[2] Basically, we should view these problems as two-for-the-price-of-one types of problems, though unfortunately, on exams, you will not get double points for getting these problems correct.

We can do some examples as follows:

Example #1 An object (height 8 cm) is located 5 cm to the left of a + 10D lens, which itself is located 10 cm to the left of a + 6.67D lens. Calculate the position of the final image and its magnification (relative to the original object).

[2]We will do some examples later in this section that deals with a lens system where the intermediate image will form to the RIGHT of the second lens/mirror.

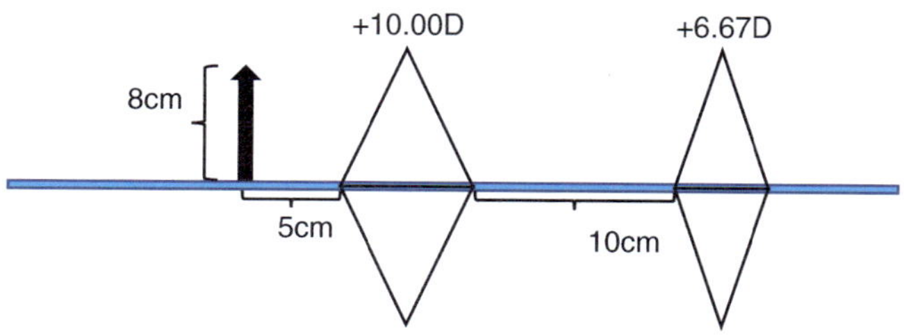

Fig. 15 Lens system for an object (height 8 cm) located 5 cm to the left of a + 10D lens which itself is located 10 cm to the left of a + 6.67D lens

Answer: Start off by drawing out this lens system to get our bearings (Fig. 15). Note: The figure is not drawn to scale (but who cares!).

We will begin by ignoring the second lens and dealing with the first lens. We can use our familiar equation: $U + D = V$

$$U + D = V \rightarrow U = 100 / -u = 100 / -5 = -20$$

$$-20 + 10 = -10 \rightarrow v = 100 / V = 100 / -10$$
$$= -10\,\text{cm to the LEFT of the} + 10D\,\text{lens}$$

$$m = U / V = -20 / -10 = +2$$

V is negative, so our first image is a virtual image; m is positive, so we have an upright image; and $|m| > 1$, so our image is magnified (2×) to a size of 16 cm.

Now, we can redraw the lens system using the first image as the "new" object, eliminating the first lens (and original object) and now dealing with the second lens (Fig. 16).

We can again use our $U + D = V$ equation as follows:

$$U + D = V \rightarrow U = 100 / -u = 100 / -20 = -5$$

$$-5 + 6.67 = 1.67 \rightarrow v = 100 / V = 100 / 1.67$$
$$= 60\,\text{cm to the RIGHT of the lens}$$

$$m = U / V = -5 / 1.67 = -3$$

V is positive, so the second image is a real image. m is negative, so the second image is inverted. Finally, $|m|$ is >3, so the second image is 3× the size of the first image.

This is where it gets slightly tricky. It is tempting to use the 2× from the first lens system and add it to the 3× for the second lens system for a total of 5× magnification (and apply that to our 8 cm object for a final magnification size of 40 cm). You can be sure that one of the wrong answer choices will have this number shown!

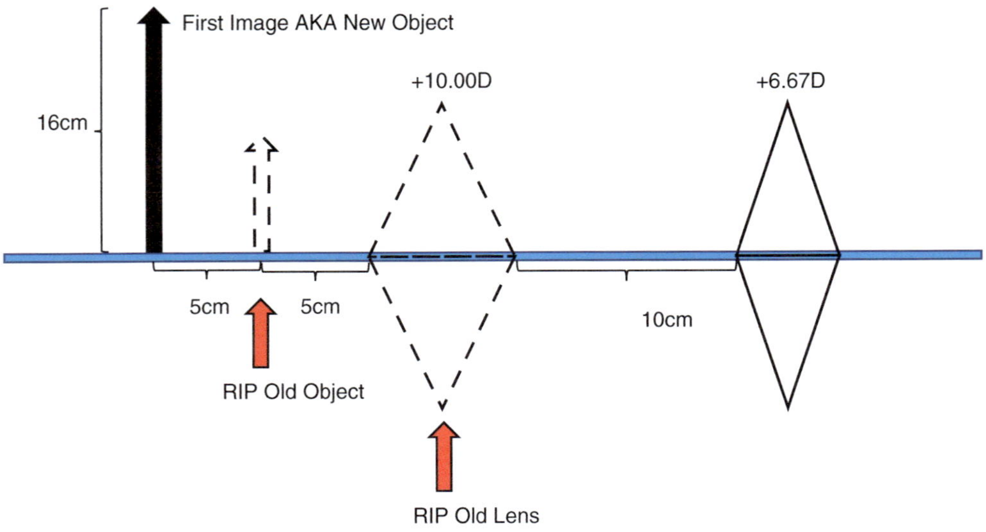

Fig. 16 Intermediate image formed by the first lens will be located 10 cm to the left of the first lens. This lens will be our "new object" (solid black arrow) that is 20 cm to the left of the +6.67D lens. We can safely ignore the first object and the first lens at this time (dotted arrow and dotted diamond, respectively)

But for the total magnification of a lens system, we have to **MULTIPLY** the individual magnifications of each lens. In other words, the total magnification is not (2 + 3 = 5×), but rather it is 6× magnification (2×*3×). Therefore, the final image size is 8 × 6 = 48 cm.

Example #2 A 20 cm object is located 10 cm to the left of a −10D lens, which itself is located 35 cm to the left of a + 15D lens. Calculate the position of the final image and its magnification.

Answer: We can skip to the chase. You can draw out the lens system on your own if you wish. But again, we have to deal with each lens separately as follows:

$$u = -10\,\text{cm}$$

$$U = 100/-u = 100/-10 = -10$$

$$U + D = V$$

$$-10 + (-10) = V = -20$$

$$v = 100/V = 100/-20 = -5\,\text{cm to the LEFT of the first lens}$$

$$m = U/V = -10/-20 = +1/2$$

V is negative, so our first image is again a virtual image. *m* is positive, so the first image is upright. However, |*m*| < 1, so the first image is half the size of the original object (first image is 10 cm in size).

Now, we can repeat these shenanigans for the second lens as follows:

$$u = -40\,\text{cm}\left(\text{note, we can also write this as } u' \text{ to keep the two lens systems separate}\right)$$

$$U = 100/-u = 100/-40 = -2.5$$

$$U + D = V$$

$$-2.5 + 15 = +12.5$$

$$v = 100/V = 100/12.5 = 8\,\text{cm to the RIGHT of the second lens}$$

$$m = U/V = -2.5/12.5 = -0.2$$

V is positive, so our second image is a real image. m is negative, so the second image is inverted (relative to both the original object and the first image). Finally, |*m*| is <1, so we again have minification of the first image (aka the second object).

The total magnification is 0.5 × 0.2 = 0.1× magnification. Therefore, the final image is 2 cm (aka 1/10th the size of the original object).

Example #3 An object is located 20 cm to the left of a + 15D lens, which itself is located 20 cm to the left of a + 14D mirror. Where is the final image in relation to the original object?

Answer: Again, take a minute to draw out the lens and mirror system to get your bearings. We will use the $U + D = V$ equation (as if there was any other equation to use!) and deal with the lens first and then the mirror second. We must be careful to make sure we follow the rules for lenses and mirrors appropriately as follows:

$$U + D = V$$

$$U = 100/-u = 100/-20 = -5$$

$$-5 + 15 = +10$$

$$v = 100/V = 100/10 = 10\,\text{cm to the RIGHT of the lens, } 10\,\text{cm to the LEFT of the mirror.}$$

$$m = U/V = -5/10 = -1/2$$

V is positive, so our first image is a real image. m is negative, so we have an inverted image. Finally, $|m| < 1$, so our image is minified.

Now, we can deal with the mirror as follows:

$$U + D = V$$

$$U = 100/-u = 100/-10$$

$$-10 + 14 = +4$$

$v = 100/V = 100/4 = 25$ cm to the LEFT of the mirror (note that this positive V for mirrors means that the image will form to the LEFT of the mirror!).

$m = U/V = -10/4 = -2.5$. The image is inverted (relative to this second object/first image, so it is actually upright relative to the first object), has 2.5× magnification (compared to the first image), and is real (positive V).

The final image is 25 cm to the LEFT of the mirror; therefore, it is 15 cm from the original object.

Just for kicks: The total magnification of this system is 1.25× (Total mag = −1/2 * −2.5).

Advanced Topics

Intermediate Images to the Right of Lenses and Mirrors (Positive U)

We spent this entire chapter talking about how U and u are almost always negative. And you, dear, naïve reader, believed us! Now we are going to give you an exception to this rule in case: If given multiple lens or mirror systems, we previously discussed that the image from the first lens/mirror becomes the object for the second lens and so on. In the examples we did so far, the intermediate images have always ended up to the left of the second lens/mirror, so we could proceed with business as usual and continue to use our $U + D=V$ equation.

But if that first image is to the **right** of the second lens/mirror, we have a positive U and a positive u. We can still use our $U + D=V$ equation, but we have to account for this object being in the "right spot" (i.e., to the right of the lens/mirror) and make sure we keep U/u as positive. Confused? Take a moment to punch a pillow or squeeze a stress ball, and then we can do some examples.

Reminder: U can only be positive if the "object" is formed by another lens/mirror. Natural objects will always have negative vergence (negative U).

Example #1 An object is 25 cm to the left of a + 5D lens, which is 67 cm to the left of a + 1D lens. Where is the image?

Answer: We can start off by drawing this out (Fig. 17).
For now, ignore the second lens and focus on the +5D lens.

$$u = -0.25\text{m} \ (u \text{ is still negative here}) \text{ or } -25\,\text{cm}$$

$$U = 100/-u = 100/-25 = -4 \ (\text{object vergence})$$

$$U + D = V$$

$$-4 + 5 = V = +1 \ (\text{image vergence})$$

$$v = 100/V = 100/1 = 100\,\text{cm} \ (\text{image distance}) \text{ to the RIGHT of the first lens}$$

So far so good. The image from the first lens is 1 m to the right of the first lens. But unfortunately, that also means it is 33 cm to the right of the second lens! Since we have our object to the right of the lens, our u (and U) for this second lens has to be **positive**. This is the only time u will be a positive number.

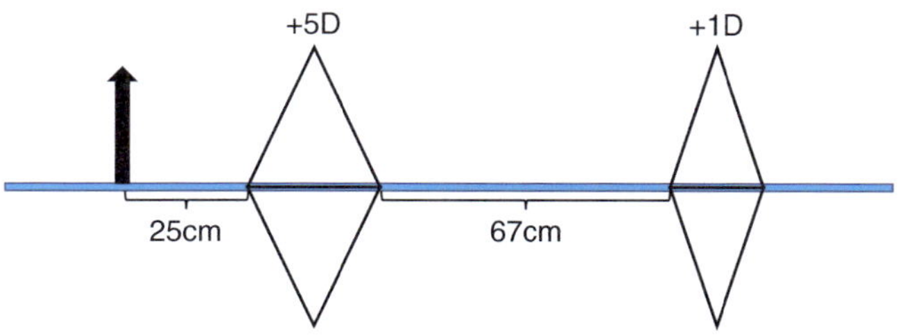

Fig. 17 Lens system for an object located 25 cm to the left of a + 5D lens which itself is located 67 cm to the left of a + 1D lens

$$u = +0.33\text{m}\ (u \text{ is positive because the object is to the right of the second lens}) \text{ or } 33\,\text{cm}$$

$$U = 100 / u = 100 / 33 = 3\ (\text{object vergence})$$

$$U + D = V$$

$$3 + 1 = V = 4\ (\text{image vergence})$$

$$v = 100 / V = 100 / 4 = 25\,\text{cm}\ (\text{final image distance in relation to the second lens})$$

The final image is 25 cm to the right of the second lens. It is 92 cm (67 cm + 25 cm) to the right of the first lens. It is 117 cm to the right of the object (25 cm + 67 cm + 25 cm). The answer could be any of these choices depending on what the test gives you as a multiple-choice answer.

Example #2 An object is 50 cm to the left of a + 3 lens, which is 75 cm to the left of a + 4 mirror. Where is the image?

Take a minute to draw out the lens and mirror system to get your bearings. For now, ignore the mirror and start with the +3D lens only.

$$U + D = V$$

$$U = 100 / -u = 100 / -50 = -2$$

$$-2 + 3 = V = 1\ (\text{image vergence})$$

$$v = 100 / V = 100 / 1 = 100\,\text{cm to the right of the lens}$$

But wait, this is now 25 cm to the RIGHT of the mirror as well!

Insert moment of screaming into the void here

This becomes the new object distance for the mirror and is a positive number. Once again, this is the rare exception to the rule that U and u are negative.

$$u = 0.25\text{m}\ (u \text{ is positive because the object is to the right of the mirror}) \text{ or } 25\,\text{cm}$$

$$U = 100 / u = 100 / 25 = 4\ (\text{object vergence})$$

$$U + D = V$$

$$4 + 4 = V = +8\ (\text{image vergence})$$

$$v = 100 / V = 100 / 8 = +12.5\ (\text{image distance})$$

The final image is 12.5 cm to the LEFT of the mirror. Remember for mirrors, a real image (positive v) is to the left of the mirror.

Index of Refraction Effects

Thus far, when we have done $U + D = V$ problems, and we have mainly used $U = 1/-u$ (or $U = 100/-u$) because we have made the assumption that the object is in air. Since air has an index of refraction of 1.0, we can do the calculation as such. However, if they are devious enough to give a problem where the object or the image is in a different medium (such as water), then we have to use the *index of refraction* of that medium as our numerator. For example, if an object immersed in water is located 66 cm in front of a + 7D lens whose back surface is exposed to air, where is the image (Fig. 18)?

$$u = -66\ \text{cm}$$

$$\text{However, } U = (-1.33 / 0.66 \text{ OR } -133 / 66) = -2$$

$$U + D = V$$

$$-2 + 7 = V = +5$$

$v = 100/5 = 20$ cm to the right of the lens. Note that we can use 100 as our familiar numerator since this image is formed in air.

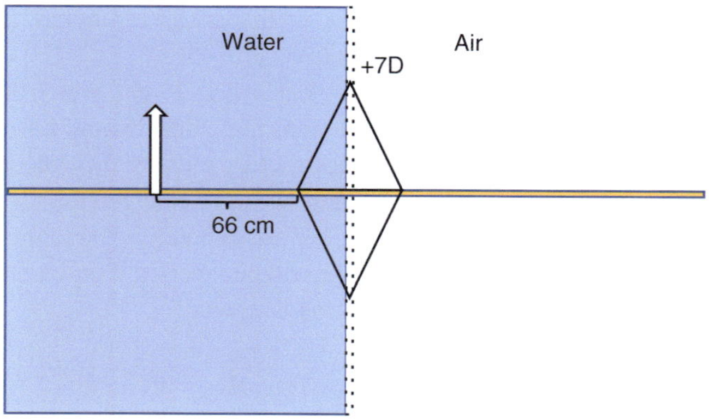

Fig. 18 If an object immersed in water is located 66 cm to the left of a + 7D lens whose back surface is exposed to air, where is the image?

Similarly, we can do an example if the object was in air, but the image was formed in water: Suppose that an object in air was located 25 cm to the left of a + 6D lens and on the other side of the lens is water. Where is the image?

$$u = -25\,\text{cm}$$

$$U = 100 / -u = 100 / -25 = -4$$

$$U + D = V$$

$$-4 + 6 = V = 2;$$

however, $v = 1.33/2 = 0.67$ m or 67 cm to the right of the lens. Note that we cannot simply use 100/2 = 50 cm as the answer.

Common Pitfalls

A few and somewhat random pieces of advice to close out this chapter are as follows:

- The nice thing about getting math-heavy optics problems is that it is a multiple-choice test. If you make a mistake converting 1/6 m into 16.7 cm, you will come up with a wrong answer that is not an answer choice and you can go back and fix your problem. The tricky wrong answers are the ones where they give you an answer choice that fits your incorrect answer due to a math error.
- Make sure U and u are negative unless you are dealing with 2 lenses or a lens and mirror. In this case, check to see if the intermediate image (aka the second object) has a positive or negative U.
- You may want to brush up on your reciprocals. A common mistake made by many trainees is getting the "math" wrong, even though they set up the equations correctly.
- It is often easier to work in centimeters to do the math. However, if the answer choices are given in meters, make sure you convert centimeters to meters for the calculations.

Practice Questions

1. A 2-meter-tall object is 25 cm to the left of a + 3D converging lens. Where is the image? How tall is it? Is it real or virtual? Is it upright or inverted?
2. Now the 2-meter-tall object is 50cm to the left of the same +3 converging lens. Where is the image? How tall is it? Is it real or virtual? Is it upright or inverted?
3. Now the 2-meter-tall object is 50cm to the left of a −3D diverging lens. Where is the image? How tall is it? Is it real or virtual? Is it upright or inverted?
4. A 3-meter-tall object is 33cm to the left of a +5 mirror. Where is the image? How tall is it? Is it real or virtual? Is it upright or inverted?
5. Now the 3-meter-tall object is 10cm to the left of the same +5 mirror. Where is the image? How tall is it? Is it real or virtual? Is it upright or inverted?
6. Now the 3-meter-tall object is 25cm to the left of a −4D mirror. Where is the image? How tall is it? Is it real or virtual? Is it upright or inverted?
7. An object is 33cm to the left of a +6D lens, which is 67cm to the left of a +4D lens. Where is the final image?
8. An object is 33cm to the left of a +4 lens, which is 67cm to the left of a +7 lens. Where is the final image?
9. An object is 33 cm to the left of a +5D lens, which is 25 cm to the left of a −6D lens, which itself is located 50 cm to the left of a +11D lens. Where is the final image located? What is the orientation of the final image? What is the magnification of the final image?
10. An object is 10cm to the left of a +15 lens, which is 70cm to the left of a +4 mirror. Where is the image? What is the magnification of the final image?
11. An object is 20cm to the left of a +6D lens, which is 75cm to the left of a +6D mirror. Where is the image? What is the magnification of the final image?
12. How far from a +60D lens should an object be placed in order to form an image onto a screen that is located 2 cm to the right of the lens?
13. An object is placed to the left of a −5D lens at an unknown distance. If an image is formed to the left of the lens at the midpoint between the object and the lens, where is the object?
14. If you are given a +2.00D lens and a +3.00D lens, how far apart must they be placed so that an object at infinity forms an image 1 meter to the right of the second lens?
15. Suppose you are an emmetrope and you are examining a patient who is a −8D myope. If you hold an ophthalmoscope 2.5cm from the patient's cornea, how much additional power must be dialed into the ophthalmoscope in order to allow for inspection of the retina?

Bonus: What if you are a −3D myope? What if you are a + 3D hyperope? Assume you are not wearing any spectacle correction.

Answers

1. This is a straightforward question testing our knowledge of the reduced vergence/simple lens formula. Remember that $U + D = V$ and $m = U/V$.

$$u = -0.25\text{m or } -25\,\text{cm}$$

$$U = 100 / -25 = -4$$

$$U + D = V$$

$$-4 + 3 = V = -1$$

$$v = 100 / V = 100 / -1 = -100$$

The image is therefore 100 cm (or 1 meter) to the LEFT of the lens.

It is virtual because v is negative.

$$m = U / V = -4 / -1 = 4$$

The image is magnified 4×, so this image is (2 m × 4 = 8) 8 m tall. It is upright because m is positive. The resulting object and image would look like Fig. 19.

2. This again is testing our knowledge of the RVF. You can draw the object–lens system out if you wish, but we can skip to the math as follows:

$$u = -0.50\text{m or } -50\,\text{cm}$$

$$U = 100 / -u = -2 \left(\text{make sure } u \text{ and } U \text{ are negative}\right)$$

$$U + D = V$$

$$-2 + 3 = V = 1$$

$$v = 100 / V = 100$$

The image is 100 cm (or 1 meter) to the RIGHT of the lens. It is real because v is positive.

$$m = U / V = -2 / 1 = -2$$

The image is magnified 2×, so this image is 4 m tall. It is inverted because m is negative.

In the first question, the object was at 25 cm, which is within the focal length of the lens (+3D lens would have focal length of 33 cm). Notice that by moving the object outside of the lens' focal length, we have changed the virtual image into a real image. We are still getting a magnified image, but this new image will be inverted (compared to the image formed in question #1).

3. $u = -0.50\text{m or } -50\,\text{cm}$

$$U = 100 / u = 100 / -50 = -2 \left(\text{make sure } u \text{ and } U \text{ are negative}\right)$$

$$U + D = V \rightarrow -2 + -3 = V = -5$$

$$v = 100 / V = 100 / -5 = -20\,\text{cm} \left(\text{or} -0.2\text{m}\right)$$

The image is 20 cm to the left of the lens. It is virtual because v is negative.

$$m = U / V = -2 / -5 = 0.4$$

The image is minified 0.4×, so this image is 0.8 m tall. It is upright because m is positive. The resulting object and image would look like Fig. 20.

4. This is again a question that tests our knowledge of the RVF. However, we are dealing with mirrors, so remember the rules we have previously discussed!

$$u = -0.33\text{m or } -33\,\text{cm}$$

$$U = 100 / u = 100 / -33 = -3 \left(\text{make sure } u \text{ and } U \text{ are negative}\right)$$

$$U + D = V$$

$$-3 + 5 = V = +2$$

$$v = 100 / V = 100 / 2 = 50\,\text{cm}$$

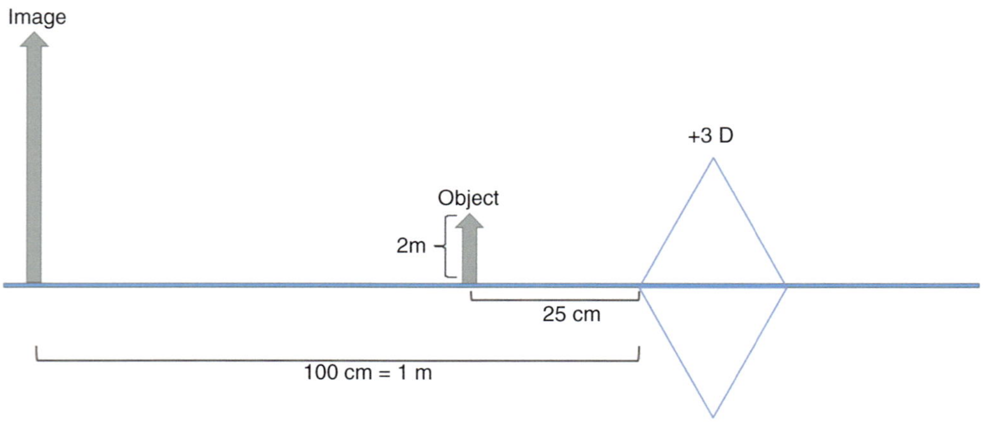

Fig. 19 Object–lens system and resulting image for a 2-meter-tall object located 25 cm to the left of a + 3D lens

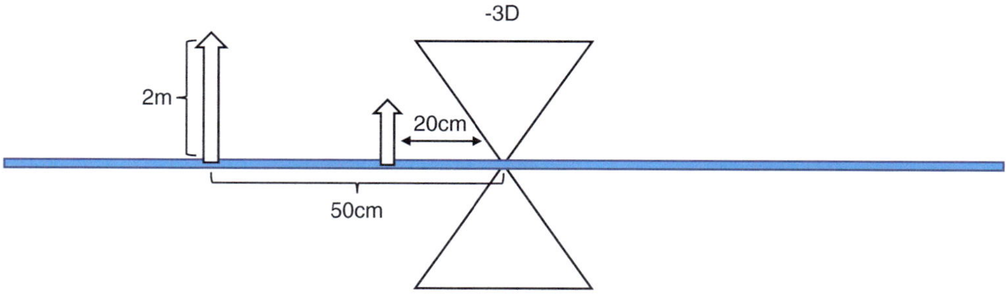

Fig. 20 Object–lens system for a 2-meter-tall object located 50 cm to the left of a −3D lens

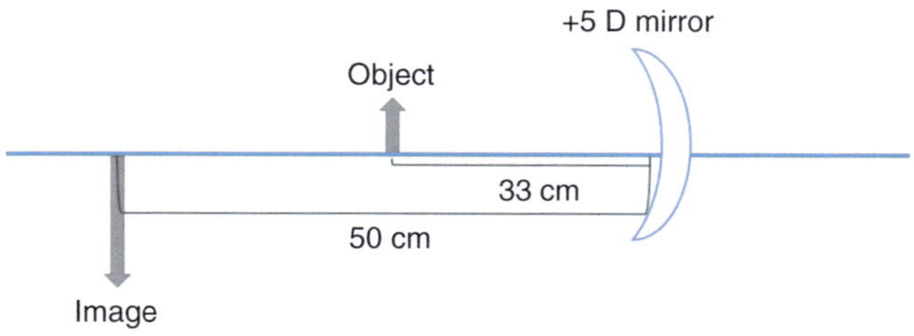

Fig. 21 Object–mirror system for an object located 33 cm to the left of a + 5D mirror. The resulting image will be 50 cm to the left of the mirror (location), inverted (orientation), 1.5× magnified (size), and real (type)

Because we are dealing with mirrors, a positive V (v) means that the image will form to the LEFT of our concave mirror. The image is 50 cm to the LEFT of the mirror. It is real because v is positive.

$$m = U / V = -3 / 2 = -1.5$$

The image is magnified 1.5×, so this image is 4.5 m tall. It is inverted because m is negative. The resulting object/image mirror system would look like Fig. 21.

Notice that the focal length of this mirror would be at 20 cm (100/5 = 20 cm) and the radius of curvature would be at 40 cm to the left of the mirror, respectively. This object is located between f and r (Case #3 as discussed in Section C, positive (concave mirrors). Our resulting image follows the "LOST" rules for this case: The image forms to the left of r (location); it is inverted (orientation); magnified (size); and real (type).

5. Use our familiar $U + D = V$ formula and remember our rules for mirrors as follows:

$$u = -0.10 \text{ m or } -10\,\text{cm}$$

$$U = 100 / u = -10 \text{ (make sure } u \text{ and } U \text{ are negative)}$$

$$U + D = V$$

$$-10 + 5 = V = -5$$

$v = 100/V = 100/5 = -20$ cm or -0.2 m. Because we are dealing with mirrors, a negative V (v) means that the image will form to the RIGHT of our concave mirror. The image is 20 cm to the RIGHT of the mirror. It is virtual because v is negative.

$$m = U / V = -10 / -5 = 2$$

The image is magnified 2×, so this image is 6 m tall. It is upright because m is positive. The resulting object/image mirror system would look like Fig. 22.

Notice that the object lies between the focal point (to the right of the focal point, which is 20 cm) and the mirror, this is, Case #5 as discussed in Section C, positive (concave) mirrors. Our resulting image is formed to the right of the mirror (location); it is upright (orientation); magnified (size); and virtual (type).

6. From the question stem, we know that this is a convex mirror so we can call upon our "VERMIN" mnemonic to help answer some of the questions asked. For image location, we will still need to use the $U + D = V$ formula as follows:

$$u = -0.25\text{m or } -25\,\text{cm}$$

$$U = 100 / -u = 100 / -25 = -4$$
$$\text{(make sure } u \text{ and } U \text{ are negative)}$$

$$U + D = V$$

$$-4 + -4 = V = -8$$

$v = 100/V = 100/-8 = -12.5$ cm or -0.125 m. Because we are dealing with mirrors, a negative V (v) means that the image will form to the RIGHT of our convex mirror. The image is 12.5 cm to the right of the mirror. It is virtual because v is negative.

$$m = U / V = -4 / -8 = 0.5$$

The image is minified 0.5×, so this image is 1.5 m tall. It is upright because m is positive. Note that our math confirms our "VERMIN" mnemonic rules. The resulting object–mirror system would look like Fig. 23.

7. Since this is our first complex lens system problem in this problem set, we should draw this out (Fig. 24).

It helps to tackle each lens separately. For now, ignore the second lens—pretend it does not exist! Let us start with the first lens.

$$u = -0.33\text{m} = -33\,\text{cm}$$

$$U = 100 / u = -3$$

$$U + D = V$$

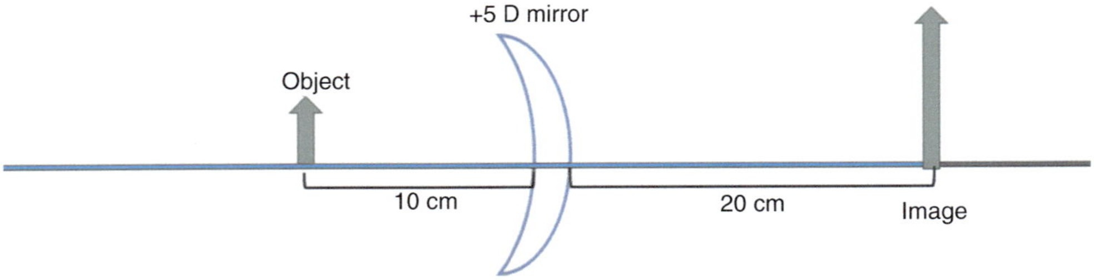

Fig. 22 Object–mirror system for an object located 10 cm to the left of a + 5D mirror and its resulting image. The image is 20 cm to the right of the mirror (location), upright (orientation), 2× magnified (size), and virtual (type)

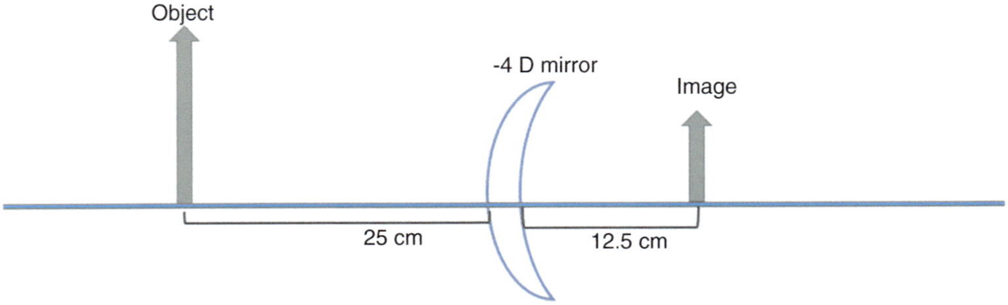

Fig. 23 Object–mirror system for a 3-meter-tall object located 25 cm to the left of a −4D mirror. Notice the location of the image obeys the "VERMIN" rule

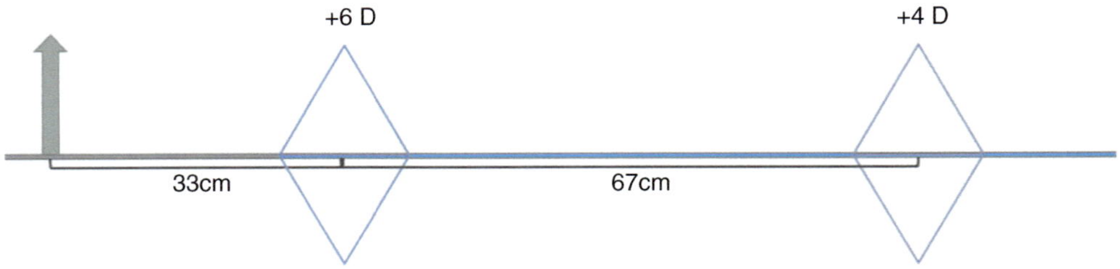

Fig. 24 Complex object–lens system for an object located 33 cm to the left of a + 6D lens which itself is located 67 cm to the left of a + 4D lens

$$-3+6=V=+3$$

$$v=100/V=100/3=33\,\text{cm or }0.33\,\text{m}$$

The image from the first lens is 33 cm to the right of the first lens. This means it is roughly 33 cm to the left of the second lens as well. We could also use 34 cm, but the math is going to be about the same. This becomes our new object distance. Now, we can ignore the first lens and deal with the second lens only (again, they won't give us double the points for solving this problem on an exam…).

$$u=-0.33\,\text{m}=-33\,\text{cm}$$

$$U=100/u=-3$$

$$U+D=V$$

$$-3+4=V=+1$$

v = 100/V = 100 cm or 1m. The final image is 1 meter to the right of the second lens.

Note this question did not ask us anything about the magnification, orientation, etc., of either image, so we will let sleeping dogs lie.

8. We can skip to the part where we just solve the problem for this one. Of course, if you wish, you can take a minute to draw out the lenses to get your bearings.

First, we can deal with the first lens.

$$u=-0.33\,\text{m}=-33\,\text{cm}$$

$$U=100/u=100/-33=-3$$

$$U+D=V$$

$$-3+4=V=1$$

v = 100/V = 100 cm or 1m. This means that the image from the first lens is 100 cm to the right of the first lens, which also unfortunately means that it is roughly 33 cm to the **right** of the second lens. This becomes our new object distance. This is the one of those rare times that u and U are positive.

Now, we have to deal with the second lens, keeping in mind that u is POSITIVE. It may help to draw a "+" sign in front of the u/U to make sure we keep our signs straight.

$$u=+0.33\,\text{m or }+33\,\text{cm}$$

$$U=100/u=+3$$

$$U+D=V$$

$$+3+7=V=+10$$

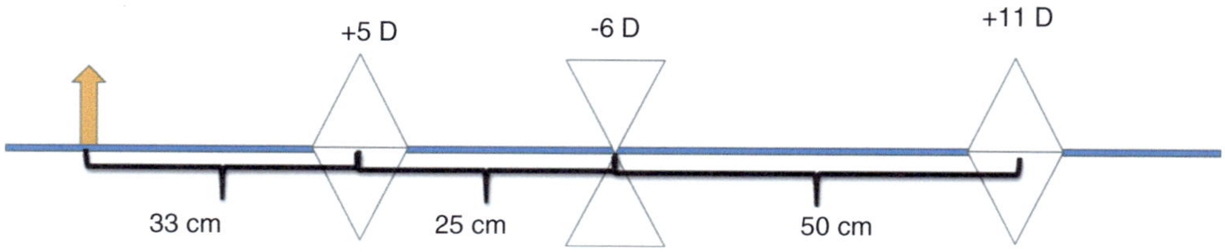

Fig. 25 Multiple lens system for an object located 33 cm to the left of a + 5D lens, which itself is located 25 cm to the left of a −6D lens, which itself is located 50 cm to the left of a + 11D lens. Two intermediate images with unique characteristics will form as detailed in the text

$v = 100/V = 100/10 = 10$ cm or 0.1m. Since V(v) is positive, the final image will be 10 cm to the RIGHT of the second lens.

9. Hopefully, this will be as tricky as exam problems will get. This is basically making us solve three $U + D = V$ problems. We will do our usual math, but we can point out a few interesting findings in terms of the image quality and location (both intermediate and final images).

We can draw this one out (Fig. 25) as follows:

Now, we have to solve for each lens as follows:

First Lens System:

$$U = 100 / -33 = -3$$

$$U + D = V$$

$$-3 + 5 = +2$$

$v = 100/V = 100/2 = 50$ cm to the right of the first lens, which would be 25 cm to the right of the second lens (yikes—we have to deal with another positive u!).

Second Lens System (Positive u!)

$$U = 100 / 25 = +4$$

$$U + D = V$$

$$+4 + -6 = -2$$

$v = 100/-2 = 50$ cm to the left of the second lens, which would be 100 cm to the left of the third lens (still following??)

Third Lens System

$$U = 100 / -100 = -1$$

$$U + D = V$$

$$-1 + 11 = +10$$

$v = 100 / 10 = 10\,\text{cm}$ to the RIGHT of the third lens.

As for the orientation, we can name the object as "Leonardo" to help sort out the resulting mess as follows:

- The image formed by the first lens system was real and inverted. We can name this image as "Donatello." Donatello is inverted compared to Leonardo.
- The image formed by the second lens system was virtual; we will name this image as "Raphael."
  - Raphael is inverted relative to Donatello, so it is upright relative to Leonardo.
- The image formed by the third lens system is real (because V was positive); we will name this image as "Michelangelo."
  - Michelangelo is inverted relative to Raphael
  - Raphael is upright relative to Leonardo
  - Therefore, Michelangelo is inverted relative to Leonardo as well.

As a result, the final image is upright relative to the original object. Undoubtedly, that was confusing, so we should confirm mathematically using our total magnification calculations below because the math never lies.

Remember that total magnification is the product of the magnification formed by each lens system.

For the first lens system: $m = U/V = -3/2 = -1.5$

For the second lens system: $m = U/V = 4/-2 = -2$

For the third lens system: $m = -1/10 = -0.1$

Total magnification = $(-1.5) * (-2) * (-0.1) = -0.3$ (this math is somewhat difficult, but can be done without a calculator).

The final image is inverted and 30% the size of the original object, thus proving that Michelangelo is inverted relative to Leonardo as well.

If you got this problem correct, congratulations, a wise sensei rat wishes he could give you three points for solving three $U + D=V$ problems, but unfortunately, we cannot.

10. We can solve this problem similar to the previous two problems that dealt with multiple lens systems.

We can draw this out if we wish. Otherwise, we can skip to solving the problem as follows:

First, we start with the lens.

$$u = -0.10\text{m} = -10\,\text{cm}$$

$$U = 100 / u = 100 / -10 = -10$$

$$U + D = V$$

$$-10 + 15 = V = +5$$

v = 100/V = 100/5 = 20 cm or 0.2m. The image from the first lens is 20 cm to the right of the first lens. This means it is roughly 50 cm to the left of the mirror. This becomes our new object distance.

Now, we deal with the mirror as follows:

$$u = -0.5\text{m} = -50\,\text{cm}$$

$$U = 100 / u = 100 / -50 = -2$$

$$U + D = V$$

−2 + 4 = V = + 2 (because V is positive, the image will form to the LEFT of the mirror)

$$v = 100 / V = 100 / 2$$
$$= 50\,\text{cm or } 0.5\text{m to the LEFT of the mirror}$$

The magnification of the final image will be the product of the magnification of each lens/mirror system as follows:

Lens magnification: m = U/V = − 10/5 = −2

Mirror magnification: m = U/V = − 2/2 = −1

Total magnification: (−2) * (−1) = +2. The final image will be upright and will be double the size of the original object.

11. We can solve this problem similar to the previous problem. Again, if you find it helps, you may wish to draw out the object, lens, and mirror.

First, we start with the first lens.

$$u = -0.20\text{m} = -20\,\text{cm}$$

$$U = 100 / u = 100 / -20 = -5$$

$$U + D = V$$

$$-5 + 6 = V = +1$$

v = 100/V = 100/1 = 100 cm or 1m. The image from the first lens is 100 cm to the right of the first lens. This means it is 25 cm to the right of the mirror (oh for crying out loud!). This becomes our new object distance. This is again one of those times that u and U are positive.

Now, we deal with the mirror as follows:

$$u = +0.25\text{m} = +25\,\text{cm}$$

$$U = 100 / u = 100 / 25 = +4$$

$$+4 + 6 = V = +10$$

v = 100/V = 100/10 = 10 cm or 0.1m (because V is positive, the image will form to the LEFT of the mirror). The final image is 10 cm to the left of the mirror.

The magnification of the final image will be the product of the magnification of each lens/mirror system as follows:

Lens magnification: m = U/V = −5/1 = −5

Mirror magnification: m = U/V = 4/10

Total magnification: (−5) * (4/10) = −2. The final image will be inverted and double the size of the original object.

12. This is yet another way of asking the same $U + D = V$ concept. In this case, we are asked to solve for u.

Since we know that v is 2 cm, we can calculate V as follows: 100/v = 100/2 = 50.

Now, we can plug this into our $U + D = V$ equation.

$$U + 60 = 50$$

$$U = -10, \text{which means } u = 100 / U = 100 / -10 = -10.$$

The object should be placed 10 cm to the left of the +60D lens.

13. This is yet another twist on the $U + D = V$ concept. Since we know that the image is formed to the left at a location between the object and the lens, this must be a virtual image. Also, since we are given a minus lens, it is more likely that we are dealing with a virtual image.

The image distance (v) is one-half the object distance (u). This means that $v = 0.5u$.

Now, we have to solve for U and V as follows:

$$V = 1 / v = 1 / (0.5u)$$

$$V = 2U$$

Now, we can use the U+D=V formula, setting $V = 2\,U$

$$U + D = 2U$$

$$U + (-5) = 2U$$

$$U = -5 \text{ and therefore } V = -10.$$

u = 100/U = 100/ − 5 = − 20. Therefore, the object is located 20 cm to the left of the lens. (The image will be located 10 cm to the left of the lens).

14. This problem seems to be a mouthful and a bit confusing. First draw out what the stem is asking (Fig. 26).

This problem is also confusing because we need to start with the second lens system in order to figure out what is happening with the first lens system.

For second lens system, we know that:

$$U_2 + D_2 = V_2$$

$$U_2 + 3 = 1$$

So U_2 must be −2, which would make u_2 100/−2 = −50. This means that the second object, which is the first image formed by the first lens, must be located 50 cm to the left of the second lens.

Now, we know that $V1 = U2$, but this $V1$ is positive because the image is forming to the right of the first lens. So, now we will set $V1 = +2$.

For the first lens system, the light is coming from infinity, so U_1 $100/\infty = 0$. This means that for all intents and purposes, we can ignore U_1 altogether.

We can solve now for the first lens system as follows:

$$U + D = V$$

$$0 + 2 = V = +2$$

$$v = 100 / V = 100 / 2 = 50\,\text{cm to the right of the first lens.}$$

This means that given a light source originating from infinity, the two lenses should be placed 1 meter (100 cm) apart in order to form an image 1 m to the right of the second lens.

15. The easiest thing to do here is to just get a 90D lens and use a slit lamp or a 20D lens and use an indirect to examine the posterior segment. Unfortunately, they are forcing us to use the ophthalmoscope, but we should realize that this is basically a "Vergence Along a Lens System" type of problem.

Let us draw out the description of the question stem so that we have a visual understanding of what is happening (Fig. 27).

For this myopic patient, light rays "leaving" the eye will form an image located at the far point of the eye where they will converge. This will form a real image of the eye (that will be so dim that no one can really "see" it) at 100/8 = 12 cm in front of the eye. If we are holding the scope at 2.5 cm, then the light rays have only traveled 2.5 cm of the total 12.5 cm, so there is still 10D of vergence that we need to account for. Therefore, 100/10 = −10D dialed into the ophthalmoscope in order to be able to view the retina.

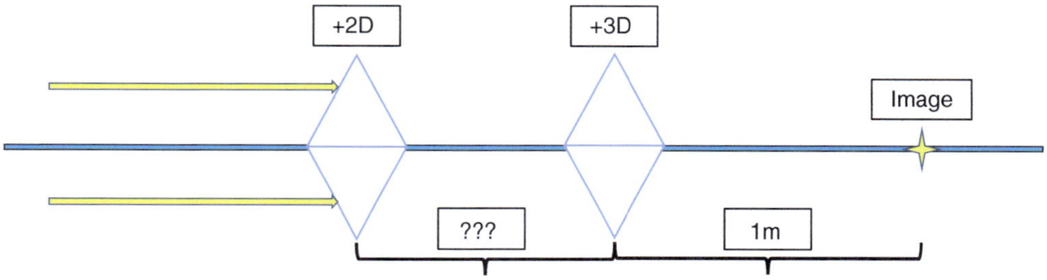

Fig. 26 How far apart must a + 2D lens and a + 3D lens be placed in order to form an image 1 meter to the right of the second lens?

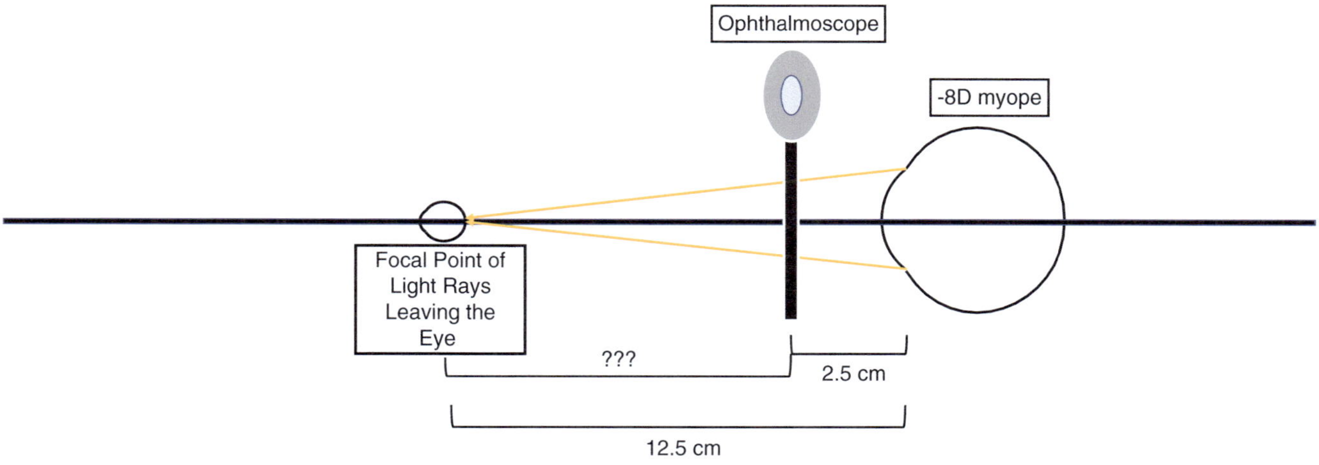

Fig. 27 How far from the cornea should an ophthalmoscope be held for a patient who is a −8D myope?

As a follow-up, if you, as the examiner, are a −3D myope and not wearing your glasses, you get to use your −3D myopia to your advantage. Therefore, you only need to dial in an additional −7D into the ophthalmoscope. However, if you are a + 3D hyperope and not wearing your glasses, you have to compensate for your hyperopia. Therefore, an additional −13D will need to be dialed into the ophthalmoscope.

Power of Lenses in Different Media

Kamran M. Riaz

Objectives

- To understand how a lens may have a different power based on the medium in which it is located
- To learn how to calculate the power of a refractive surface
- To discuss how different indices of refraction can affect the power of a lens
- To briefly discuss the Lensmaker's Formula
- To define the Power of a Lens in Different Media Equation (PLDME) and its application to solve problems

Introduction

Apologies in advance, but the topics discussed in this chapter are often confusing. Depending on which textbook or resource you consult, you may read a dozen different explanations, examples, and even varying terminology used to refer to this concept. Perhaps this is why this topic is confusing to so many trainees—we cannot even agree on standard terms to discuss this![1] In order to make our discussion relevant for examination purposes, we are going to use our own terminology (which admittedly is adding new terms) that we think is a bit more descriptive and simplified. As always, we will comment on clinical relevance whenever and wherever appropriate.

We can take a minute to recap what we have done so far: In the previous two chapters, the reduced vergence formula (aka, the Simple Lens Formula, $U + D = V$) was used to calculate many components of a lens (or mirror) system, including the power of the lens in question. However, a clinically relevant (and often testable) effect occurs when we change the refractive index when light rays undergo refraction. For example, recall from Chap. 1 when we stated that incoming light rays undergo refraction at the air-tear film interface. Thus, the effective power of a lens depends on the index of refraction of a given medium. By convention, we assume that air is the medium for most lenses encountered in Object-Lens problems; thus, a plus-power lens that has +10D written on its side will have +10D of power when held in air, but the power of this lens will change if placed in a different medium, such as water, silicone oil, or even chocolate sauce.

Fun fact: IOLs are manufactured such that the numerical power of the IOL written on the box (e.g., +20D IOL) means that the IOL will have +20D of power when bathed in aqueous ($n = 1.33$). However, the power of this +20D IOL will be much different if held in air ($n = 1.00$). The next time you have a chance to come across a (preferably expired, unusable) IOL, look through the IOL both underwater and in air. The IOL power in air is *much stronger* (more plus) than its power underwater.

We can also apply this concept to another area of relevance in ophthalmic optics. One of the reasons that the cornea has greater plus power than the crystalline lens is because light enters the cornea from the air at the **air–tear film** ($n = 1.00$ to $n = 1.33$) interface. The crystalline lens has much lesser "power," partly because the light passes from an aqueous-to-lens medium ($n = 1.33$ to $n = 1.409$, though much debate exists about the exact value, including the central and peripheral regions of the lens) as it passes from the anterior chamber to the lens.

Before we continue further, an aside is necessary here. In Ophthalmic Optics, the term "Lens Maker Equation" may be used to reference the Simple Lens Formula.[2] However, in physics optics (the kind you may still have PTSD about

[1] Don't get us started on the confusion between "meridian" and "axis" when it comes to describing astigmatism. We will save this misery for Chap. 10, "Spherocylindrical Lenses".

[2] For example, some texts refer to the lens maker's equation as a precursor equation used to calculate the simple lens formula.

K. M. Riaz (✉)
Dean McGee Eye Institute, University of Oklahoma, Oklahoma City, OK, USA

K. M. Riaz et al. (eds.), *Optics for the New Millennium*, https://doi.org/10.1007/978-3-030-95251-8_5

when you think back to your undergraduate physics classes), the term "lens makers' formula/equation" has an entirely different meaning. In physics optics, the "lens maker's formula/equation" is used to describe the relationship between 4 components of a lens: the radii of curvature (front surface and back surface), refractive index, lens thickness, and focal length. In essence, by calculating the focal length, one can determine the true effective power of the lens. The equation is easier for thin lenses because lens thickness can be ignored; however, for thick lenses, the lens thickness is significant and must be taken into account. Clinically, we have to deal with thick lenses, while in Geometric Optics, we will work with thin lenses unless otherwise specified. We will briefly discuss this version of the Lens Maker Formula at the end of the chapter, and we will use the abbreviation "LMF" when referring to it. It is unlikely that this version will appear on tests because the math required to calculate this is extremely difficult to do without a calculator, so you can take some comfort in this fact!

Therefore, for this chapter, we will focus on the ophthalmology-relevant version of determining the power of a lens in different media. To further assist with clarity, we will refer to this as "PLDME" (Power of a Lens in Different Media Equation) when referring to the equation and concepts necessary for exams and clinical practice. Of course, one could argue that this nomenclature is making it even more confusing, but we believe that this terminology is helpful for clarity and distinction purposes.[3]

Calculating the Refractive Power of a Spherical Surface

The refractive power of a spherical surface can be calculated using the wonderfully yucky equation:

$$D_s = \frac{n' - n}{r}$$

In this equation, n will refer to the medium with the *lower index of refraction* (usually air), and n' will refer to the medium with the *higher index of refraction*. In addition, r will refer to the radius of the refractive spherical surface; however, its value in the equation is represented **in meters**.[4] Usually, the radius of a refractive surface is measured in centimeters or millimeters. Therefore when we place that number in the above equation, we will often use a decimal that has a disgusting appearance, rendering the math nearly impossible without a calculator. Again, we can sense a theme here: Because of the complex math, this type of calculation problem is unlikely to appear on tests. Instead, we should know that the primary determinant of the "functional" power of the lens when we change the media is due to the change in the indices of refraction.

In Ophthalmic Optics, the cornea is a common spherical surface that we encounter frequently. Therefore, while we should not waste valuable brain cells on memorizing r values for different refractive spherical surfaces, one number that should be committed to memory is that the corneal curvature radius is .007 m. This may seem difficult to remember, but you may recognize that this number (007) is also the code number for the most famous spy in her Majesty's Secret Service.

Nonetheless, we can learn a few key points from the above equation. First, assuming r is constant or relatively small, the power of a refractive surface *primarily depends* on the change between the indices of refraction. Specifically, the greater the difference between the two indices of refraction, the greater the power of the refractive surface. Therefore, a plus power lens will have more power in water or chocolate sauce than its power in air because of the value of $(n' - n)$. Second, because r is constant (or relatively small), we can combine two of these equations into a Frankenstein equation that becomes the PLDME.

We can now see how this equation can help us determine the corneal refractive power in air vs. the corneal refractive power underwater. Again, people, if you decide to submerge your head underwater to test your corneas' power underwater, be sure to remove any and all contact lenses!

If we want to know the power of the cornea in air vs. the power of the cornea in water, we can use the above equation and plug in the following numbers:

Corneal Refractive Power in Air (Air–Tear Film Interface)

$$D_s = \frac{n' - n}{r} = \frac{1.33 - 1.00}{0.007} = 47.14\text{D}$$

Corneal Refractive Power in Water:
(Cornea–Water Interface)

$$D_s = \frac{n' - n}{r} = \frac{1.37 - 1.33}{0.007} = 5.7\text{D}$$

Even if we use 1.376 as the corneal refractive index, the corneal refractive power in water would be approximately +6.57D. Would you ever have to calculate this on a test? No! The math is too hard. Nevertheless, understanding this helps to explain, for example, why we do not see well underwater: The cornea has significantly *lower refractive power underwater* as compared to an air medium. In essence, *we become significantly far-sighted underwater* because the cornea cannot sufficiently refract light to hit the retina as it is able to do in air. In order to see underwater, we would have to generate significant, additional plus power (e.g., by accommodation) to overcome this barrier; thus, a high/pathologic myope may have an easier time seeing underwater as compared to an

[3]We apologize that we could not come up with a better acronym or mnemonic, however!

[4]Remember, many optics formulas are technically in meters, but we often work in centimeters to make the math easier.

emmetrope or hyperope (the latter would have the most difficulty).

Suppose the superhero king of Atlantis (whose name we cannot mention lest we incur the wrath of copyright lawyers), who is emmetropic underwater, decides to visit us surface dwellers. What will his refractive error be on the surface?

Answer: Our superhero king of Atlantis likely has incredibly powerful corneas and/or crystalline lenses that can bend light rays underwater. Therefore, if he is *emmetropic* underwater, he will be significantly *myopic* on the earth's surface. He may end up needing −40 to −50D contact lenses in order to see us surface dwellers. The fact that he does not need glasses or contact lenses on dry land is perhaps, in this author's belief, the most fascinating of all the superhero's powers and should have been explored in the movie's plot much more deeply.

A similarly fascinating real-life example has been documented and reported among the semi-nomadic Moken people who have lived for generations in boats or stilted dwellings along the coast of Thailand.[5] Moken children can gather shellfish and other food from the ocean floor as deep as 75 feet (23 meters). Even though children have more accommodative ability than adults, as optics nerds, we should ask ourselves: *How are these children able to do this?*

Researchers have observed that Moken children can maximally constrict their pupils (less than 2 mm-think back to our discussions on diffraction and the Airy disc in Chap. 1) and can accommodate past the known limits of human performance (up to 15–16D accommodation). Thus, they can overcome the hyperopia encountered by most human beings underwater! Interestingly, as these children grow older, they "age out" of this underwater diving task, as they eventually lose this ability of "super-accommodation" and the diving job is passed on to younger children. With intense training, other children of different ethnic backgrounds may similarly achieve this level of underwater vision.[6]

Returning to the less exciting world of Ophthalmic Optics, we can use the same equation to calculate the refractive power of the **back surface** of the cornea:

Refractive Power of the Back Surface of the Cornea:

$$D_s = \frac{n' - n}{r} = \frac{1.37 - 1.33}{0.007} = 5.7\text{D}$$

However, we have to ask ourselves is the power of the back surface +5.7D or −5.7D? We can take a closer look at the back surface of the cornea (Fig. 1).

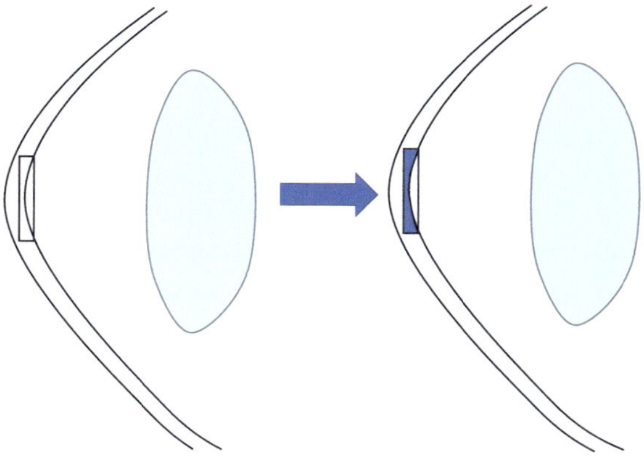

Fig. 1 The back surface of the cornea most closely resembles a concave lens, thereby giving it minus power

We can see that the back surface of the cornea has *minus power* that must be subtracted from the plus power of the front surface of the cornea. Therefore, the net power of the cornea will be less than the >47 D of power that we calculated earlier. This calculation shows the average net refractive power of the average human cornea as ~42-43D. Admittedly, we have employed some shortcuts, so the math does not exactly match up.[7] The main lesson here is that the net refractive power of the cornea is the difference between the front surface (positive power) and the back surface (negative power). Clinically, this is important when dealing with eyes that have undergone previous laser refractive surgery, especially for correction of myopia. In these eyes, since the procedure flattens the anterior cornea, keratometry and biometry devices will measure the anterior cornea and assume a fixed-ratio between anterior and posterior corneal power when calculating the corneal power. This often leads to the biometry device measuring falsely steeper-than-real corneal power measurements, leading to a lower-than-needed IOL power and potential hyperopic surprise.[8]

[5]Gislen A, Dacke M, Kroger RH, etc. Superior underwater vision in a human population of sea gypsies. Current Biology 2003;13(10):833–6.

[6]Gislen A, Warrant EJ, Dacke M. Visual training improves underwater vision in children. Vision Research 2006;46(20):3443–60.

[7]We have intentionally left the math simple here and taken some significant shortcuts to highlight the more important teaching points mentioned in the text. A more strenuous and accurate calculation of this can be done in several ways. One way is to take the Gullstrand eye's anterior corneal power (approximately 48.8D)—posterior corneal power (−5.8D) to arrive at approximately 43D. The magical number of 1.376 has been used historically for the refractive index of the cornea. With more accurate methods of measuring the refractive index, we now know that the various layers of the cornea themselves have their own refractive index. For example, the epithelium is approximately 1.400, Bowman's layer is approximately 1.380, the stroma is approximately 1.369, and the endothelium is approximately 1.373. Other methods have indicated a refractive index of the entire tear-film/cornea complex ranging from 1.423 to 1.436. In summary, the refractive index of the tear-film/cornea complex varies significantly from patient to patient, but may be actually much higher than previously thought. See Patel S, Tutchenko L. The refractive index of the human cornea: A review. Cont Lens Anterior Eye. 2019 Oct;42(5):575–580.

[8]See Chap. 26, "Preoperative Optics for Cataract Surgery", for more information.

The Power of a Lens in Different Media Equation (PLDME)

The Power of a Lens in Different Media Equation (PLDME) is simply a comparison of the power of a refractive surface (in this case, a lens) based on the media in which it is placed. The PLDME allows us to eliminate the *r* (and its associated complex math) and use the differences in the indices of refraction to determine the functional power of a lens based on the medium we are measuring.

The PLDME used in ophthalmic optics is as follows:

$$\frac{D_{\text{medium1}}}{D_{\text{medium2}}} = \frac{(n_{\text{lens}} - n_{\text{medium1}})}{(n_{\text{lens}} - n_{\text{medium2}})}$$

D_{medium1} = the power of the refractive surface (or lens) in the first medium

D_{medium2} = the power of the refractive surface (or lens) in the second medium

We can see from the PLDME that if we know the power of a lens in a given medium (e.g., air, with $n = 1.00$), then we can calculate the power of that same lens in a different medium as long as we know the index of refraction of (1) the lens and (2) the new medium.

#ProTip: When setting up this equation, be careful that you match up the power of the lens in a given medium in the same row as the corresponding index of refraction. For example, be careful that you maintain the power of the lens in medium1 and place the index of refraction of medium2 in the same row. The math involved in solving these equations should be relatively simple for test purposes. If you find yourself struggling with the math, pause for a minute and ensure you have not accidentally placed your numbers in the wrong spot.

The index of refraction of most materials should not be committed to memory and will likely be given to you on an examination. However, you may wish to know a few commonly used indices of refraction as shown in the table below that we have simplified (rounded) to two decimals for easier memorization[9] (Table 1):

Let us do a few examples of typical PLDME questions.

Table 1 Values of common indices of refraction encountered in ophthalmic optics

Medium	Index of refraction (*n*)
Air	1.00
Water/aqueous/vitreous	1.33
Cornea	1.376
Crystalline lens	1.386–1.406

[9]Source: Emsley HH (ed), *Visual Optics, 5th Edition, Volume 1: Optics of Vision*, 1953, Butterworth-Heinemann, pp. 336–403.

Example #1

If an IOL made of PMMA ($n = 1.49$) has a power of +16D when measured in aqueous, what is the power of this IOL in air?

$$\frac{D_{\text{medium1}}}{D_{\text{medium2}}} = \frac{(n_{\text{lens}} - n_{\text{medium1}})}{(n_{\text{lens}} - n_{\text{medium2}})}$$

Answer

Begin by using the PLDME:

In this case, we can set medium$_1$ as air and medium$_2$ as aqueous. In general, it is easier to solve these problems by having the numerator end up as the larger number, so whenever possible, *set the medium with the lower index of refraction as medium$_1$*.

$$\frac{D_{\text{medium1}}}{D_{\text{medium2}}} = \frac{(n_{\text{lens}} - n_{\text{medium1}})}{(n_{\text{lens}} - n_{\text{medium2}})} = \frac{D_{\text{air}}}{D_{aq}} = \frac{(n_{IOL} - n_{\text{air}})}{(n_{IOL} - n_{aq})}$$

$$\frac{D_{\text{air}}}{16} = \frac{(1.49 - 1.00)}{(1.49 - 1.33)}$$

$$\frac{D_{\text{air}}}{16} = \frac{(0.49)}{(0.16)} \approx 3$$

$$D_{\text{air}} = (3)(16) = 48 \text{ diopters in air}$$

Example #2

If a pair of prescription swimming goggles made from plastic ($n = 1.44$) has −2D of power in air, what is the power of the goggles in water? Bonus points: What is the flawed premise of this question?

Answer

Once again, use the PLDME:

$$\frac{D_{\text{medium1}}}{D_{\text{medium2}}} = \frac{(n_{\text{lens}} - n_{\text{medium1}})}{(n_{\text{lens}} - n_{\text{medium2}})}$$

As mentioned previously, for consistency, we can set up the PLDME such that the numerator ends up being the higher number. Therefore, we can place the numbers associated with the medium with the lower index of refraction in the top row.

$$\frac{D_{\text{medium1}}}{D_{\text{medium2}}} = \frac{(n_{\text{lens}} - n_{\text{medium1}})}{(n_{\text{lens}} - n_{\text{medium2}})} = \frac{D_{\text{air}}}{D_{\text{water}}} = \frac{(n_{\text{goggles}} - n_{\text{air}})}{(n_{\text{goggles}} - n_{\text{water}})}$$

$$\frac{-2}{D_{\text{water}}} = \frac{(1.44 - 1.00)}{(1.44 - 1.33)} = \frac{(0.44)}{(0.11)}$$

$$-2 / D_{\text{water}} = 4$$

$$D_{\text{water}} = -2/4 = -0.5 \text{ diopters in water}$$

To answer the bonus portion of the question, we have to ask ourselves: Does this mean that if we use these goggles underwater, the −2D goggles will only have a power of −0.5D? If yes, then why did we spend all this money on prescription goggles if they will be underpowered? Moreover, do we intentionally need to over-minus the goggles to have the required −2D of power underwater?

This is one of those favorite questions that senior attendings may ask as a rite of passage to younger ophthalmologists. The answer to this is both yes and no. The goggles are constructed such that the power is on the *inside* surface of the goggles. This maintains an air–tear film interface between the back of the goggles and the swimmer's eyes. Therefore, as long as the goggles are properly worn and no water gets into the space between the back of the goggles and the swimmer's eyes, the goggles will maintain their −2D of power "underwater." However, if water gets inside the goggles, the air-tear film interface has been replaced with a water-water interface. When the swimmer tries to use the goggles, they will only have –0.5D of power "in the water." Note the semantic difference between "underwater" and "in the water" that makes all the difference on whether you will correctly answer the senior attending's question of the day.

Example #3

A +27D IOL is constructed of a novel material (n = 1.69). You perform successful cataract surgery on a patient with silicone oil (n = 1.37) and place the IOL in the capsular bag. A few days later, the patient experiences trauma. You note that the IOL has fallen into the posterior chamber on examination. What is the effective power of the IOL at this time?

Answer

First of all, why are we worrying about optics when this patient likely needs surgery to get the IOL out of the posterior chamber and avoid the risk of further problems, including retinal detachment and/or blindness? Second, this novel material for the IOL is a terrible choice because the greater the index of refraction, the higher the chances of other problems, such as dysphotopsias, though it is likely very thin and thus easily foldable and injectable through a smaller incision. Third, let's go ahead and solve this problem using the PLDME:

$$\frac{D_{\text{medium1}}}{D_{\text{medium2}}} = \frac{(n_{\text{lens}} - n_{\text{medium1}})}{(n_{\text{lens}} - n_{\text{medium2}})} = \frac{D_{\text{aqueous}}}{D_{\text{vitreous}}} = \frac{(n_{IOL} - n_{\text{aqueous}})}{(n_{IOL} - n_{\text{vitreous}})}$$

$$\frac{27}{D_{\text{vitreous}}} = \frac{(1.69 - 1.33)}{(1.69 - 1.37)} = \frac{(0.36)}{(0.32)}$$

$$D_{\text{vitreous}} = 27/(9/8) = 24\text{D of power}\,(+3\text{D hyperopic shift})$$

Therefore, during the (hopefully) short time between the initial exam and surgical intervention, the patient will have a +3D hyperopic shift, and we can take solace that we figured this out using the magical powers of the PLDME.

Lens Maker's Formula (Physics Optics)

As stated previously, this type of problem is unlikely to appear on examinations because of the difficult calculations required to solve it. The Lensmaker's Formula (LMF) is used to construct a lens with a specified focal length.[10] Since a lens has two curved surfaces (anterior and posterior), if we know the index of refraction, lens thickness, and radius of curvature (in centimeters) of each surface, we can calculate the focal length of that particular lens. Basically, a thick lens requires us to factor in the fact that light rays will get refracted in three different places. Figure 2 shows a typical thick convex lens.

The power of the front surface, back surface, index of refraction, and lens thickness can be used to calculate the focal length.

We can then take the inverse of the focal length to calculate the power.

The LMF is[11]:

$$D = \frac{1}{f} = (n-1)\left[\frac{1}{R_1} - \frac{1}{R_2}\right]$$

[10] Some texts will refer to this as lens maker's equation. We have chosen to use the term lens maker's formula since the BCSC also uses the term lens maker's equation, albeit as a reference to the simple lens formula. All very confusing!

[11] Technically, this is the LMF for a thin lens. The LMF for thick lenses in air is even more complicated: $D = 1/f = (n-1)\,[1/R_1 - 1/R_2 + [(n-1)d]/[nR_1R_2]]$. That is one disgusting equation, and thus, it is even more unlikely that this will appear on examinations.

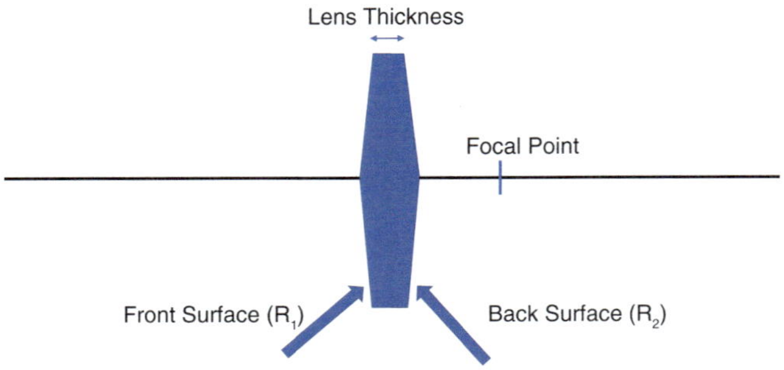

Fig. 2 In a thick convex (converging, positive power) lens, the power of the lens is determined by the front radius of curvature, back radius of curvature, index of refraction, and the thickness of the lens. This can be used to calculate the focal length, and these variables can be combined into the LMF equation

A convex lens (such as the cornea or crystalline lens) will have a positive value for R1 and a negative value for R2. A concave lens will have a negative value for R1 and a positive value for R2. If the question does not explicitly state whether the lens is convex or concave, looking at the R1 and R2 values can help determine what type of lens we are encountering.

Hopefully, the LMF will never appear on an examination. But in case it does:

Example

If the refractive index of a lens is 1.6, the front radius of curvature is 10 cm, and the back radius of curvature is −15 cm, what is the focal length of this lens? What is the power of this lens?

Answer

We will start by writing out the LMF, filling in the given variables, and solving for the unknown variable:

$$D=\frac{1}{f}=(n-1)\left[\frac{1}{R_1}-\frac{1}{R_2}\right]=(1.6-1)\left[\frac{1}{10}-\frac{1}{-15}\right]$$
$$=(0.6)\times(0.1+0.0666)$$
$$=(0.6)\times(0.1666)=0.1$$
$$\text{So } f=1/0.1=10\,\text{cm (focal length)}$$
$$\text{So } D=1/f=1/.1=+10\text{D}$$

Practice Questions

1. What is the power of a lens in air with a refractive index of 1.8 and a radius of curvature of 10 cm? What is the same power of this lens in water?
2. What is the refractive index of a lens with radius of curvature of 5 cm that has a power of +15D in air?
3. What is the radius of curvature of a lens with a refractive index of 1.66 that has a power of +6D in water?
4. What is the radius of curvature of a lens with an index of refraction of 1.5 and a power of +8D when measured in air?
5. If a lens is made of a material (n = 1.5) and has a power of +21D when submerged in acetone (n = 1.35), what is the power of this lens in air?
6. If a lens made of a material (n = 1.44) has a power of +40D in air and a power of +20 in an unknown liquid, what is the index of refraction of this unknown liquid?
7. A lens of an unknown index of refraction is determined to have a power of +80D in air and +20D in water. What is the index of refraction of this lens?
8. Suppose you examine a patient's biconcave snorkeling glasses of unknown power. You note that the front surface has a radius of curvature of 5 cm, the back surface has a radius of curvature of 10 cm, and the index of refraction is 1.5. What is the power of the glasses in air versus underwater?

Answers

1. Answer: Use the equation for calculating the power of a refractive surface, making sure we convert the radius of curvature into meters.

$$D_s=\frac{n'-n}{r}=\frac{(1.8-1.0)}{0.1}=\frac{0.8}{0.1}=+8\text{D in air}$$
$$=\frac{(1.8-1.33)}{0.1}=\frac{0.47}{0.1}=+4.7\text{D in water}$$

2. Answer: This is a twist on the familiar equation for calculating the power of a refractive surface, except this time, we are asked to solve for n'. We can set up our equation as follows:

$$D_s=\frac{n'-n}{r}\quad n'=(D_s\times r)+n=(15\times0.05)+1$$
$$=1.75$$

3. Answer: This is a third twist on the familiar equation for calculating the power of a refractive surface, except this time we are asked to solve for r. We can use our equation as before:

$$D_s=\frac{n'-n}{r}\quad r=\frac{(n'-n)}{D_s}=\frac{(1.66-1.33)}{6}=\frac{0.33}{6}=0.055$$

The radius of curvature for this lens would be 5.5 cm.

4. Answer:

$$D_s=\frac{n'-n}{r}=\quad r=\frac{(n'-n)}{D_s}=\frac{(1.5-1.0)}{8}=0.0625\text{m}$$
$$=62.5\,\text{mm}$$

5. Answer: This is a relatively straightforward PLDME question:

$$\frac{D_{\text{medium1}}}{D_{\text{medium2}}}=\frac{\left(n_{\text{lens}}-n_{\text{medium1}}\right)}{\left(n_{\text{lens}}-n_{\text{medium2}}\right)}=\frac{D_{\text{air}}}{D_{\text{acetone}}}=\frac{\left(n_{\text{lens}}-n_{\text{air}}\right)}{\left(n_{\text{lens}}-n_{\text{acetone}}\right)}$$

$$\frac{D_{\text{air}}}{21}=\frac{(1.5-1.00)}{(1.5-1.35)}=(21)(0.5/15)=21\times3.333=+70\text{D in air}$$

6. Answer: This is a bit of a twist on the PLDME equation. We are given the two different powers, as well as one index of refraction of a medium, along with the index of refraction of the lens. We can set it up as follows:

$$\frac{D_{\text{medium1}}}{D_{\text{medium2}}}=\frac{\left(n_{\text{lens}}-n_{\text{medium1}}\right)}{\left(n_{\text{lens}}-n_{\text{medium2}}\right)}=\frac{D_{\text{air}}}{D_{\text{liquid}}}=\frac{\left(n_{\text{lens}}-n_{\text{air}}\right)}{\left(n_{\text{lens}}-n_{\text{liquid}}\right)}$$

$$\frac{40}{2}=\frac{(1.44-1.00)}{\left(1.44-n_{\text{liquid}}\right)}=1.44-n_{\text{liquid}}=\frac{0.44}{2}$$

$$n_{\text{liquid}}=1.44-0.22=1.22$$

7. Answer: The complexity of this problem was admittedly beyond the scope of what would be encountered on typical examinations. Nonetheless, we have seen how the PLDME concept can be tested in various situations. Fun fact: the index of refraction of silicone is 1.39–1.43, so maybe this lens is made of silicone-like material?

$$D_{\text{air}}/D_{\text{water}}=\left(n_{\text{lens}}-n_{\text{air}}\right)/\left(n_{\text{lens}}-n_{\text{water}}\right)$$

$$80/20=\left(n_{\text{lens}}-n_{\text{air}}\right)/\left(n_{\text{lens}}-n_{\text{water}}\right)$$

$$80\left(n_{\text{lens}}-1.33\right)=20\left(n_{\text{lens}}-1.00\right)$$

$$80*n_{\text{lens}}-106.4=20*n_{\text{lens}}-20$$

$$60*n_{\text{lens}}=86.4$$

$$n_{\text{lens}}=(\text{approximately})\ 1.44$$

8. Answer: This problem requires us to combine our knowledge of concepts discussed in the previous chapters (thick lenses) and concepts from this chapter. We can simplify the thick lens equation (see Chap. 3) into one that primarily requires us to compare the power of this lens in air versus underwater. Since the question stem tells us the glasses are "biconcave," we know that we are dealing with minus-power lenses: Power of the snorkeling glasses in air:

D = (n2–n1) * [(1/R1) + (1/R2)]
= (1.5–1.0) * [(100/–5) + (100/–10)]
= (0.5) * (–30) = –15D

Now we can calculate the power of the snorkeling glasses underwater, using the shortcut that we only have to account for the difference in the indices of refraction: 1.5–1.33 = 0.17. Now we can multiply 0.17 and –30: 0.17 * –30D = –5.1D (approximately –5D) underwater. Finally, we have seen several examples of glasses, lenses, and IOLs changing from air to water. As a rule of thumb, the power in air is approximately three times stronger than the power of the lens in water.

Lens Effectivity

Kamran M. Riaz

Objectives

- To understand how moving a lens closer to the eye and away from the eye can change its effective power
- To define the far point and near point for myopic and emmetropic eyes
- To apply the principles of lens effectivity to clinical examples of eyeglasses and contact lenses

Introduction

We have previously discussed that the dioptric power value of a lens relies on many factors, such as the radii of curvature, index of refraction, and lens thickness. For example, if you hold it in front of your eye, a +10D lens will have +10 diopters of power based on these previous factors. One assumption made here is that the lens is held at a certain distance from the eye (known as the *vertex distance*, which will be important in our discussion on glasses) to maintain this dioptric power. In other words, we have to hold the +10D lens at a fixed distance from the eye in order for that +10D lens to behave like a + 10D lens.

The concept of lens effectivity states that if we hold the lens closer or farther away from the eye (i.e., if we change the vertex distance), that +10D lens may now have "effectively" different powers. By altering the vertex distance, we can cause a lens with a given power to effectively have a different power. We will see how this will serve as a foundation for later discussions on glasses and contact lenses.

Lens Effectivity

To understand the concept of lens effectivity, imagine that we are dealing with Pinocchio as our test patient. He has been telling lots of lies recently (such as telling people that optics is fun and exciting), so his nose is quite long these days. Imagine that if we place glasses on this liar's nose, we have quite a bit of room to move the lenses forward (down along the nose, away from the eye) and backward (up the nose, closer to the eye). We can visualize this nomenclature in the following figure – we apologize that we could not fork over the big bucks to get the actual picture of Pinocchio from his corporate masters, so instead, we will have to imagine that the horizontal line in the figure below is his "nose" (Fig. 1).

When we move lenses toward the eye or away from the eye, we have "effectively" changed the lens' power. In other words, the lens is "behaving" like a lens with a different power. We can see how this works for Pinocchio with both plus- and minus-power lenses.

Plus Lenses

Moving a plus lens **forward** (down along the nose, away from the eye) will <u>increase</u> its effective plus power. Therefore, a +3D lens may "behave" like a +4D lens when Pinocchio moves the lens away from his eye. If we want him to have eyeglasses with +3D of "effective" power, then we will have to decrease the power of the lens if he moves it down along his nose. This is an important rule for clinical practice: in order to maintain the desired distance correction, a plus lens will have to be *decreased* in power if it is moved forward (i.e., if the vertex distance increases). Or we could just tell him to stop telling lies so that we do not have to worry about this effectivity nonsense! (Fig. 2).

Moving a plus lens **backward** (up along the nose, toward the eye) will <u>decrease</u> its effective plus power. Therefore, our same +3D lens may "behave" like a +2D lens when Pinocchio moves the lens closer to his eye. If we want him to have eyeglasses with +3D of "effective" power, we will have to increase the power of the lens if he moves it up along his nose. Now that we told him to stop telling lies, we have to deal with this problem (Fig. 2). This example is a corollary to the above rule for clinical practice: to maintain the desired distance correc-

K. M. Riaz (✉)
Dean McGee Eye Institute, University of Oklahoma, Oklahoma City, OK, USA

K. M. Riaz et al. (eds.), *Optics for the New Millennium*, https://doi.org/10.1007/978-3-030-95251-8_6

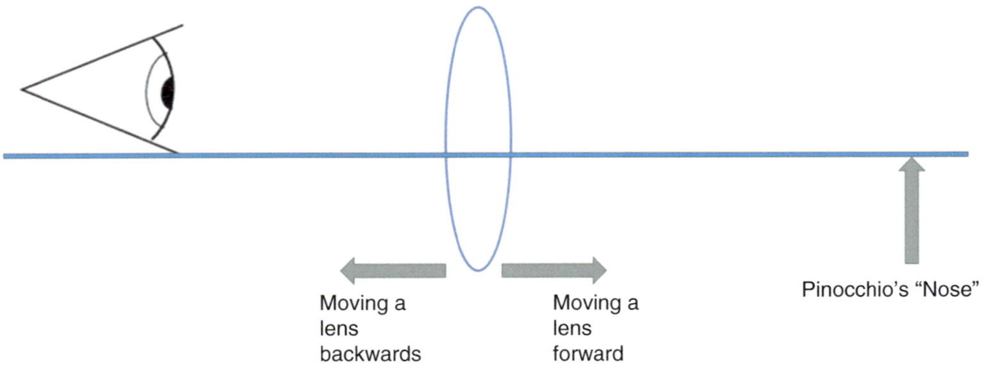

Fig. 1 Visual representation of terminology used in discussions of lens effectivity. Moving a lens "forward" means moving it away from the eye, and moving a lens "backward" means moving it closer to the eye

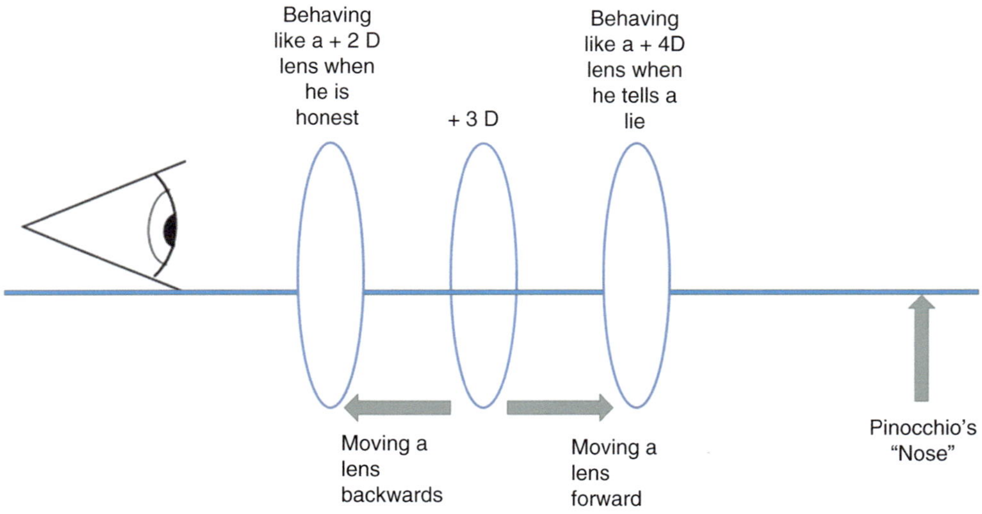

Fig. 2 Moving a plus lens away from the eye will increase its effective plus power. Moving a plus lens toward the eye will decrease its effective plus power

tion, a plus lens will have to be *increased* in power if it is moved backward (i.e., if the vertex distance decreases).

Using these two principles, we can understand why a hyperope patient will have to wear higher powered (i.e., higher number) contact lenses than their glasses. Because we have moved the lens closer to the eye, we have to increase the power of the needed contact lens.

Minus Lenses

Moving a minus lens **forward** (down along the nose, away from the eye) will decrease its effective minus power. We can think of this scenario as similar to the plus lens in that the minus lens will also gain more effective plus power the further it moves away from the eye. Therefore, a −3D lens will "behave" like a −2D lens if pushed forward down along the nose. If we want Pinocchio to have −3D of "effective" power, we will have to increase the power of the lens if he reverts to telling lies and the eyeglasses end up further away from the eye (Fig. 3).

This example helps explain why presbyopic myopes often slide their glasses down along their noses for real-life purposes. By doing this, they weaken their myopic prescription glasses (i.e., adding plus power) and essentially give themselves "reading glasses" to help with their near vision needs.

Moving a minus lens **backward** (up along the nose, closer to the eye) will increase its effective minus power. If Pinocchio stops telling lies and the −3D lens moves closer to his nose, it may "behave" like a −4D lens. If we want him to have −3D of "effective" power, then we will have to decrease the power of the lens if he moves it closer to his eye (Fig. 3).

For real-life purposes, this helps explain why an under-corrected myope will often push his/her glasses up along their nose and closer to the eye – they are (unconsciously) using the concept of lens effectivity to increase the "effective" minus power of their eyeglasses.[1]

[1]As an additional "why should I care about this" point of relevance, understanding the concept of lens effectivity serves as a useful foundation for understanding *effective lens position* (ELP) for IOL calculations. We can deduce that if an IOL sits more anterior (closer to the cornea), it will have effectively less power, causing a more myopic-than-intended refractive outcome. Similarly, if the IOL sits more posteriorly, it will have effectively more power, causing a more hyperopic-than-intended refractive outcome. This concept also has relevance for other scenarios, such as why we have to adjust the power of an IOL if it is placed in the sulcus. See Chap. 28 "Intraoperative Optics", Intraoperative Optics for Cataract Surgery for more information.

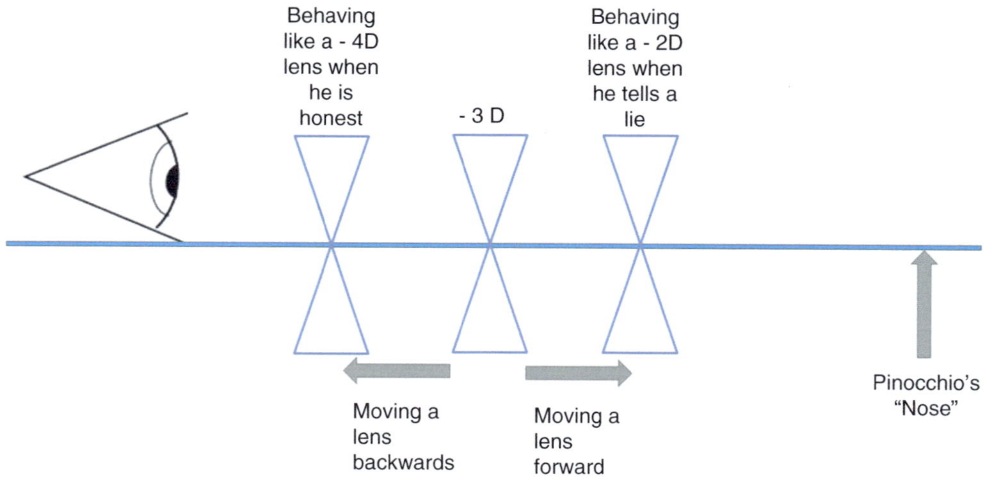

Fig. 3 Moving a minus lens away from the eye will decrease its effective minus power (and give it more plus power). Moving a minus lens closer to the eye will increase its effective minus power

This concept can be easily understood for those readers who may be myopic by using themselves as an example. We imagine a fair number of you reading this book may be myopic – for you emmetropes out there, sorry! For myopes who wear both glasses and contact lenses, the power of the glasses is usually "more minus" than the power of the contact lens. For example, a myope who wears −6D glasses may only need −5.50D contact lenses – because the "lens" (contact lens) is closer to the eye, less effective power is needed.

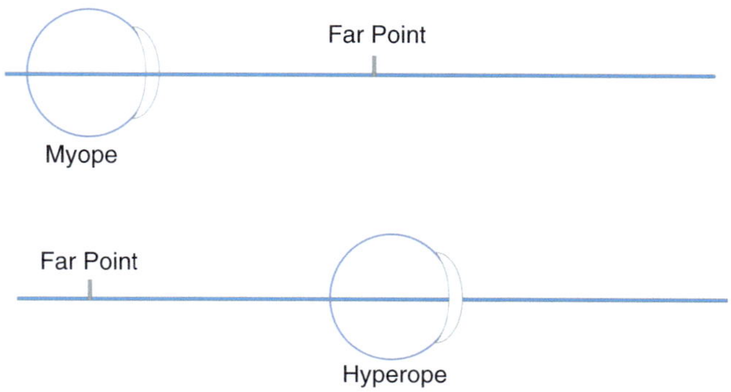

Fig. 4 For myopes, the far point is located in *front* of the eye. For hyperopes, the far point is located *behind* the eye

The "CAP" Mnemonic

The "Closer Add Plus (CAP)" mnemonic is useful for both minus- and plus-power lenses. This mnemonic helps us remember that regardless of the lens (whether it is a plus lens or a minus lens), the **c**loser we move the lens toward the eye, we must **a**dd **p**lus power to the lens to maintain the desired "effective" power of the lens. In both the plus- and minus-powered lenses examples above, we saw that moving the lens closer to the eye requires us to add more plus power to the lens. This is easily understood for the plus lens: simply add more plus power to the plus lens; however, for the minus lens, "adding plus power" means we have to decrease the minus lens power. You may want to read this several times as it may initially seem counter-intuitive.

The Far Point for Myopic and Hyperopic Eyes

The **far point** is a term used to describe "what is the farthest point that the eye can see without glasses (and without any accommodation)". We will discuss far point and near point in greater detail in Chap. 9 Accommodation and Presbyopia, but we can use this definition for now.

The far point will be located in front of the eye for a myope. This intuitively is easier to understand because, in these eyes, there is too much plus power present in the eye: either the axial length is too long (axial myopia), or the corneal power is too strong (refractive myopia). Myopic patients can see targets located at the far point (or closer) with good clarity.

For a hyperope, the far point will be located behind the eye. Admittedly, this is hard to understand or visualize for a hyperope, so we should discuss this further. In the hyperopic eye, parallel light is refracted (by the cornea and lens) but does not come to a focus at the retina; it will finally converge to a focal point behind the retina (Fig. 4) which we will term as the far point. Therefore, when the light hits the retina, since it is still converging, it will produce a blurry image. The hyperopic eye must generate additional plus power (accommodation) or use plus-power glasses to "bring the light forward" so that light rays converge on the retina.

For the hyperope, bringing the object closer worsens the blurriness because this creates additional negative vergence at the cornea, which requires additional plus power. This explains why young patients with low amounts of hyperopia (e.g., 1–3D hyperopia) don't need glasses as teenagers and young adults: they can generate the needed plus power through natural accommodation. These patients may present in their late 30s/early 40s with complaints of blurry vision worse at near compared to distance as they can no longer generate the needed accommodation (latent hyperopia).[2]

As we will see in the next section, we will need to know how to use the far point when dealing with vertex distance problems.

Applying Lens Effectivity to Glasses and Contact Lenses

As we hinted at in the previous section, we can use this principle to help us understand why the power of glasses and contact lenses, especially with higher prescriptions (whether myopic or hyperopic), is often very different.

When we prescribe glasses, we assume a fixed distance between the eye and the glasses (known as the **vertex distance**) that is accounted for in the eyeglass prescription. In our previous Pinocchio discussions of him telling lies or being truthful, we were simply changing the vertex distance of the glasses and therefore needing to change the power of the glasses.[3]

For clinical purposes, when we change from glasses to contact lenses (and vice versa), we are basically changing the focal length of the lens based on the presence or absence of the vertex distance. Remember that the focal length of a lens can be calculated by $F = 1/D$ (or $F = 100/D$ to work in centimeters). For example, a +5D lens will have a focal length of 20 cm or 0.2 m.

When we change from *glasses to contact lenses*, we have to **subtract the vertex distance**. This should make sense because the contact lens sits on the cornea, so there is no vertex distance to factor.

When we change from *contact lenses to glasses*, we have to **add the vertex distance** because now the lens is away from the eye, so we have to account for the vertex distance. As an aside, we often assume a given vertex distance (e.g., 12.5 mm) when performing these calculations clinically. However, for higher refractions and/or unique facial anatomy, changes in vertex distance can significantly affect the patient's tolerance and satisfaction with the prescribed glasses.[4]

If we are given problems that ask us to calculate the power of glasses from the power of contact lenses (or vice versa), we basically have to get the focal lengths of each to match up. The trick is to make sure we account for the vertex distance. Many trainees are confused about whether we should add or subtract the vertex distance depending on whether we are dealing with a plus- or a minus-power lens. If we simply maintain the signed values at all times, we can apply the above rules inclusive of both lenses. We can do some examples to reinforce these points.

Example #1

If a patient wears +10D glasses with a vertex distance of 10 mm, what power contact lenses should be ordered?

A. +9 D
B. +10.5D
C. +10.75D
D. +11 D
E. +11.25 D

Answer: Suppose we are given this problem on an exam, and we have a brain freeze, forgetting all the Pinocchio discussions and whatnot. We can at least eliminate wrong answer choices by simply remembering that hyperopes will need "more plus power" in their contact lenses (because of the "CAP" mnemonic). Therefore, we can at least eliminate answer choice A and increase our chances of getting this problem correct.

But we should not live life by simply guessing. We want to actually solve the problem and feel that we have accomplished something meaningful today. In order to solve this problem, we need to figure out what is the focal length of the glasses first:

$$f_{\text{glasses}} = 100 / D = 100 / 10 = 10\,\text{cm}$$

Since we are going from glasses to contact lenses, we have to subtract the vertex distance:

$$f_{CTL} = f_{\text{glasses}} - \text{vertex distance}$$

$$f_{CTL} = 10\,\text{cm} - 1\,\text{cm} = 9\,\text{cm}$$

$$P_{CTL} = 100 / 9 = +11.1\text{D}$$

Therefore, we will need to order +11D contact lenses (Answer Choice D).

[2]See Chap. 21, Clinical Problems with Optics and Refractive Manifestations for more information on latent hyperopia

[3]Knowledge of the vertex distance is also helpful surgically. For example, the ASCRS IOL Calculator for Eyes with Prior Myopic LASIK/PRK requires information about the pre-LASIK/PRK vertex distance to improve accuracy in some of the generated formulas. If the vertex distance is unknown, the calculator defaults to 12.5 mm. Of course, this information is not absolutely necessary for this calculator as other formulas, such as the Barrett True-K No History Method, can generate relatively accurate predictions without this information. We point this out to merely emphasize how vertex distance affects our daily practice as ophthalmologists. See https://iolcalc.ascrs.org/wbfrmCalculator.aspx

[4]See Chap. 16 Construction of Glasses: Ophthalmologists as Opticians for more information.

Example #2

What power eyeglasses are needed for a patient who wears −8D contact lenses? Assume a vertex distance of 14 mm.

A. −7.50D
B. −8.00D
C. −8.50D
D. −8.75D
E. −9.00D

Answer: E. Again, suppose we are given this problem on an exam, and we forget everything we have previously discussed. Since we are dealing with minus-power lenses, the further we move the lens away from the eye, we will need more minus power to maintain the effective −8D of correction. Therefore, we can safely eliminate answer choices A and B.

Now for the actual math here. Since we are going from contact lenses to glasses, we have to add the vertex distance, making sure that we maintain the signed values at all times:

$$f_{CTL} = 100 / -8 = -12.5\,\text{cm}$$

$$f_{\text{glasses}} = f_{CTL} + \text{vertex distance}$$

$$f_{\text{glasses}} = -12.5\,\text{cm} + 1.4\,\text{cm} = -11.1\,\text{cm}$$

$$P_{\text{glasses}} = 100 / -11.1\ \text{cm} \approx -9\text{D}$$

Example #3

Suppose a +4D hyperope is given a +3D lens. How far in front of the eye must she hold it to see clearly at distance?

Answer:

This question is a repackaging of the concepts we have discussed thus far: all we have to do is figure out the focal lengths of the eye and the lens so that this +3D lens can "behave" like a +4D lens

$$f_{\text{lens}} = 100 / 3 = 33\,\text{cm}$$

$$f_{\text{eye}} = 100 / 4 = 25\,\text{cm}$$

Now we have to match up the focal distances:

$$\text{Vertex distance} = 33\,\text{cm} - 25\,\text{cm} = 8\,\text{cm in front of the eye}$$

Practice Questions

1. Suppose Pinocchio is a myope who is fully corrected with −8D glasses at a vertex distance of 15 mm. If he were to start telling lies again such that his vertex distance became 25 mm, what is the power of the new glasses needed?
2. Given the same problem above, what if the vertex distance was changed to 5 mm? What is the power of the new glasses?
3. Given the same problem above, what if we wanted to prescribe him contact lenses (i.e., the vertex distance became zero)?
4. Suppose Pinocchio is now a hyperope fully corrected with +10D glasses with a vertex distance of 10 mm. What power eyeglasses are needed if the vertex distance is changed to 20 mm?
5. Given the same problem above, what if the vertex distance was changed to 5 mm? What is the power of the new glasses?
6. Given the same problem above, what if we wanted to prescribe him contact lenses (i.e., the vertex distance became zero)?
7. What power contact lenses are needed for a patient who wears +12.5D glasses with a vertex distance of 13 mm?
8. What power contact lenses are needed for a patient who wears −6D glasses with a vertex distance of 16 mm?
9. Suppose a patient is fully corrected for her refractive error with a +7D lens with a 10 mm vertex distance; how far in front of the previous location of the +7D lens should a +5D lens be placed in order to fully correct her refractive error?

Answers

1. Basically, we have to figure out how the change in vertex distance will affect the power of the lens that is needed. We can draw this out as shown in Fig. 5.

   Before he started telling lies, Pinocchio's far point of the eye was (Fig. 5a)

   $$\text{Myopic Far Point} = f_{\text{glasses}} + \text{vertex distance} = (100/8) + 1.5 = 12.5 + 1.5 = 14\,\text{cm}$$

   Now we basically need to find the focal length of the new glasses: 14 cm – 2.5 cm = 11.5 cm (Fig. 5b).

$$\text{Power of the new glasses}: 100 / 11.5 \approx -8.7\text{D}$$ (−8.75D glasses since glasses can only be made in 0.25D steps)

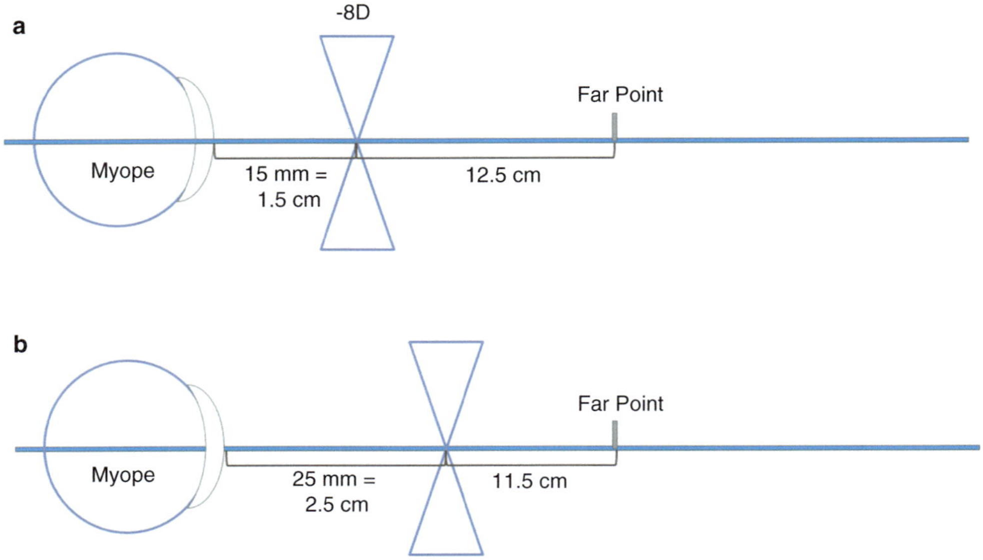

Fig. 5 Figure for Practice Problem #1. Calculation of eyeglass power needed with increased vertex distance for myope. Figure 5a displays the power of the eyeglasses (-8D) with 15 mm vertex distance. Figure 5b displays the new vertex distance (25 mm) that can be used to calculate the power of the new glasses

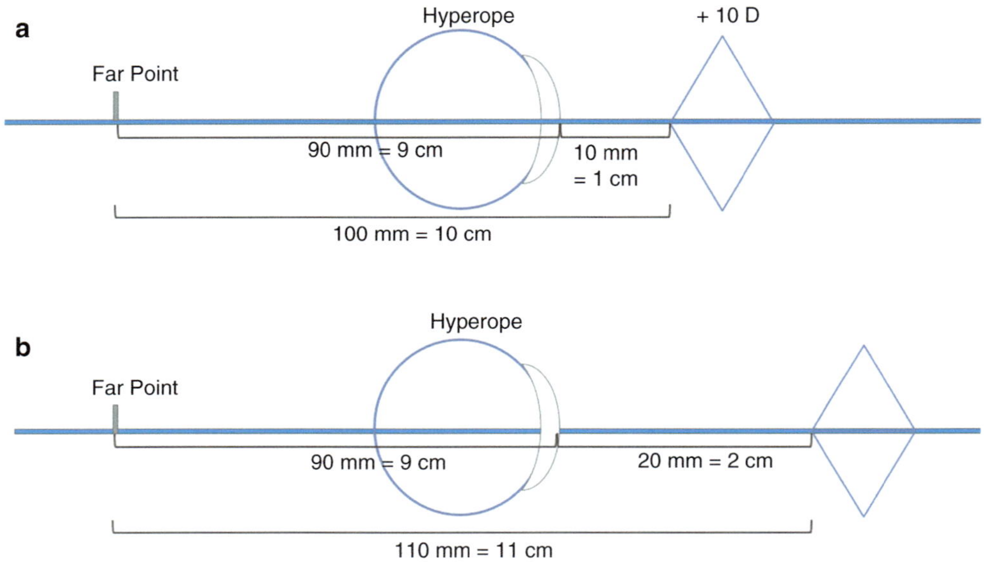

Fig. 6 Figure for Practice Problem #4. Calculation of eyeglass power needed with increased vertex distance for hyperope. Figure 6a displays the far point of the eye as determined by the +10D eyeglasses and 10mm vertex distance. Figure 6b displays the new vertex distance (20 mm) that can be used to calculate the power of the new glasses

2. We can modify our calculations from the previous problem to find the new focal length of the glasses: 14 cm – 0.5 cm = 13.5 cm.

$$\text{Power of the new glasses}: 100/13.5 = -7.41\text{D} \left(\approx 7.5\text{D}\right)$$

3. Now we simply have to take the focal length (14 cm) and find the power of the contact lens:

$$\text{Power of the contact lens}: \\ 100/14 = 7.14\text{D} \approx -7\text{D contact lens}$$

Notice that in problems 2 and 3, as we moved the glasses closer to the eye (until it became a contact lens), the "minus" power of the glasses continued to decrease (i.e., became more plus) in line with our "CAP" mnemonic.

4. Since we are dealing with a hyperope, we need to account for the far point being "behind" the eye (Fig. 6a).

$$\text{Hyperopic Far Point} = f_{\text{glasses}} - \text{vertex distance} \\ = \left(100/10\right) - 1\,\text{cm} = 10 - 1 = 9\,\text{cm}$$

Now we need to basically find the focal length of the new glasses: 9 cm + 2 cm = 11 cm (Fig. 6b).

$$\text{Power of the new glasses}: 100/11 \approx +9\text{D}$$

5. We can modify our calculations from the previous problem to find the new focal length of the glasses: 9 cm + 0.5 cm = 9.5 cm.

Power of the new glasses: 100/9.5 = +10.5D. Again, this makes sense as it follows our "CAP" mnemonic. We will need stronger "plus" power in the eyeglasses as we move them closer to Pinocchio's eyes.

6. Now we simply have to take the focal length (9 cm) and find the power of the contact lens:

$$\text{Power of the contact lens}: 100/9 = +11\text{D}$$

7. We can start off again by locating the far point of the eye. In this case, 100/12.5 = 8 cm or 80 mm behind the eye (since we are dealing with a hyperope). This also takes into account our 13 mm vertex distance (Fig. 7a).

   Now since we are going from glasses to contact lenses, we can *subtract* our vertex distance: 8 cm – 1.3 cm = 6.7 cm (or 67 mm).

   Now we can find the power of the contact lens using this "new" focal length: 100/6.7 = 14.92D (≈ +15D contact lens) (Fig. 7b).

8. We can start off by locating the focal length of the glasses (Fig. 8a):

$$f_{\text{glasses}} = 100/D = 100/-6 = -16.6\,\text{cm}$$

   Since we are going from glasses to contact lenses, we have to subtract the vertex distance, making sure we maintain the signed values (Fig. 8b):

$$f_{CTL} = f_{\text{glasses}} - \text{vertex distance}$$

$$f_{CTL} = -16.6\,\text{cm} - 1.6\,\text{cm} = -18.2\,\text{cm}$$

   $P_{\text{CTL}} = 100/-18.2 = -5.5\text{D}$. Again, this follows our previous examples with minus-power contact lenses and glasses because our contact lens power is "more plus"

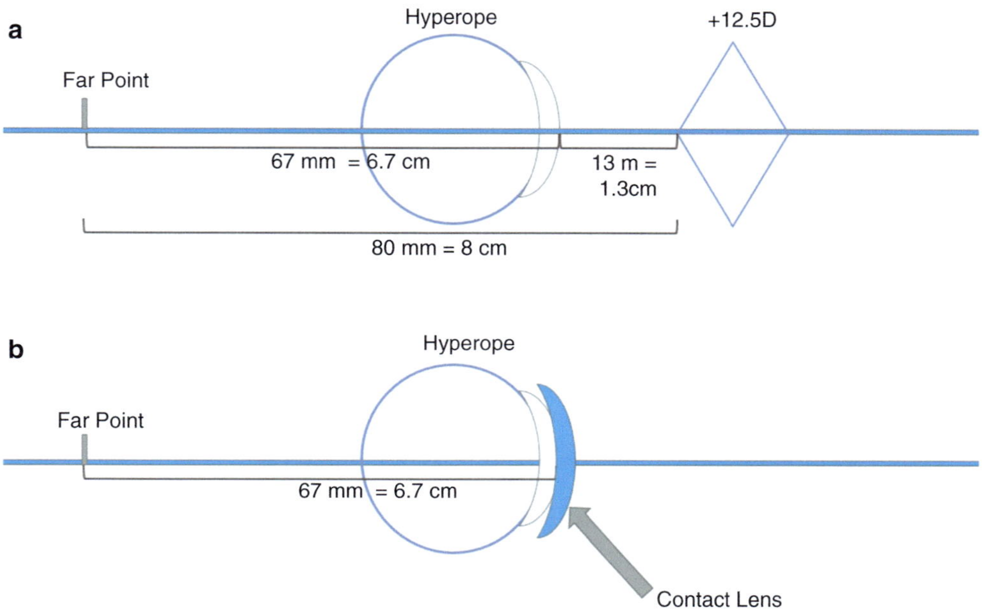

Fig. 7 Figure for Practice Problem #7. Figure 7a displays how using the +12.5D glasses and 13 mm vertex distance can be used to find the far point of the eye. Figure 7b shows the contact lens power can be calculated

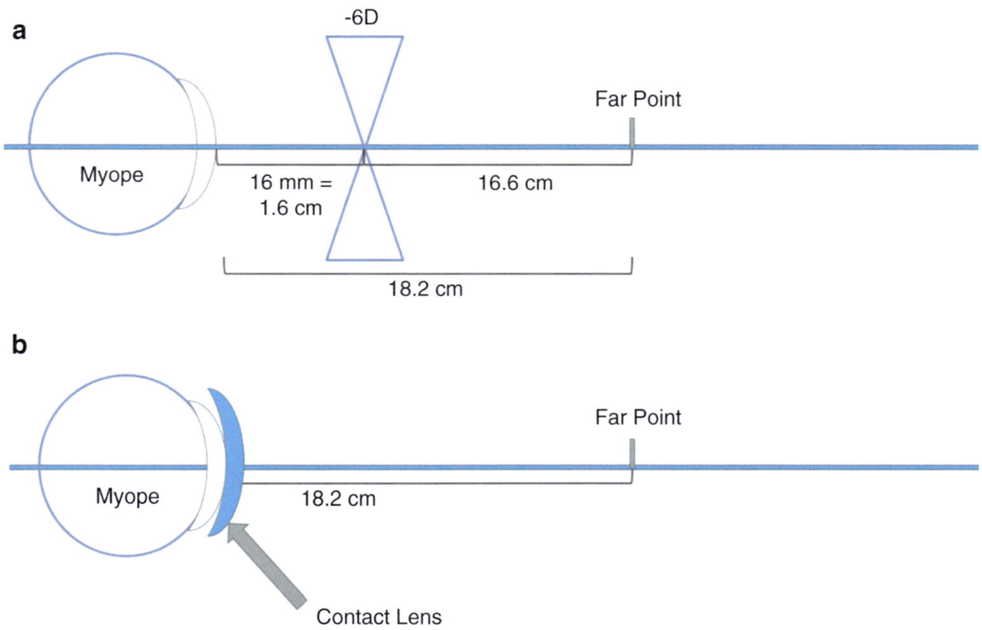

Fig. 8 Figure for Practice Problem #8. When given an eyeglass prescription power with vertex distance (Figure 8a), the contact lens power can be calculated (Figure 8b)

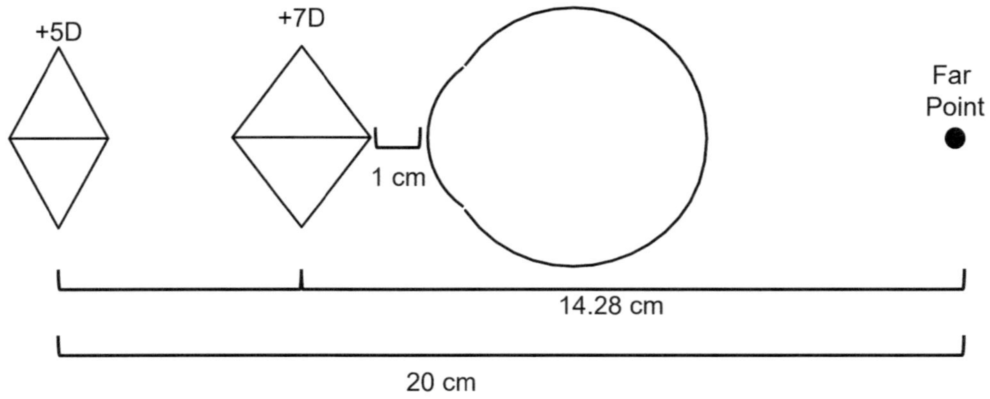

Fig. 9 Figure for Practice Problem #9. Calculation of vertex distance based on different spherical lens power

(i.e., less minus power) than our eyeglass prescription.

9. We can start by first finding the far point for this patient. We can ignore the vertex distance because the question does not ask how far from the cornea we have to place the new +4D lens, but rather how far from the original +7D lens.

Far point: 100/7 = 14.28 cm from the lens behind the eye (Fig. 9).

Next, we need to find the far point for a + 5D lens: 100/5 = 20 cm.

Finally, we can subtract these two numbers: 20–14.28 = 5.72 cm in front of where the +7D used to be, aka 6.72 cm in front of the cornea.

Schematic Eye

Daniel Wee

Objectives
- To understand the history of Gullstrand's model eye
- To understand how the Reduced Schematic Eye is used to calculate problems that test this concept on written exams

Introduction

The schematic eye ("Reduced Schematic Eye" (RSE)) is a topic that seems intimidating and confusing, but it is actually a simplified model of an eye used in ophthalmic optics. The official definition is that the RSE is a model that represents the basic optical features of a real eye. This allows us to create ray tracings to determine sizes of retinal lesions, scotomas, or blind spots. In our case, it is a simple geometry math problem using two congruent triangles that is a common question on written exams.

Some useless information that will likely never show up on exams: the schematic eye was invented by Dr. Allvar Gullstrand (1862–1930), a Swedish ophthalmologist who developed the model eye to better study refraction and optical images in the eye. Fascinatingly enough, he self-taught himself geometric and physiological optics! He was awarded the Nobel Prize in Physiology or Medicine in 1911 (must have been a slow year) for his work.[1] Fun fact: he remains the only ophthalmologist to ever receive the Nobel Prize. Tragically, Dr. Charles Kellman, the inventor of phacoemulsification technology, never received a Nobel Prize. While the good Dr. Kellman's legacy remains inventing a device that has restored vision to millions of people worldwide, the good Dr. Gullstrand's legacy remains inventing a (inaccurate) model of the eye that is required learning for ophthalmology trainees worldwide.

[1] "Allvar Gullstrand Biographical". https://www.nobelprize.org/prizes/medicine/1911/gullstrand/biographical/. Accessed December 22, 2019.

Model of the Reduced Schematic Eye

The RSE relies upon certain assumptions to simplify the optical properties of the human eye (Fig. 1). It should be noted that in modern optics, especially for cataract and refractive surgery, many of the assumptions of the RSE are inaccurate and have since been replaced with other models and principles. Nonetheless, the RSE remains a useful starting foundation to later study these advanced topics.

- The RSE assumes that the eye only has a single refractive point (n, the nodal point) that combines the cornea, aqueous, and lens into a simplified refractive location.
- Another assumption is that the only two indices of refraction are air ($n = 1.00$) and water/aqueous ($n = 1.33$).[2]
- The refractive power of the eye is +60D.
- The anterior focal point is 17 mm (determined by $F = 1/60 = 16.7$ mm ≈ 17 mm) in front of the cornea.
- The nodal point is 5.5 mm behind the cornea.
- The axial length of the eye is 22.5 mm.

As stated previously, the nodal point (n) is simply a fancy term used for the point in the eye where all light rays entering or leaving the eye do not deviate (Fig. 2). We can see how incoming light rays, regardless of their incoming angle, will pass through the nodal point as if the cornea did not exist (Fig. 2).

For the purposes of exams, just think of the nodal point as the part of the eye that allows us to draw two triangles to get our correct answer. The more important number to remember is the distance from the nodal point to the retina (F'), which is 17 mm. This number has to be memorized because

[2] The index of refraction of the cornea is closer to 1.376; aqueous is 1.336; crystalline lens is 1.386–1.406 (outer-inner layers); and vitreous is 1.337.

D. Wee (✉)
Center for Sight, Stockton, CA, USA

K. M. Riaz et al. (eds.), *Optics for the New Millennium*, https://doi.org/10.1007/978-3-030-95251-8_7

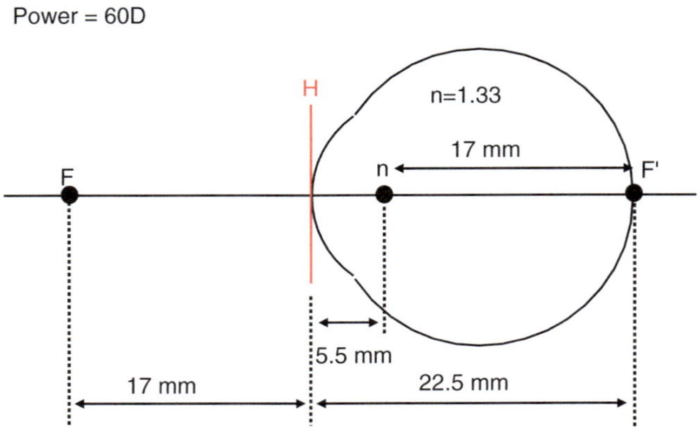

Fig. 1 The Reduced Schematic Eye (RSE). Note that the nodal point (*n*) that is used for ray tracing is located inside the eye. Also note that the distance from the nodal point to F′ is 17 mm. This number must be committed to memory

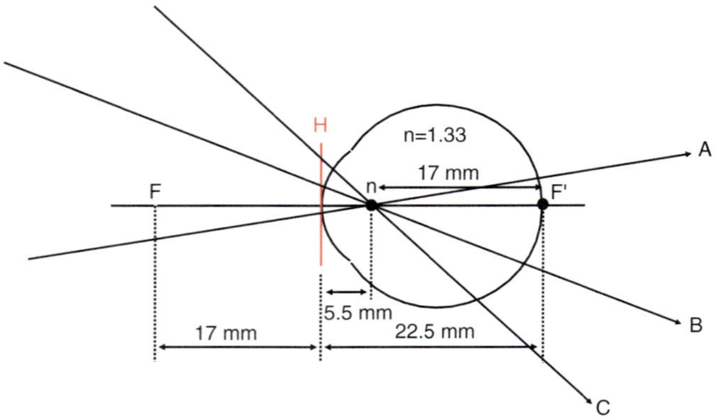

Fig. 2 Incoming light rays (A, B, and C) will all pass through the nodal point (*n*) as undeviated light rays as if the cornea did not exist

it will never be given to you on the exam! If you can remember 17 mm, it is a simple geometry problem.[3] It is also worth noting that the distance from the cornea to the nodal point is 5.5 mm as that may come up in test questions as well.

For most RSE problems, we can safely ignore the 5.5 mm as the distance of the target from the eye is usually in meters; therefore, the 5.5 mm does not contribute much to the distance. For example, if the question states that the tangent screen is located 4 meters away, then the true distance from the nodal point is 4005.5 mm, but using 4000 mm is "close enough" and makes the math easier. However, for problems wherein the target is much closer to the eye (e.g., an ophthalmoscope held "*x*" cm from the eye), then 5.5 mm may need to be taken into account.

[3]A useful mnemonic here is to remember that the chromosome for the NF-1 gene in neurofibromatosis is located on chromosome 17. How does this help you may ask? It is highly likely that you remember "chromosome 17" from way back in medical school days, so that number 17 is somewhere in your brain. So you can now apply that useful number to optics (or you can use this optics moment to remember a useful chromosome number that may come up on exams!).

Ray Tracing with the Reduced Schematic Eye

We can use our RSE model to create another model using our knowledge of undeviated light rays, the nodal point, and this magical number of 17 mm to create a simplified model comparing two congruent triangles (Fig. 3).

Notice that we have eliminated the anterior focal point as well as the distance from the nodal point to the cornea (5.5 mm).

When comparing similar triangles, it is vital that we compare **similar** parts of the triangle. In other words, how we set up the comparison ratio is extremely important because if we end up comparing the height of one triangle to the base of the other triangle, it will lead to some very difficult math – and more importantly, the wrong answer. We can be reasonably certain that one of the wrong answer choices given on exams will be a calculation obtained by simply setting up the comparison ratio wrong!

#Protip: If you have started your calculations and encounter some strange, disgusting numbers, then you may want to stop and ask yourself if you have plugged in the numbers correctly.

Therefore, set up the calculations as either:

Choice #1 (Math will usually be easier) - Compare the height and base of one triangle to the height and base of the other triangle:

$$\text{Height}_1 / \text{Base}_1 = \text{Height}_2 / \text{Base}_2$$

Choice #2 (Also possible, but math may be trickier) – Compare the height of one triangle with the height of the other triangle and compare that to the base of one triangle with the base of the other triangle:

$$\text{Height}_1 / \text{Height}_2 = \text{Base}_1 / \text{Base}_2$$

Using this construct, test questions will basically ask us to determine one of the missing components in this comparison ratio by giving us two numbers; the third number is always 17 mm!

The other thing to keep in mind is that it will make things easier to use **millimeters** as our preferred unit of measurement. Again, recall that 17 mm (Neurofibromatosis I chromosome!) is already in millimeter notation, so it will help to convert the other numbers that will be given to us into millimeter notation to keep our calculations consistent. Finally, pay attention to the answer choices as they may be given in millimeter, centimeter or even meter notation.

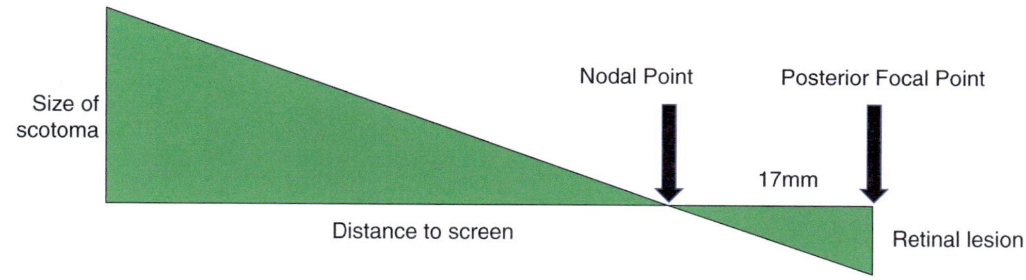

Fig. 3 The RSE can be further simplified into a geometry problem comparing two similar triangles using the nodal point and its distance to the posterior focal point (17 mm)

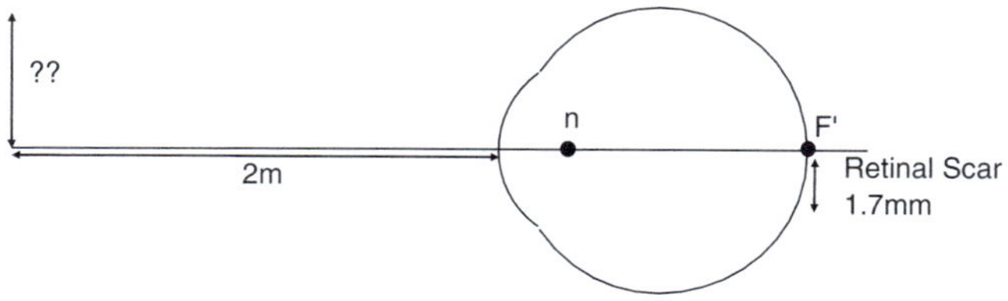

Fig. 4 First figure for practice question 1: What is the size of a scotoma measured 2 m away from the eye caused by a 1.7 mm retinal scar?

Practice Questions

1. What is the size of a scotoma measured 2 m away from the eye caused by a 1.7 mm retinal scar (Fig. 4)?
2. What is the size of a retinal hemorrhage causing a 30 cm scotoma on a screen when measured 1 m from the eye?
3. A 3.4 mm retinal scar causes a 40 cm scotoma on a screen. How far is the screen from the eye?
4. A patient has a macular lesion of unknown size that corresponds to a blind spot of 2.5 cm when viewed at a screen placed 0.1 m away. How big is the macular lesion?
   A. 4.25 mm
   B. 0.425 mm
   C. 4.25 cm
   D. 42.5 mm
5. How far away must a tangent screen be placed from a patient who has a 1 mm scotoma to manifest 150 times its size?
6. Using the model eye, calculate the size of the image formed by a 3 mm retinoscope pinhole on the patient's retina if the scope is held 51 cm from the nodal point of the patient's eye.
7. Using the RSE as a model, suppose we are told that the location of the second principal plane is 1.6 mm behind the anterior corneal surface. If a patient views an object at infinity, how far away from the anterior corneal surface will the image be formed?
8. What is the size of a 2.55 mm retinal hemorrhage if viewed by an emmetropic examiner using an ophthalmoscope held 2 cm from the patient's eye?

Answers

1. Remember, the 17 mm distance from the nodal point to the retina is not going to be given to you.

   Let us set this up as two congruent triangles and convert 2 mm to 2000 mm. We can redraw the figure as a comparison of two similar triangles (Fig. 5).

   $$\text{Height}_1(Y)/\text{Base}_1 = \text{Height}_2/\text{Base}_2$$

   $$Y/2000\,\text{mm} = 1.7\,\text{mm}/17\,\text{mm}$$
   $$Y/2000\,\text{mm} = 0.1\,\text{mm}$$

   The scotoma is 200 mm or 20 cm or 0.2 m (depending on what units the answer choices may have) in size.
2. We can go ahead and set up our congruent triangles, taking care to place the given numbers in their appropriate locations.

   Now we can go ahead and plug in the numbers accordingly. This is little trickier because we have units in m, cm, and mm. Let us make the problem a little easier by converting all the units to mm, as seen in Fig. 6.

   $$Y/17\,\text{mm} = 300\,\text{mm}/1000\,\text{mm}$$
   $$Y/17\,\text{mm} = 0.3\ \text{mm}$$
   $$Y = (0.3\,\text{mm})(17\,\text{mm})$$
   $$Y = 5.1\,\text{mm}$$

   The retinal hemorrhage is 5.1 mm in diameter.
3. By now, we should be in a bit of a rhythm, setting up our familiar congruent triangles (Fig. 7).

   $$\text{Height}_1/\text{Base}_1 = \text{Height}_2/\text{Base}_2$$

   This time we are solving for *X*. Let us convert the 40 cm to 400 mm.

   $$400\ \text{mm}/\text{x} = 3.4\,\text{mm}/17\,\text{mm}$$
   $$400\,\text{mm}/\text{x} = 0.2\,\text{mm}$$

   $X = 2000$ mm or 200 cm or 2 m in front of the eye.

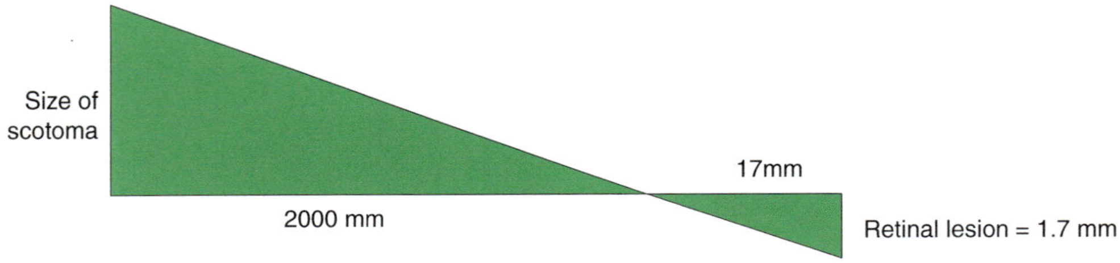

Fig. 5 Second figure for practice question 1: Note the use of a similar triangles schematic to solve for the size of the scotoma

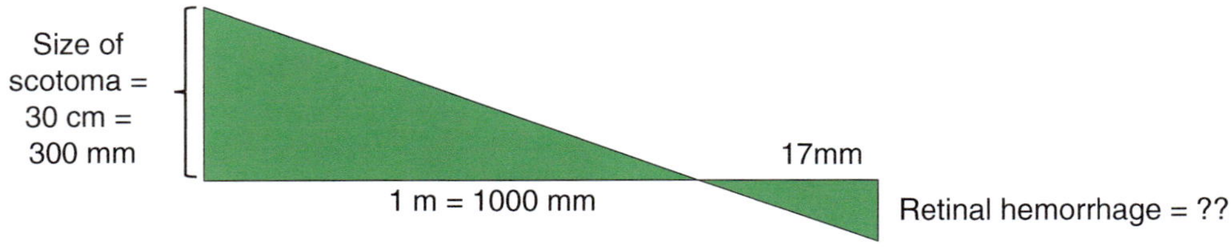

Fig. 6 First figure for practice question 2: What is the size of a retinal hemorrhage causing a 30 cm scotoma on a screen when measured 1 m from the eye?

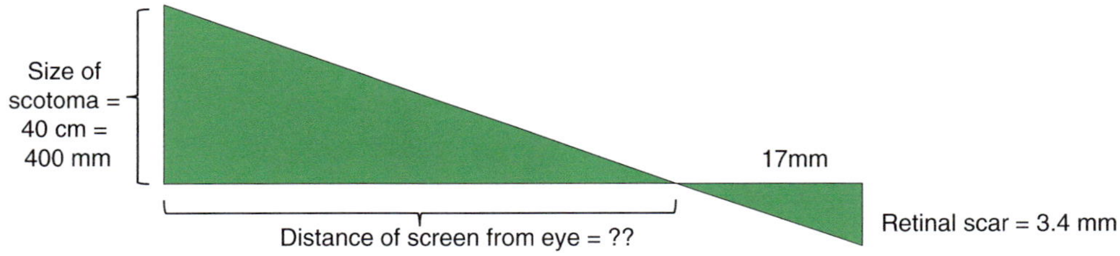

Fig. 7 The similar triangles schematic can again be used to solve for the unknown variable: the distance of the screen from the eye

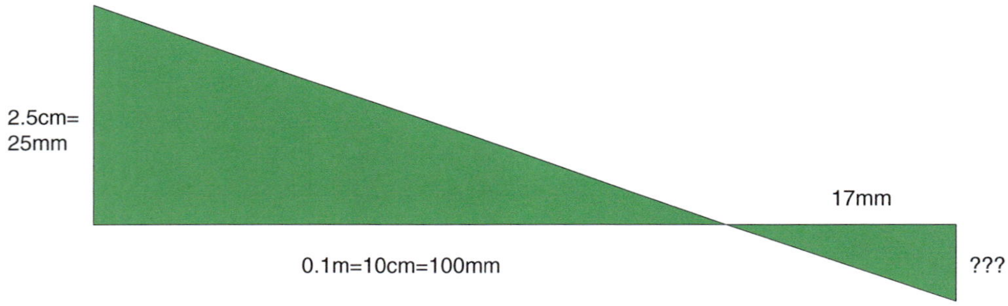

Fig. 8 The similar triangles schematic can again be used to solve for the unknown variable: the size of the macular lesion

4. A. This is a great example of a problem where the given units are all different (note the centimeter and meter notation in the stem). On an exam, one may be short pressed on time so we can see how easy it is to make a mistake in the calculations. This is why developing a habit to work in the same unit will make our calculations easier.

   Again, start by converting everything to millimeter notation and drawing out the congruent triangle diagram (Fig. 8).

$$\text{Height}_1 / \text{Base}_1 = \text{Height}_2 / \text{Base}_2$$

$$X / 17\,\text{mm} = 25\,\text{mm} / 100\,\text{mm}$$
$$X / 17\,\text{mm} = 1/4\,\text{mm}$$
$$X = 4.25\,\text{mm}$$

5. This is a convoluted way of asking the same concept we have been doing thus far.

   We can again set up our schematic eye equation as:

$$\text{Height}_1 / \text{Base}_1 = \text{Height}_2 / \text{Base}_2$$

   We basically have to solve for Base_2:

$$1\,\text{mm} / 17\,\text{mm} = 150\,\text{mm} / \text{x}$$
$$\text{x} = 2550\,\text{mm} = 2.55\,\text{meters away}$$

6. Start off by converting all the units to mm notation and draw out our familiar similar triangles diagram (Fig. 9).

$$\text{Height}_1 / \text{Base}_1 = \text{Height}_2 / \text{Base}_2$$

   This time we are solving for × (Height_2)

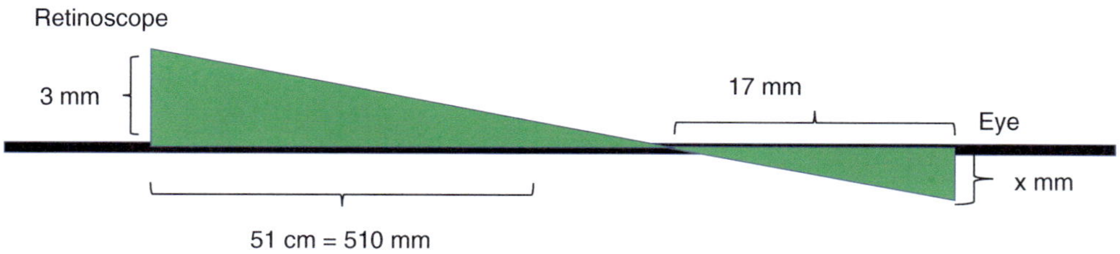

Fig. 9 The similar triangles schematic can again be used to solve for the unknown variable: the size of the 3 mm retinoscope pinhole cast onto the patient's retina when held 51 cm from the nodal point of the patient's eye

$$x(\text{Height2}) = (\text{Height}_1 / \text{Base}_1)(\text{Base}_2)$$
$$= (3/510) * (17) = 51/510 = 0.1\,\text{mm}$$

Note: we could have used 515.5 mm in place of 510 mm if we wanted to be more accurate as to the "true" distance of the ophthalmoscope from the nodal point. This would incur a slightly more difficult calculation:

$$\text{Height}_1 / \text{Base}_1 = \text{Height}_2 / \text{Base}_2$$

This time we are solving for (Height_2)

$$(\text{Height2}) = (\text{Height}_1 / \text{Base}_1)(\text{Base}_2)$$
$$= (3/515.5) * (17) = 0.0989\,\text{mm}$$

Notice that this answer is essentially the same as 0.1 mm.

7. This is a bit of a tricky problem that requires us to combine our knowledge of the RSE along with our old friend $U + D = V$. We know that the object is at infinity, so we can set $U = 0$. We also know that the index of refraction of vitreous is 1.336. This gives us:

$$U + D = V$$
$$0 + 60 = V = 60$$

$V = 1.336/v$, as we have to account for the new index of refraction.

Thus, $v = 1.336/60 = 0.0223$ m or 22.3 mm.

Now we can add: 1.6 mm + 22.3 mm = 23.9 mm behind the anterior corneal surface, which is "close" to the typical axial length of an average (emmetropic) eye.

8. This is a similar problem to the ones that we have done before. The one caveat is because the ophthalmoscope is held relatively close to the patient's eye; we have to factor in the 5.5 mm distance between the anterior cornea and the nodal point.

We can again set up our schematic eye equation as:

$$\text{Height}_1 / \text{Base}_1 = \text{Height}_2 / \text{Base}_2$$

We basically have to solve for Height_2; however, Base_2 cannot simply be 20 mm. We have to factor in the 5.5 mm and use 25.5 mm instead.

Now we can solve: $\text{Height}_2 = (\text{Height}_1 / \text{Base}_1) * \text{Base}_2 = (2.55/17) * (25.5) = 3.825$ mm.

Had we not factored in the 5.5 mm, we would have instead gotten:

$$\text{Height}_2 = (\text{Height}_1 / \text{Base}_1) * \text{Base}_2 = (2.55/17) * (20) = 3.0\,\text{mm}$$

Notice that this 0.825 mm difference is significant because we are working in much smaller distances as compared to the tangent screen problems previously.

Magnification and Telescopes

G. Vike Vicente

Objectives

- To define, understand, and calculate the various kinds of magnification (transverse[linear], axial, and angular)
- To define and understand how the two main types of telescopes (Astronomical [Keplerian] and Galilean) work
- To appreciate clinical relevance of magnification of telescopes in clinical and surgical practice

Introduction

Ahoy Optics mateys! To help make this chapter easier to understand and remember, we will periodically slip into a "pirate voice" so that the image of a pirate using a telescope will help us conceptualize some important concepts and examples. If a German spectacle maker in the seventeenth century can understand telescopes, so can you! (see Hans Lippershey).[1]

Argg! Here we go.

Telescopes work by combining a series of lenses or curved mirrors to improve and enlarge our visualization of distant objects. Therefore, to understand telescopes we first need to understand magnification. There are four types of magnification we will discuss: Transverse Magnification (aka Linear Magnification), Axial Magnification (aka Longitudinal Magnification), Angular Magnification, and Magnification from a Simple Magnifier.

After discussing magnification, we will then discuss the two main types of telescopes, as well as their clinical, surgical, and testable relevance: Astronomical (Keplerian) & Galilean. Just like pirates, we ophthalmologists are surrounded by telescopes in our daily practices.

Magnification

Transverse Magnification

Transverse magnification (aka linear magnification) is similar to the magnification we discussed when doing lens and mirror systems.[2] We have previously introduced this formula, $M = U/V = v/u$ ("big MOVIE, little view" mnemonic), when discussing object-lens-mirror systems.[3] Recall that we can use either the sizes or the distances between the object and the image to calculate the magnification.

To continue this discussion, we can use similar triangles to give us more background to calculating transverse magnification.

Remember the bilge-sucking law of similar triangles, bucko? We can compare the height and the base of a given triangle with the height and the base of another similar triangle (Fig. 1).

$$\frac{X_1}{Y_1} = \frac{X_2}{Y_2}$$

Suppose we wanted to calculate the height of the image (X_2), we can simply rearrange the above equation as: $X_2 = (X_1{}^*Y_2)/Y_1$

[1] Hans Lippershey. https://en.wikipedia.org/wiki/Hans_Lippershey. Accessed March 27, 2021.

[2] Technically, linear magnification refers to the magnification of the area of an image relative to the area of an object along an optical axis. We have thus far only addressed the height of an object. But suppose we had an object that measured 3 cm ×5 cm with 2× transverse magnification. This would give us an object with dimensions of 6 cm × 10 cm. Therefore, the linear magnification would go from 15 cm² to 60 cm², a fourfold increase in image area. To keep things simple for the purposes of ophthalmic optics, we will consider transverse magnification and linear magnification to be the same thing.

[3] See Chaps. 3 and 4, if you need to review this.

G. V. Vicente (✉)
Clinical Pediatrics and Ophthalmology Georgetown University Hospital, Washington, DC, USA

Eye Doctors of Washington, Chevy Chase, MD, USA
e-mail: vvicente@edow.com

K. M. Riaz et al. (eds.), *Optics for the New Millennium*, https://doi.org/10.1007/978-3-030-95251-8_8

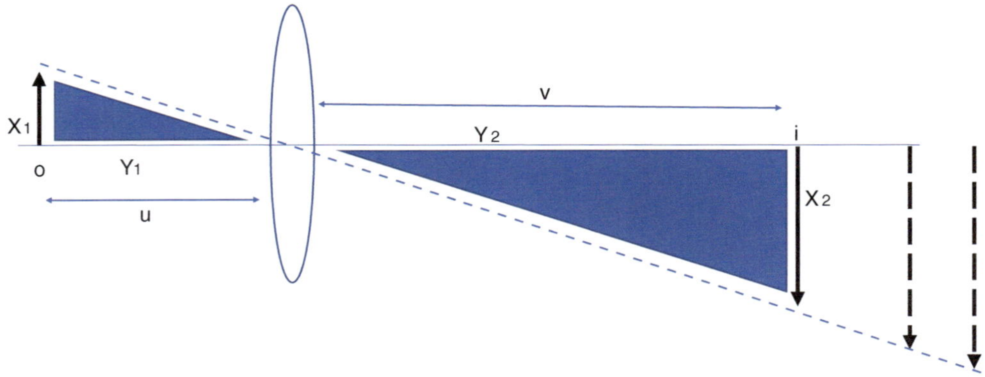

Fig. 1 Using the law of similar triangles, we can use object/image height OR object/image distance from the lens to calculate more information about the lens system, including information about magnification

The vertical height difference between the object (X_1) and the image (X_2) (i.e., the transverse magnification) will be proportional to the distance between the object (u) and the image (v) from the lens. Notice how a larger (v) or Y_2 will give a larger image, as seen in the dashed arrows to the right. We can use this relationship between the **SIZES** of the object and image to calculate transverse magnification.

Similarly, if we know the **DISTANCES** of the lens to an object (u) and from the lens to an image (v), we can calculate the magnification by using the following formula:

$$\text{Transverse Mag} = \text{image distance} / \text{object distance} = v / u.$$

On exams, we may be asked to determine the transverse magnification of a lens system solely based on distances or sizes, without any information about the lens power. Let us do some examples that test this concept.

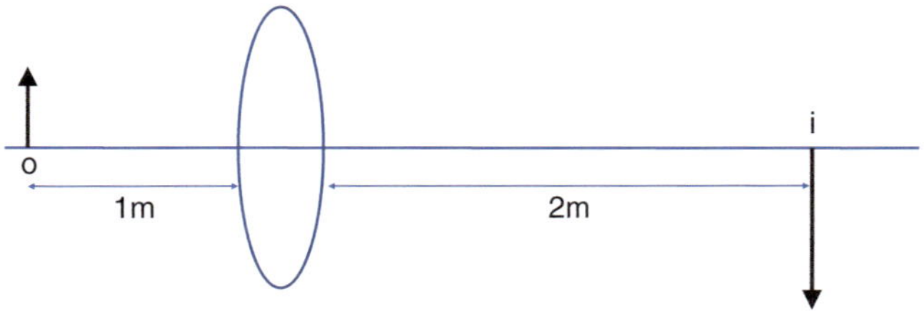

Fig. 2 What is the transverse magnification of an object 1 m away from a convex (+) lens, if the image is 2 m away?

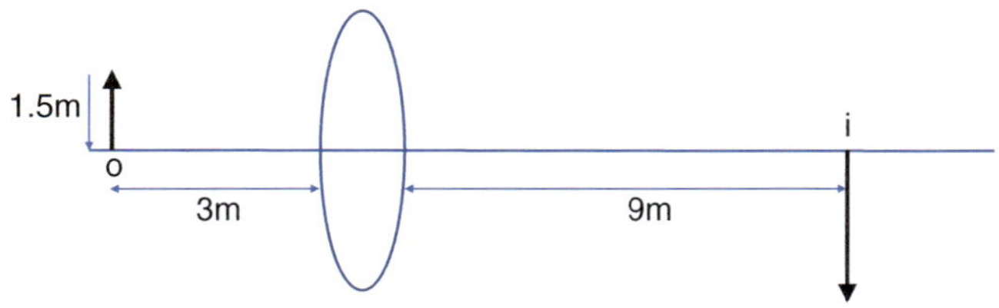

Fig. 3 If a 1.5 m tall object is 3 m from a lens, and the image is formed 9 m to the right of the lens, how large is the image?

Example #1 (Fig. 2)

Transverse Magnification = v/u = 2m/1m = 2×

Arrrg!!. See ye landlubbers, magnification is not that tough! Notice how we did not need any information about the object or image height in order to calculate the magnification. Similarly, if we are only given information about the object and image heights without any information about object and image distances, we can still calculate the magnification of the system.

Example #2 (Fig. 3)

Transverse Magnification = v/u = 9m/3m = 3×.

The image will be 3 × 1.5 m = 4.5 m tall.

Notice again that we did not need to know the power of the lens to solve this equation! Of note, we assumed this was a plus lens because the question stem stated that the image formed to the right of the lens.

Example #3 (Fig. 4)

First, we notice that since this is a concave lens system, the image will likely form to the LEFT of the lens. When we enter our distance values into our now-familiar equation:

Transverse Magnification = v/u = 0.5/1m = 0.5

Notice that if the absolute value of the *magnification is less than 1*, then the image will be *minified*. In this case, the image is 50% (1/2) size of the object.

Example #4

A 2-m tall object is 3 m away from a lens and the image is 1 m away. What is the size of the image?

$$\text{Transverse Magnification} = v / u = 1\text{m} / 3\text{m} = 0.33\times$$

The image will be 2 m x 0.33 = 0.66 m. Notice we did not draw the object, lens, and image in this example showing that you can solve these problems without drawing it out as well. Initially, it may help to draw them out if you are just getting your sea legs under you on this pirating adventure of telescopes in ophthalmology.

Example #5

Shiver me timbers, let us complicate things just a wee bit, shall we?

What if we have more than one lens (Fig. 5)?

In order to solve these two lens systems, we again will start off by ignoring the second lens and directing our attention to the first lens. We can first calculate the magnification of the first lens (Mag1), and then the magnification of the second lens (Mag2). The final magnification of this lens system will be the **PRODUCT** (not the sum!) of Mag1 * Mag2. This is a key point to remember for exam purposes because it is very likely that one of the wrong answer choices will be one that has the sum of Mag1 and Mag2, and picking that would be like dancing the hempen jig!

Start off by solving for the first lens (Fig. 6).

Applying the formulas $U = -1/u$ and $U + D = V$:

$$U = -1/0.166\text{m}\left(\text{OR} -100/16.6\right) = -6\text{D}.$$

$$U + D = -6\text{D} + 8\text{D} = +2\text{D} = V,\ v = 1/V = 1/2\left(\text{OR}\,100/2\right) = 0.5\,\text{m}\left(\text{or}\,50\,\text{cm}\right)$$

Magnification of first image = $U/V = 6/2 = 3\times$. (We could also use Mag = $v/u = 50/16.6$, which should give us the same answer with slightly more difficult math).

After having determined that the magnification from the first lens (Mag1) is 3×, we can now solve for the second lens (Fig. 7).

Applying the formulas $U = -1/u$ and $U + D = V$:

$$U = -1/0.1\text{m} = -10\text{D}.$$

$$U + D = -10\text{D} + 14\text{D} = +4\text{D} = V,\ v = 1/V = 1/4\text{D} = 0.25\text{m} = 25\,\text{cm}.$$

$$\text{Magnification of second image}\left(\text{Mag2}\right) = U/V = 10/4 = 2.5\times$$

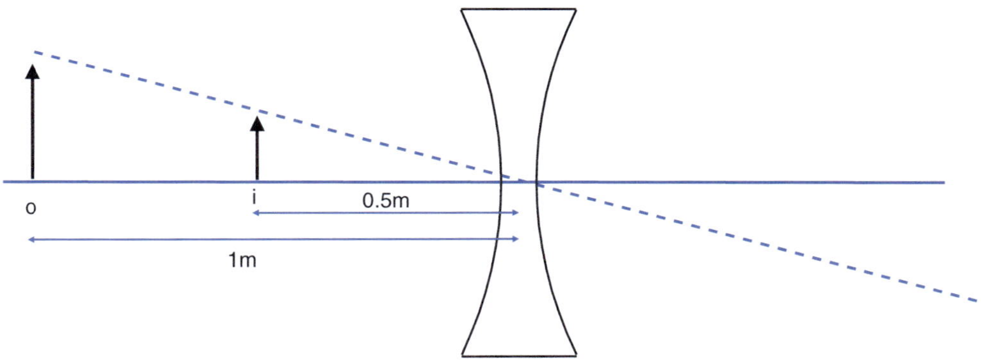

Fig. 4 What is the transverse magnification of an object 1 m away from a concave lens, if the image is 0.5 m from the lens?

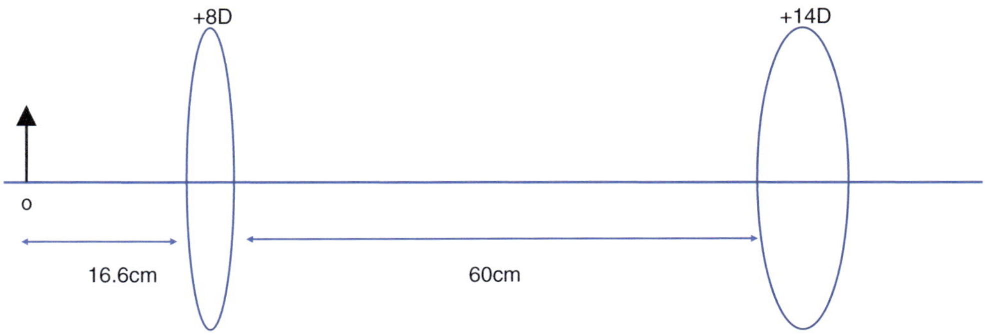

Fig. 5 What is the final image magnification of an object that is located 16.6 cm to the left of a + 8D lens, which itself is located 60 cm to the left of a + 14D lens?

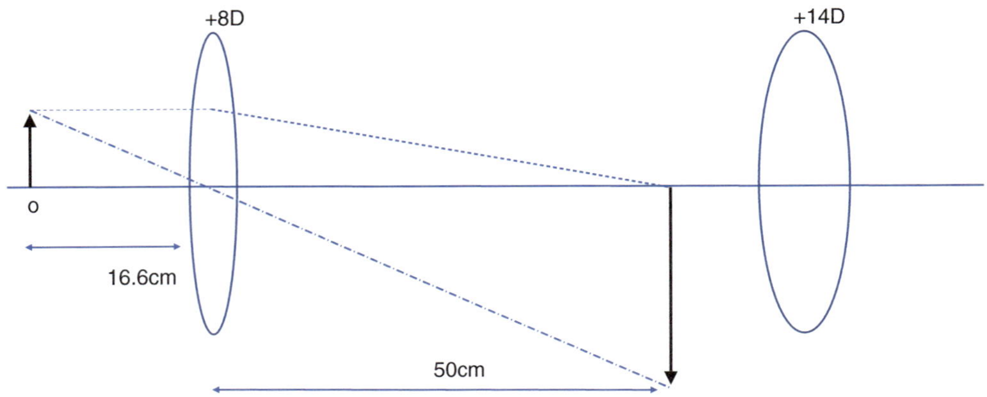

Fig. 6 An inverted image is formed 50 cm to the right of the first lens

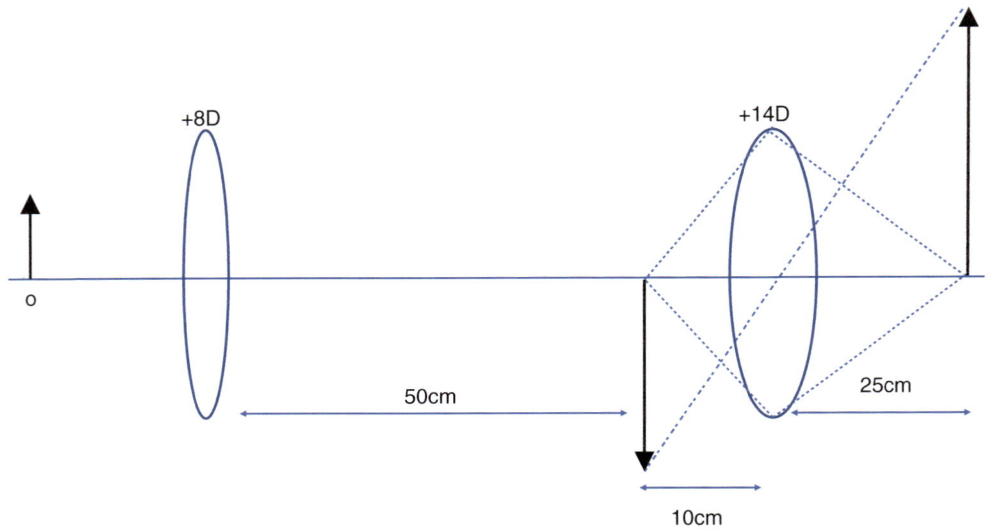

Fig. 7 An upright image is formed 25 cm to the right of the second lens

Since the first lens system has a transverse magnification of 3× (Mag1), and the second lens system has a transverse magnification of 2.5× (Mag2), the magnification of the final image compared to the original object will be the *product* of the Mag1 and Mag2: Mag1 × Mag 2 = 3 * 2.5 = 7.5× total magnification. Note that the sum of Mag1 and Mag 2 (5.5×) is not correct.

Suppose that the problem had stated that the object was 10 cm in size and we were asked to calculate the final size of the image, we would calculate the image size as 10 cm × 7.5× (total magnification) = 75 cm.

Axial Magnification (aka Longitudinal Magnification)

Now that we have discussed transverse magnification, we can bring a spring upon'er and move onto other types of magnification, such as Axial Magnification (also known as the armpit of optics).

Axial magnification describes the magnification along an axis **between two conjugate points**. Simply put, it is the change of depth along the axis; it is basically the square of transverse magnification:

$$M_{\text{axial}} = \left(M_{\text{transverse}}\right)^2$$

Why do we care about axial magnification? Blimey, because clinically, it will cause distortion of 3D images. For example, it can exaggerate the height of a retinal detachment viewed by indirect ophthalmoscopy. This helps offset the loss of some stereoacuity caused by the indirect ophthalmoscope's effect on pupillary distance (Fig. 8).

We can see how the math works here: if we assume a pupillary distance (PD) of the examiner to be 60 mm, when the examiner looks through the binocular eyepiece, the effective PD is reduced to 15 mm (Fig. 9), thereby reducing stereopsis by a factor of 4-fold (60/15). Our good matey, axial magnification of the aerial image compensates for this reduction.

For example, if we are using a 20D lens (and assume 60D as the power of the eye[4]), the transverse magnification will be:

[4]This is the power of the Reduced Schematic Eye. See Chap. 7, "Schematic Eye" for a review.

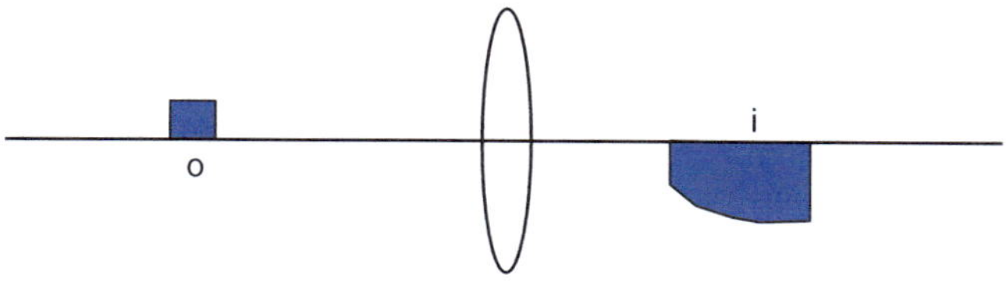

Fig. 8 The depth of the object is exaggerated by axial magnification

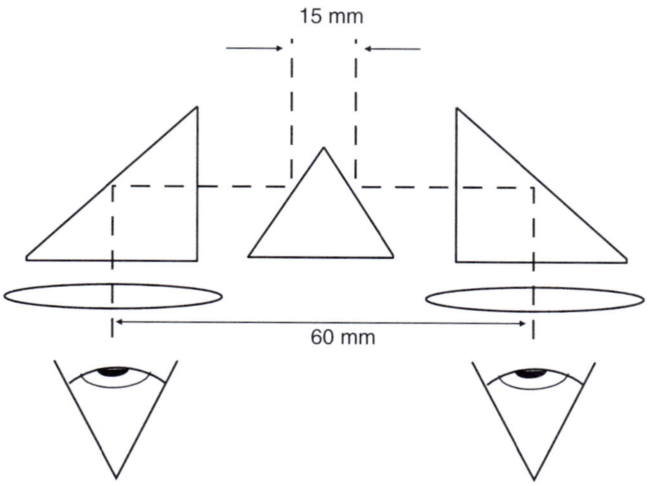

Fig. 9 Optics of an indirect ophthalmoscope. Notice how prisms are used to reduce the effective pupillary distance by a factor of approximately four

Transverse magnification = Power of eye / Power of lens = 60D/20D = 3× magnification

Now, we can calculate the axial magnification:

$$M_{\text{axial}} = \left(M_{\text{transverse}}\right)^2 = (3)^2 = 9 \times \text{magnification}$$

As stated above, the eyepieces will reduce the PD and therefore reduce the field of depth by a factor of 4×. Therefore, the final magnification will be 9×/4× = 2.25×. Therefore, the retinal detachment will be magnified by a factor of 2.25× when viewed through a 20D lens, thereby making it easier to see on clinical exam and detect the retinal detachment before our patient heads down to Davy Jones' locker!

Let us do one more example: suppose that an object is located at an unknown distance from an unknown lens and it forms an image to the right of the lens at a distance that is four times the distance of the object from the lens. What is the transverse magnification? What is the axial magnification?

At first glance, me hearties, we may wish to skip this treacherous island and move on to finding other treasures. But if we pause for a moment, we will realize that this problem is simply testing previously discussed concepts in a roundabout (and needlessly complicated) manner.

From the question stem, we can see that the image distance (v) from the lens is four times the distance of the object from the lens (u). This means that transverse magnification is 4×. Therefore, the axial magnification is $(4\times)^2$ = 16× magnification.

Angular Magnification

This type of magnification is used with objects and images located at infinity, such as scouring the horizon for friendly or enemy ships. Recall that an object at any distance will subtend a certain angle in the observer's visual field, even when viewed with the naked eye. In other words, it will occupy some portion of the observer's visual field (e.g., a few arcseconds or arcminutes), even though it may be very small. When looking at an object through an optical instrument, that object will also occupy some portion of the observer's visual field. Angular Magnification is simply the ratio of the image when seen with an optical instrument (e.g., telescope, microscope, etc.) to the image when not seen with an optical instrument. Recall that with any telescope, the vergence of incoming light rays is zero, and the vergence of light rays exiting the telescope is also zero.

Although the distances and sizes may be infinitely large and hard to measure, they have a finite angular size; thus, angular magnification relies on angles not distances.

Angular Magnification = $\theta_{\text{out}}/\theta_{\text{in}}$, where θ_{out} is the angle formed with the telescope and θ_{in} is the angle formed without the telescope.

Why bother with angular magnification? Why not just use transverse magnification and keep life simple? The problem is that transverse magnification is only applicable when lenses produce real images; when we use an optical instrument with eyepiece (such as a microscope, telescope, etc.), we are actually viewing virtual images without true "linear dimensions"; thus, we have to rely on angular magnification as a workaround. Furthermore, transverse magnification will only give us a small percentage of the size of the object (i.e., minification), whereas angular magnification will give us true magnification.

For example, suppose we told our coxswain to go up the crow's nest to look at the moon to calculate our location in the ocean. When he looks up at the moon with the naked eye, it subtends an angle of approximately 0.5°. When he uses his binoculars (we are modern pirates, after all), the moon will appear to subtend an angle of 5°. Therefore the angular magnification is 5/0.5 = 10× magnification, meaning that the image of the moon formed on the retina when looking through the binoculars is ten times larger than the image of the moon formed on the retina when looking with the naked eye.

Here is another example: suppose that we now tell our trusty coxswain (who is still up in the crow's nest) to look for neighboring ships on the horizon. He sees a ship off in the distance but does not know how far away this ship is, not to mention whether this is a friendly or enemy ship. Suppose that he only had a + 2D lens (Fig. 10a). Using the $U + D = V$ equation, we can make $U = 0$, making $D = V$; the ship would therefore cast an image 50 cm to the right of the +2D lens. This image would be inverted and would have nearly no magnification ($M = U/V = \approx 0/2 = \approx 0$). Our coxswain would not be able to see the ship!

Suppose that we also gave our coxswain an additional +20D lens and he has been paying attention to our nightly optics lectures given after dinner to boost our crew's morale (Fig. 10b). He could then hold the +20D lens at a distance of 5 cm to the right of where the image is forming (50 cm) and create a telescope of 55 cm. Even though the image of the ship will be inverted, he will enjoy the benefit of magnification 10×, so hopefully he will be able to see the ship! Also note that if we used stronger lenses for the eyepiece, we would get more magnification and the length of the telescope would also become smaller (e.g., +40D lens as eyepiece will give 20× magnification and the length of the telescope would be only 52.5 cm). Our coxswain tells us this is a friendly ship, so we have no need to hoist the black flag and we can continue our discussions on magnification.

Magnification From a Simple Magnifier

A simple magnifier takes advantage of angular magnification by bringing the image of the object closer to the eye (in the form of an enlarged virtual image) than the eye can normally focus. The standard close focus distance is taken at 25 cm – whoever came up with this number and agreed to it should be made to walk the plank!

We can use trigonometry to compare these two angles: Θ_{lens} & $\Theta_{25\text{cm}}$ and calculate the angular magnification caused by the lens… but we have no time to do any fancy calculations. We can run a rig (use a shortcut) by using our knowledge of the lens powers to give us an easier calculation:

$$\text{Angular Magnification} = \frac{\Theta_{\text{lens}}}{\Theta_{25\text{cm}}} = \frac{\left(\tan^{-1} 0\right)/f}{\left(\tan^{-1} 0\right)/25\,\text{cm}} = \frac{25\,\text{cm}}{f} = \frac{D}{4}$$

(For Simple Magnifier)

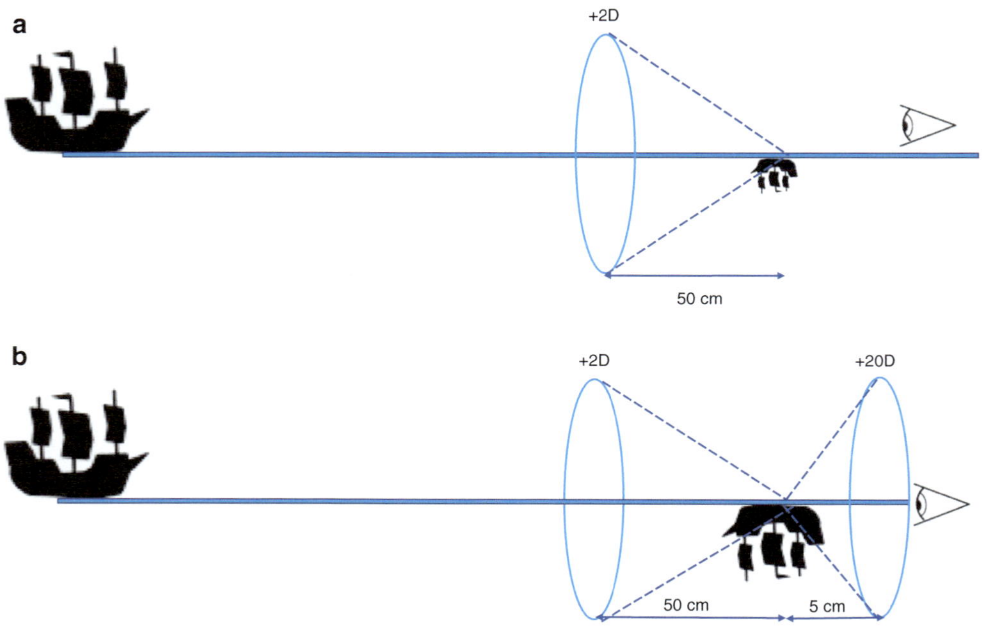

Fig. 10 (**a**) Notice the transverse magnification given by a + 2D lens for an object located close to infinity is very minimal. (**b**) When a second lens is introduced (i.e., +20D lens), the first image of the ship is magnified 10× due to angular magnification (Images are not drawn to scale)

Angular magnification for a simple magnifier = $D/4$. In other words, angular magnification for a simple magnifier simply relies on taking the power of the lens and dividing it by 4. If our coxswain was using a + 40D lens and wanted to see his map, he could hold it 25 cm from the map and get 10× (40/4) magnification.

Let us apply this to a clinical, instead of pirating, scenario. You are at the hospital doing inpatient rounds, and your portable slit lamp is out of batteries. If you need to look for infiltrates around the corneal abrasion of a patient, you wish that you had a magnifying glass with you. But wait, you do have a magnifying glass, the 20D lens! If you used the 20D lens as a simple magnifier, how much angular magnification would it have at 25 cm?

Angular Magnification = $D/4$ = 20/4 = 5×. This means that if you held the 20D lens 25 cm away from the patient's cornea, you would be able to take advantage of the 5× magnification to check for a possible infiltrate. Yes, the image will be inverted, but we can work around that as needed.

It may be helpful to apply this to another scenario: how much angular magnification is provided by a direct ophthalmoscope when looking at a patient's optic nerve? Remember the direct ophthalmoscope uses the optics of the patient's eye as ~60D (assuming that the patient is emmetropic) (Fig. 11).

Angular Magnification = $D/4$ = $60D/4$ = 15×. The optic nerve looks 15 times larger than the original optic nerve if the ophthalmoscope was held at 25 cm.

We can now use our understanding of magnification, especially angular magnification, to describe the magnification produced by telescopes.

Telescopes

Astronomical (Keplerian) and Galilean Telescopes

There are two types of telescopes that we must know for ophthalmic optics: Galilean and Keplerian (also known as Astronomical). Each telescope is constructed by putting together two lenses, termed as the *eyepiece* (i.e., the lens closest to your eye) and the *objective* (i.e., the lens closest to the object of interest). Heave ho, and understand the differences between these two lenses before proceeding further!

Both telescopes (Fig. 12) will involve using a positive lens as the *objective* lens. The two telescopes therefore only differ in the type of lens used in the *eyepiece*. Additionally,

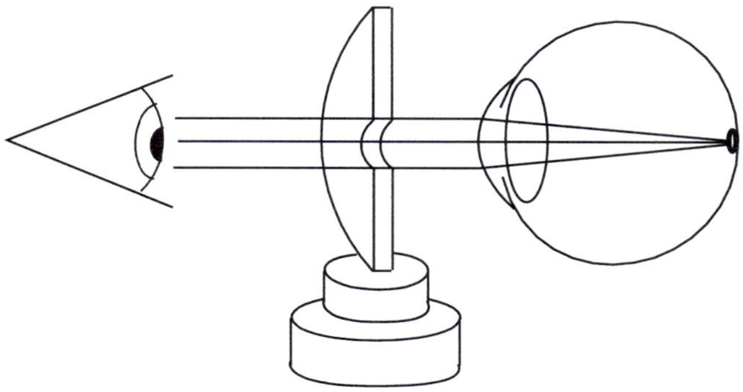

Fig. 11 Using the direct ophthalmoscope as a simple magnifier. When held 25 cm from the patient's eye, the image of the optic nerve will be 15 times larger (60/4 = 15)

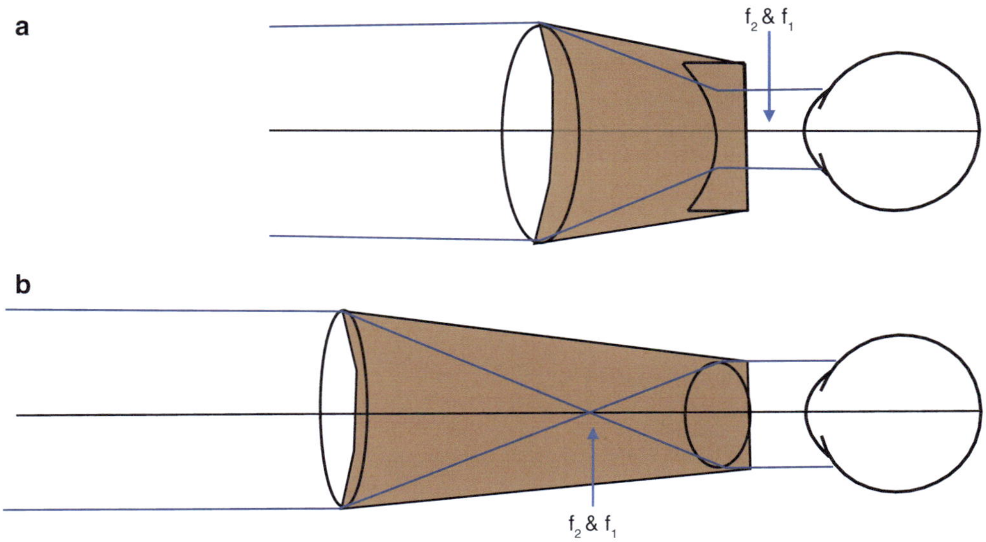

Fig. 12 Both Keplerian and Galilean telescopes will use a plus power lens as the objective. Figure 12a is a Galilean telescope with a negative lens as its eyepiece. Figure 12b is a Keplerian telescope with a plus lens as the eyepiece. Telescopic Magnification = $-(D_{\text{eyepiece}}/D_{\text{Objective}})$

both types of telescopes will require that the quantitative value of the *eyepiece* is higher than the *objective* in order to give any magnification. If the quantitative value of the *eyepiece* is lower than the *objective*, then we will inadvertently see a minified image.

A Galilean telescope will use **a negative lens** as its eyepiece and it will create an **upright** magnified image. The primary focal point of the (minus) eyepiece lens (f_1) will align with the secondary focal point of the (plus) objective lens (f_2).[5]

A Keplerian (astronomical) telescope will use **a positive lens** as its eyepiece and it will create an **inverted** magnified image. The primary focal point (f_1) of the eyepiece will coincide with the secondary focal point (f_2) of the objective. This will be located at a point between the objective and the eyepiece.

To summarize, for both types of telescopes:

- The secondary focal point (*f*2) of the *objective* lens must coincide with the primary focal point (*f*1) of the *eyepiece* lens.
- The eyepiece lens will be a higher numerical power value than the objective lens.
- They both are examples of *afocal systems*, meaning that vergence in = zero, vergence out = zero.
- The distance between the two lenses must be the **sum** of their focal points.

Many privateers often get confused about which telescope is which. Avast ye, a helpful mnemonic is as follows:

- Keplerian (astronomical) telescopes have a positive eyepiece and a positive objective and will yield inverted images.
  - Mnemonic: Write it out as "**A**s + ronomical":
    - The "+" will help you remember that it uses two "+" lenses.
    - **A** will remind you that you will get an "ass-backwards" (inverted) image.
- Galilean telescopes will have a negative eyepiece and a positive objective and will yield upright images.
  - Mnemonic: "**G**alileo was a **good (upright) guy** (upright image) despite all the **negative people** around him (**negative eyepiece**)".

Clinical Examples of Astronomical and Galilean Telescopes

In our previous example, our coxswain's telescope (made with a + 20D eyepiece and +2D objective) was an astronomical telescope. One may think that unless we were pirates or astronomers, we do not need to learn about telescopes because we never use them. Wrong...

Fun fact: The slit lamp is basically a Keplerian (astronomical) telescope that uses inverting prisms (Porro-Abbe prism) to re-invert the inverted image (and therefore making it upright).[6] This means that every time we use the slit lamp to examine the patient, we are just like pirates using telescopes! Similarly, most modern binoculars and even operating microscopes are advanced, modified Keplerian telescopes with similar inverting prisms. Finally, during fundus examination with a + 20/+28D lens, we are using an astronomical telescope setup - this is why the fundus image is inverted.

As for Galilean telescopes: most surgical loupes are a type of Galilean telescope as they use a minus powered eyepiece and a plus powered objective to give us an upright (and magnified) image.[7] For fundus examination, if we do not have access to our usual +90D lens, we can use a Hruby (−55D) lens (which is attached to some slit lamp models) to examine the optic nerve and macula. The lesson here is that even if we despise the optics of telescopes, we are using telescopes daily in clinical and surgical settings.

Magnification of Telescopes

The magnification for both telescopes can be calculated by recalling our discussion on angular magnification and making a small modification. Instead of using the incoming and outgoing angles, we can simply use the power of each lens to determine the magnification given by a telescope. Therefore, old salt, our modified formula is:

$$\text{Telescopic Magnification} = -\left(D_{\text{eyepiece}} / D_{\text{Objective}}\right)$$

This formula should be committed to memory. Notice the (−) sign, which will create an upright image for the Galilean telescope and an inverted image for the Keplerian

[5]The location of primary and secondary focal points is always confusing for trainees and is worth a review here. Remember that the primary focal point (F_1) is to the LEFT of a plus lens and to the RIGHT of a minus lens. To be specific, F_1 for a plus lens is defined as the location at which light originates (in a divergent fashion) and strikes the lens such that the light rays exit in a parallel fashion (forming an image at infinity). For a minus lens, F_1 is defined as the location at which incoming light is directed, via an imaginary extension of incoming light rays, to emerge from the lens in parallel fashion. The secondary focal point (F_2) is to the RIGHT of a plus lens and to the LEFT of a minus lens. To be specific, F_2 for a plus lens is the location at which incoming parallel light rays will converge to form an image. We have been primarily referring to this F_2 as the "focal point" when doing $U + D = V$ problems. For minus lenses, F_2 is the location at which incoming parallel light rays, via imaginary extension, appear to converge; recall that these light rays will actually *diverge* after striking the minus lens.

[6]See Chap. 17, Optical Instruments for more information regarding the optics of the slit lamp.

[7]Surgical loupes that use an astronomical telescope (and inverting prisms) are also available.

telescope. So even if you forget the above silly mnemonic from the previous section, mathematically, you should be able to determine that Galilean telescopes will give upright images and Keplerian telescopes will give inverted images. Finally, notice how this magnification formula bears some similarity to, but differs from, the transverse magnification formula.

Construction of Telescopes for Exam Problems

A subtopic of telescope construction, especially for exam problems, involves knowing how far apart to place the two lenses in order to construct a useful telescope. As stated above, the distance between the two lenses must be the **sum** of their focal points, regardless of whether we are dealing with a Keplerian or a Galilean telescope:

$$F_{\text{lens1}} + F_{\text{lens2}} = \text{distance between the two lenses for construction of telescope}$$

Again, it is helpful to use "cm" notation when calculating focal points as you will likely be given the power of the lenses in diopter values.

For example: if given a + 5D and a − 10D lens, how far apart must the lenses be placed in order to create a functional Galilean telescope?

$$F_{\text{lens1}} + F_{\text{lens2}} = (100/5) + (100/-10) = 20 + (-10) = 10\,\text{cm apart}$$

Notice how a Galilean telescope will often be shorter? It would be pretty cumbersome to operate when looking through a long telescope and pretty scary to operate on an inverted image (unless, of course, you are doing retinal surgery).

Another example: if given a + 16D lens and a + 4D lens, how far apart must the lenses be placed in order to create a functional Keplerian (astronomical) telescope?

$$F_{\text{lens1}} + F_{\text{lens2}} = (100/16) + (100/25) = 16.6 + 4 = 20.6\,\text{cm apart}$$

Notice that if we instead used a − 16D lens as the eyepiece and a + 4D lens as the objective, we can form a Galilean telescope. The lenses can now be placed 16.6 – 4 = 12.6 cm apart. We can therefore note that the "length" of a Galilean telescope is usually shorter than a Keplerian telescope, especially when considering lens combinations that differ only in the signed (positive/negative) value of the eyepiece lens. This is one reason why most surgical loupes utilize a Galilean telescope construction.

Sample Telescope Problems

Example #1

What is the magnification of a telescope if one end consists of a − 50D lens and the other end consists of a + 20D lens? How far apart are the lenses?

First, we can determine what kind of telescope this is by looking at the values of both lenses. Given that we have a minus lens (−50D) and a plus lens (+20D), this must be a Galilean telescope. We can then calculate the magnification using our formula:

Telescopic Magnification = − ($D_{\text{eyepiece}}/D_{\text{Objective}}$) = − (−50/20) = + 2.5 × magnification. The positive value of 2.5× confirms that the telescope will give us an upright image.

Now we have to figure out how far apart these lenses are before we are made to walk the plank:

$$F_{\text{lens1}} + F_{\text{lens2}} = (100/20) + (100/-50) = 5 + (-2) = 3\,\text{cm}$$

This "length" of a telescope, 3 cm, may be quite similar to how some surgical loupes may be constructed.

Example #2

What is the magnification of a telescope that is constructed with a + 20D lens and a + 4D lens? How far apart must the lenses be placed?

First, we can determine what kind of telescope this is by looking at the values of both lenses. Given that we have two plus lenses (+20D and +4D), this must be a Keplerian (astronomical) telescope. We can then calculate the magnification using our formula:

Telescopic Magnification = − ($D_{\text{eyepiece}}/D_{\text{Objective}}$) = − (20/4) = − 5 × magnification. The negative value of −5× confirms that the telescope will give us an inverted image.

Now we have to give no quarter and figure out how far apart these lenses must be placed:

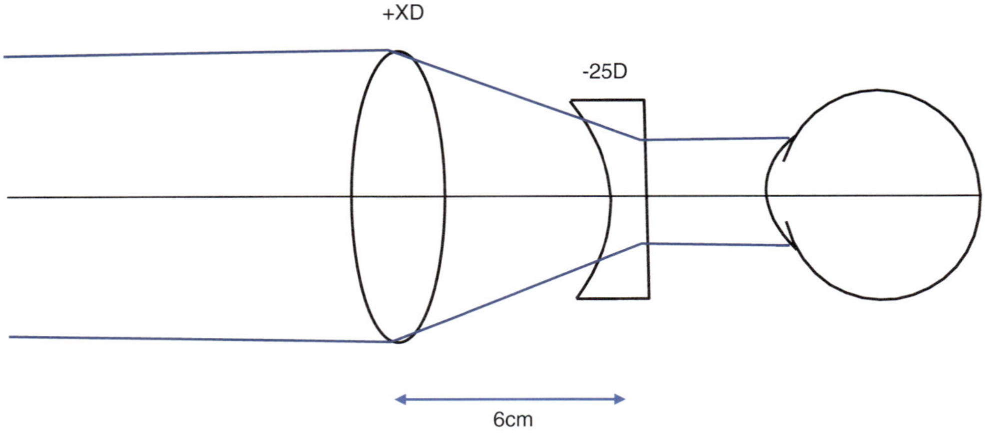

Fig. 13 What is the power of the objective lens?

$$F_{\text{lens1}} + F_{\text{lens2}} = (100/20) + (100/4) = 5 + 25 = 30\,\text{cm}$$

Remember that the minus sign indicates an inverted image and does not imply minification.

Example #3
A second level type of problem that may be asked based on the above concepts is as follows: if the eyepiece of a functional astronomical telescope has a power of +10D and is located 43 cm from an objective lens of unknown power, what is the power of the objective lens?

We can start off by first calculating the focal length of the eyepiece: $F_{\text{eyepiece}} = (100/10) = 10$ cm. Since the lenses are 43 cm apart, we can now subtract 10 cm from 43: 43–10 = 33 cm. The unknown objective lens has a focal length of 33 cm. Therefore, the power of the unknown lens is: $D_{\text{objective}} = 100/33 = +3$ D. For the sake of completion, this telescope will give a − 10/3 = −3.33× magnification.

Example #4
If we are given a − 25D lens and an unknown power lens to create a functional telescope such that the lenses are 6 cm apart, what is the power of the unknown lens? What is the magnification of this telescope? (Fig. 13)

We know that this must be a Galilean telescope since we are given a minus lens (which must therefore be the eyepiece lens). The focal length of this lens is: $F_{\text{eyepiece}} = 100/-25 = (-)4$ cm.

The distance between the two lenses is: $F_{\text{lens1}} + F_{\text{lens 2}} = 6 \rightarrow -4 + F_{\text{lens 2}} = 6$

$$F_{\text{lens 2}} = 10\,\text{cm} \rightarrow D_{\text{objective}} = 100/10 = +10\text{D}$$

$$\text{Telescopic magnification} = -\left(D_{\text{eyepiece}} / D_{\text{Objective}}\right) = -(-25/10) = 2.5 \times \text{magnification}$$

Clinical Examples and Scenarios Involving Telescopes

While we have previously mentioned some examples of telescopes in daily ophthalmic practice, we can focus on several examples and scenarios that may have significant clinical implications on how we care for patients.

The Over-Minused Myope

This is a common clinical scenario, especially when trying to refract a young myopic patient. Suppose that we have successfully refracted a young myopic patient down to the 20/15 line. When deciding between two lenses at this line, the patient may favor the more minus lens as he/she may feel that the letters look "clearer or sharper". However, the patient may or may not realize during the refraction that the letters will also become smaller – more likely, he/she may come back to your office unhappy with the new glasses that you have given them, complaining that "everything looks smaller".

Why is this happening? Recall that young patients, especially young myopic patients, are able to accommodate much easier than older patients.[8] This means that they are able to generate extra "plus" power inside their eyes. As a result, they will end up requiring more "minus" power in their glasses – hence the common clinical teaching phrase, "myopes eat minus", which means that myopic patients will gladly favor more and more minus power during a manifest refraction because they are accommodating (and therefore

[8] We will discuss accommodation in more detail in the next chapter.

generating plus power inside the eye). This is why a cycloplegic refraction is crucial in young patients, especially when prescribing glasses for significant refractive errors or evaluating patients for laser refractive surgery. A duochrome test can also be used for these patients but does not have the same impact as a cycloplegic refraction.

Why are we discussing this in the context of telescopes? Recall in the previous section we defined a Galilean telescope as having a minus lens as the eyepiece and a plus lens as the objective. In the case of our over-minused myope, the patient is generating extra plus power (through accommodation) inside the eye (forming the "eyepiece" of the telescope) and is looking through a minus lens outside the eye (forming the "objective" of the telescope). In other words, the patient is basically looking at the world through a **reverse Galilean telescope**; therefore, instead of giving the patient a magnified image, as would be seen through a regular Galilean telescope, the reverse Galilean telescope will give the patient a minified image. However, the image will still be upright. The patient may still feel that the image is clear and sharp; however, the minification of the image may be bothersome (Fig. 14).

Therefore, by definition, any patient wearing a myopic prescription in his/her glasses is looking at the world through a reverse Galilean telescope. For the sake of completeness (and you may have guessed this, dear privateer!), any patient wearing a hyperopic prescription in his/her glasses is looking at the world through a regular Galilean telescope – hence, he/she may feel the world is magnified. More on this in the examples below...

Aphakic Magnification

When wearing glasses, hyperopes will experience a magnification effect because they are looking at the world through a Galilean telescope. Aphakic patients, for the sake of this discussion, are basically extreme hyperopes and therefore will experience significant magnification.

To understand this better, we should first review internal refractive errors (Fig. 15). It is almost as if patients with aphakia or high hyperopia have an internal imaginary −12.5D lens at their nodal point that diverges light behind the retina. If you want to make a resident more cautious about not breaking the posterior capsule during cataract surgery, make them see what it is like to have aphakia. To do this you could remove their crystalline lens or place a secondary −12.5D IOL in the sulcus. (Make sure the resident signs an informed consent first and any other necessary paperwork to ensure you do not get sued for this madness). Or ask them to look through a − 12.5D loose lens, which is probably safer and less lawsuit inducing.

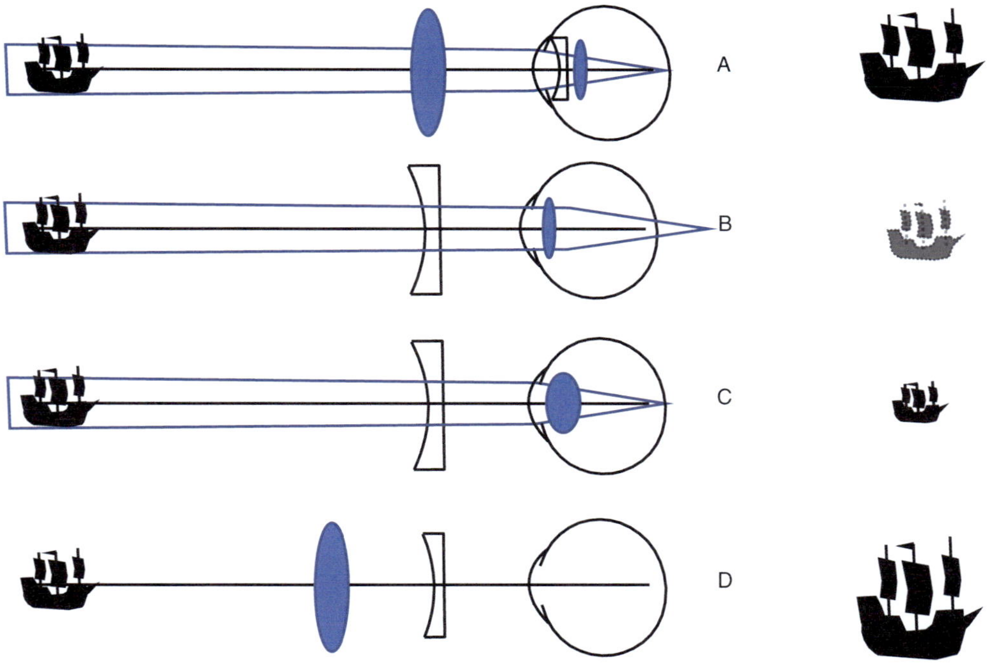

Fig. 14 Comparison of magnification for a patient with hyperopia who has an internal negative refractive error (Fig. 14a), an over minused patient (Fig. 14b), over minused patient who is accommodating to see clearly (Fig. 14c), and a regular Galiean telescope (Fig. 14d). Note that when wearing glasses, the myope will see the world through a reverse Galilean telescope, whereas the hyperope will see the world through a regular Galilean telescope. The image seen by the patient is on the far right

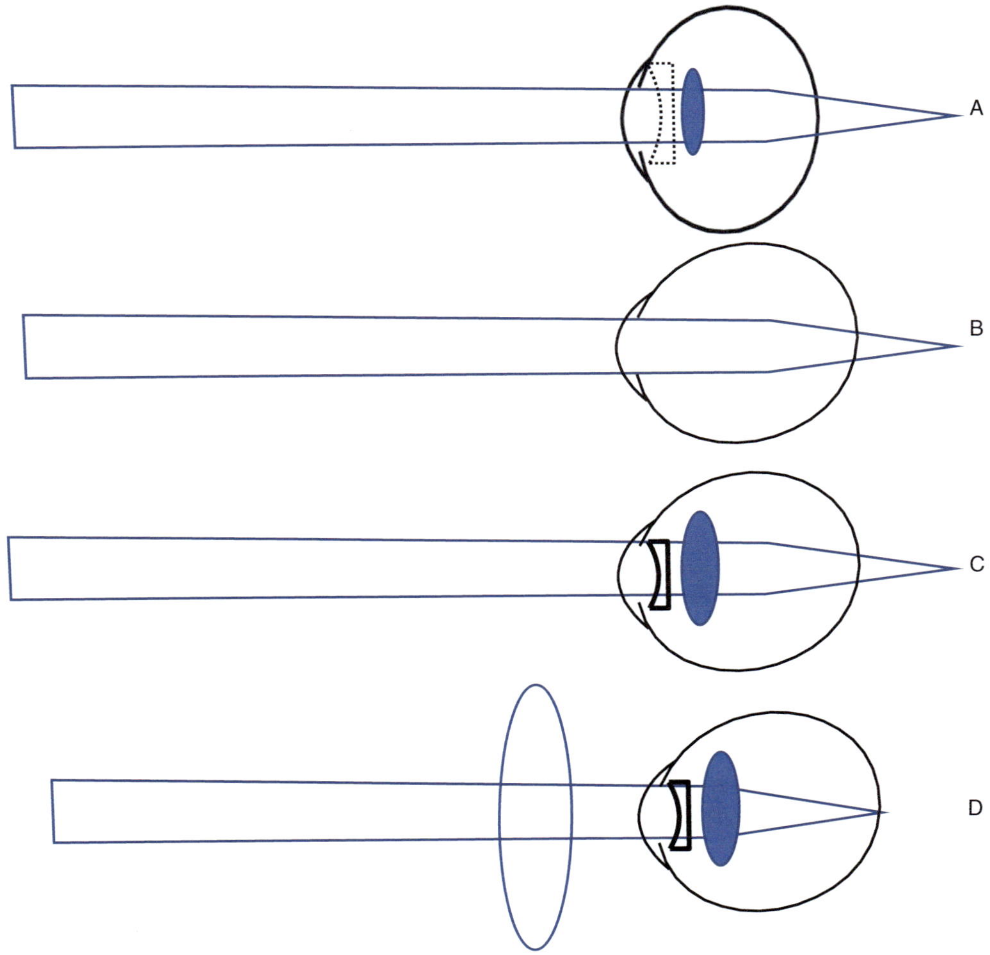

Fig. 15 Internal refractive errors for high hyperopes, bad residents, and aphakic patients. Figure 15a shows a patient with high hyperopia, with an imaginary divergent lens ~ a negative internal refractive error. Figure 15b shows a patient with aphakia. Figure 15c illustrates a bad resident with an actual −12.5D piggyback lens. Figure 15d illustrates same resident with a + 10D spectacle lens

In order to see clearly, both the patient with aphakia and the resident with a − 12.5D piggyback lens would need a + 10D spectacle lens. The −12.5D lens is basically the "eyepiece" lens and the +10D spectacle lens is now the "objective" lens. This lens arrangement would therefore create a Galilean telescope.

The magnification of this telescope would be:

$$\text{Telescopic Magnification} = -\left(D_{\text{eyepiece}} / D_{\text{Objective}}\right) = -\left(-12.5/10\right) = 1.25\times = 25\% \text{ magnification.}$$

As a side note, this may also have some relevance when performing cataract surgery on a long-standing hyperope. As these patients have been viewing the world through their "Galilean telescope eyeglasses", they may have gotten used to the world being larger – in other words, the magnification caused by the glasses may be "normal size" to them. If planning for a postoperative target of plano (or minimal myopic target), it is important to batten down the hatches before surgery and discuss with the patient that he/she may feel that the world is "smaller" postoperatively. Many patients eventually adjust to this change in size over time, but initially, they may complain that their perception of their environment is different. This may be frustrating to the scallywag practitioner because objectively, these patients may test extremely well in the office in terms of visual acuity. These patients may require extra counseling through the immediate postoperative period until they can adjust to the "new size" of the world, which may take up to 6 months to occur.

Interestingly enough, the same phenomenon is not seen with long-standing high/pathologic myopes who achieve plano after cataract surgery. One would think that these patients may complain that the world looks "larger" after cataract surgery, but these patients tend to tolerate the increased size perception of the world much better than their hyperopic counterparts. Perhaps these patients are so happy that they can see without glasses after cataract surgery that the increased size of objects is a minor issue?

Anisometropia and Aniseikonia

#Pro tip: These two terms are favorite questions for senior attendings to quiz trainees about, so learn them well, me hearties!

In our previous discussions of magnification, we learned that myopic glasses will minify the world (reverse Galilean telescope) and hyperopic glasses will magnify the world (Galilean telescope). The power of the spectacles will determine how much magnification or minification will take place. As a rule of thumb, ordinary spectacle lenses will change the size of the retinal image by approximately 2% per diopter power at 12 mm vertex distance.

For example, a hyperopic patient wearing +7D lenses in both eyes at 12 mm will see images ~14% larger than they appear to an emmetropic patient. Similarly, a myopic patient wearing −5D lenses in both eyes at 12 mm will see images ~10% smaller as compared to an emmetropic patient. If you have a significant refractive error and wear glasses, you can test this yourself by looking at your thumb up close with and without your glasses, and you will see that your thumb will appear to have a different size (e.g., if you wear a myopic prescription, the size of your thumb will be *slightly larger* without glasses as compared to with glasses).

Despite the extent of the refractive error in both eyes, as long as the quantitative value of the refractive error is within 3 D between each eye, the patient will not experience any subjective image size distortions. In other words, both our +7D OU hyperope and −5D OU myope will not report any major issues with their perception of image sizes when they wear their glasses because the refractive error in each eye is similar.

However, problems arise when the quantitative refractive error between each eye is more than 3D: this is the very definition of **anisometropia**. Anisometropia is mainly a problem on paper: that is to say that simply having a refractive error difference between two eyes of ≥3 D is not the main problem. The bigger problem is that anisometropia leads to a far greater problem: **aniseikonia**, which is the difference in *size perception* due to anisometropia. Aniseikonia is a far worse problem to have. Most adult patients can only tolerate about a 6–7% size difference between the two eyes.[9]

Imagine that anisometropia is an average pirate, but he works for the dreaded Edward Teach, aka "Blackbeard" himself. We should be more afraid of aniseikonia (Blackbeard) than anisometropia (the average pirate)!

[9]This is the classic textbook teaching. The authors have noted patients in their respective clinical practices who could not tolerate even 2D anisometropia in their glasses, and others who can easily tolerate 6-7D anisometropia.

For pediatric patients, this is not a problem to prioritize as compared to correcting the full refractive error in each eye to prevent amblyopia. Therefore, for young kids, we should always give the full cycloplegic refraction for each eye. For example, a 3-year-old patient who needs +2D OD and −2D OS must be given the full cycloplegic refraction; we should not worry about anisometropia and aniseikonia in this situation. Blackbeard and his pirate show mercy to children and only prey upon adults! See Chap. 23, Pediatric Optics, for more information about anisometropia and aniseikonia in the little buccaneer population.

We can highlight these two concepts with two common clinical scenarios:

Clinical Scenario #1

You have just prescribed a pair of glasses to your 30-year-old patient two weeks ago. The patient returns complaining about the new glasses: "Doctor, with the new glasses you prescribed, I can see really well with one eye open at a time, but I cannot tolerate the glasses with both eyes open because I see two images. What should I do? I am a pirate so should I just wear a pirate patch over one eye permanently, or be referred to a strabismus expert?"

The first thing we should do is to check the previous manifest refraction from two weeks ago and now check the new glasses that our pirate patient is wearing. We should also check to make sure there is not any undetected strabismus (!). Suppose the clinical exam, including EOM exam, is unremarkable, and we notice the following:

- Manifest refraction (two weeks ago): OD −2.00 sph, OS: +3.00 sph.
- New glasses (checked with lensmeter): OD: −2.00 sph, OS: +3.00 sph.

Our pirate patient is unfortunately suffering from a mistake that we should have caught two weeks ago. Notice that the refractive error between the two eyes is approximately 5D (anisometropia); this is likely causing aniseikonia.

We can calculate how much aniseikonia is present using our previously discussed rule of thumb for aniseikonia:

- Right lens: −2D. Images look 4% smaller.
- Left lens: +3D. Images look 6% larger.

Total aniseikonia: 10% size difference between the two eyes. To be specific, when wearing the glasses, the patient will feel that images seen by the right eye will be approximately 10% smaller than the images seen by the left eye.

What can we do for our patient, besides telling him to find a new line of work because pirating is not really a good long-term career?

There are several therapeutic options in this scenario:

A. Compromise on Visual Acuity: We can issue lenses for each eye that are closer in power. For example, we could give a − 1D lens OD and +1.5D lens for OS. This will make the net refractive error difference between the two eyes as 2.5D, which may be a bit more tolerable. The patient may not end up 20/20 in each eye with this new prescription but may be 20/happy as he will not have to deal with aniseikonia anymore.
B. Reduce Vertex Distance: By bringing the glasses closer to the corneal plane, we can help minimally reduce some of the magnification/minification effects of each lens. This may be hard to do on every patient due to other factors such as facial anatomy, deep set eyes, long eyelashes, etc.
C. Contact Lenses: This would probably be the best long term, nonsurgical option for the patient. By eliminating any vertex distance, we will also decrease the magnification experienced by the patient.
D. Refractive Surgery: If the patient is a good candidate for refractive surgery, this could be offered, especially after a contact lens trial.
E. Tell the patient their brain will adapt over time (at least 2–3 months), or until the next resident comes on rotation. Remember, younger patients can adapt to aniseikonia, so it is possible that our young 30-year-old pirate may have success with the tincture of time.

Clinical Scenario #2

A 65-year-old patient named Anne Bonny presents to your office for a second opinion. She underwent cataract surgery in her right eye with another provider two weeks ago and is extremely unhappy with her vision. She states that she was told to remove her eyeglass lens from her right eye and continue to wear the glasses for her left eye's visual needs. She complains that this is totally unacceptable for her pirating career, which she hopes to eventually retire from in a few more years.

On exam: Visual acuity, OD, sc: 20/20 Visual acuity, OS, cc: 20/20

Manifest refraction: OD – plano; OS: −5.00 sph (20/20).

Why is our patient unhappy?

This is a potentially common clinical scenario that can happen without proper discussion with patients with significant refractive errors prior to cataract surgery. We can see that there are 5D of anisometropia postoperatively that is likely causing aniseikonia, with the pseudophakic right eye seeing images approximately 10–15% larger than the phakic left eye.

What should have been done? Prior to surgery, the surgeon should have discussed with the patient that this may happen if she elected to target plano in the surgical eye and delayed surgery (and continued to wear glasses) in the phakic eye. If the patient wished to only have surgery in the right eye, then her options could have been:

(a) Proceed with surgery in the right eye only with a myopic target of approximately −2.50D to avoid anisometropia/aniseikonia postoperatively. This target of −2.50 also allows approximately ±0.50D of inaccuracy in the final refractive error so that the patient may end up between −2D and −3D in the surgical eye.
(b) Proceed with surgery in the right eye only and target plano, but counsel the patient that she will likely need to wear a contact lens in the phakic left eye to avoid anisometropia/aniseikonia issues.

It looks like this naughty referring surgeon did not have this discussion with the patient. What can be done now? Given that it has only been two weeks, we have several options that we can provide the patient:

(a) Contact lens for the phakic left eye, as discussed above.
(b) Intraocular lens exchange for the right eye for a more myopic target within the limits of anisometropia, as discussed above. Since it has only been two weeks since the first surgery, it should be relatively easy to exchange the IOL, but this would require an additional, second (unnecessary) surgical procedure.
(c) Piggyback IOL for the right eye: Since we want to make the right eye more myopic, we can use a plus power piggyback IOL placed in the sulcus to induce myopia. Assuming that there is a hydrophobic acrylic IOL in the bag (these are the most popular IOLs available) and there is good capsular integrity (especially of the anterior capsule), a three-piece IOL of a different material (e.g., silicone or collamer) can be placed in the sulcus to make the patient more myopic. To determine the power of the piggyback IOL, online calculators or software may be used.[10] Otherwise, a rule of thumb for inducing more myopia after cataract surgery is:
    - Hyperopic error: Piggyback IOL power = −1.5× desired refraction.
    - Myopic error: Piggyback IOL power = −1.0× desired refraction.

    In this case, we would use the hyperopic error calculation (because even though we have ended up plano, we have ended up more hyperopic than needed). So if we wanted to now make the patient −3D in her pseudopha-

[10] IOL power calculations piggyback lens. https://www.doctor-hill.com/iol-main/piggyback.htm. Accessed March 27, 2021.

kic eye, we will calculate: −1.5× −3D (desired refraction) = +4.5D power for the piggyback IOL.

(d) Proceed with cataract surgery in the left eye to make both eyes have minimal difference of intereye refractive error (i.e., target the phakic eye to have the same refractive error as the pseudophakic eye). Per CMS guidelines, anisometropia and aniseikonia after cataract surgery of the first eye are acceptable indications to proceed with cataract surgery of the second eye and should be covered by the patient's insurance.[11] Specifically, current guidelines state "if cataract extraction is performed due to anisometropia, the medical record must substantiate the presence of significant aniseikonia secondary to anisometropia arising from the first cataract extraction with IOL implant. The medical record must reflect that the aniseikonia is visually significant to the patient by documenting the patient's subjective complaints and must also document that anisometropia is present by determination of the refractive error in both eyes after the first cataract surgery." In other words, me mateys, even if you plan to only do cataract surgery after training, you cannot escape knowledge of anisometropia/aniseikonia!

(e) Offer the patient refractive surgery in the phakic eye to decrease the intereye refractive error. This may be a reasonable option especially with young patients (20–40 year olds) who require early cataract surgery due to trauma or steroids in one eye only, and have a relatively clear lens in the other eye. The costs of refractive surgery for anisometropia, however, must still be borne by the patient and will likely not be covered by insurance.

Knapp's Rule

Knapp's Rule states that if we have a patient with pure axial anisometropia (i.e., one eye has a longer axial length than the fellow eye), then an equal image size can be achieved on both retinas (i.e., we can eliminate anisometropia and aniseikonia) by giving each eye a spectacle lens placed at the anterior focal point of the eye, which is about 15–16 mm in front of the cornea. According to this rule, we would not have to use contact lenses for axial aniseikonia - we can solve all anisometropia/aniseikonia issues by simply increasing the spectacle vertex distance by a few millimeters.

However, in clinical practice, Knapp's Rule unfortunately does not account for other anatomical factors, such as stretched photoreceptors and reduced retinal element density; therefore, these patients will still have clinically significant aniseikonia which can decrease binocular and subjective vision.[12] In addition, patients may have aniseikonia due to other functional (sensory), physiologic, and/or neurologic conditions. In clinical practice, contact lenses are almost always better for all types of symptomatic aniseikonia, regardless of etiology. A 15–16 mm vertex distance is also a bit longer than the usual vertex distance (12–13 mm), so unless our patient was Pinocchio telling lies, this may be a difficult pair of glasses to construct and wear.[13] Therefore, while Knapp's Rule sounds good on paper, we do not see "aye to aye" with its clinical performance. Yes, we saved that joke for the very end, even though it would have been the easiest joke to make throughout the chapter.

We would like to end this telescope chapter with some humor and some poetry:

Patient: "Doctor every time I close my eyes; I see pink elephants."

Doctor: "Have you ever seen a psychiatrist?"

Patient: "No doctor, only pink elephants."

"There are stars whose radiance is visible on Earth though they have long been extinct. There are people whose brilliance continues to light the world even though they are no longer among the living. These lights are particularly bright when the night is dark. They light the way for humankind." — Hannah Senesh

Practice Questions

1. What is the magnification of a Keplerian telescope consisting of a + 2D objective lens that is located 83 cm from a + 3D eyepiece lens? (Fig. 16)
2. Where would you place the −10D eyepiece of this Galilean telescope? (Fig. 17)
3. Where would you place the +10D eyepiece of this Keplerian (astronomical) telescope if you are given a + 4D as the objective lens?
4. If an object is located 50 cm to the left of a + 6D lens which itself is 35 cm to the left of a + 12D lens, what is the final transverse magnification? (Fig. 21)
5. For the previous problem, what is final angular magnification?
6. What is the axial magnification if we are given a lens system that has an image height of 4 cm and object height of 1 cm?
7. A 9-year-old patient presents to your office for low vision consultation. His best corrected visual acuity is 20/350. If the patient needs a telescope to help him see

[11] Local coverage determination (LCD): Cataract extraction (L33954). https://www.aao.org/assets/e7b872ad-a76c-4f13-8525-d03a622bfb45/636396238727070000/cgs-l33954-cataract-surgery-updated-07062017-with-effective-dates-10012016-pdf?inline=1. Accessed December 4, 2019.

[12] Kramer P, Shippman S, Bennett G, Meininger D, Lubkin V. A study of aniseikonia and Knapp's law using a projection space eikonometer. Binocul Vis Strabismus Q. 1999;14(3):197–201.

[13] See Chap. 6, "Lens Effectivity".

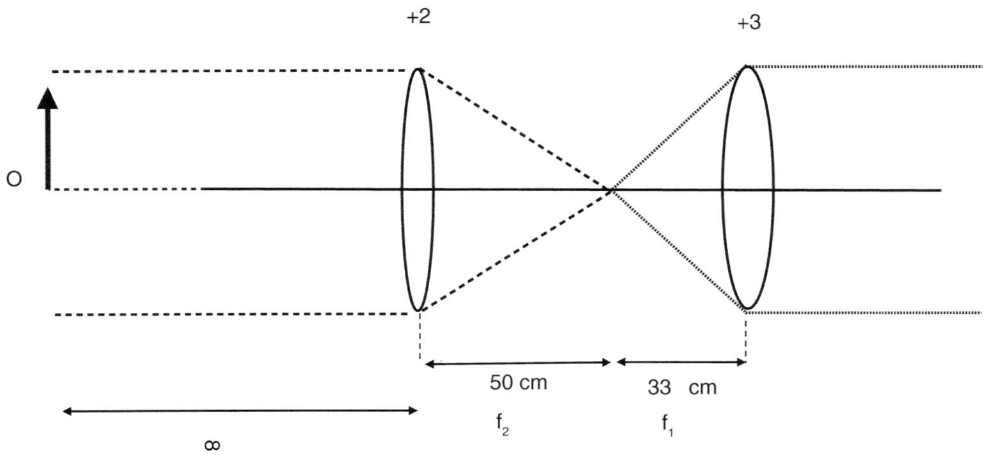

Fig. 16 Figure for practice question #1: What is the magnification of a Keplerian telescope consisting of a + 2D objective lens that is located 83 cm from a + 3D eyepiece lens?

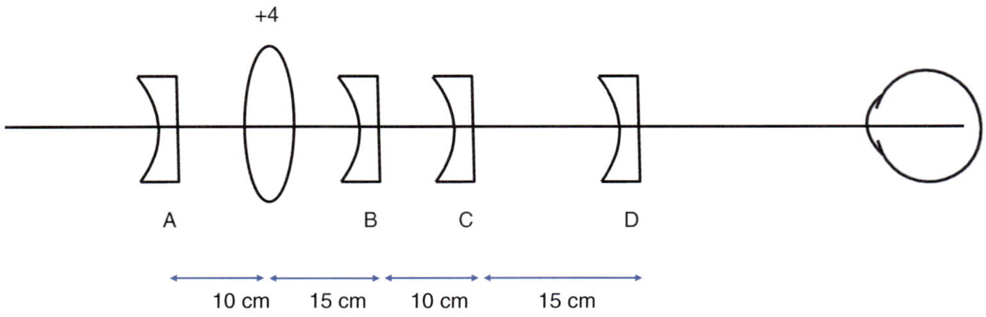

Fig. 17 First figure for practice question #2: At which location should a − 10D lens be placed to form a working Galilean telescope?

the blackboard in school, much magnification is needed in order for him to be able to read the 20/70 line from 20 feet away?

8. Suppose that you are given the following three lenses: −9D lens, +3D lens, and a + 2D lens. If you are told you must place two lenses into two slots in a lens stand (Fig. 23) in order to make a functional Galilean telescope, which two lenses will you choose and in which slots will you place these two lenses?
9. Suppose we have three bumbling pirates stranded on a desert island: Larry (emmetrope), Curly (a + 4D hyperope), and Moe (a − 4D myope). Our three heroes are now shipwrecked on an island with nothing more than a + 16D lens and a + 8D lens. As they attempt to construct a telescope, what folly will ensue? Who will have the "best" telescope?
10. Your elderly patient, Cal Icojack, comes in for his annual exam. He proudly shows you a telescope from his "youthful days" that he used to sight ships on the horizon. He now wants to be able to use it to sight his home computer. The monitor is 50 cm away from where he sits at his home office desk. You note that the telescope is constructed with a − 50D and +10D lens. How can you modify the telescope length to help him with his home computer needs?

Answers

1. Angular Magnification = − ($D_{\text{eyepiece}}/D_{\text{Objective}}$) = −(3/2) = −1.5×. This tells us that we will get an inverted image (minus sign) with 1.5× magnification.
2. In order to create a functional telescope, the secondary focal point (F_2) of the objective lens (the +4D lens) must coincide with the primary focal point (F_1) of the eyepiece −10D lens. For Galilean telescopes, the eyepiece must be between the objective lens and its secondary focal point.

   We can calculate the secondary focal point (F_2) of the objective lens: 100/4 = 25 cm.

   We can now calculate the primary focal point (F_1) of the eyepiece lens: 100/10 = 10 cm.

   Now we can add (F_1) + (F_2) = −10 + 25 = 15 cm distance between the two lenses.

   So we should place the −10D lens at location B (See Fig. 18).
3. In order to create a functional telescope, the secondary focal point (F_2) of the objective lens (the +4D lens) must coincide with the primary focal point (F_1) of the eyepiece +10D lens. For Keplerian telescopes, the eyepiece must be to the right of the focal point of the objective lens.

We can calculate the secondary focal point (F_2) of the objective lens: 100/4 = 25 cm.

We can now calculate the primary focal point (F_1) of the eyepiece lens: 100/10 = 10 cm.

Now we can add $(F_1) + (F_2) = 10 + 25 = 35$ cm distance between the two lenses (Fig. 19).

Notice how this problem is different from the previous one! Be careful to keep your plus and minus signs properly aligned when doing these calculations (Figs. 20).

4. First, we must solve for the transverse magnification of the first lens (+6D).

$$U + D = V \rightarrow U = 100 / -50 = -2$$

$$-2 + 6 = 4 = V \rightarrow v = 100 / 4 = 25\,\text{cm to the right of the lens}$$

$$\text{Mag1} = v / u = 25 / -50 = -0.5 \quad \text{OR} \quad U / V = -2 / 4 = -0.5$$

The first image is minified (50% size of the object) and inverted (due to the minus sign and also because this is a Keplerian (astronomical) telescope).

Next, we must solve for the transverse magnification of the second lens (+12D)

$$U + D = V \rightarrow U = 100 / -10 = -10$$

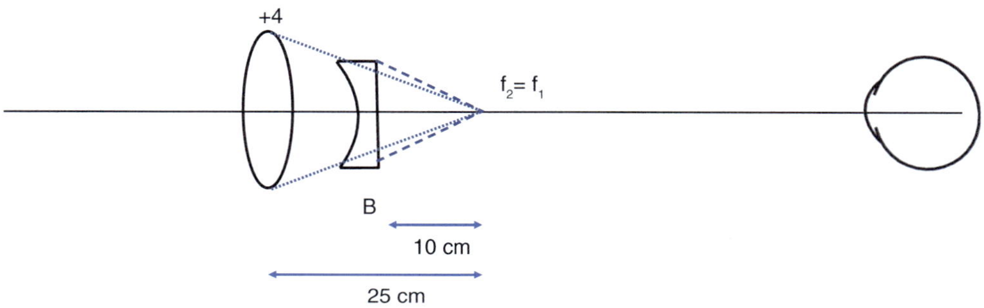

Fig. 18 Second figure for practice question #2: By placing the −10D lens at location B, the secondary focal point of the objective lens will match the primary focal point of the eyepiece lens, thereby forming a working Galilean telescope

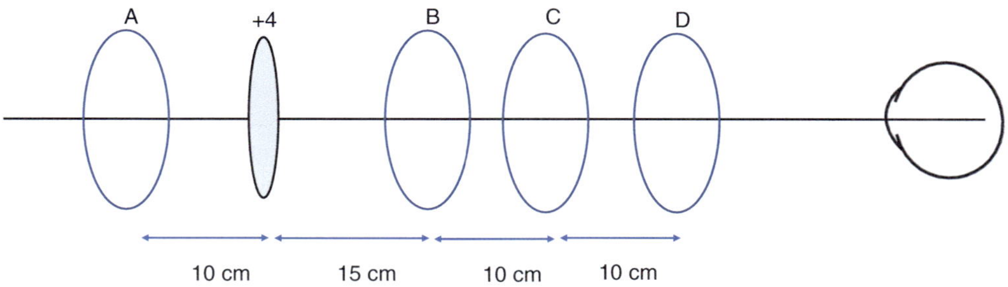

Fig. 19 First figure for practice question #3: Where would you place the +10D eyepiece of this Keplerian telescope if you are given a + 4D as the objective lens?

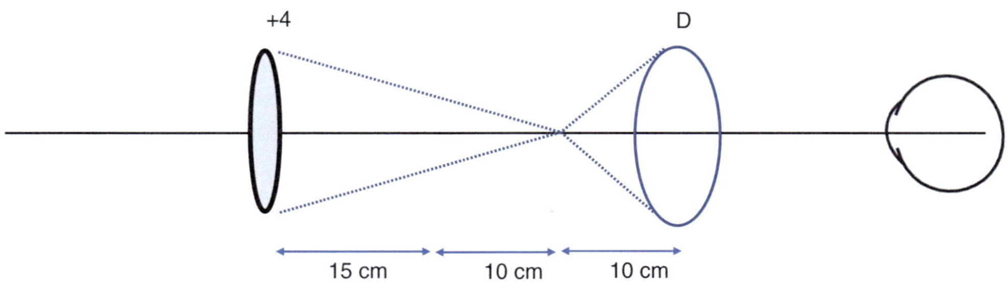

Fig. 20 Second figure for practice question #3: By placing the +10D lens at location D, the secondary focal point of the objective lens will match the primary focal point of the eyepiece lens, thereby forming a working Keplerian (astronomical) telescope

$$-10+12=2=V \rightarrow v=100/2=50\,\text{cm to the right of the second lens}$$

$$\text{Mag2} = v/u = 50/-10 = -5 \quad \text{OR} \quad U/V = -10/2 = -5$$

The second image is magnified: it is five times the size of the first image. It is inverted relative to the first image, which itself is inverted to the object. Therefore, the second image is UPRIGHT compared to the object.

The final transverse magnification = Mag1*Mag2 = 0.5*5 = 2.5×. Therefore, the final image is 2.5 times the size of the original object. Again, note that the final magnification is the PRODUCT of the individual magnification of each lens system (Fig. 22).

5. Angular Magnification $= -\left(D_{\text{eyepiece}} / D_{\text{Objective}}\right)$
$= -\left(12/6\right) = -2$

6. We may be tempted to simply plug in the values for magnification as $m = i/o = 4/1 = 4\times$ magnification. But this would only give us the transverse magnification. In order to calculate the axial magnification, we have to square the transverse magnification:

$$4^2 = 16 \times \text{magnification}.$$

7. When we have a specific line that we want the patient to be able to read, we can determine the magnification necessary by taking the best corrected visual acuity (20/350) and dividing that by the desired line of visual acuity:

$$\text{BCVA } 20/350 \rightarrow \text{desiring to see the } 20/70 \text{ line} = 350/70 = 5 \times \text{magnification needed.}$$

Bonus points: we could construct a Galilean telescope that gives us 5× magnification. For example, we could use a − 20D lens and a + 4D lens to give us 5× magnification. We can then use our formula for calculating the focal length distance between the two lenses:

$F_{\text{lens 1}} + F_{\text{lens 2}}$ = (100/ − 20) + (100/4) = − 5 + 25 = 2 0 cm apart. This would create a Galilean telescope that can fit comfortably in a patient's hand.

8. Since we are told we need to make a Galilean telescope, we can see we only have one minus lens (−9D), so that lens must be the eyepiece. We can consider using either the +3D lens or the +2D lens as the objective to give us 3× and 4.5× magnification, respectively. In order to figure out which of these two lenses to use, we can use our formula for calculating the distance between the two lenses:

$$F_{\text{lens1}} + F_{\text{lens2}} = (100/-9) + (100/3) = -11 + 33 = 22\,\text{cm}$$

$$F_{\text{lens1}} + F_{\text{lens2}} = (100/-9) + (100/2) = -11 + 50 = 39\,\text{cm}$$

Looking at the lens stand we can see that the total length of the lens stand is 30 cm. Therefore, even though the +2D lens would give us more magnification, we cannot use the +2D lens for this lens stand.

The slots are arranged such that the distance between slot A and slot C is 22 cm. Therefore, we will place the −9D lens into **slot A (eyepiece)** and the +3 lens into **slot C (objective)** to make our Galilean telescope.

9. Answer: This is a problem that tests our knowledge of constructing telescopes in combination with the observer's refractive error. We can have each of our "stooges" constructs his telescope and see what happens:

For Larry: Since he is an emmetrope, the +16D eyepiece will function as a + 16D eyepiece. He can use both lenses to make an astronomical telescope: 16/8 = 2× magnification. The telescope can be made with the two lenses held (100/16 = 6.25 and 100/8 = 12.5) → 6.25 cm + 12.5 cm = 18.75 cm apart.

For Curly: Since he is a hyperope, he will end up "using" 4D from the eyepiece to correct his refractive error. For him, the +16D eyepiece will function as a + 12D eyepiece. Thus, his astronomical telescope will be: 12/8 = 1.5× magnification. The telescope can be made with the two lenses held (100/12 = 8.3 and 100/8 = 12.5) → 8.3 cm + 12.5 cm = 20.8 cm apart.

For Moe: Since he is a myope, he gains an additional 4D from his refractive error to "add" to the eyepiece. For him, the +16D eyepiece will function as a + 20D eyepiece. Thus, his

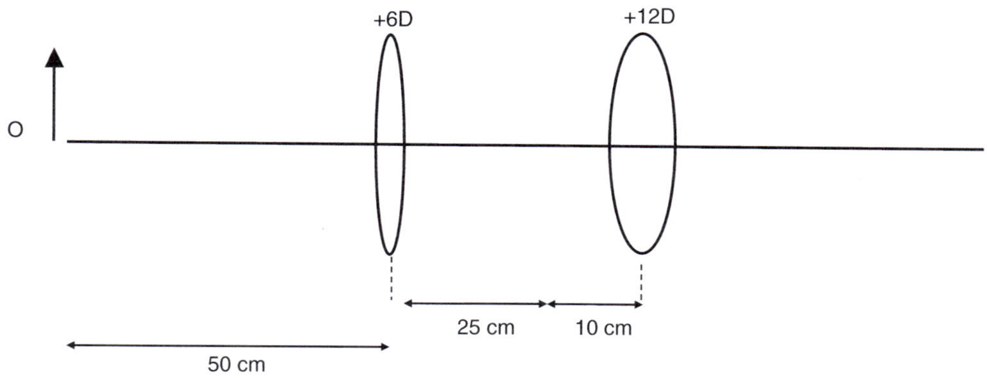

Fig. 21 First figure for practice question #4: If an object is located 50 cm to the left of a + 6D lens which itself is 35 cm to the left of a + 12D lens, what is the final transverse magnification?

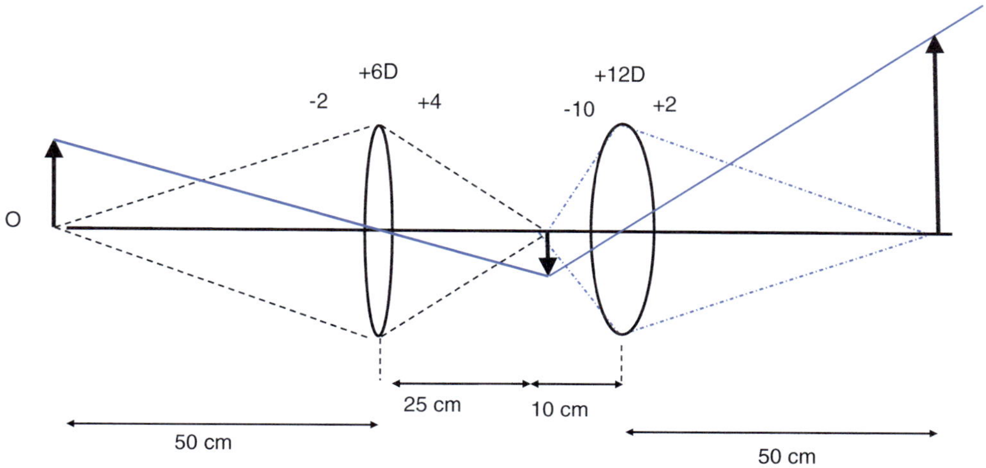

Fig. 22 Second figure for practice question #4: The $U + D = V$ equation can be used to determine the magnification of each lens system. The final magnification is the product of the individual magnification of each lens system

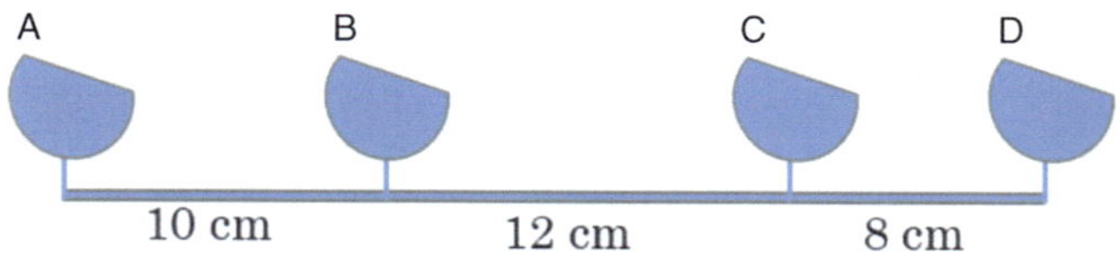

Fig. 23 Diagram for practice question #8: Suppose that you are given the following three lenses: −9D lens, +3D lens, and a + 2D lens. If you are told you must place two lenses into two slots in a lens stand in order to make a functional Galilean telescope, which two lenses will you choose and in which slots will you place these two lenses?

astronomical telescope will be 20/8 = 2.5× magnification. The telescope can be made with the two lenses held (100/20 = 5 cm and 100/8 = 12.5) → 5 + 12.5 = 17.5 cm apart.

Therefore, Moe will be able to construct the "best" telescope as it will have the most magnification and the lenses can be held the closest together; however, as you can imagine, each of our friends will argue and fight over which telescope is the best.

10. First, we should realize that this is a Galilean telescope yielding 5× magnification. In order for him to use this telescope to sight objects at distance, we can simply calculate the length of the telescope by finding the focal lengths of the eyepiece (−50D lens) and the objective (+10D). The focal length of the eyepiece is 100/−50 = −2 cm; the focal length of the objective lens is 100/10 = 10. The tube length of the telescope is −2 + 10 = 8 cm total length.

In order to see objects at 50 cm, the "effective power" of the objective lens must be modified. In order to see at 50 cm, a + 2D lens will be needed; therefore, we have to subtract 2D from the objective lens. The new objective lens power effectively will be: 10–2 = 8D. The focal length of the objective lens now becomes 100/8 = 12.5 cm.

Now we can calculate the length of the modified telescope by adding the focal length of the eyepiece and "new" objective lens: −2 + 12.5 = 10.5 cm.

Accommodation and Presbyopia

G. Vike Vicente

Objectives

- Describe the anatomical and physiological mechanisms of the eye during accommodative and nonaccommodative states
- Define key concepts such as far point, near point, range of accommodation, and amplitude of accommodation
- Define and describe presbyopia and how it relates to accommodation
- Highlight differences in the clinical presentation of presbyopic myopes versus presbyopic hyperopes
- Understand how the loss or lack of accommodation can present in various clinical scenarios

Introduction

Accommodation is one of those terms that you may hear about when older patients and attendings lament about how much they miss it. For our younger readers, you may not be able to fully appreciate losing accommodation as you very likely have a great deal of accommodation still present. Accommodation allows the eye to maintain a clear image of an object of interest as its distance varies.

Before we even define accommodation, let us first discuss the concept of internal refractive errors as it will serve as a useful foundation. An internal refractive error can be thought of as either an "extra minus" lens in the eye of a hyperope, or an "extra plus lens" in the eye of a myope. This will cause incoming light rays from infinity to fall behind or in front of the retina, respectively (Fig. 1).

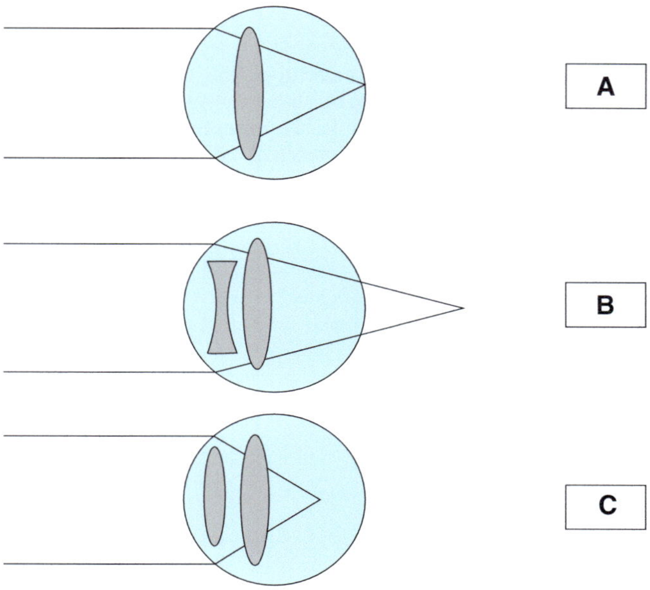

Fig. 1 In an emmetropic eye (Panel A), no refractive error is present and thus all incoming light rays from infinity will land directly on the retina. In a hyperope (Panel B), there is an "extra minus lens" that causes incoming light rays to fall behind the retina. In a myope (Panel C), there is an "extra plus lens" that causes incoming light rays to fall in front of the retina

For our hyperopic patient (remember our general theme: unfortunate are the hyperopes…), his/her eye will have to adjust – i.e., accommodate – to bring these light rays a bit more "forward" to fall on the retina. Therefore, a hyperopic patient will have to use accommodation even to see distance objects (i.e., incoming light rays from infinity). As a basic definition, we can think of accommodation as the changes that the eye must make in order to bring light rays "forward" onto the retina.

Since we are fancy eye doctors, we should now bring in the formal definition. **Accommodation** is the ability of the eye to change its focus from distant to near objects (and vice versa) by changing the shape of the crystalline lens through the contraction or relaxation of the ciliary muscle for near vision and far vision, respectively.[1]

G. V. Vicente (✉)
Clinical Pediatrics and Ophthalmology Georgetown University Hospital, Washington, DC, USA

Eye Doctors of Washington, Chevy Chase, MD, USA
e-mail: vvicente@edow.com

[1] There are several other theories regarding the etiology and mechanics of accommodation but we are going to skip those academic discussions and use this definition for the bulk of our discussion.

K. M. Riaz et al. (eds.), *Optics for the New Millennium*, https://doi.org/10.1007/978-3-030-95251-8_9

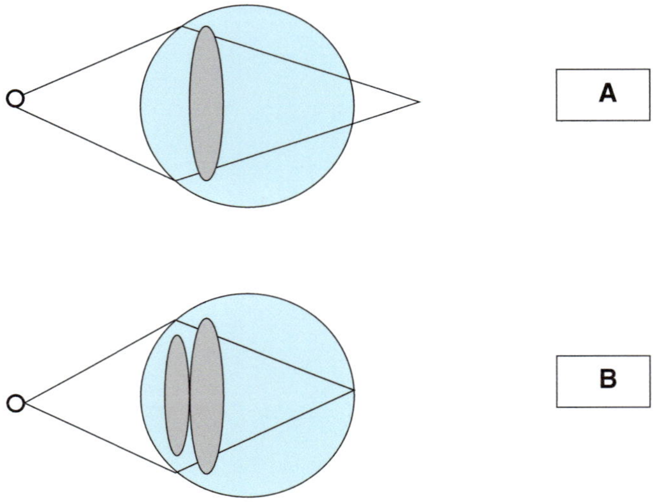

Fig. 2 For light rays at near, an emmetropic patient (Panel A) will also have to accommodate. However, because the myopic patient (Panel B) has an "extra plus lens" in the eye, he/she will not have to accommodate and will be able to easily see near objects as well

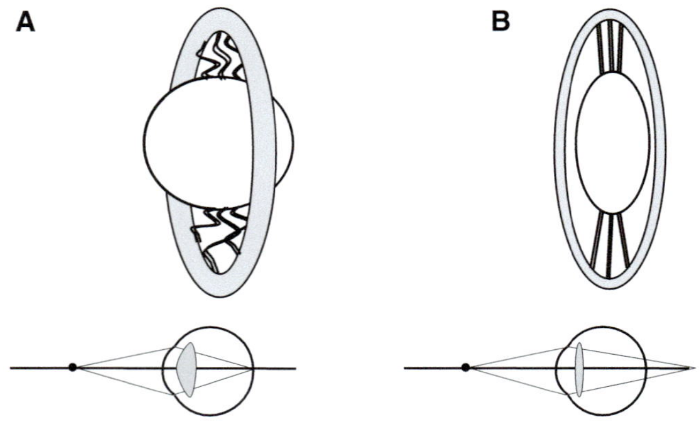

Fig. 3 Panel A shows an exaggerated schematic of a contracted ciliary muscle, relaxed zonules, and a more convex lens (tennis ball shape). Panel B shows a relaxed ciliary muscle, stretched zonules, and a flatter lens with less refractive power (tight drum shape)

Things are a bit different when we are dealing with incoming light rays from near (Fig. 2). Our poor hyperopic patient will have to accommodate even more, that is a given, but now our emmetropic patient will also have to accommodate since light rays from a near object will fall behind the fovea. Our myopic patient will have an advantage here because his/her myopia will function as "extra accommodation" and will allow the eye to focus on a near target.

During accommodation (Fig. 3), the ciliary muscle contracts, which in turn *loosens the zonules* around the crystalline lens. This increases the convexity of the crystalline lens (i.e., the lens becomes more spherical like a tennis ball). The anterior surface will be much more spherical than the posterior surface. The net result is increased plus power. The pupil will simultaneously constrict during the process of accommodation.

When the ciliary muscle relaxes for distance vision, the *zonules will tighten* around the crystalline lens. This causes the lens to flatten (i.e., the lens becomes shaped like a frisbee or a tight drum - those of you went to percussion summer camp, c'mon admit, can appreciate this analogy). The net result is decreased plus power. The pupil will simultaneously become larger as accommodation is relaxed.

A potentially useful mnemonic: when we throw a frisbee in the distance, the lens looks like a frisbee; when we want to hit a tennis ball that is incoming, the lens looks like a tennis ball. An animation of accommodation, including changes that occur to the shape of the pupil, can be seen in this supplementary online video (LINK HERE: https://gph.is/g/Z2mJgw8).

Hyperopia and Accommodation

Let us explore the concept of accommodation a bit further using our poor hyperopic patient as an illustrative example.

There are five types of hyperopia that one should commit to memory:

- Absolute Hyperopia: The least amount of plus power (either in glasses or accommodation) that a hyperope has to have in order to see anything at distance.
- Manifest Hyperopia: The maximum amount of plus power (either in glasses or accommodation) that a hyperope can accept without experiencing blurring (i.e., becoming myopic). In other words, this is the most plus power that an undilated hyperope will accept. Remember, he/she will still be generating some accommodation even when checking the manifest hyperopia.
- Facultative Hyperopia: Difference between absolute hyperopia and manifest hyperopia.
- Cycloplegic Hyperopia: The total amount of hyperopia that is actually present in the patient's eye. When the patient is cyclopleged, he/she cannot generate any plus power on his/her own, so the cycloplegic hyperopia will be more than the absolute or manifest hyperopia. Teenage/young adult hyperopes will not be able to tolerate the cycloplegic hyperopia initially if given as an eyeglass prescription (see Chap. 21, Clinical Problems with Optics and Refractive Manifestations). To review, a pediatric patient must be given the full cycloplegic refraction to avoid the risk of amblyopia.
- Latent Hyperopia: Difference between manifest and cycloplegic hyperopia.

We can use an imaginary patient example to make this easier to understand. Suppose a patient requires +2.00D to see at distance; manifest refraction reveals she will tolerate up to +3.50D; cycloplegic refraction is +5.00D.

In this case:

- Absolute hyperopia: +2.00D
- Manifest hyperopia: +3.50D

- Facultative hyperopia: Manifest – Absolute → +3.50 – +2.00 = +1.50D
- Cycloplegic hyperopia: +5.00D
- Latent hyperopia: Cycloplegic – Manifest → +5.00 – +3.50 = +1.50D

We can see that a hyperope *always* has to use some accommodation to see anything at a distance. Therefore, when he/she wants to focus up close, there is less accommodative ability remaining, explaining why these patients have problems with near vision.

Definitions

For written exams, a few more definitions must be committed to memory in order to be able to solve accommodation problems.

- **Presbyopia** is the loss of accommodation due to loss of lens elasticity. The loss of accommodation continues to increase as we age. Several subtypes are of academic interest:
  - **Incipient Presbyopia**: Similar to an "incipient cataract", a patient may have some signs/symptoms of presbyopia (such as mid-late 30s), but may be able to function quite well and not need any reading glasses.
  - **Functional Presbyopia**: As the name suggests, this is when presbyopia begins to cause symptoms to the patient. By definition, patients will benefit from and/or require reading glasses for near work.
  - **Absolute Presbyopia**: With aging, eventually no accommodative ability remains.
  - **Nocturnal Presbyopia**: This may overlap with incipient presbyopia. Increased pupil size in low-light conditions may cause an apparent decrease in accommodative ability. When tested during daytime or bright light conditions, these patients function well and have normal accommodative ability.
- **Accommodative Insufficiency** has similar symptoms to presbyopia but is due to other factors such as concussions, intracranial processes such as meningitis or neoplasms. It may be a transient or permanent process. It may also occur in down syndrome around elementary school age.
- **Accommodative Excess** is due to ciliary muscle spasm and may occur in any patient regardless of refractive error. This may be due to excessive near work, uncorrected hyperopia or astigmatism, anticholinesterases, or iridocyclitis. This is also known as spasm of accommodation. The clinical implications of this will be discussed in more detail in Chap. 21, Clinical Problems with Optics and Refractive Manifestations.
- **Far Point** is the point on the visual axis that is conjugate to the retina with *accommodation completely relaxed*. In other words, think of this as: "How far can the eye see when not using any accommodation?"
- **Near Point** is the point on the visual axis that is conjugate to the retina with accommodation fully active. In other words, think of this as: "How close can the eye see when fully using accommodation?"
- **Amplitude of Accommodation (AOA)** is the maximum capacity of the lens to accommodate. The AOA value, in addition to measuring how awesome some of you were in medical school, is expressed in diopters.[2] It can be measured by the near point of accommodation, accommodation rule (aka RAF Rule) or method of spheres.
- **Range of Accommodation (ROA)** is the extent of clear vision when the patient is accommodating. It is expressed as the distance between the near and far points and therefore its value is given in units of measurement (such as centimeters).

Accommodation and Refractive Errors

Let us discuss the relationship between accommodation and refractive errors. We introduced this concept briefly with the theoretical hyperopic patient earlier in the chapter but let us consider how a given refractive error can affect accommodation.

A useful analogy here is to think of accommodation (which is expressed in diopters) as "money in the bank". When we want to see up close, we have to spend some of this money in the bank.

We can think of myopia as "extra money" in the bank. Since the myope does not have to accommodate to see at distance, he/she has extra accommodation (extra money in the bank) to view objects up close.

We can therefore think of hyperopia as "less money" in the bank. Since the hyperope has to accommodate to see at distance, he/she has less accommodation (less money in the bank) to view objects up close.

The emmetropic patient has his/her amplitude of accommodation to spend – therefore, he/she has no additional or less money in the bank.

We can quickly review how the far point and near point are different for an emmetrope, hyperope, and myope.

Emmetrope All light rays from infinity will fall directly on the retina when the patient is not accommodating. Therefore, the far point is infinity. When the emmetrope fully accommodates, the AOA is basically the near point.

[2] None of the authors were AOA and we still sometimes wonder how we got into Ophthalmology.

Hyperope All light rays from infinity will fall behind the retina when the hyperope is not accommodating. Therefore, the far point is behind the eye - the exact distance is essentially the refractive error. For example, a + 3 hyperope will have a far point of 33 cm behind the retina. The hyperope's near point is basically the AOA minus the hyperopic refractive error.

Myope All light rays from infinity will fall in front of the retina when the myope is not accommodating. Therefore, the far point is in front of the eye - the exact distance is the refractive error. For example, a − 3 myope will have a far point of 33 cm in front of the eye. The myope's near point is the AOA plus the myopic refractive error.

Let us use some examples to further highlight this:

The Hyperope

Suppose we have a patient who has 4D of hyperopia and 8D amplitude of accommodation (AOA). What is the near point? What is the range of accommodation (ROA)?

Answer: We are told that the patient has 8D AOA ($8 in the bank). This patient must spend 4D of accommodation ($4 from the bank account) just to bring distant light to focus onto the retina. The far point (without using additional money from the bank account) will be 25 cm behind the eye (Fig. 4). This means that only 4D of accommodation ($4 left in the bank account) is left to see up close. When the patient uses this remaining 4D, the near point can be calculated as 100/4 = 25, or 25 cm. The ROA for this patient is infinity to 25 cm.

This patient is able to focus on a page as close as 25 cm.

The Myope

Suppose we have a patient who has 4D of myopia and has 8D AOA. What is the near point? What is the ROA?

Answer: Things are a bit different for our myopic friend here as compared to our previous example with our hyperopic friend. In order to see at distance, the myope does not have to dip into the bank account to accommodate at all. However, the myope's far point is limited; it is basically the refractive error. Therefore, the farthest that the myope can see is 100/4 = 25 cm, which is the far point (Fig. 5). However, when our myopic friend wants to see up close, he/she not only has the full 8D AOA ($8 in the bank account), but also the 4D of myopia can be thought of as an additional 4D AOA (additional $4 in the bank account). Therefore, the myope *actually has 12D AOA* ($12 in the bank account). Now when focusing up close, he/she can use all 12D; the near point can be calculated as 100/12 = 8.3 cm. The ROA for this patient is 25 cm to 8.3 cm, or 16.7 cm.

When our myopic friend wears his glasses, he/she is not able to use the additional 4D of accommodation; only the 8D AOA is available. Therefore, the near point is 100/8 = 12.5 cm. When he/she takes off the glasses, the near point is 100/12 = 8.3 cm. This helps explain why presbyopic myopes might take off their glasses when reading (see the next section for more on this topic).

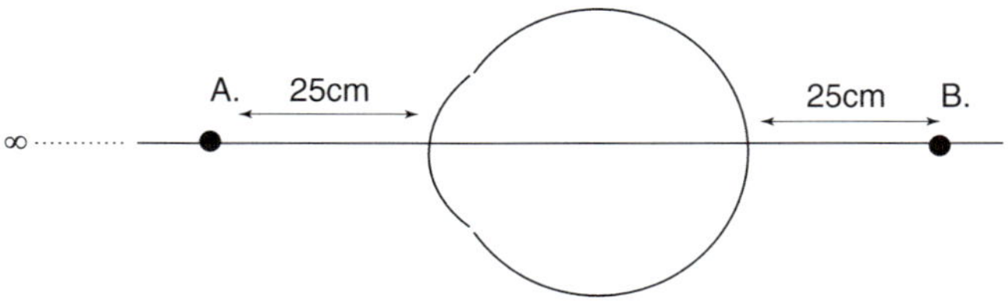

Fig. 4 A 4D hyperope with 8D of accommodation. The far point (without accommodation) will be 25 cm behind the eye at point B. The near point (using the remaining 4D of accommodation) will be at 25 cm (Point A). The range of accommodation is from infinity to 25 cm

The Emmetrope

Suppose we have a patient who is emmetropic and has 8D AOA. What is the near point? What is the ROA?

Answer: For our emmetropic friend, the far point is infinity (Fig. 6). Theoretically, light rays from a distance should fall onto the retina without our friend having to dip into the bank account. When focusing up close however, the emmetrope can use 8D AOA ($8 in the bank account). Therefore, the near point is 100/8 = 12.5 cm. The ROA is infinity to 12.5 cm (Fig. 6).

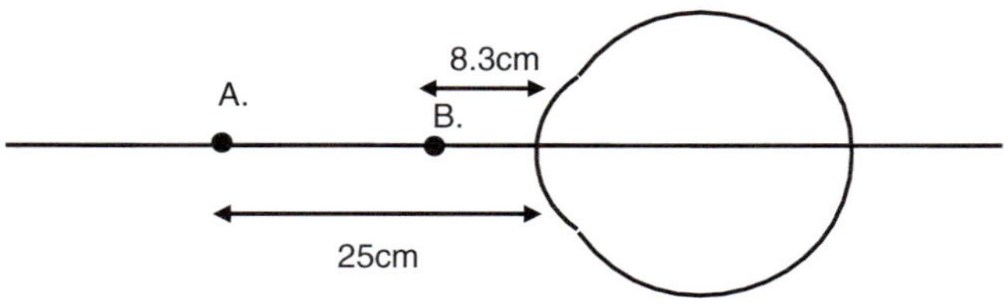

Fig. 5 A 4D myope with 8D of AOA. The far point will be at 25 cm (Point A). The near point will be at 8.3 cm (Point B). The ROA is the distance between the two: 25 – 8.3 = 16.7 cm

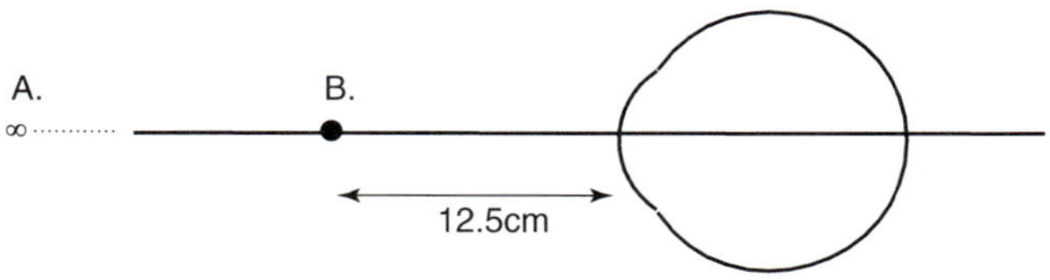

Fig. 6 An emmetrope with 8D of AOA. The far point will be at infinity (Point A). The near point will be equivalent to the AOA: 100/8 = 12.5 cm (Point B). The ROA is from infinity to 12.5 cm

The Cyclopleged Emmetrope

Suppose we have a patient who is an emmetrope, has a bit too much time (and curiosity) on his/her hands, and decides to put in a bunch of atropine drops because of some viral challenge video he/she saw online. What is the far point, near point, and ROA?

Answer: In addition to smacking this patient upside the head for doing this silly challenge, we can determine that the far point is still infinity. However, because of the atropine on board, this patient can no longer accommodate. As a result, the near point will also be at infinity. In order to see anything up close, the patient will need, in addition to a lecture about the perils of following online challenge videos, reading glasses to see up close until the atropine wears off.

Accommodation in Presbyopic Myopes and Presbyopic Hyperopes

This is a subtopic that deserves its own section because many students are often confused when encountering this topic. In the previous section, we stated that myopia functions as an extra accommodation ("extra money in the bank"). However, we made a broad assumption that we must now address: we assumed that the myope was not presbyopic and therefore had a healthy amount of natural accommodation left.

But what happens when our myopic friend ages? Eventually, as with all things in life, there comes a time to pay the piper.

Suppose we have a 45-year-old patient who is a − 8D myope. He has been wearing −9D glasses (let us assume 14 mm vertex distance) for a slight overcorrection, −8D contact lenses, and presents with complaints of headaches and strain when he wears his contact lenses for reading his cell phone (at 25 cm) as compared to when he wears his glasses. Why is this patient unhappy? The short answer: he probably has to accommodate *more* with his contacts as compared to his glasses. Whereas previously he could easily generate this additional accommodation needed with his contact lenses, now he is struggling to generate that additional accommodation.[3]

But why is this? Let us compare the amount of accommodation needed with glasses versus contact lenses. We can calculate this using our good old friend: $U + D = V$. Do not worry too much about the math: it is highly unlikely you will have to ever calculate this on an exam, but we wanted to show you the math to prove this concept (Fig. 7).

[3] We are making an assumption that the patient was not over-minused his whole life, otherwise a simpler solution would be to give him his correct ("underpowered") prescription.

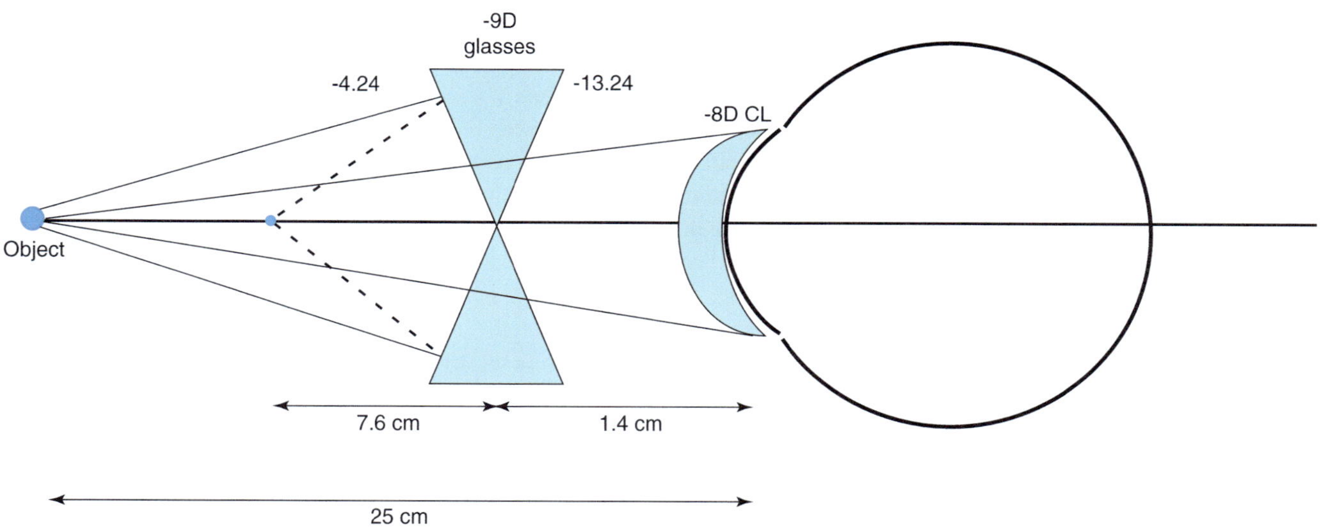

Fig. 7 Calculation for accommodation needed for a − 8D myope who wears −9D glasses (14 mm vertex distance) and − 8D contact lenses when wanting to see an object at 25 cm

Accommodation Needed with Glasses

$$U = -100/u = -100/(25\,\text{cm} - 1.4\,\text{cm}) = -100/23.6\,\text{cm} = -4.24$$

$$U + D = V \rightarrow -4.24 + -9 = -13.24 \rightarrow v = 100/V = 100/-13.24 = -7.6$$

Now for the patient to see this object (that has "gone through" the glasses):

$$u = 7.6 + 1.4 = 9\text{ cm}$$

$$U = -100/u = -100/9 = 11\text{D}$$

So, the patient has to generate 11 D of accommodation in order to see this object at 25 cm. We know that the patient is basically able to use 8D of myopia as extra accommodation ($8D extra in the bank), so he only has to generate 3D of accommodation on his own.

Additionally, a myopic patient wearing minus power glasses enjoys beneficial prismatic effects in the reading position. Recall that minus lenses act like a base-in prism when the eyes converge for near tasks; this means less convergence is required, and near vision tasks are easier. This advantage is lost when the myope wears contact lenses.

Accommodation Needed with Contact Lenses

We can again use $U + D = V$ (Fig. 7):

$$U = -100/u = -100/25 = -4$$

$$U + D = V \rightarrow -4 + -8 = -12$$

The patient now has to generate 12 D of accommodation in order to see the same object at 25 cm when he is wearing his contact lenses. He is still able to generate 8D accommodation because of his myopia, but now he has to generate an additional 4D of accommodation on his own.

Therefore, he is probably experiencing headaches and strain because he has to generate an additional 1D of accommodation when wearing his contact lenses as compared to wearing his glasses. This is actually a common clinical scenario that myopes may complain about as they reach presbyopic age, especially if their day job requires a lot of close work. They may find they do well in situations with contact lenses with mainly distance viewing (such as driving, playing sports, and weekend activities not requiring a lot of close work), but may start to have gradual difficulties with near tasks.

How can we help a contact lens wearing presbyopic myope? Possible solutions include:

- Wearing single vision glasses for full myopic correction (i.e., they get to use the extra accommodation gained with the glasses)
- Wearing contact lenses that are slightly underpowered (i.e., he could wear contact lenses such that residual −1D myopia is remaining in order to gain an advantage for near work)
- Switching to monovision or multifocal contact lenses
- Using reading glasses for close work activities while wearing the full contact lens correction
- Surgical options for presbyopia (beyond the scope of this chapter)

We can add another level of nuance (and possible confusion). In the previous example, we assumed that our presbyopic myope friend was wearing soft contact lenses. However, if he was wearing a rigid gas permeable contact lens (RGPCL), the mid-peripheral optic zone creates vaulting in the mid-periphery through that section due to the tear film. The tear film of a RGPCL has some "plus power" (as compared to clinically negligible power of a soft contact lens tear film) that may help a myopic patient with near vision tests. See Chap. 13 "Contact Lenses for Written Exams", for more information.

Conversely, unlike presbyopic myopes, presbyopic hyperopes may paradoxically enjoy wearing contact lenses because they will actually have to accommodate less with their contact lenses on as compared to their glasses. The "math" involved in this is the opposite of the math presented above for the myope.

Other Miscellaneous Notes About Accommodation

We can end our discussion on these topics with a few miscellaneous points, in no particular order:

- Our accommodative ability decreases throughout life; it does not start suddenly at 40. Emmetropes notice it around this age because this is usually when it affects our working or reading distance; some patients may

Table 1 Amplitude of accommodation by age

Age (years)	Donders	Duane (mean)	Hofstetter (probable)
10	14	13.4	15.5
15	12	12.6	14
20	10	11.5	12.5
25	8.5	10.2	11
30	7.0	8.0	9.5
35	5.5	7.3	8
40	4.5	5.9	6.5
45	3.5	3.7	5
50	2.5	2.0	3.5
55	1.75	1.3	2
60	1.0	1.1	0.5
65	0.50	1.1	0.5
70	0.025	none	none

notice it earlier or later since AOA varies from patient to patient. Have you ever heard a patient complain: "Doctor, ever since I turned 40, I have been using those over the counter reading glasses. They ruined my eyes, now I'm 50 and can't read anything anymore!" You can safely reassure these patients that this is simply a natural process that is taking place: congratulate them on getting older and reassure them that this is not a pathological change.

- As we age, the lens stiffens. The nerves and ciliary muscles are still working normally but the lens is not as flexible as it used to be. The main reason for the loss of accommodation is therefore the hardening of the crystalline lens.
- Several landmark papers and studies have been published in the literature regarding the AOA expected with changes in age (Table 1).[4] However, because the methods used in these papers varied, they cannot be used as a be-all/end-all guide to definitively "know" the AOA in a given patient. However, they can be useful guides to appreciate how AOA changes with age. Do not memorize these numbers!
- When giving reading correction for presbyopes, in general, you want them to still use one-half of their AOA, so you would prescribe them the other one-half of their AOA. For example, if a patient is found to have AOA of 3D, you would still want him/her to use 1.5D, so you should prescribe +1.5D reading add. This allows patients to use some of their AOA while keeping some AOA in reserve, analogous to splitting the budget between a saving and spending account.

[4]Modified from: Optometric Clinical Practice Guideline: Care of the Patient with Presbyopia, 2010. https://my.ico.edu/file/CPG-17%2D%2D-Presbyopia.pdf. Accessed July 4, 2021.

Practice Questions

1. A + 3D hyperope has 5D of amplitude of accommodation. Where is his near point?
   A. 0.2 m
   B. 0.15 m
   C. 0.5 m
   D. 0.3 m

2. A hyperopic patient wears +3.0D glasses for driving and can maintain near focus at 10 cm without glasses. What is her amplitude of accommodation?
   A. 3D
   B. 7D
   C. 10D
   D. 13D

3. An uncorrected myope has a far point at 1.0 m and a near point at 20 cm. What is her amplitude of accommodation?
   A. 1D
   B. 4D
   C. 5D
   D. 6D

4. A 50-year-old patient presents to your office inquiring about reading glasses. You measure her AOA as 3D. The patient wants to be able to read at 33 cm. What power reading glasses should be given to this patient?
   A. +1.00 D
   B. +1.50 D
   C. +2.00 D
   D. +2.50 D

5. A 65-year-old patient presents to your office inquiring about reading glasses. You determine that with +2.50D reading glasses, he can read at 25 cm comfortable. Which of the following values is a reasonable estimate of his AOA?
   A. 1.5 D
   B. 2.5 D
   C. 3.0 D
   D. 3.5 D

6. An 85-year-old patient comes to your office inquiring about reading glasses. She likes to read the newspaper at 25 cm but feels that her current +3.00D reading glasses are inadequate. Her AOA is 0.5D. How much additional power should you add to her reading glasses?
   A. +0.25 D
   B. +0.50 D
   C. +0.75 D
   D. +1.00 D

Answers

1. Answer: C. Since the patient has to use 3D of AOA to see anything at distance, he only has 2D ($2 left in the bank) of accommodation left to use for near vision. 100/2 or 1/2D = 50 cm or 0.5 m.
2. Answer: D. When the patient is uncorrected, it takes 3D for the patient to see clearly far away. The patient is able to focus from infinity all the way to 10 cm uncorrected. This takes 10D of accommodation to go from infinity to 10 cm. Therefore, the patient must have started with 13D of accommodative amplitude, 3D to see at distance +10D to bring the near point to 10 cm.
3. Answer: B. If the far point is 1.0 m then the patient must have −1D of myopia. The near point is 20 cm, the reciprocal of 20 cm = 5D. To go from 1D to 5D they must have accommodated another 4D.
4. Answer: B. We can start of by first determining how much add power is needed to read at the desired reading distance: 100/33 = 3D. We are told that she has 3D AOA. Therefore, we want her to continue using one-half of this AOA (1.5D), so we must prescribe an additional +1.50D in the form of reading glasses.
5. Answer: C. In order to read comfortably at 25 cm, this patient will need +4D of accommodation through some combination of his own abilities and his reading glasses. Currently, he is using +2.50D "help" from his reading glasses, so he is using +1.5D on his own. Doubling this value gives us +3.0D as a reasonable estimate of his AOA. Of course, there are much better ways to measure AOA objectively – such as Step 1 scores, number of MS3 clerkship honors, etc. (sorry, we had to!).
6. Answer: C. In order to read at 25 cm, she will need 4D of help, either from her reading glasses or her AOA. Since her AOA is 0.5D, she really can use 0.25D (at most), so she will need +3.75D in her reading glasses. Therefore, her current reading glasses will need an additional +0.75D of power.

Spherocylindrical Lenses

Kamran M. Riaz

Objectives

- To introduce nomenclature used to describe spherocylindrical lenses and keratometry measurements
- To clarify two key definitions used with spherocylindrical lenses: meridian and axis
- To discuss clinical relevance of these terms as it pertains to streak retinoscopy, keratometry measurements, and astigmatism correction
- To understand how to use spherocylindrical notation to solve clinical and testable refraction problems
- To understand how to use power crosses to solve clinical and testable refraction problems
- To revisit Prentice's Rule to solve advanced problems involving spherocylindrical lenses

Introduction

Dante Alighieri (1265–1321) was a famous Italian poet and political theorist of the late Middle Ages who wrote the *Divine Comedy*, which is considered one of the greatest literary achievements of his time. In this epic poem, Dante, possibly under the influence of recreational substances, describes his imaginary journey through various places of the afterlife, including his journey through *Inferno* (Hell). He reported that the following phrase is inscribed over the gates of Hell:

Lasciate ogne speranza, voi ch'intrate (Abandon all hope ye who enter here).

It is fitting that as we embark upon this journey through spherocylindrical lenses, especially when dealing with spherocylindrical notation (SC notation) and power crosses (PC notation), we also can imagine that we are passing into a realm through a door with the same quote inscribed above.

This topic arguably causes much angst and stress to trainees, mainly because no one can seem to agree on terminology and how to speak about a particular teaching point under the topic. Even published articles and podium presentations are filled with authors and speakers using these terms interchangeably (and sometimes wrongly!) The problem is astigmatism itself[1]: how do we speak about it related to the cornea, lenses, streak refractions, and the surgical correction of astigmatism? The idea of a cylindrical lens, especially in regards to "axis" and "meridian", and how this relates to corneal astigmatism and the actual "power" exerted by the cylindrical lens is confusing.

After figuring out astigmatism and spherocylindrical lens nomenclature, we may feel trapped with the two additionally challenging topics of SC Notation and PC Notation. The key is to realize that both methods are used to arrive at the same answer. Both methods can determine eyeglass prescription power for clinical and testable scenarios, especially based on streak refraction results. These methods are likely remnants of days past when clinicians lacked phoropters, autorefractors, and wavefront aberrometers, and perhaps when these technologies become more mainstream, this topic may lose its relevance. It is also possible that you may find yourself in a situation, such as a rare occasion in clinic or while serving in a medical mission, when you may lack access to your favorite toys and may have to rely on these older methods. Alternatively, you may need to know this material simply to get through your exams.

In Dante's epic story, he eventually finds his way out of *Inferno*. In our story, we hope to do the same.

[1]The next time your patient tells you, "Doc, I got a huge problem, they told me I got this here "stigmatism", what can you do to fix it?" you can silently nod to yourself: yes, you and me both, pal.

K. M. Riaz (✉)
Dean McGee Eye Institute, University of Oklahoma, Oklahoma City, OK, USA

K. M. Riaz et al. (eds.), *Optics for the New Millennium*, https://doi.org/10.1007/978-3-030-95251-8_10

Nomenclature and Definitions

This topic is often confusing because definitions and nomenclature vary among textbooks (and subsequent discussions among ophthalmologists!). Studying this can be very frustrating because you may find it used differently in another textbook when you think you have understood a particular term. This is like standing in line for hours to buy an Apple iPhone® and then realizing you only have an Android® charger (or vice-versa, depending on where your allegiances lie!)

We should first discuss a few important terms to help us navigate this Inferno.

Keratometry Measurements

We need to define several terms that we will use consistently throughout this chapter. We can start with our familiar friend, the cornea, and simplify its shape as a circle. While a circle has 360 degrees, we need a term to refer to the point of interest in this "circle." The term *meridian* is simply a term used to refer to a location on this corneal circle. Technically, while there are an infinite number of meridians in the cornea, we will limit these to 360 meridians.[2] Of course, we know that the cornea is not an actual circle; most patients have corneas with orthogonal, symmetrical astigmatism, so the corneal shape is more like an oval. Thus, there is a flat (longer) side and a steep (shorter) side of this oval, which we can term the *flat meridian* and the *steep meridian*, respectively. As a simplification, we can consider that the flat meridian is 90° away from the steep meridian in a cornea with regular astigmatism.[3]

When we perform keratometry (K) measurements, we are generally given two numbers of corneal power – for our purposes in this chapter, the corneal power measurements also give us information about the location of the flat meridian and the steep meridian. For example, suppose we have a patient with K measurements of 43.00 × 45.00 @ 85. We know from these readings that the steep meridian is located at 85°; therefore, the flat meridian is located 90° away (at 175°). This cornea has the shape of a horizontal football such that the center is getting ready to hike it to the quarterback (with-the-rule (WTR) corneal astigmatism).[4]

For this cornea with 2D keratometric astigmatism, we can ask the following question: *how can we correct this corneal astigmatism when using (1) glasses, (2) corneal incisions, (3) toric IOLs, and (4) laser refractive surgery*. We will deal with the first situation in this chapter and the other three situations in the next chapter.[5]

In order to help this patient (and assuming zero lenticular astigmatism), we will need to prescribe cylindrical correction to neutralize the corneal WTR astigmatism with a cylindrical lens. But how should we orient this eyeglass lens?

Cylindrical Lens: Axis Meridian and Power Meridian

Before we discuss cylindrical lenses, let us review spherical lenses. Recall that a pure spherical lens will focus any incoming light ray, regardless of its entrance location on the lens (i.e., regardless of the meridian of the lens), onto a single focal point behind the lens (Fig. 1). For example, any incoming light ray that enters a +1D lens from infinity will focus at the focal point 1 m behind the lens.

A spherocylindrical lens has different powers in different locations (meridians) in the lens. Light rays that pass through this lens will focus on more than one focal point (astigmatism). We will discuss these concepts in greater detail in the following sections. The focal point locations for light rays entering a spherical lens (Fig. 2, Panel a) and spherocylindrical lens (Fig. 2, Panel b) differ significantly. For example, a spherocylindrical lens with power of +1.00 + 2.00 × 90 will focus incoming light at two focal points: 1 m and 0.33 m (33 cm) behind the lens.

We can describe cylindrical or spherocylindrical lenses by their axis and power. We primarily care about only two terms related to these lenses:

- Axis Meridian (AM): This is the degree (meridian) in which the cylinder's long side is oriented. We will use the

[2] As a nerdy nomenclature point: the cornea has no "axis". It is incorrect to use the term, for example, in cataract surgery when deciding to place a main incision at a given location to reduce corneal astigmatism as "operating at the steep axis", which unfortunately has been used in numerous published papers and podium presentations. The correct term is "operating at the steep meridian". See: Rosen E. Axis or meridian? J Cataract Refract Surg. 2011 Oct;37(10):1743

[3] This simplification breaks down for irregular corneas such as postrefractive corneal ectasia, keratoconus, and postpenetrating keratoplasty. For the purposes of this introductory discussion, we will assume the cornea has a symmetrical shape (regular astigmatism). For corneas with irregular and nonorthogonal astigmatism, one "half" of the cornea is not a perfect mirror reflection of the other "half". Thus, flat and steep meridians are not necessarily 90° away from one another.

[4] See Chap. 11, "Astigmatism", for a more detailed discussion of these concepts.

[5] For those readers who want to anxiously know, we can summarize as follows. Regarding corneal incisions, the main incision can be placed superiorly (at 85°); if using a temporal main incision, paired limbal relaxing incisions can be made centering at 85° – various nomograms exist for the degree length for these incisions. Regarding toric IOLs, the IOL should be placed with its markings at 85° in order to exert power 90° away (at the 175-degree meridian). Finally, when considering laser refractive surgery, given that ablation is typically done in minus cylinder, the laser will ablate the steeper section of the cornea (along the 85-degree meridian) to flatten it.

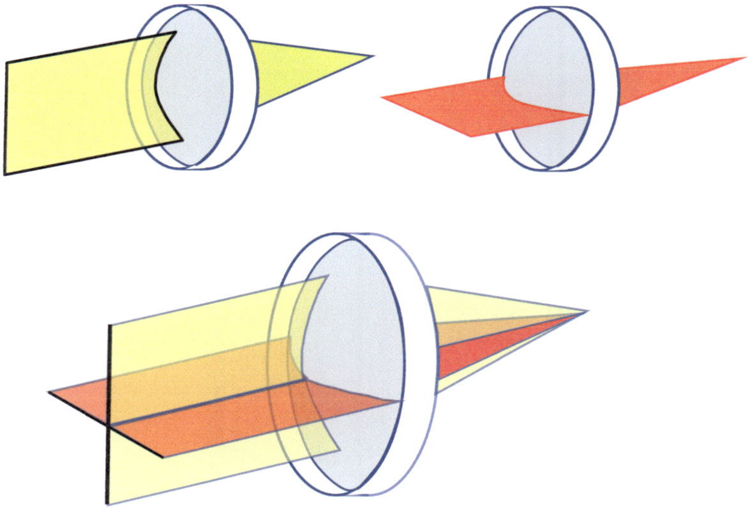

Fig. 1 All incoming light rays that refract through a pure spherical lens will focus at a single point. Notice that the entrance location of the yellow and red light rays differs by 90°, but they both are focused on the same focal point behind the lens

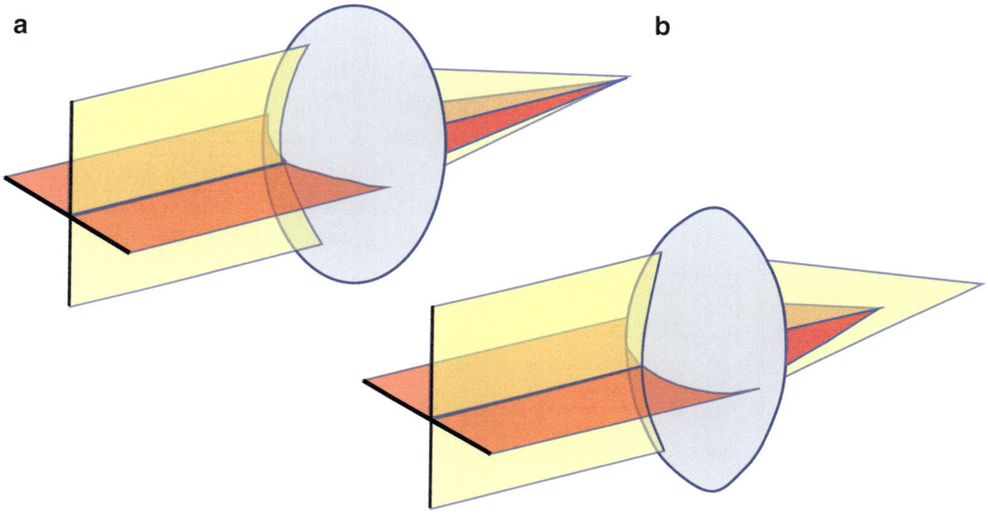

Fig. 2 Comparison of spherical and spherocylindrical lenses. All incoming light rays that pass through a spherical lens (Panel **a**) will be focused to a singular focal point. Incoming light rays passing through a spherocylindrical lens (Panel **b**) will be focused at two distinct focal points. Notice that light along the vertical meridian (flat meridian) is less refracted and converges at a further point

term "IN" to indicate the meridian location of this cylindrical lens. The AM is also the meridian (location) at which a line will form by light rays passing through the cylindrical lens – this latter quality of the AM confuses many trainees.

- Power Meridian (PM): This is the degree (meridian) at which the cylinder is having an effect. We will use the term "AT" to indicate the meridian location of where the cylindrical power is "acting at."

AMs and PMs are easier to understand with a pure cylindrical lens, such as plano +2.00 × 90. Since this is a cylindrical lens, we can envision it like a soda can (Fig. 3). The AM (green line) refers to the meridian in which the cylinder is placed "IN"; in this case, this is 90°. The PM (red line) refers to the meridian at which the cylindrical power is having an effect "AT"; in this case, this is actually 180°.

Notice that the AM and PM are 90° apart in the above example. This concept works for any cylindrical lens, regardless of the value of its AM. Even if the lens was placed in an oblique orientation, the PM will still be 90° away. For example, if we had a plano +2.00 × 45 cylindrical lens, the AM is located in the 45° meridian, and the PM is located at the 135° meridian (Fig. 4).

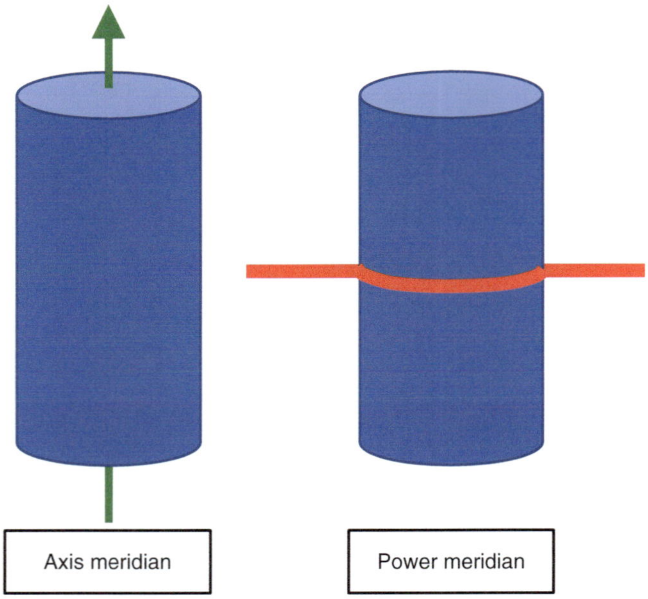

Fig. 3 A cylindrical lens is defined by its axis meridian (green line), which indicates the orientation of the "longer" side of the cylinder. The power meridian indicates where the cylindrical lens's power is "acting at" (red line). The axis meridian and power meridian are always 90° apart

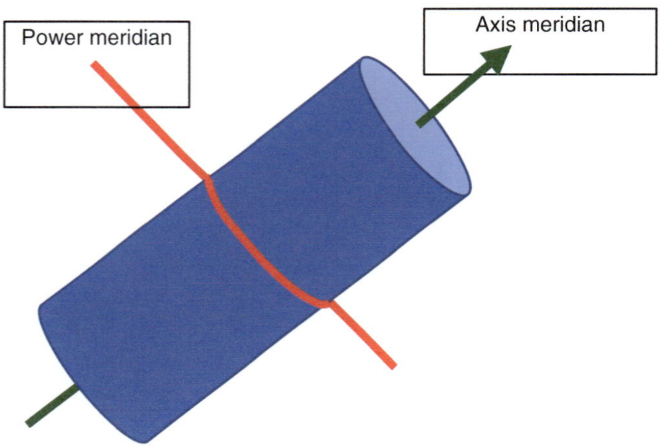

Fig. 4 Axis and power meridians for a plano +2.00 × 45 cylindrical lens. Note that the axis meridian and power meridians are located 90° away, despite the lens having an oblique axis meridian

Cylindrical Lenses: What Happens to Incoming Light Rays?

Note: This section, in particular, is often confusing for trainees because it seemingly contradicts what was introduced in the previous section.

We have just discussed how a cylindrical lens can be used to correct astigmatism: the lens exerts its power *AT* the PM. However, what is happening with the incoming light ray is a slightly different story. In this subtopic, many trainees get lost in the Inferno.

The first key learning point is that *incoming light ray(s) parallel to the AM will not be refracted*. They will not form any focal point or line!

The second key learning point is that *incoming light ray(s) perpendicular to the AM* (i.e., *parallel to the PM) will get refracted by the curvature of the lens (PM)*. They will form a focal point/line ***parallel*** to the AM (Fig. 5).

As a point of clarification, each individual light ray will form a *focal point*. Since numerous light rays enter the lens at a given location, they will form a *focal line*. These will form at a location parallel to the AM (Fig. 6). This concept is understandably confusing, especially on a first-time read of this material. Now do you see why we are in the Inferno?

A cylindrical lens could compensate for the corneal astigmatism of a patient with K readings 43.00 × 46.00 @ 90 (Fig. 7, Panel a). In other words, a lens with its axis (meridian) IN 90° will exert power AT the 180-degree (power) meridian to strengthen the 43D at this location by an extra 3D to equal the 46D at the 90-degree meridian (Panel a). Supplementary hyperopic sphere (Fig. 7, Panel b) and myopic sphere (Fig. 7, Panel c) can be added to the cylinder power based on the refractive error of a given patient.

Please take a minute to re-read the above to make sure you understand it correctly. As much as we want to escape the Inferno, there are several important landmarks to conceptualize clearly--otherwise, we will get even more lost later.

Eyeglasses: Sphere and Cylindrical Lenses

We can tie the previous discussions together by using eyeglass prescriptions involving sphere and cylinder correction as a starting point of reference.

For example, if we are given the prescription for the right eye: −6.00 + 2.00 × 90.

This prescription notation means that +2.00 D of cylinder has been placed IN the 90-degree axis meridian (AM) in order to ACT AT the 180-degree power meridian (PM).

However, because glasses are typically made in minus cylinder, if we were to write such a prescription, our optical shop friends would technically make a pair of glasses such that there is actually a minus cylinder placed in the 180-degree AM. This cylinder acts at the 90-degree PM to direct incoming light to form a horizontal line at 180°.

There is astigmatism throughout the entire lens, but we can think of there being only −6D of power at the 90-degree PM. If the patient looks purely up and down from the optical center, only −6D of power must be considered. We have a slightly different story at the 180-degree meridian. Since we

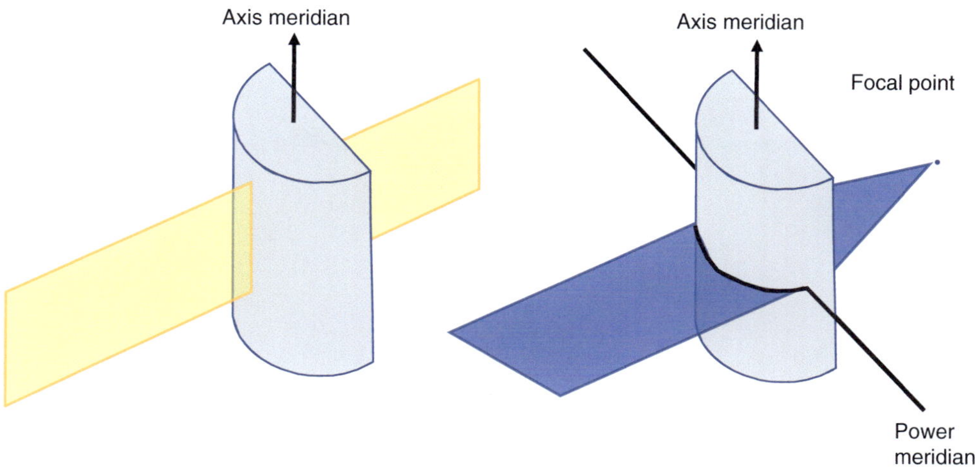

Fig. 5 Incoming light rays parallel to the axis meridian will not be refracted, and they will not form a focal point (or focal line). Incoming light rays perpendicular to the axis meridian (i.e., parallel to the power meridian) will be refracted by the curvature of the lens. Light at this plane will form a focal point/line, which is parallel to the axis meridian. The figure above could represent a cylindrical lens (plano +2.00 × 90). Incoming light that passes through this lens would be refracted as described above

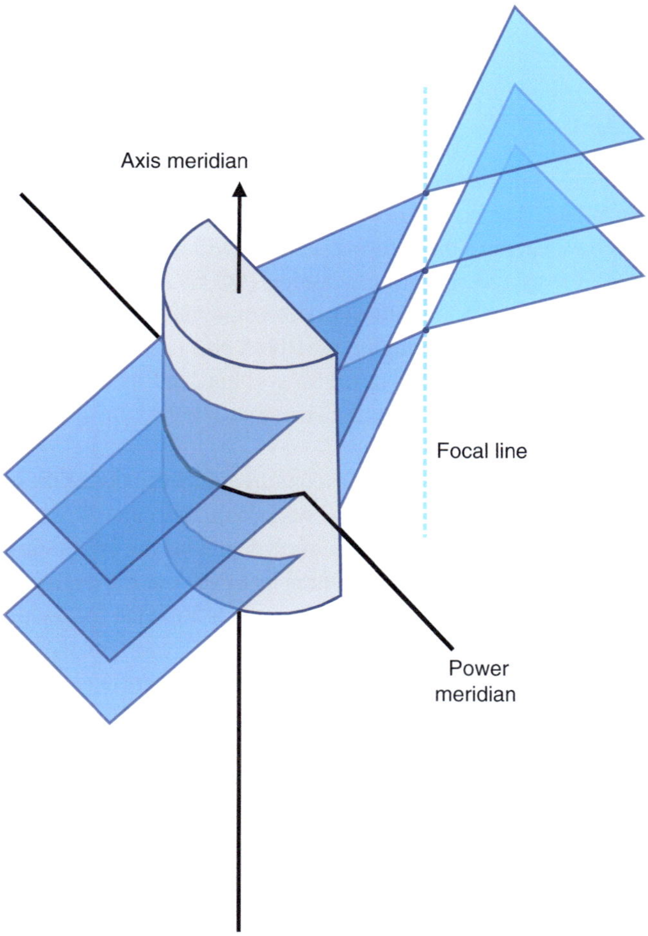

Fig. 6 A focal line is formed by light entering the cylindrical lens at the power meridian

have placed +2D cylinder in the 90-degree AM to ACT AT the 180-degree PM, we have a total of −6 + 2 = −4D of total power at the 180-degree meridian. If that patient looks purely right or left of the optical center, we have to now consider −4D of power. Later in the chapter, we will explore this concept further when we revisit "Prentice's Rule, Part II".

For a patient who requires the above prescription, we can assume that her K measurements (assuming zero lenticular astigmatism) could be: 44.00 × 46.00 @ 90. This means there are 2 D of cylinder AT the 90-degree meridian (WTR astigmatism). Therefore, we have to place 2 D of plus-cylinder IN the 90-degree AM to ACT AT the 180-degree PM (and make it 2 D stronger to equal the 90-degree meridian).

Streak Retinoscopy

Streaking a patient with purely spherical refractive error is relatively straightforward. The same power lens can neutralize the reflex in all directions.[6] However, most patients will require some cylindrical correction as well. Different power lenses will be needed to neutralize the reflex, primarily in meridians located 90° from each other.

Note that some texts and resources will use "when you streak at 90 degrees" when discussing streak results or constantly flip between "at" and "in" nomenclature. In clinic, senior attendings may say, "when you streak in this 90-degree axis…" Again, the nomenclature is somewhat confusing. Some may even argue that having to do 20 streak refractions in a row is a level of punishment within the Inferno.

Both expressions are (hopefully) trying to convey the same message: when we place the streak with a hand-held

[6] See Chap. 15, "Glasses in Clinical Practice", for a more detailed discussion of streak refraction.

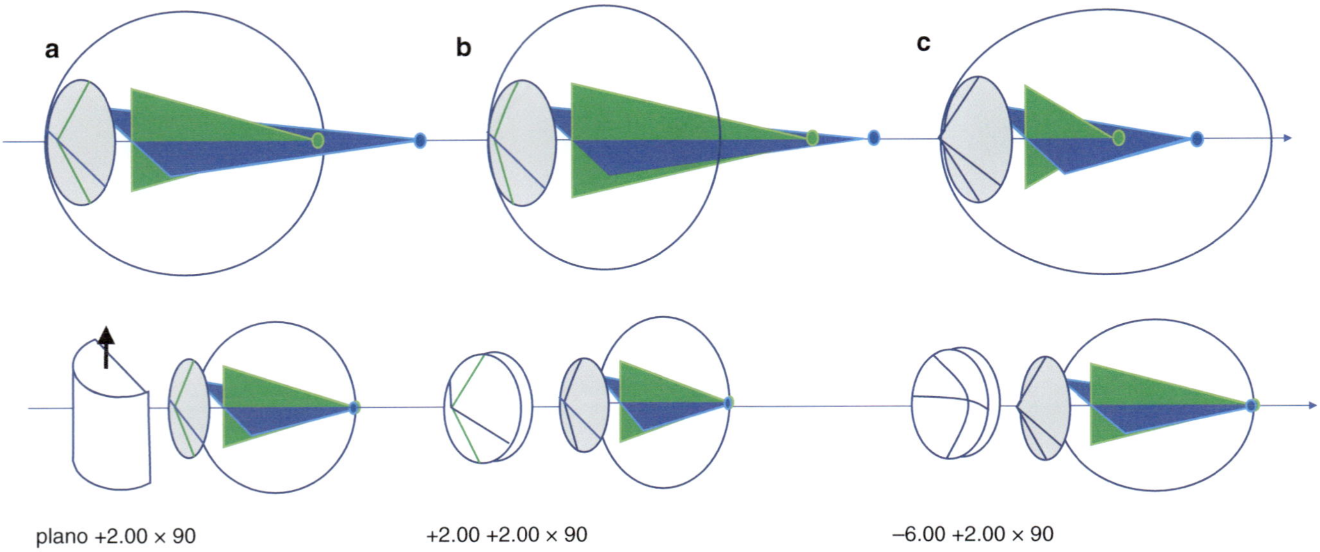

Fig. 7 Corneal (keratometric) astigmatism and cylindrical lens correction. All three panels have a patient with a cornea that is steeper at 90° and flatter at 180°. For example, the keratometry measurements may be 43.00 × 46.00 @ 90 for all three panels. In Panel **a**, an upright cylindrical lens (plano +2.00 × 90) with its axis meridian at 90° will help a patient with astigmatism see better. In Panel **b**, a plus-power spherocylindrical lens (e.g., +2.00 + 2.00 × 90) will help a patient with hyperopic astigmatism. In Panel **c**, a minus-power spherocylindrical lens (e.g., −6.00 + 2.00 × 90) will help a patient with myopic astigmatism

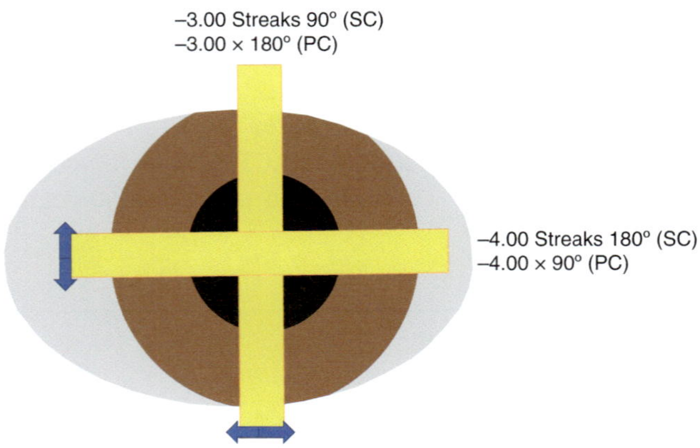

Fig. 8 Streak refraction results for the clinical scenario presented in the text. Notice the nomenclature used to refer to the degree of the streak. The streak results can then be used for either SC notation or PC notation

lens of some power in the 90-degree AM (oriented vertically), we can neutralize with/against motion because the lens is exerting an effect at the 180-degree power meridian.

In order to keep things (hopefully) a bit less confusing, we will use the term "STREAKS the x DEGREE" in order to avoid using the terms of "axis" and "meridian" when discussing streak results. In our previous example, we will instead refer to it as "STREAKS the 90 degree", and the results of that streak should be clear.

Why is this important? Do we enjoy making new names for things that do not need new names? Hopefully, we will see how keeping these terms separate will allow us to work in either spherocylindrical notation (SC notation) or power cross notation (PC notation) to determine the necessary eyeglass prescription. Imagine that both SC notation and PC notation are two different highways that lead us out of the Inferno, so we have to make sure that we get our bearings and directions straight![7]

We can use a streak retinoscopy to compare both of these highways (SC notation and PC notation). Note that SC notation requires us to work in the same degree as the orientation of the streak; PC notation requires us to work at the degree at which the streak is exerting its power. We hope the following examples make these points clearer.

Clinical scenario of streak retinoscopy results (Fig. 8)

- If we move the retinoscope with the streak horizontally oriented and move it up and down (vertically), and the reflex neutralizes with a −4.00 D sphere, we can think of this as "−4.00D STREAKS the 180 degree (SC notation)" or "−4.00 × 90 (PC notation)".

[7] Over the years, trainees have suggested other shortcuts for each of these methods that help them arrive at the correct answer(s) as well. We have chosen here to teach the more commonly employed methods, with each step spelled out, that we have used to teach this topic over the years. As you read this, if you come up with shortcuts that work for you, that is awesome! As long as you get out of the Inferno, we do not care which road(s) you take.

- If we move the retinoscope with the streak vertically oriented and we move it side to side (horizontally), the reflex neutralizes with a −3.00 D sphere. We can think of this as "−3.00 D STREAKS the 90 degree (SC notation)" or −3.00 × 180 "(PC notation)".

There are several ways to take the results of streak retinoscopy and translate them into eyeglass prescriptions. We can now discuss how we can use both SC notation and PC notation to arrive at the same answer.

In general, SC notation works well if you feel comfortable (or enjoy) doing math, like seeing every "step" of the calculation and do not like drawing things out. PC notation works well if you do not like doing math and prefer drawing things out. We will not judge you on which method you take! We just want you to get the answer right (i.e., escape the Inferno).

In order to use either SC or PC notation, we must first determine how to orient the streak results. One way that may be helpful is to think of the streak results as "mini lenses" that we can combine to arrive at the "final lens". If you are given a streak refraction, think of the "SC Lens" written with the axis meridian (i.e., the same degree in which the streak was placed in); the "PC Lens" power is located 90° away from the streak results (i.e., at the power meridian).

Returning to our example, −4.00D streaks the 180 degree and −3.00D streaks the 90 degree:

- SC Lens Power: −4.00D × 180 AND −3.00D × 90
  - Add a "plano" sphere lens in front to further differentiate
  - Rewrite this as: plano − 4.00 × 180 AND plano − 3.00 × 90
- PC Lens Power −4.00D × 90 AND −3.00D × 180
  - For our PC lenses, we are going to write our streak results showing the meridian at which the lens is exerting its power (power meridian).

In the next section, we will work with SC notation; in the section after that, we will work with PC notation.

Spherocylindrical Notation (SC Notation)

Consider the following example: You perform a streak retinoscopy on a patient. A +2.00D lens streaks the 80 and −4.25D lens streaks the 170. We will ignore the working distance for this first example (Fig. 9).

We can use these results to write out our initial SC notation "mini lenses". Note: some texts may also refer to these "mini lenses" as *cross cylinder notation*.

$$\text{Since} + 2.00\ \text{STREAKS 80:SC Lens 1} = +2.00 \times 80\ \left(\text{aka plano} + 2.00 \times 80\right)$$

$$\text{Since} - 4.25\ \text{STREAKS 170:SC Lens 2} = -4.25 \times 170\ \left(\text{aka plano} - 4.25 \times 170\right)$$

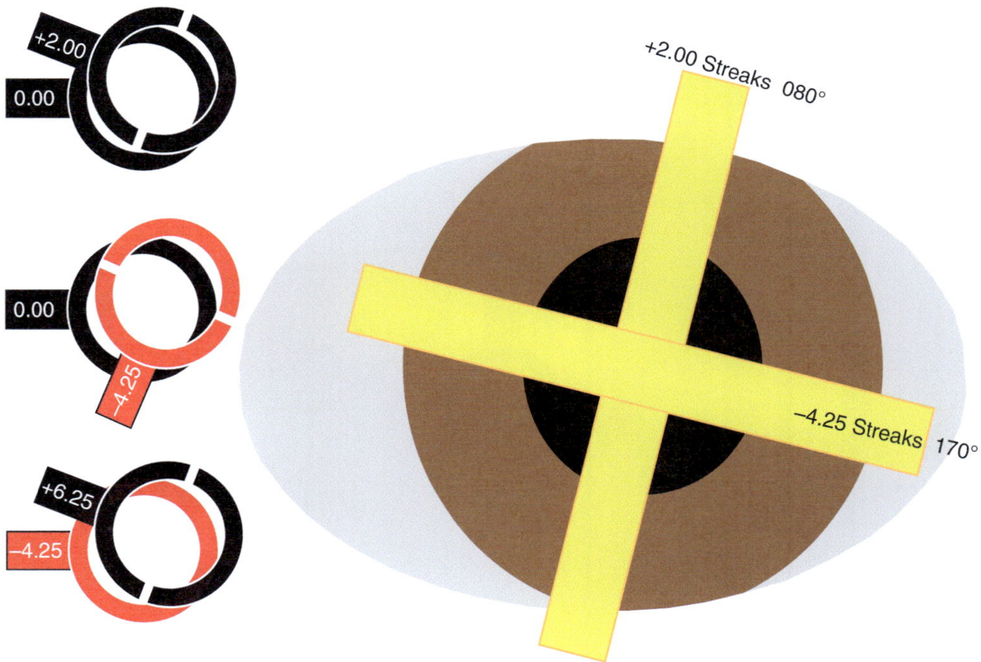

Fig. 9 Streak refraction results: +2.00 STREAKS the 80 and −4.25 STREAKS the 170

Now we can convert Lens 1 to minus cylinder format and Lens 2 to plus cylinder format:

$$\text{Lens 1: plano} + 2.00 \times 80 = \ +2.00 - 2.00 \times 170 \ (\text{minus cylinder format})$$

$$\text{Lens 2: plano} - 4.25 \times 170 = \ -4.25 + 4.25 \times 80 \ (\text{plus cylinder format})$$

Next, we can *algebraically combine* the two notations with the *same axis*; we can use either the two plus cylinder format lenses or the two minus cylinder format lenses. Note, we *must not* try to combine two lenses with different axis notation; otherwise, we will get the wrong answer and remain trapped in the Inferno.

If we took the plus cylinder format lenses:		plano + 2.00 × 80
	(+)	−4.25 + 4.25 × 80
	==========================	
	Final MRx:	−4.25 + 6.25 × 80

We would get the same result if we combined the two lenses in minus cylinder format, and we could check our work by converting that result to plus cylinder format:

	Plano − 4.25 × 170
(+)	+2.00 − 2.00 × 170
=====================	
Final MRx:	+2.00 − 6.25 × 170

We can convert this result to plus cylinder format to check our work: −4.25 + 6.25 × 80.

This second calculation confirms that we can use either the plus cylinder lenses or the minus cylinder lenses to get the same final MRx result. Speaking of the MRx, this is certainly a lot of cylinder! We should make sure our patient does not have a corneal ectasia, or if this is a post-keratoplasty patient, it might be time to cut some sutures.

Let us do another example, but this time we have to incorporate the *working distance*. We want the patient to be able to focus at infinity (or at least at a far enough distance to avoid the terrifying monsters of the Inferno) and not at our retino-

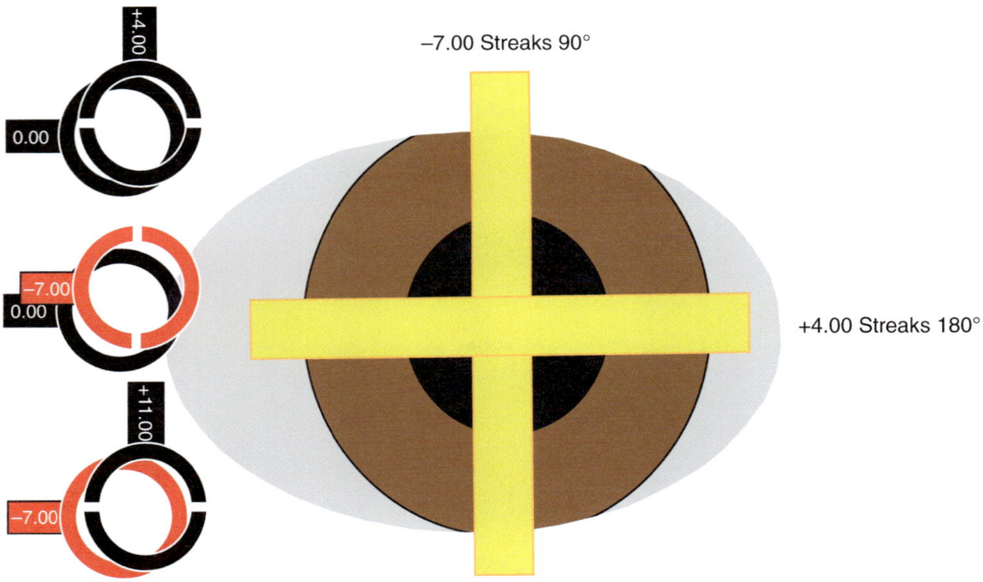

Fig. 10 Streak refraction results: −7D STREAKS the 90 and +4D STREAKS the 180 with a working distance of 67 cm

scope (Fig. 10). Suppose that a −7D lens streaks the 90 and a +4D lens streaks the 180. *Assume a working distance of 67 cm.*

We can again use SC notation to determine the final eyeglass prescription, but this time, we must consider our working distance. We can proceed similarly to the previous example and save the working distance adjustment until the end.

$$\text{SC Lens 1: } +4.00\times 180 = \text{plano} + 4.00\times 180 = (\text{minus cylinder}) + 4.00 - 4.00\times 90$$

$$\text{SC Lens 2: } -7.00\times 90 = \text{plano} - 7.00\times 90 = (\text{plus cylinder})\ -7.00 + 7.00\times 180$$

We can then pick the two prescriptions in the same axis notation and combine them.

plano + 4.00 × 180	plano − 7.00 × 90
+ −7.00 + 7.00 × 180	+4.00 − 4.00 × 90
================	==============
−7.00 + 11.00 × 180	+4.00 − 11.00 × 90

Now that we have our initial results, we have to adjust for working distance (67 cm): Since the working distance is 67 cm, we can determine how much "extra" spherical correction we have to add using the D = 100/f formula, where f is our focal length in centimeters (or working distance, in this case). Therefore, 100/67 = 1.5. For all these working distance problems, we have to *ADD ADDITIONAL MINUS (SPHERE) POWER*, so we have to add an additional −1.5D spherical correction; it is crucial that we do not adjust the cylinder or axis values at this time. Notice the nomenclature that we have specified above: trainees often get confused by the terminology used in clinics, such as "subtract sphere from the refraction" or "take away sphere from the refraction".

When we add an additional −1.5D sphere:

- Final spectacle prescription: −8.50 + 11.00 × 180 +2.50 −11.00 × 90.[8]

Bonus Tip When solving these problems, you may want to look ahead at the answer choices and see what notation (plus cylinder or minus cylinder) is present. This strategy will help you to pick which lenses you will combine accordingly. Alternatively, suppose you chose to combine the two minus cylinder lenses, and the answer choices are listed in plus cylinder format; you can just convert your minus cylinder notation answer into plus cylinder notation. You do not have to start from scratch all over.

We can do one more example using SC notation: a +4.00D lens streaks the 135 and a +6.50D lens streaks the 45. What is the required prescription if the *working distance is 50 cm* (Fig. 11)?

Based on these streak refraction results, we can generate our SC lenses:

$$\text{SC Lens 1: } +4.00\times 135 = \text{plano} + 4.00\times 135 = +4.00 - 4.00\times 45$$

$$\text{SC Lens 2: } +6.50\times 45 = \text{plano} + 6.50\times 45 = +6.50 - 6.50\times 135$$

Now we can algebraically combine two lenses of our choosing in the same axis notation:

$$+4.00 - 4.00\times 45$$
$$\text{plano} + 6.50\times 45$$
$$= = = = = = = = = = = = = = =$$
$$+4.00 + 2.50\times 45$$

Even though we have calculated the +4.00 + 2.50 × 45, we are not done yet - this may likely be a "distractor" answer choice because we have not yet factored in the working distance. Given that the working distance is 50 cm, we have to add an additional 100/50 = −2D to the above result. Hence, the final prescription is +2.00 + 2.50 × 45.

Power Crosses (PC Notation)

Just like SC notation, power crosses can be very confusing. Some texts may refer to this as an "Optical Cross" or "Optical Power Cross".[9] Power crosses are nothing more than a schematic way of describing trial lenses. It may help to remem-

[8] Note that this is a very strange refraction and this patient, with significant ATR astigmatism seen in the plus-cylinder refraction notation, may actually have a corneal ectasia causing the ATR such as pellucid marginal degeneration present! So, while we are monkeying around with this refraction, we should also make sure to get topography on our fictional patient and ensure we are not missing a vision-threatening corneal disease.

[9] Note that a power cross is *not the same* as an axis cross, which will be discussed in the next section.

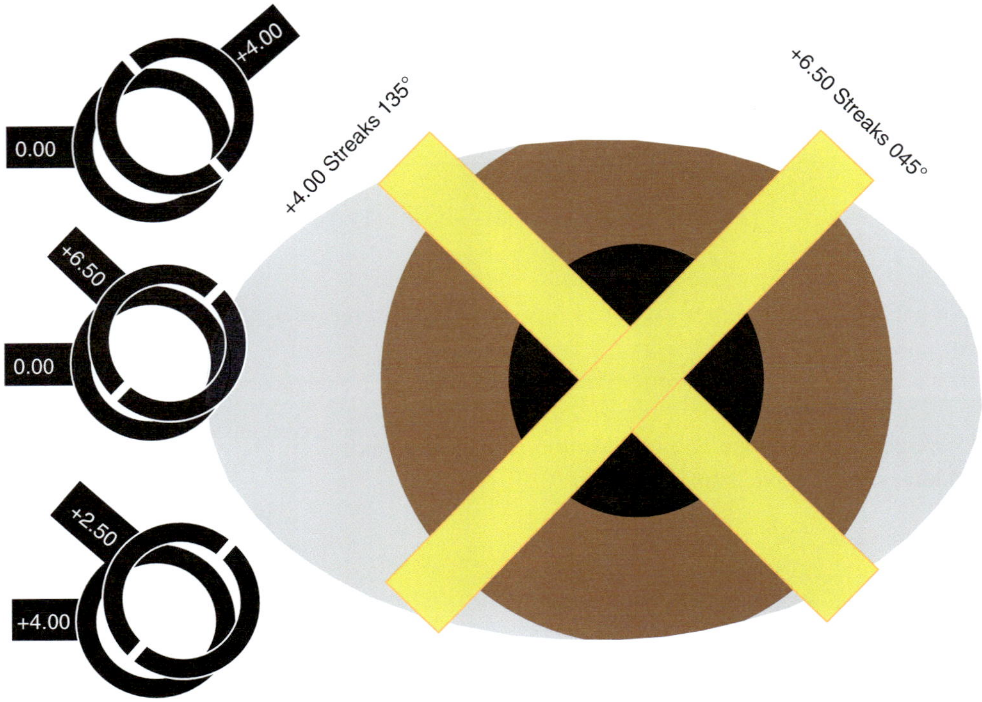

Fig. 11 Streak refraction results: a +4.00D lens STREAKS the 135 and a +6.50D lens STREAKS the 45. The working distance is 50 cm

ber that the purpose of power crosses is to ultimately yield an eyeglass prescription (in addition to making your life miserable). Whereas SC notation depends on a fair amount of math, as seen in the previous section, power crosses rely on far less math and much more visualization. Depending on your learning style, you may find that power crosses make more sense and are easier to work with, so long as your drawings are correctly oriented.

Defining the Power Cross

For starters, let us define a power cross. A Power Cross is a visual representation showing us *where* a cylindrical lens's power is ACTING at. If we have a +3.00 × 90 lens, its axis meridian (AM) is 90°, and its power meridian (PM) is 180°. In other words, this lens will exert power 90° away from the AM. In the figure below, we can map out the orientation (AM, green arrow) versus the power (PM, red arrow) visually using a power cross (Fig. 12). The power cross basically shows us the meridian at which the lens is exerting power (i.e., *where* the lens power is acting at).

Here is another slightly offensive but hopefully unforgettable visual mnemonic to help us remember this point. Imagine as you are trying to get out of Inferno, you are encountering all sorts of monsters and demons trying to stop you from escaping. You decide to give them the middle finger. Now think of your middle finger as the AM, but the "power" (effect) of this gesture is acting 90° away (PM) (Fig. 13).

Similarly, if we are given a +3.00 × 180 cylindrical lens, we can determine that the lens has been placed such that its long side is in the 180-degree AM, but it will exert its power at the 90-degree PM. We can show this on a power cross (Fig. 14).

We can do one more example:

If we are given a cylindrical lens with a power of −3.00 × 90, how can we represent this lens as a power cross?

Since −3.00D has been placed IN the 90-degree AM to exert power AT the 180-degree PM, we can show this on a power cross (Fig. 15).

Using the Power Cross

Now that we have defined them, let us do some streak retinoscopy problems using power crosses (PC). The most significant difference is how we set up our PC based on retinoscopy results, which is the *exact opposite of how we set up our SC notation lenses.*

Example #1 A +4.00D lens STREAKS the 135°, and a +6.50D lens streaks the 45°. Ignore the working distance (for this problem).

If we want to use SC notation, we will start with +4.00 × 135 and +6.50 × 45. However, since we want to work with PC notation, we have to set it up differently. Remember that the +4.00D exerts its power AT 45°, and the +6.50D exerts its power AT 135.

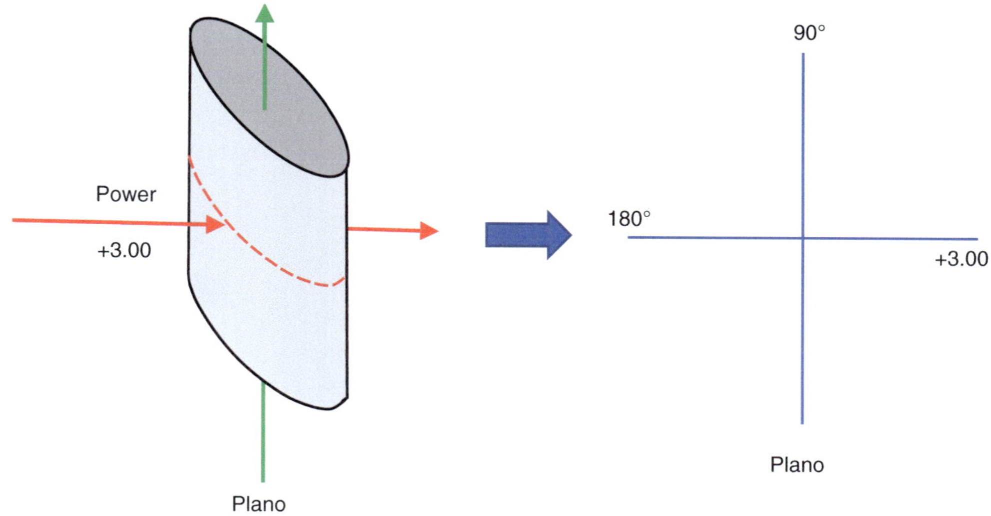

Fig. 12 Visual representation (left panel) of a +3.00 cylindrical lens placed in the 90-degree meridian (AM, green arrow). This lens will exert its power at the 180-degree meridian (PM, red arrow). A power cross (right panel) shows us the meridian at which the lens is exerting power (PM)

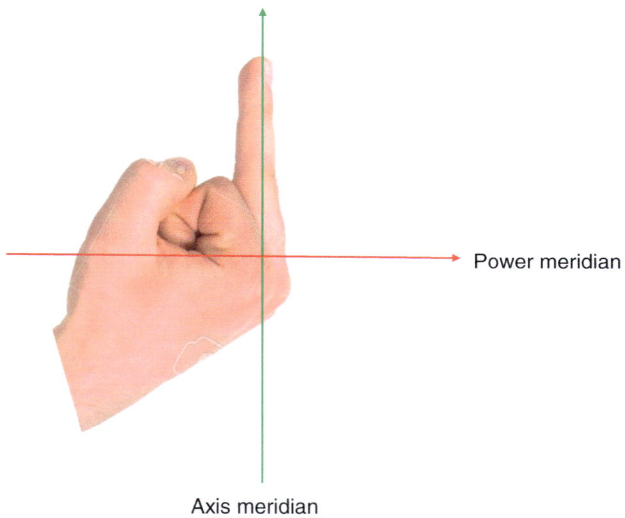

Fig. 13 The middle finger is placed in the 90-degree meridian (axis meridian, green arrow) but is exerting its power at the 180-degree meridian (power meridian, red arrow)

Our PC must show that the +4.00D is connected with the 45-degree meridian, and +6.50D is connected with the 135-degree meridian. We can draw the PC based on these results (Fig. 16).

Once we have our PC, we can now use this diagram to calculate the eyeglass prescription. There are several ways to do this, but one technique is to use a method we have termed the "Double Arches" (apologies to the world's largest fast food restaurant chain, please do not sue us…) Method (DAM).[10] The DAM simply requires you to know how to draw and do some basic addition and subtraction; it may also help you to avoid choosing the wrong axis in your zeal to get the answer. There are three steps to this method:

1. Pick a lens as your **starting sphere** (either one is fine). Usually, starting with the more "minus" lens will allow you to work in plus cylinder notation.
2. Then ask yourself, "How much do I have to add/subtract to this lens to "equal" the other lens". Draw your *first arch* to connect the two lenses. This value is the **cylinder portion** of the eyeglass prescription.
3. Draw your *second arch* that connects this second lens to the adjacent axis. This value is the **axis portion** of the eyeglass prescription. Note, because it is a double arch, *you cannot cross over 180° for the axis* but must instead jump over 90° to get the axis. Feel free to celebrate at this time.

Going back to our above PC example, we can determine the eyeglass prescription using the DAM (Fig. 17).

Applying the DAM to our PC:

1. Suppose we selected +4.00D as our **starting sphere**.
2. Then we can ask ourselves, "How much do we have to *add/subtract* to +4.00 to get to +6.50?" (Arch 1). In this case, it would be +2.50D; this is the **cylinder portion** of the prescription.
3. Then draw the second arch to obtain the axis for the prescription (45). The second arch allows us to make sure we pick "45" instead of accidentally choosing "135".
4. The final eyeglass prescription is: +4.00 + 2.50 × 45.

We could have also used +6.50D as our starting sphere and used the DAM to arrive at the same prescription in minus cylinder notation (Fig. 18).

[10]This acronym may also represent how you are feeling at this point in the chapter.

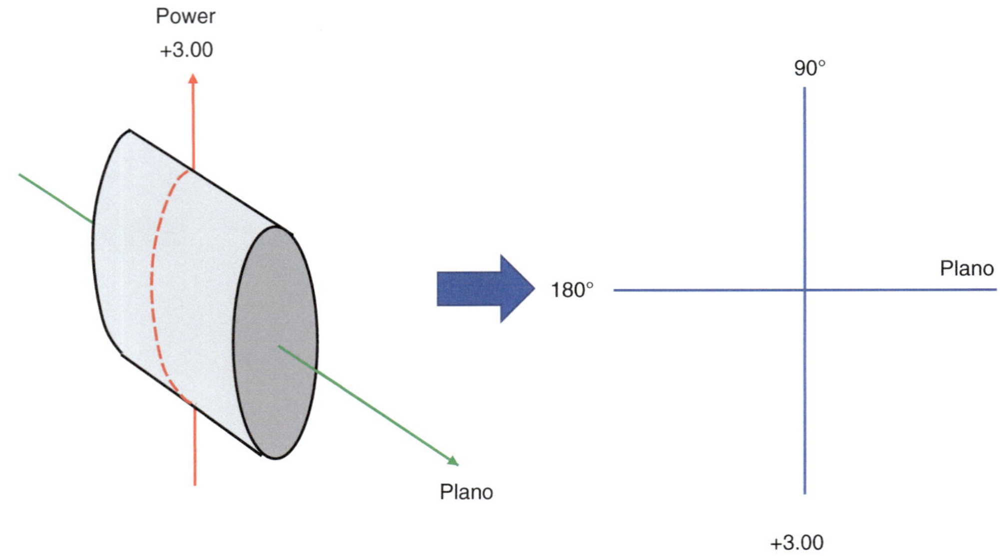

Fig. 14 Visual representation (left panel) of a +3.00 × 180 cylindrical lens. This lens will exert its power at the 90-degree power meridian. A power cross shows that the lens has +3D power at 90° (right panel)

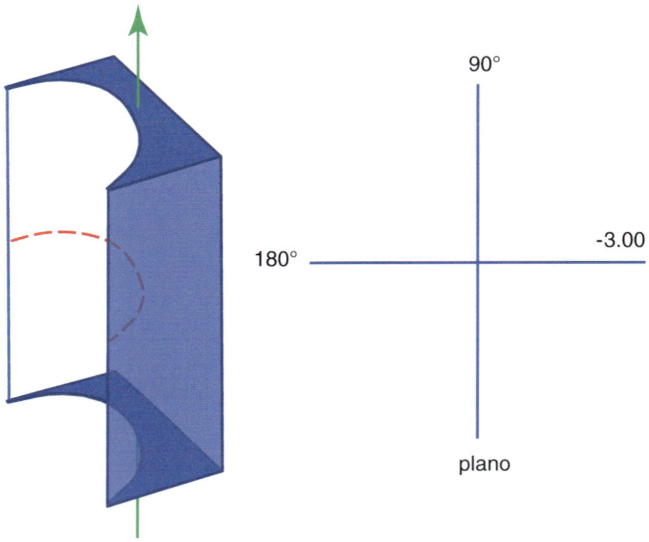

Fig. 15 Power cross for a cylindrical lens −3.00 × 90. Note that this lens has zero power at the 90-degree meridian and −3D power at the 180-degree meridian

DAM applied:

1. The +6.50D is chosen as the **starting sphere**.
2. Then we ask ourselves, "How much do we have to add/subtract to +6.50 to get to +4.00?" In this case, it would be −2.50D for the **cylinder portion** of the prescription.
3. Then draw the second arch to give **axis** of the prescription (135).
4. The final eyeglass prescription is: +6.50 – 2.50 × 135.

Note: we could have also converted either result into the opposite cylinder format to get the answer.

Example #2 We will factor in the working distance this time.

Suppose we perform a streak refraction with the following results: a +3.00D lens streaks the 150°, and a +5.00D lens streaks the 60°. If the working distance is 67 cm, what is the final refraction?

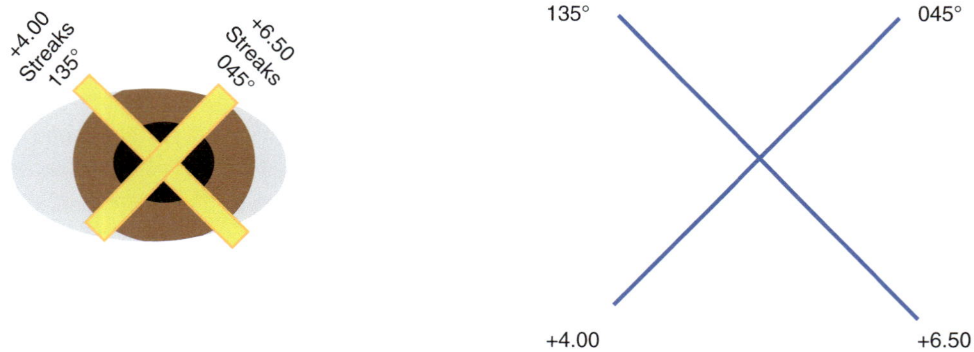

Fig. 16 Power cross drawn from the streak refraction results: +4.00D lens STREAKS the 135° and a +6.50D lens STREAKS the 45°

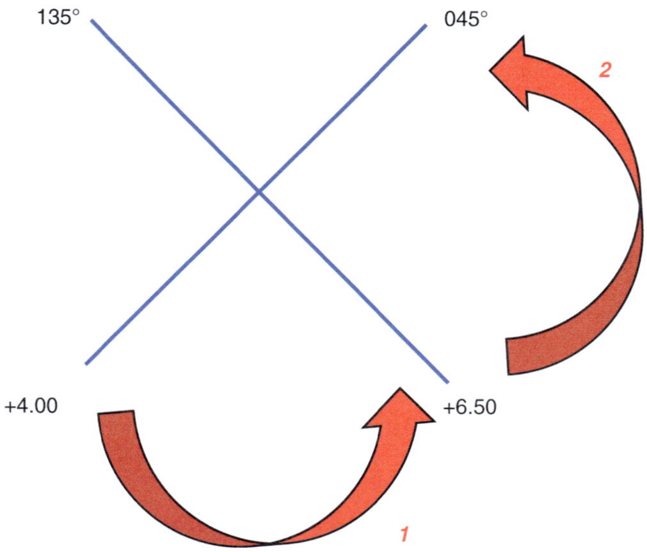

Fig. 17 After setting up a power cross, the Double Arches Method can be used to calculate the final eyeglass prescription. First, pick one of the two spheres as the starting lens; it is recommended to choose the "more minus lens" to work in plus cylinder notation, though this is not a must. Next, draw the first arch to the second sphere and determine how much we must add or subtract to arrive at this second sphere value. This value will be the cylinder power. Third, draw a second arch to the adjacent axis for the axis portion of the prescription. Note that it is crucial to choose a starting lens and proceed in a stepwise fashion taking care to draw the double arches correctly to avoid picking the wrong axis value in the final eyeglass prescription

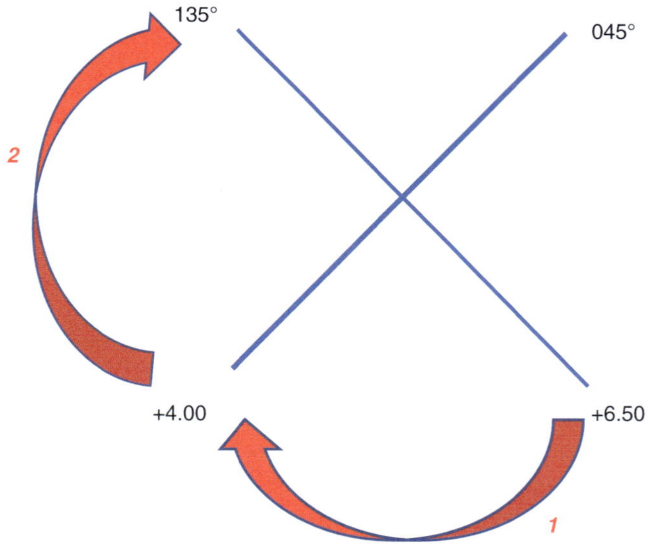

Fig. 18 The DAM can be used for the previous PC above using the +6.50D lens as the starting lens. Note that this result will yield an eyeglass prescription in minus cylinder format

We know that the +3.00D lens exerts its power AT the 60-degree meridian, and the +5.00D lens exerts its power AT the 150-degree meridian. We can draw our PC to show this relationship (Fig. 19).

We can then use the DAM (Fig. 20).

The steps of the DAM are:

1. Select +3.00D as our **starting sphere** (the more minus of the two spheres).
2. Then we can ask ourselves, "How much do we have to add/subtract to this starting sphere to get to +5.00?" In this case, it would be +2.00D, which would be the **cylinder portion**. Draw our first arch.
3. Then we can draw a second arch to the **axis** (60).
4. The refraction would be: +3.00 + 2.00 × 60, but are not finished yet!
5. Now factor in the working distance of 67 cm (additional −1.5D sphere) for the final eyeglass prescription: +1.50 + 2.00 × 60.

Notice that if we had chosen the +5.00D as our starting lens, we could still apply the DAM, but our result would be in minus cylinder: +5.00 − 2.00 × 150. Factor in the working distance (additional −1.5D sphere), and the final prescription would be: +3.50 − 2.00 × 150.

Reconciling SC Notation and PC Notation

We can also prove to ourselves that we can use SC notation and PC notation interchangeably, taking care to follow the rules of each, and get the same result. Again, we just need to find any road that will lead us out of the Inferno.

Applying SC Notation and PC Notation to Same Streak Refraction

Looking back at the first example we used for SC notation, we can now use PC notation to get the same result.[11]

In that example (Fig. 9), the streak results were: +2.00D STREAKS the 80 and −4.25D STREAKS the 170. When we did SC notation, we set the SC lenses as +2.00 × 80 and −4.25 × 170.

For power crosses, we have to "flip" these lens results since the +2.00D is acting at the 170-degree meridian and the

[11] #ProTip. You can use one method and then use the other to "check your work" for extra practice.

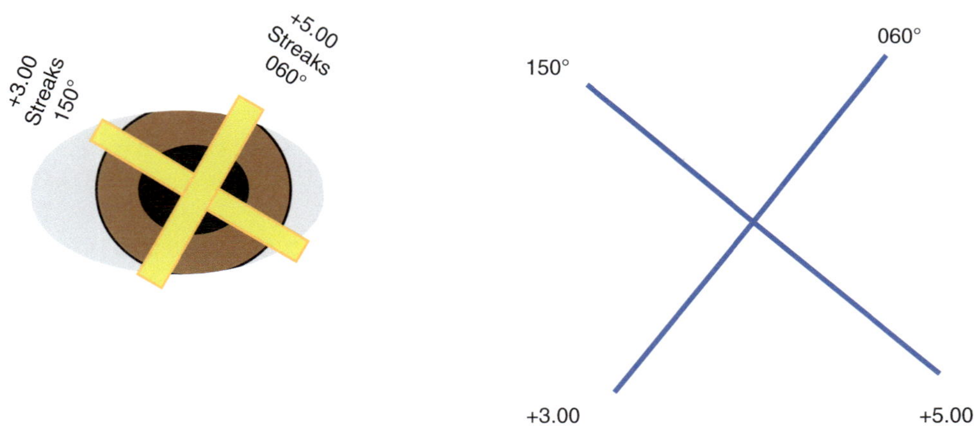

Fig. 19 Power cross indicating the +3.00D lens is exerting its power at the 60-degree meridian, and the +5.00D lens is exerting its power at the 150-degree meridian

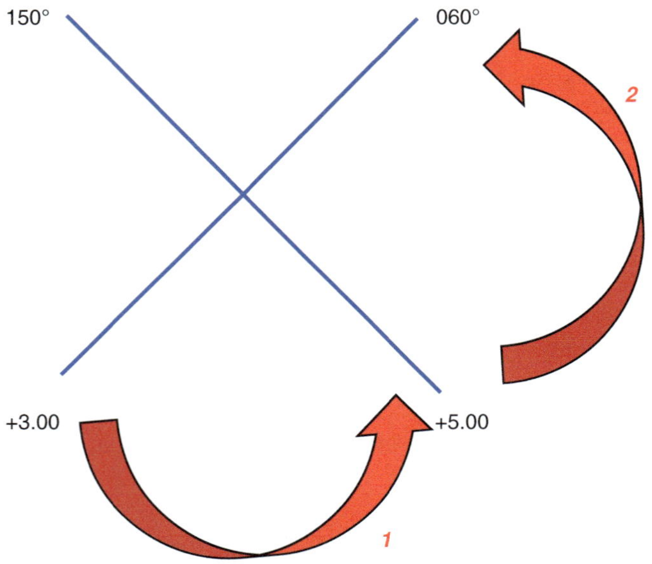

Fig. 20 Double Arches Method applied to the power cross derived in Fig. 19

−4.25D lens is acting at the 80-degree meridian. We can use this information to draw our PC (Fig. 21).

We can then use the DAM to determine the eyeglass prescription (Fig. 22).

1. Choose −4.25D as the **starting sphere**.
2. Then we have to draw an arch to +2.00 and ask ourselves, "How much do we have to add/subtract to −4.25 to get to +2.00?" In this case, it would be +6.25D, which is the **cylinder** of the eyeglass prescription.
3. Then draw a second arch to yield the **axis** of the eyeglass prescription (80).
4. The final prescription would be: −4.25 + 6.25 × 80.

This answer is the same result that we calculated with SC notation. We will pause here while you celebrate, recover from having your mind blown, or some combination thereof.

Miscellaneous Topics

Another way these problems may be presented is by giving you two "cylindrical lenses" and asking you to express these problems in SC notation, PC notation, or as an eyeglass prescription.

Example: A patient can see well by combining two trial cylindrical lenses: +2.00 × 120 and −2.25 × 30. Ignoring the working distance, determine the needed eyeglass prescription.

A. SC Notation: Make the "SC lenses" directly from the cylinder lens notation

   Plano +2.00 × 120 and Plano – 2.25 × 30

   (convert first lens to minus cylinder and second lens to plus cylinder)

   +2.00 − 2.00 × 30 and −2.25 + 2.25 × 120

   (then add either pair of lenses in the same axis notation)

   Eyeglass prescription: −2.25 + 4.25 × 120 OR +2.00 − 4.25 × 30.

   Note: This may also be written as: "−2.25 with +4.25 × 120" OR "+2.00 with −4.25 × 30". This notation is a slightly archaic way of speaking about an eyeglass prescription, but we will mention it here if it ever shows up unexpectedly on an examination.

B. PC Notation: We know that the +2.00D acts at the 30-degree meridian and the −2.25D acts at the 120-degree meridian. We can generate our PC and use the DAM (Fig. 23).

Fig. 21 Power cross drawn from the streak refraction results used to obtain SC notation lenses in the example from Fig. 9. Notice how the PC will differ from the SC notation in its setup but should still yield the same result

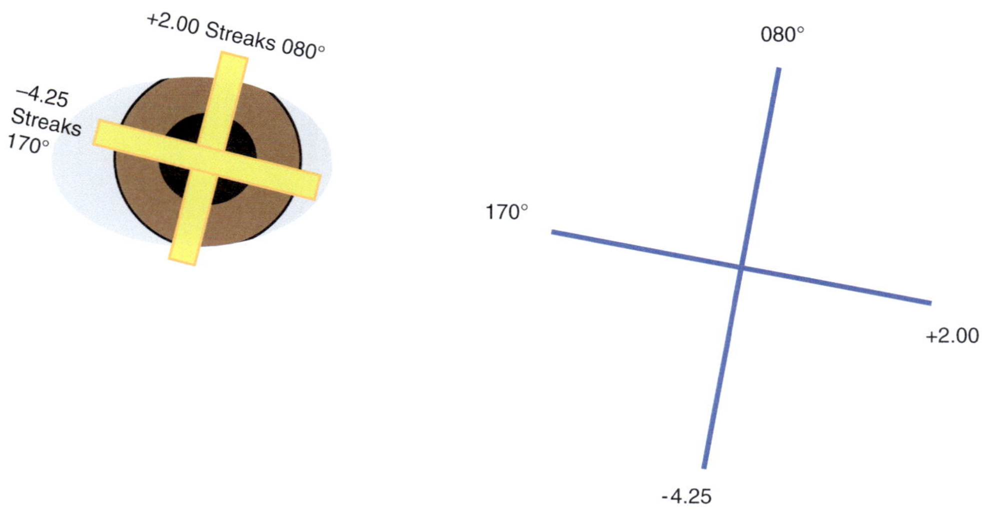

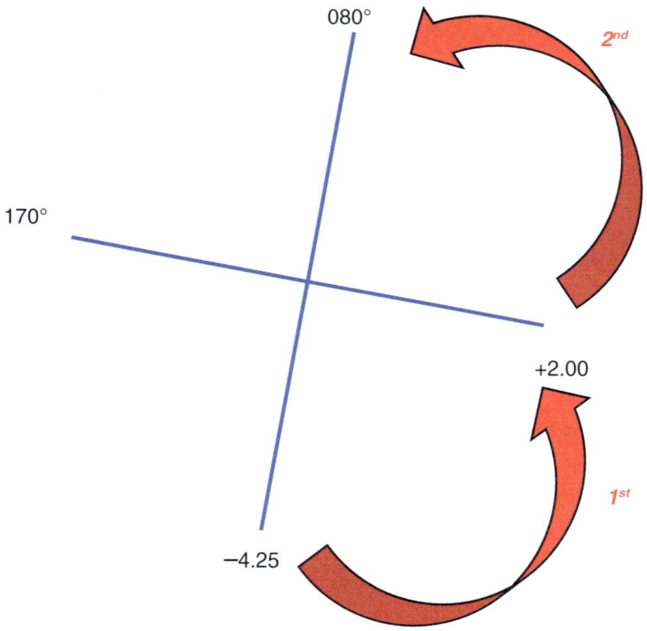

Fig. 22 The Double Arches Method can be applied to the power cross derived in Fig. 21

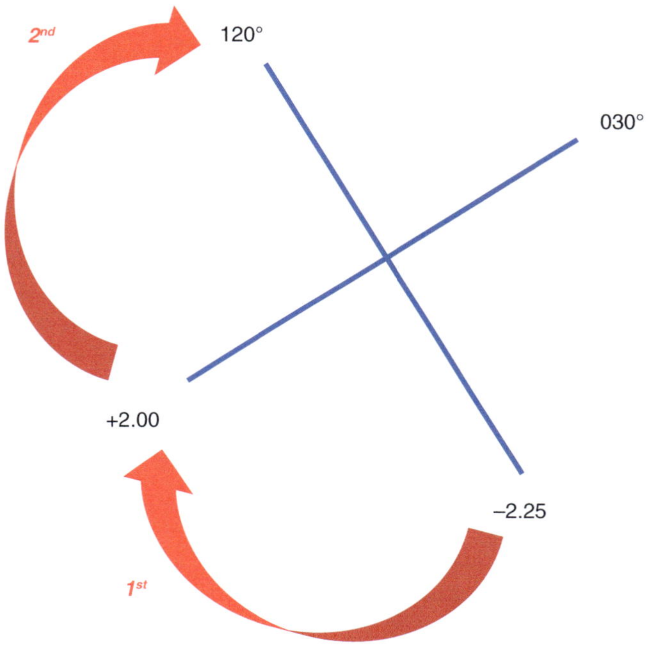

Fig. 23 The Double Arches Method can be used on the generated power cross to determine the final eyeglass prescription

Eyeglass prescription: $-2.25 + 4.25 \times 120$ OR $+ 2.00 - 4.25 \times 30$

C. Eyeglass Prescription
   1. Same with either method! Both should yield $-2.25 + 4.25 \times 120$ (plus cylinder) or $+2.00 - 4.25 \times 30$ (minus cylinder). Factor in the working distance as needed.

Finally, we can also use a given eyeglass prescription to generate a power cross. There is not much usefulness in doing this (other than to maybe generate streak refraction results as a working point to titrate a streak refraction further). However, if we were ever asked to do this, the "Telephone Method" can be used (to derive power crosses, unfortunately not useful for calling for help to escape the Inferno). Note that this method may need to be renamed in a few years because no one uses telephones shaped like this anymore!

When given a starting prescription, the Telephone Method can be used as follows:

1. Write the given prescription in the opposite cylinder format. Thus, write out the minus cylinder format directly underneath if we are given the prescription in plus cylinder format.
2. Then draw a "telephone shape" around the sphere and axis values ONLY. Ignore the cylinder values at this time.

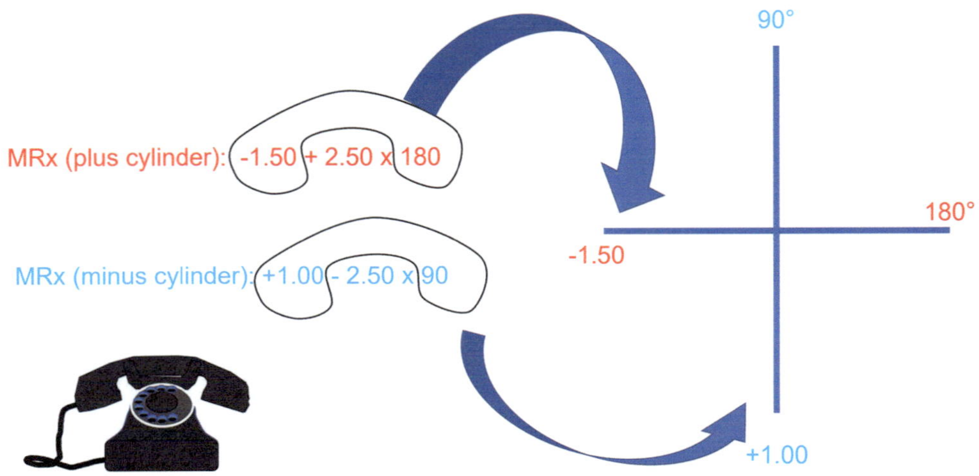

Fig. 24 If given an eyeglass prescription, we can use the Telephone Method to derive a power cross. This method involves drawing a telephone shape around the sphere and axis values to generate the power cross. A visual representation of an "ancient" telephone has been added for those readers born after the year 1990

3. Think of this "telephone shape" between the sphere and axis as the lines of the power cross.

For example, if we are given a starting prescription of −1.50 + 2.50 × 180 (Fig. 24):

1. Start by first writing out the minus cylinder format directly underneath: +1.00 − 2.50 × 90.
2. Then draw two telephone shapes around just the sphere and axis values. These can be connected to make the power cross.
3. Now we can draw the power cross.
4. Finally, you can use the DAM to check your work and see if you can get back to the starting prescription. If we have made the power cross correctly, we should be able to get back to our starting prescription.

Axis Cross

If you have thus far understood SC notation and PC notation and do not want to confuse yourself any further, feel free to skip ahead to the next section. However, if you want to learn of a potential third road that can lead you out of Inferno, then read on to learn about the axis cross. Admittedly, this method is not as popular or common, but it can still be used to derive an eyeglass prescription.

The advantage of an axis cross (compared to a power cross) is that we can take the streak refraction results and draw an axis cross without having to "cross-up" the streak results. However, if we choose to draw an axis cross, we *cannot* use the DAM to determine the final eyeglass prescription. Remember, the DAM can *only* be used for power crosses.

We can do one quick example and move on:

Suppose we perform streak retinoscopy on a patient and obtain the following results: a +1.50D streaks the 180° and a +4.00D streaks the 90°. We will ignore working distance.

The critical difference in drawing the axis cross is that we *do not have to flip* the streak refraction results. We can basically use the SC notation "lenses" as the connections of the axis cross (Fig. 25). We have also drawn a power cross next to the axis cross for comparison purposes.

If we choose to use an axis cross, we can still start by choosing either sphere as our starting sphere lens. We can also ask ourselves our familiar question: "how much do we have to add/subtract to this lens to get to the other?" In this case, suppose we chose +1.50D as our starting lens. We would have to add +2.50 to get to +4.00; therefore, the +2.50D becomes our cylinder. Now we have to choose our axis, and here is the crucial difference when using an axis cross as compared to a power cross: instead of swinging over to "180" as our axis with a "double arch", we *must remain in the +2.50D axis*, which is "90". In other words, we do *not* make a second arch as we do with our power cross.

Using the axis cross, our prescription would be: +1.50 + 2.50 × 90.

Note that we can use our PC notation as described in the previous section, generate our familiar PC, and use the DAM to get the same eyeglass prescription (right panel of Fig. 19).

Most people do not like axis crosses. Again, you do not have to work in axis cross notation if you do not understand it. Just find any road to get out of Inferno.

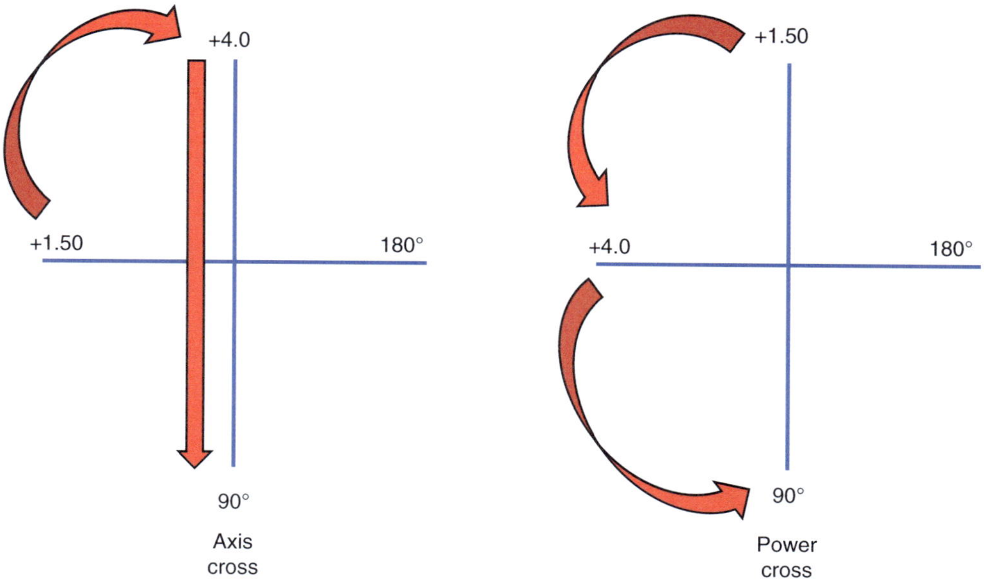

Fig. 25 Axis cross versus power cross. Streak refraction results can be used to set up the axis cross without having to flip the results. Note that the DAM *cannot* be used with an axis cross

Keratometry Readings and Eyeglasses Prescriptions

As we started off the chapter discussing keratometry readings, we can return briefly to this topic to discuss a few additional details, especially when using these measurements to generate eyeglass prescriptions. Note that this is not very clinically useful since it assumes all of the refractive astigmatism is contained within the keratometric astigmatism, but this may come up on exams.

One way to look at keratometry readings is to imagine that the flat meridian is the "little brother" and the steep meridian is the "big brother". The little brother is weaker than the big brother. A plus-cylinder lens will give the little brother additional power to equal the big brother. Similarly, a minuscylinder lens will weaken the big brother to equal the little brother.

For example, if we measure a patient's cornea and the keratometry readings are: 43.00 × 45.00 @ 95, the flat meridian (5°) is the little brother, and the steep meridian (95°) is the big brother. Now we can ask ourselves: "How much "help" should we give the little brother, using plus cylinder, to equal the stronger big brother?" Since the lower keratometry value needs cylinder "help", we need to place the plus cylinder IN the *steep* meridian so that it ACTS AT the *flat* meridian. In other words, the cylinder's axis meridian (AM) has to be parallel to the steep meridian; this will make the power meridian (PM) parallel to the flat meridian. Remember, somewhat confusingly, light rays that pass through this cylindrical lens will form a line at the AM.

For example, if we are given keratometry readings presented with a slightly different notation: 41.50 @ 30 and 44.50 @ 120,[12] we can understand these readings as follows:

- The 41.50 @ 30 is the little brother. The 44.50 @ 120 is the big brother. In this case, the big brother is stronger than the little brother by 3 D.
- In order to help the little brother, we need to give "him" +3D of cylinder power.
- We have to place +3D of cylinder IN the steep meridian (120°) so that it ACTS AT the flat meridian (30°).
- This "helping cylinder" lens can be written as: +3.00 × 120; the AM is the 120-degree meridian, and the PM is the 30-degree meridian.
- Alternatively, you could choose to work in minus cylinder notation and would need −3D to weaken the big brother. In this case, we could place the −3D of cylinder IN the flat meridian (30°) so that it ACTS AT the steep meridian (120°) to weaken it.

If we were asked to dispense an eyeglass prescription to correct this keratometric astigmatism *while maintaining a spherical equivalent of plano*, the dispensed prescription would be:

[12]Note in this presentation the flat meridian has also been indicated. In the first example, an abbreviated form was used wherein the flat meridian can be deduced as 90° away from the steeper meridian.

$$\text{Plus Cylinder}: -1.50 + 3.00 \times 120 \ (\text{or Minus Cylinder}: +1.50 - 3.00 \times 30).$$

We can do another example. If we are given keratometry values of 42.50 @ 45 and 44.50 @ 135, what is the power of the glasses that we must dispense to maintain a spherical equivalent (SE) of −1.00D?

- First, identify the little brother (42.50 @ 45) and the big brother (44.50 @ 135). In this case, the big brother is stronger than the little brother by 2D.
- In order to help the little brother, we need +2.00D to be placed IN the 135-degree (steep) meridian so that it ACTS AT the 45-degree (flat) meridian: +2.00 × 135.
- Finally, since we have to maintain the SE of −1.00D, we have to add additional minus sphere power: −2.00 + 2.00 × 135 (or: plano – 2.00 × 45).

Prentice's Rule, Part II: Spherocylindrical Lenses

Previously, on "Prentice's Rule" (see Chap. 2, "Prisms in Ophthalmic Optics"), a show that no streaming provider has picked up for a second season, we discussed how this rule applies to the change in the functional power of a lens when one looks away from the optical center. Remember that Prentice's Rule states that this change can be calculated using the formula: $P = h * D$, where h is the distance (in centimeters) from the optical center of the lens, and D is the power of the lens. In the previous discussion, all of our examples only used spherical lenses. In this section, we will discuss how to use Prentice's Rule when we are given spherocylindrical lenses.

Incorporating Cylinder Power Based on Gaze Position

For example, if we are given an eyeglass prescription: −3.00 + 2.00 × 180:

This means that +2.00D cylinder power will be *placed IN* the 180-degree axis meridian in order to *act AT* the 90-degree power meridian.

With Prentice's Rule problems dealing with spherocylindrical lenses, we have to determine the net "prism power" at a given meridian, considering the cylinder present. The key question is, when given a spherocylindrical lens, when must we incorporate the cylinder power?

Depending on which part of the lens the patient is "looking through", we must account for the cylinder (if present) in that gaze position.

We can compare the prismatic effect of spherical lenses and spherocylindrical lenses at different locations from the optical center. It is important to note a −5D sphere lens will have −5D power at all locations when measured with a lensmeter, but the prismatic effect will be different based on the distance from the optical center. For example, Fig. 26 shows the prismatic effects of a −5D lens when measured in the center of the lens as compared to its inferior portion. Notice the increasing prismatic power when the lens is measured at an increasing distance away from the optical center. Figure 27 shows a +5D lens with similar increasing prism power when measuring away from the optical center. Figure 28 shows a spherocylindrical lens (−3.00 +2.00 × 90) that has the same power throughout the lens, but the prismatic effect will be *asymmetrical*.

Some helpful rules are as follows:

- Cylinder power placed in the 90-degree axis meridian will have an effect AT the 180-degree power meridian and therefore only play a role if the patient looks to either side (left or right) of the optical center.
  - Ex: −5.00 + 1.75 × 90 = when looking up and down, only the −5D has "prism power". So, if a patient looks vertically away (up and down) from the optical center of this lens, it basically functions as a −5D lens.
- Cylinder power placed in the 180-degree axis meridian will have an effect AT the 90-degree power meridian, and therefore only play a role if the patient looks up or down relative to the optical center.
  - Ex: −5.00 + 1.75 × 180 = when looking left and right, only the −5D has "prism power". So, if a patient looks horizontally away from the optical center of this lens, it basically functions as a −5D lens.

Notice that we are conveniently only considering the sphere power in a chosen gaze direction in each of these examples. However, if the patient looks horizontally or vertically, respectively, we have to account for the cylinder power in each of the previous two examples. When considering the cylinder effect at these gaze positions, we can convert the eyeglass prescription from plus cylinder to minus cylinder notation and then apply the new "sphere" value to the new "axis meridian" to determine how much power is present.

Using our two examples from above:

- For the −5.00 + 1.75 × 90 lens, we can convert to minus cylinder: −3.25 – 1.75 × 180. Therefore, if a patient looks to the right and left of the optical center of this lens, it would basically function as a −3.25D prism lens.

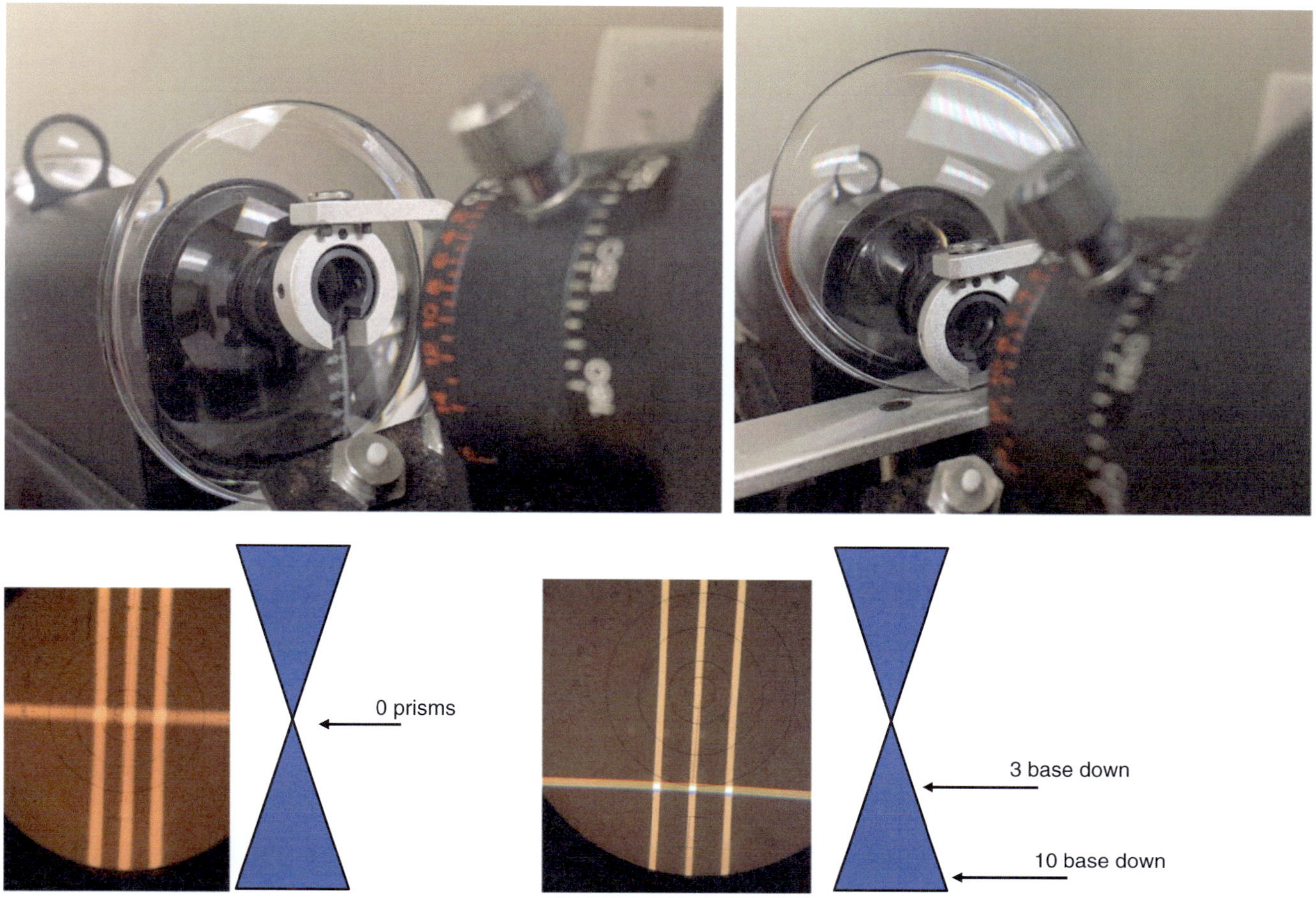

Fig. 26 How much prism power do different parts of a −5D lens have? There is no prismatic effect at the center of the lens (left panel). When measuring inferior to the optical center (right panel), there is an increasing base-down prism measured. The prismatic effect of the lens increases linearly as we increase the distance from the optical center

- For the −5.00 + 1.75 × 180, we can convert to minus cylinder: −3.25 − 1.75 × 90. Therefore, if a patient looked vertically up and down relative to the optical center of this lens, it would basically function as a −3.25D prism lens.

When doing the following problems, it may help to convert between plus cylinder and minus cylinder notation to get the desired "axis" of the eyeglass prescription depending on the gaze position. Usually, for these problems, cylinder notation will likely be in 90-degree or 180-degree form, and the patient will be looking horizontally or vertically. Other degree notations and gaze positions will require vector addition (and calculators) and will not likely be tested on examinations.

Additional Examples

Example #1

If we are given a right eye lens with a prescription of +2.50 + 1.75 × 90, what is the induced prismatic effect in each of the following circumstances?

(a) If we look 10 mm below the optical center
(b) If we look 10 mm temporal to the optical center

If we first look 10 mm below the optical center:

- When looking vertically up and down, ONLY the +2.75D is having an "effect" because +1.75D is acting at the 180-degree meridian.
- We can safely ignore the +1.75 cylinder and draw out our "functional lens" as a simple +2.50D in downward gaze (Fig. 29).

We can use our familiar Prentice's Rule equation, remembering to convert 10 mm to 1 cm: $P = hD = 1\text{ cm} \times 2.5\text{D} = 2.5$ prism diopters BU.

Now if we look 10 mm *temporal* to the optical center with the right eye:

- Because we are looking to the side, cylinder power placed in the 90-degree meridian will have an effect at the 180-degree meridian (nasal and temporal gaze), and we must account for this "prism power".

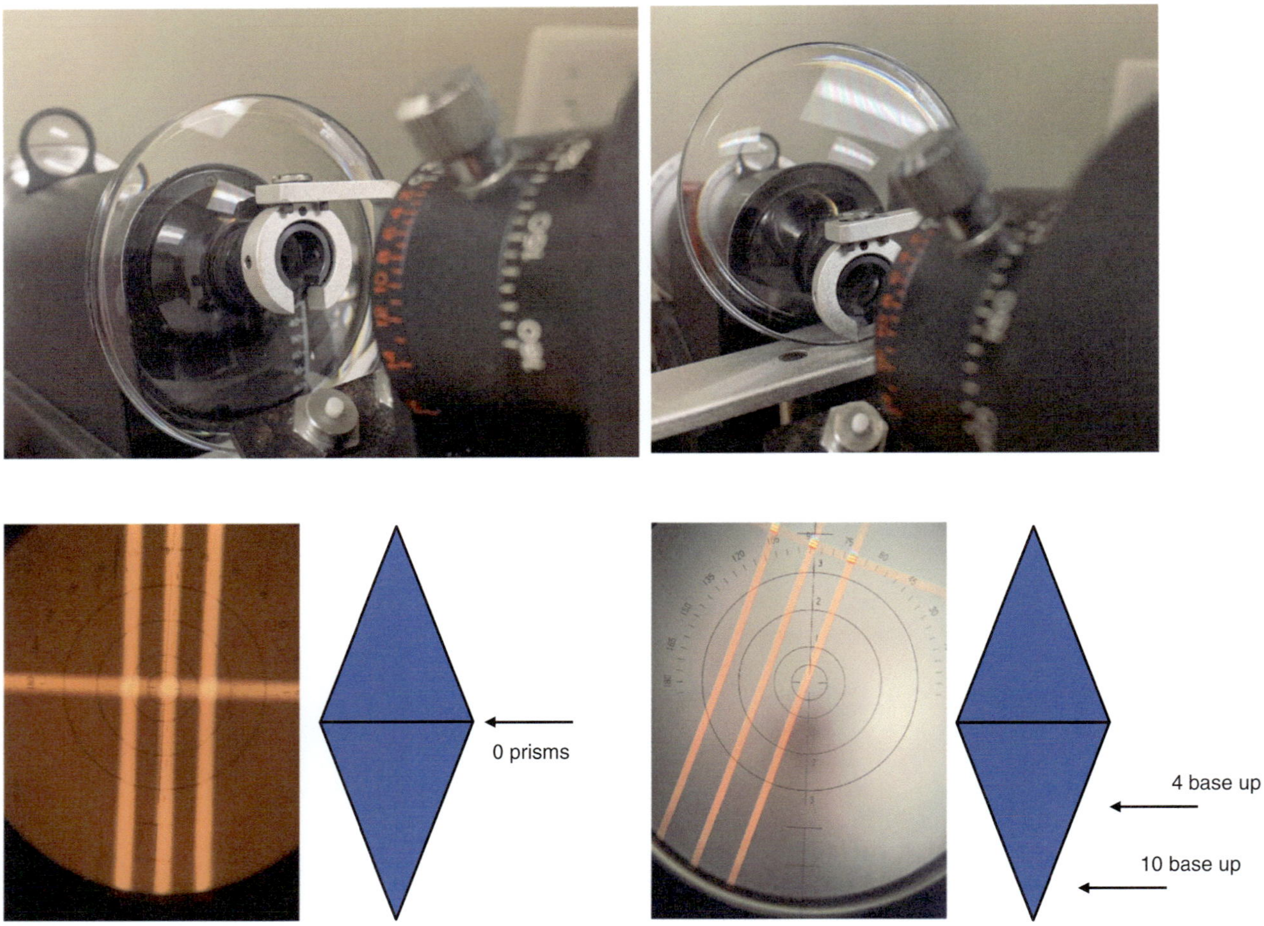

Fig. 27 How much prism power do different parts of a +5D lens have? There is no prismatic effect at the center of the lens (left panel). When measuring inferior to the optical center (right panel), increasing base-up prism is measured. The prismatic effect of the lens increases linearly as we increase the distance from the optical center

- We can convert to minus cylinder so that we have a new "sphere" power to deal with: Minus cylinder = +4.25 − 1.75 × 180.
- We can safely ignore the −1.75D cylinder and realize that this lens will basically function as a +4.25D lens when looking temporally to the optical center. This "new lens" can be drawn out as Fig. 30.

We can use Prentice's Rule once more: $P = hD$ = 1 cm × 4.25D = 4.25 prism diopters BI. Note that drawing out this lens can help from wrongly thinking there is a base-out effect. We are nearly out of the Inferno, so we do not want to make any mistakes.

Example #2
If we are given a pair of glasses with the same prescription (−1.50 + 5.00 × 90) in each lens, what is the net induced prism:

(a) When we look 8 mm inferior to the optical center (in each eye)
(b) When we look 12 mm temporal to the optical center (in each eye)

First off, why are wasting time looking off-center on a pair of glasses when we are nearly out of Inferno? Second, let us go ahead and solve this problem anyway.

Only the −1.5D has to be accounted for in inferior gaze because the +5.00D is placed in the 90-degree meridian and will only have power at the 180-degree meridian.

- In inferior gaze, only the −1.5D has an effect: we can draw these as two minus lenses with the green dots representing where we are looking relative to the optical center. This will immediately show us a BASE DOWN effect present (Fig. 31). Now we can use our Prentice's Rule equation.

- $P = hD$ = 0.8 × 1.5D = 1.2 prism diopters base down.
- There is no net prism effect because both eyes have moved "down".

In temporal gaze, if we look 12 mm temporal to the optical center of this pair of glasses (imagine that the pupillary distance of the glasses is much too small for our face), we can determine the net prismatic power:

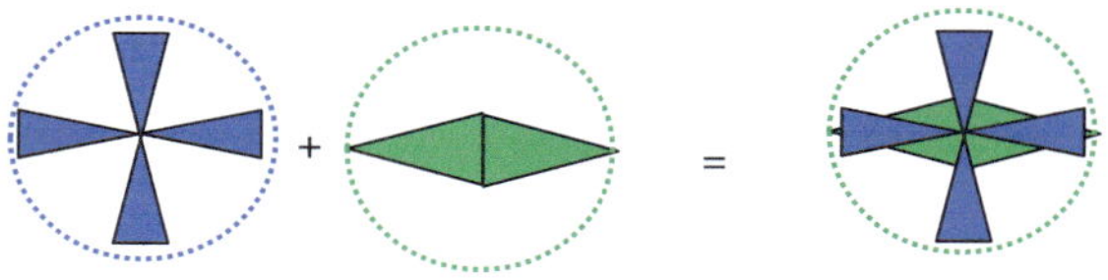

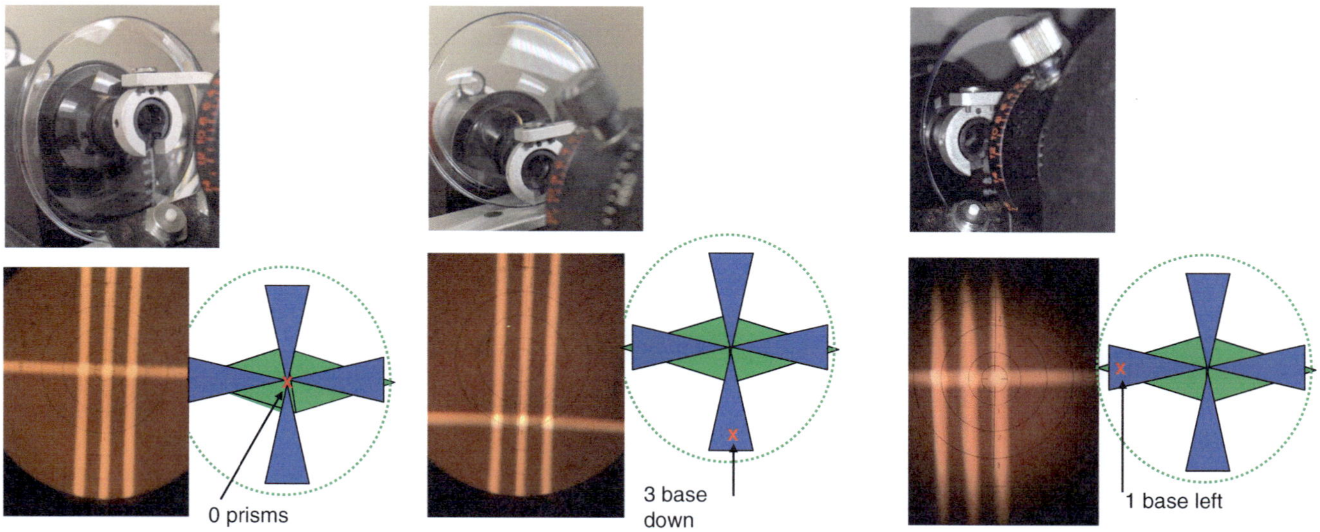

Fig. 28 How much prism power do different parts of a −3.00 + 2.00 × 90 lens have? The top panels show a −3.00D sphere lens (blue) combined with +2.00D cylinder lens (green) that has power and prismatic effect along the 180-degree meridian. There is no prismatic effect through the center of the lens (bottom left panel). The bottom-middle panel shows 3 PD base-down prismatic effect 1 cm inferior to the optical center. The bottom right panel shows 1 PD prismatic effect base left 1 cm to the left of the optical center

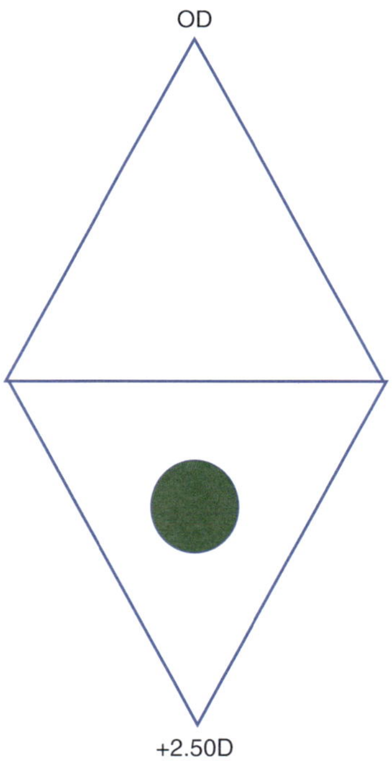

Fig. 29 In downward gaze, the +2.50 + 1.75 × 90 lens will function as a simple +2.75D spherical lens

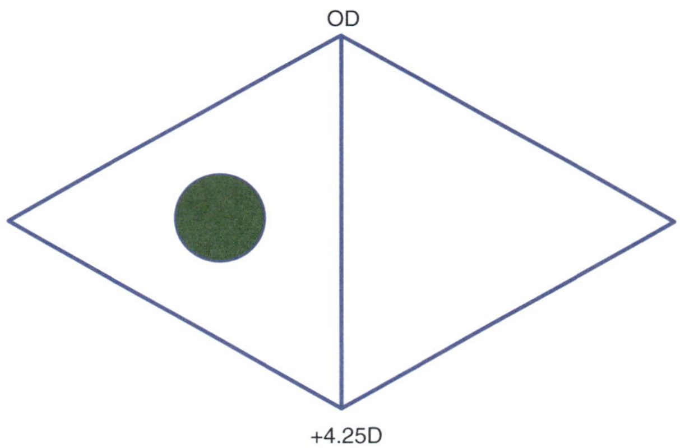

Fig. 30 In temporal gaze of the right eye, the +2.50 + 1.75 × 90 lens will now incorporate the cylinder power and function as a +4.25D lens

- First, figure out how much effect is AT the 180-degree meridian by converting to minus cylinder: −1.50 + 5.00 × 90 = +3.50 − 5.00 × 180.
- This conversion means there is +3.50D having an effect at the 180-degree meridian; when we look temporal to the optical center, we can simplify this spherocylindrical lens as a simple +3.50D lens for both eyes (Fig. 32). Notice that this "minus" lens now functions as a "plus lens" in horizontal gaze. Now we can use Prentice's Rule:

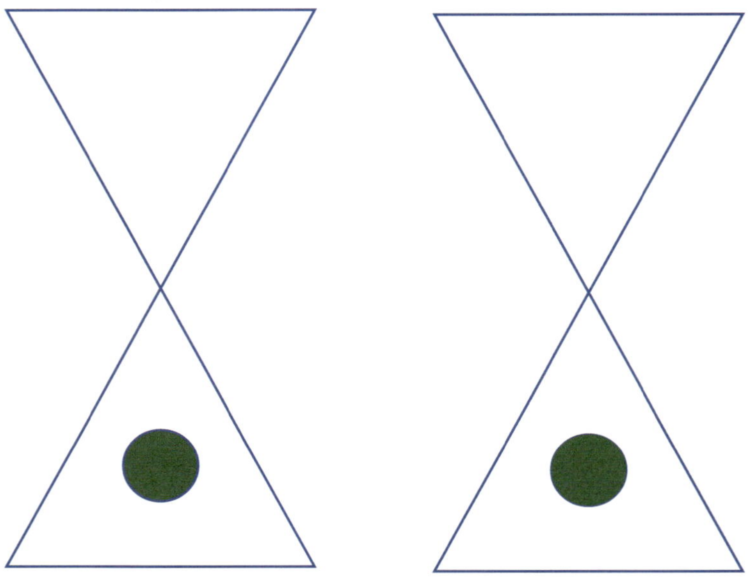

Fig. 31 In downwards gaze, this spherocylindrical (−1.50 + 5.00 × 90) lens will function as a −1.50D lens

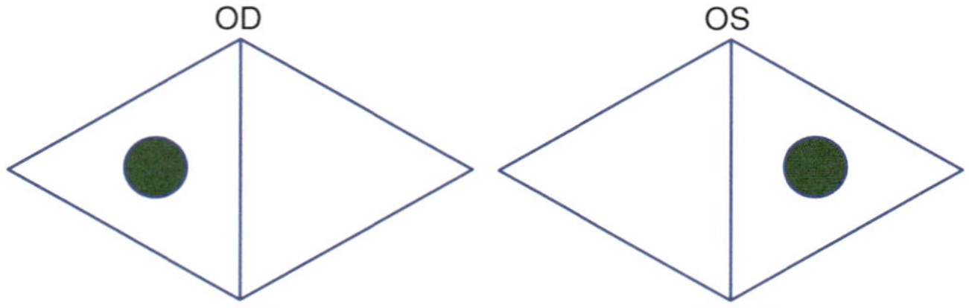

Fig. 32 This lens will function as a +3.50D lens in temporal gaze. Note that both eyes are moving toward the nose (opposite directions)

- $P = hD = 1.2$ cm × 3.5 = 4.2 prism diopters base in OU.
- Net induced prism: 4.2 + 4.2 = 8.4 PD BI.
- Both eyes move nasally, so an esotropia is induced.

Bonus Wrinkle: what if the question had asked how much prism would we have to dispense to counteract these glasses' induced prismatic effect? We would have to place 8.4 PD BO (rounded to 8.5 PD BO) in either the right or left eye

The Conoid of Sturm and Circle of Least Confusion

One last "circle" to get through before we can escape Inferno: the *Conoid of Sturm (COS)* and the resulting (and ironically named) "*circle of least confusion (COLC)*".

We can start with the COS (Fig. 33). The COS is a three-dimensional asymmetrical trumpet shape that we represent as a two-dimensional ray-tracing formed as light passes through a (sphero)cylindrical lens. To simplify our discussion, imagine that we have a spherocylindrical lens oriented like a vertical football. From our earlier discussions in this chapter, we know that incoming light rays will get refracted by the steeper portion of the lens (in this case, the horizontal meridian [power meridian]) and first form a vertical focal line parallel to the axis meridian. Incoming light rays that get refracted by the flatter portion of the lens (in this case, the vertical meridian) will later form a horizontal line parallel to that axis meridian. However, there are several other shapes and figures formed: after light rays are refracted by and exit the lens, the following lines and shapes ensue, in sequential order:

- Converging light rays (immediately behind the lens)
- Vertical focal line
- Vertical oval
- Circle (aka the COLC)
- Horizontal oval
- Horizontal focal line
- Diverging light rays

The COLC is basically the halfway point (circular cross-section) between the two focal lines on the COS (in terms of *diopters, not distance*); in practical terms, this is the smallest blur spot (i.e., the "clearest" image) that a spherocylindrical lens can make. It is a compromise between the sphere and cylinder components of a spherocylindrical lens. Thus, we can also think of the **COLC** as the *spherical equivalent*. Notice that the COLC may be closer to one of the focus lines. Again, it is NOT the average distance between the two focal points!

This concept is understandably difficult without visualization, especially in three dimensions. The following examples will hopefully reinforce this discussion.

Example #1 Suppose we have a lens with power +3.00 + 2.00 × 180. What is the orientation of the first line of

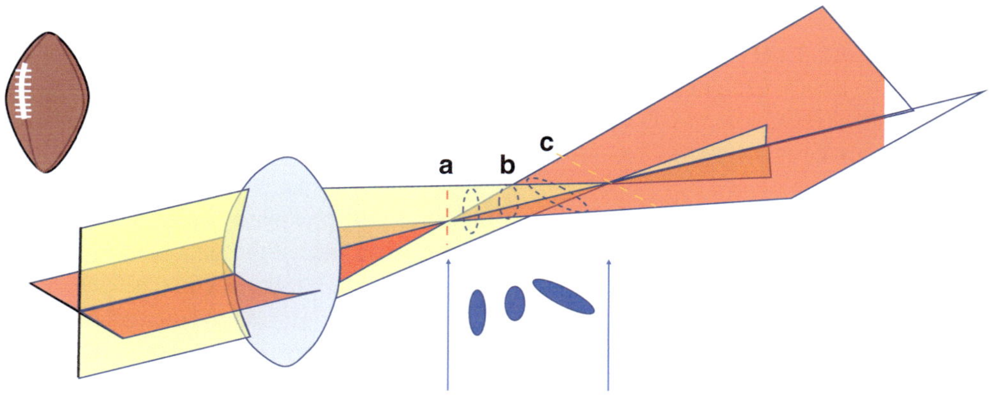

Fig. 33 The conoid of sturm can be used to indicate the figure formed by converging light rays refracted by a spherocylindrical lens. Each power meridian of the lens forms two sharp focal lines (A and C). The COLC is formed at the halfway point, B (*in terms of diopters*, not distance), between these two focal lines. Converging light has an ovoid shape between each focal line and the COLC

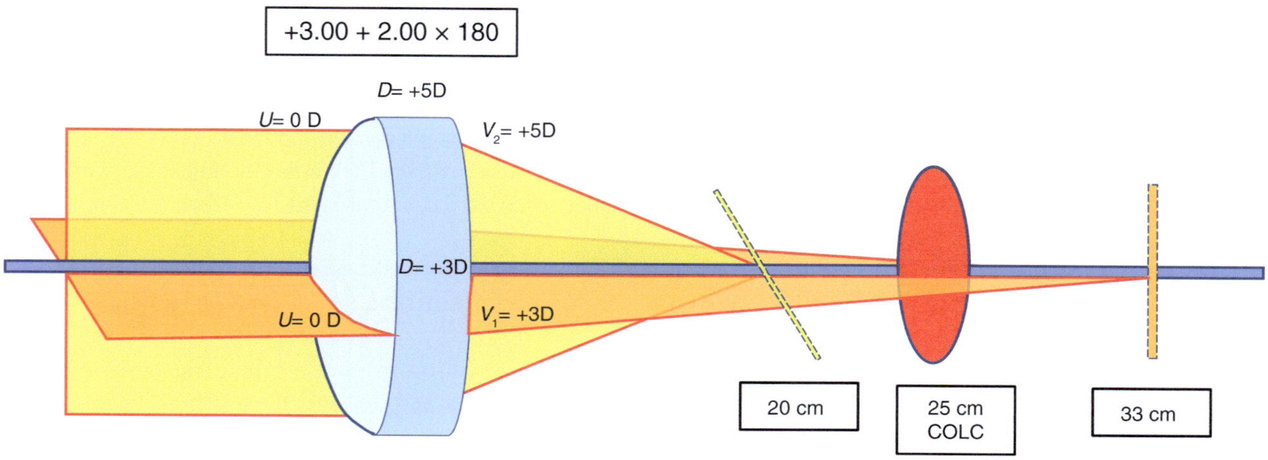

Fig. 34 Light rays that pass through a +3.00 + 2.00 × 180 spherocylindrical lens will first form a horizontal line at 20 cm (+5D) and then a vertical line at 33 cm (+3D). The COLC is formed at the halfway point of the diopters (+4D), corresponding to 25 cm right of the lens

focus? Where is the COLC? What is the orientation of the second line of focus?

We can turn to our friend (or enemy), the power cross, to help make this problem a bit easier. Using the spherocylindrical lens power, we know that this lens has +3D of power acting at the 180-degree meridian and +5D of power acting at the 90-degree meridian.

Light rays that pass through the +5D portion of the lens (vertical meridian, aka the power meridian) will form a horizontal line at 100/5 = 20 cm (horizontal meridian, aka the axis meridian). Similarly, light rays that pass through the +3D portion of the lens (horizontal meridian, aka the power meridian) will form a vertical line at 100/3 = 33 cm (vertical meridian, aka the axis meridian). The COLC will therefore be determined by the spherical equivalent: +3 + (1/2 * 2) = +4D. The focal point is 100/4 = 25 cm to the right of the lens (Fig. 34).

The horizontal and vertical focal lines will be "equally blurry" at this location, and thus the image will be the sharpest. Remember that at 20 cm, all the horizontal lines from the source object will be in perfect focus, but none of the vertical lines will be in focus; similarly, at 33 cm, all the vertical lines will be in perfect focus, but none of the horizontal lines will be in focus. The COLC is the spot where there is a compromise between the vertical and horizontal focus lines.

Why is this relevant? Suppose you find yourself on a medical mission trip and a patient with astigmatism needs a pair of glasses. Unfortunately, if you only have spherical glasses left, then a lens with the spherical equivalent similar to the patient's refraction may be a reasonable option.

Finally, note that we cannot simply take the average of the focal points to find the COLC: 20 cm + 33 cm = 53/2 = 26.5 cm. This approach is incorrect. The COLC is the halfway point in terms of **diopters**, *not distance*.

Example #2 Suppose we place an object 100 cm away from a spherocylindrical lens with the following power: +2.00 + 3.00 × 180. Where is the COLC?

By now, we should know that this lens will function like a + 2.00D at 180° and +5.00 at 90°. Unlike the previous problem, we have incoming light from a finite distance of 100 cm to the left of the lens.[13] This means that since $u = -100$ cm, $U = -1$ (divergent light). Therefore, we have to use $U + D = V$ twice:

$$-1+3=+2\text{D at }180^{\circ}, \text{ which will create a vertical line 50 cm to the right}$$

$$-1+5=+4\text{D at }90^{\circ}, \text{ which will create a horizontal line 25 cm to the right.}$$

We may be tempted to say that the COLC is the halfway point between 25 cm and 100 cm, 62.5 cm.[14] But we would be stuck in this last circle of the Inferno because we instead need to use the spherical equivalent (SE) to calculate the COLC (Fig. 35).

$$\text{The SE of this toric lens is } 2+\left(1/2^{*}3\right)=+3.50\text{D}.$$

We can "re-run" the object rays through this lens using the SE to calculate the COLC. Note that a horizontal oval will form in between the horizontal line at 25 cm and the COLC, and a vertical oval will form in between the COLC and the vertical line at 100 cm:

$$-1+3.50=+2.50,\ 100/2.50=40\text{ cm. The COLC is located 40 cm to the right of the lens.}$$

Congratulations! We have escaped the Inferno (for now). We can finish up with some practice questions and tell the stories of our adventures to future generations.

Stenopeic Slit

Note to the reader: we freely admit that this is a low-yield topic, mainly a relic of older textbooks. The stenopeic slit is an opaque trial lens with an elongated slit aperture that can be used to find a spherocylindrical refraction. This lens is likely gathering dust in a drawer in your exam lane. This technique may be helpful in patients with small pupils, lenticular opacities, and irregular corneal surface (irregular astigmatism). The examiner can place a spherical lens (minus- or plus-power) with the stenopeic slit in front of the patient's eye. The slit will minimize refractive blur in the meridian perpendicular to the slit, allowing the examiner to neutralize the refractive error in the meridian of the slit. By rotating the slit in all meridians, we can find the "least lousy" meridian. Compared to the previously mentioned streak refraction, the primary difference with the stenopeic slit technique is that the results are transcribed directly in the meridian of the slit to generate a power cross. We understand that this entire paragraph is confusing, so an example will hopefully help explain this technique further. For example, suppose we placed the stenopeic slit in the 80-degree position with a –3.00D sphere. The patient indicates that the image is still blurry, so we rotate the slit in 10-degree increments in both directions until the patient states that the image is in the best focus. Suppose the patient says the clearest image is in the 127-degree meridian with the –3.00D lens; after all, we are dealing with irregular astigmatism. We can now rotate the slit 90 degrees away to the 37-degree meridian. Suppose now the patient says the clearest image is formed with a +4.50D lens. We can interpret our tomfoolery with the steonpeic slit as follows: –3.00D @ 127 and +4.50 @ 37. We can construct our power cross such that the –3.00D is connected to 127-degrees and +4.50D is connected to 37-degrees. Now we can use the DAM to get the final refraction: –3.00 + 7.50 x 127. We do not adjust the working distance since we did not perform any streak refraction.

Practice Questions

1. Suppose you are given two cylindrical lenses: +2.50 × 90 and +1.00 × 180. Express the combined power of these lenses as a spherocylindrical lens.
2. Suppose you perform streak refraction on a patient and obtain the following results: with the retinoscope streak positioned vertically and moved horizontally, the reflex was neutralized with a −6.00 D sphere ("A −6D lens streaks the 90 degree"). With the streak positioned horizontally and moved vertically, the reflex was neutralized with a −3.50 D sphere ("A −3.50D lens streaks the 180 degree"). Assume your working distance is 50 cm. What is the final prescription to be dispensed?
3. If you perform streak refraction on a patient and obtain the following results: a + 5.50D lens streaks the 135°, and a + 2.00D lens streaks the 45°. Assume a working distance of 67 cm. What is the final prescription?
4. If you perform streak refraction on a patient and obtain the following results: a − 5.00D lens streaks the 150°, and a + 1.00D lens streaks the 60°. Assume a working distance of 67 cm. What is the final prescription?

[13] Strictly speaking, we were using the $U + D = V$ equation in example 1 as well, but since the incoming light was originating at infinity, $U = 0$.

[14] One can be fairly certain that such an answer would be given as a "distractor" answer choice on exams.

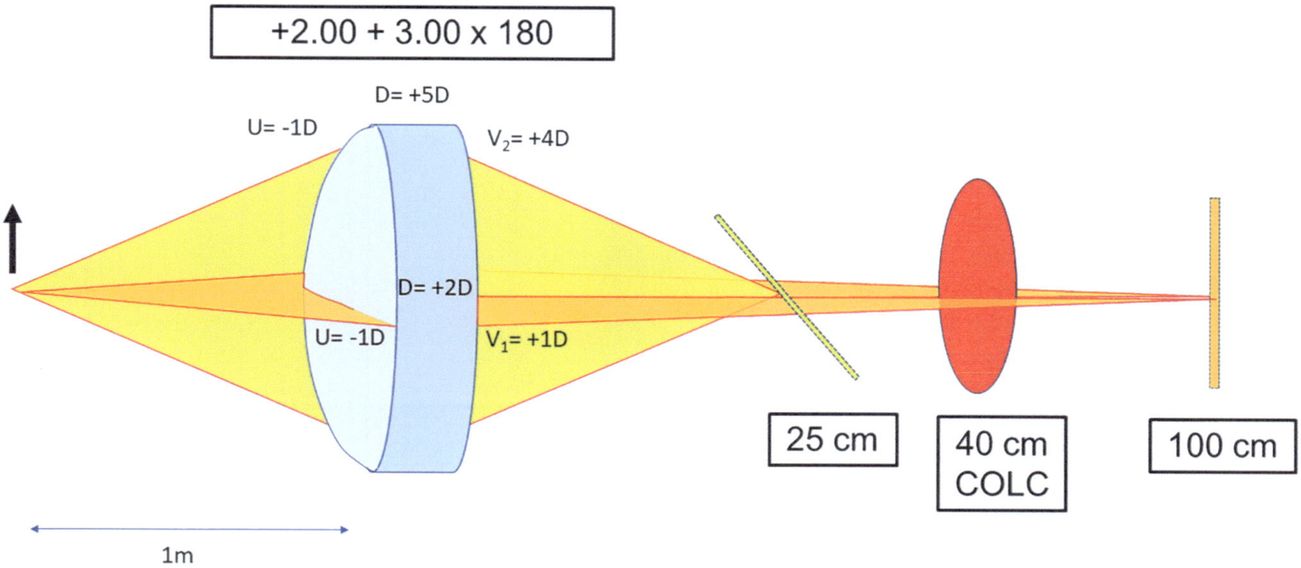

Fig. 35 Divergent light rays originate from a source object located 100 cm to the left of a +2.00 + 3.00 × 180 spherocylindrical lens. These light rays will first form a horizontal line at 25 cm (+4D) and then a vertical line at 100 cm (+1D). The circle of least confusion is formed at the halfway point of the diopters (+2.5D), corresponding to 40 cm right of the lens

5. Draw the Power Cross for the following manifest refractions:
   (a) −2.50 + 1.50 × 90
   (b) −6.00 + 2.00 × 180
   (c) −10.00 + 3.50 × 45
   (d) +4.25–2.75 × 20
6. If a patient has keratometry readings of 38.50 × 41.50 @ 60, prescribe a pair of glasses that will neutralize this astigmatism while maintaining a spherical equivalent of plano. Assume there is no lenticular astigmatism.
7. If a patient has keratometry readings of 45.25 × 47.75 @ 25, prescribe a pair of glasses to neutralize her astigmatism while maintaining a spherical equivalent of −2.50. Assume there is no lenticular astigmatism.
8. A light source falls on a spherocylindrical lens with unknown power. A line is formed at 60° on a screen placed at 20 cm right of the lens. When the screen is moved to 33 cm, the line is now at 150°.
   (a) At what distance is the circle of least confusion seen on the screen?
   (b) What is the power of the unknown lens?
9. If a patient wears the following prescription:

$$\text{OD}: +4.00+1.50\times180$$

$$\text{OS}: +2.50+2.50\times90$$

   and the original pupillary distance put into the glasses is 60 mm, what is the net prismatic effect in horizontal gaze if the patient's actual pupillary distance was 70 mm?
10. Using the above example, what would be the net prismatic effect if the pupillary distance was changed to 50 mm?
11. If a patient wears glasses with the following prescription (−2.50 + 3.50 × 90) in both eyes, how much prismatic correction must be dispensed in order to balance possible diplopia if:
    (a) The patient looks 6 mm inferior to the optical center (in both eyes)
    (b) The patient looks 10 mm nasal to the optical center (in both eyes)
12. Suppose that a monocular patient's refraction in the right eye was −4.00 + 2.00 × 180 prior to cataract surgery. Due to an error in IOL calculations, the patient ended up with postoperative refraction of +2.00 + 2.00 × 90 (hyperopic surprise). If this patient was orthoptic in the reading position, read 10 mm below the optical center prior to surgery, and continues to read 10 mm below the optical center after the surgery, how much of a postoperative prismatic deviation is now present? How can you correct this induced prismatic deviation? (The patient adamantly refuses any further surgery).
13. A cyclopleged 30-year-old patient looks at an Amsler grid located 50 cm away. He notices that the vertical lines are focused sharply when a + 3.00D sphere is held in front of the eye, and the horizontal lines are focused sharply when a + 5.50D sphere is used. What is the distance correction that should be given to this patient?
14. Given a prescription of: −4.00 + 1.00 × 90
    (a) Express this prescription in minus cylinder form
    (b) Draw the power cross for this lens

(c) Express the lens power using SC notation lenses
(d) Draw the axis cross for this lens
(e) What would your streak refraction results be if you were an emmetrope and had a working distance of 50 cm?

15. A spherocylindrical lens of unknown power refracts light originating from a source located at infinity. A line is formed at 45° on a screen placed 25 cm to the right of this lens. A second line is formed at 135° when the screen is moved to 67 cm to the right of this lens.
(a) At what distance is the circle of least confusion seen on the screen?
(b) What is the power of this spherocylindrical lens?

Answers

1. Answer: We can use either SC notation or power crosses to calculate the final power.

SC Notation Method

$$+2.50 \times 90 = \text{plano} + 2.50 \times 90 = +2.50 - 2.50 \times 180$$

$$+1.00 \times 180 = \text{plano} + 1.00 \times 180 = +1.00 - 1.00 \times 90$$

Algebraically combine either the "90" or "180" lenses. Let us choose the "90" lenses:

$$\text{Plano} + 2.50 \times 90$$
$$+1.00 - 1.00 \times 90$$
$$\text{================}$$
$$+1.00 + 1.50 \times 90$$

If we choose the "180" lenses:

$$\text{Plano} + 1.00 \times 180$$
$$+2.50 - 2.50 \times 180$$
$$\text{================}$$
$$+2.50 - 1.50 \times 180$$

Notice that we could have also derived either result by simply converting the first result (in plus cylinder) into minus cylinder and vice versa.

PC Notation

From the cylindrical lens given above, we know that the +2.50D lens is exerting its power at the 180-degree meridian, and the +1.00D lens is exerting its power at the 90-degree meridian.

We can draw the power cross and use the double arches method (DAM) (Fig. 36).

If we select +1.00D as our "starting sphere lens", we will have to "add +1.50" (which will become our cylinder) to get to +2.50D (first arch). Then we draw our second arch to 90 (which will become our axis). The final prescription will be: +1.00 + 1.50 × 90, which is the same result we calculated using SC notation. We can do the same exercise using +2.50D as our starting lens. Using the DAM, we would get a minus cylinder prescription of: +2.50–1.00 × 180.

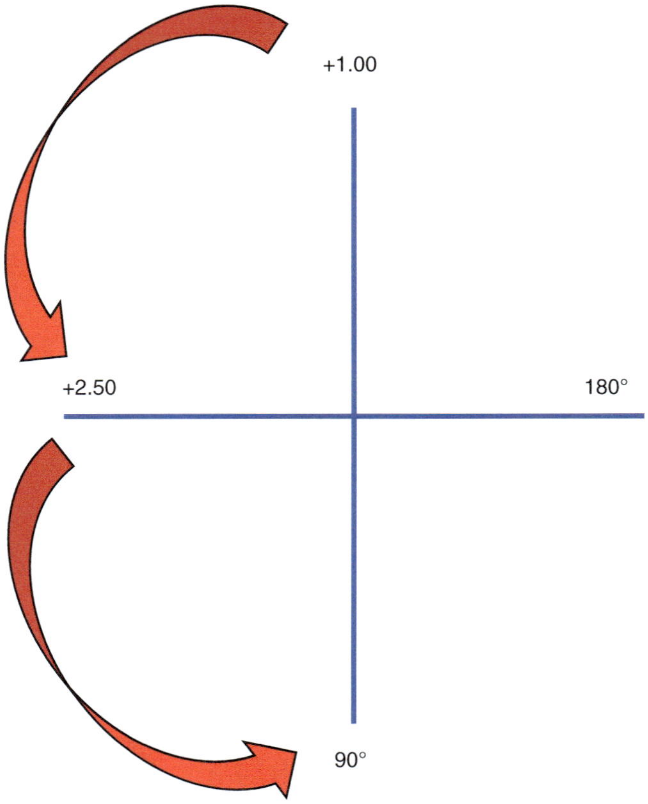

Fig. 36 Power cross and double arches method for practice question #1

2. Answer: We can use either SC notation or power crosses to calculate the final prescription. Remember that we need to an additional −2.00D of sphere in order to compensate for the working distance.

$$\textit{SC Notation}: -6.00 \times 90 \text{ and } -3.50 \times 180$$

$$-6.00 \times 90 = \text{plano} - 6.00 \times 90 = -6.00 + 6.00 \times 180$$

$$-3.50 \times 180 = \text{plano} - 3.50 \times 180 = -3.50 + 3.50 \times 90$$

Suppose we chose to combine our two "lenses" that are currently in the 180-degree axis notation:

$$-6.00 + 6.00 \times 180$$
$$\text{Plano} - 3.50 \times 180$$
$$\text{================}$$
$$-6.00 + 2.50 \times 180$$

$$\text{Add additional} - 2\text{D for working distance}: -8.00 + 2.50 \times 180$$

If we had used our other two lenses in 90-degree axis notation:

$$-3.50 + 3.50 \times 90$$
$$\text{Plano} - 6.00 \times 90$$
$$\overline{\qquad\qquad}$$
$$-3.50 - 2.50 \times 90$$

$$\text{Add additional} - 2\text{D for working distance}: -5.50 - 2.50 \times 90$$

PC Notation: We know that the –6.00D lens is exerting its power at the 180-degree meridian and the –3.50D lens is exerting its power at the 90-degree meridian. We can use this information to draw the power cross and use the DAM (Fig. 37).

Suppose we chose –3.50 as our "starting sphere lens", we will have to "subtract –2.50" (which will become our cylinder to get to –6.00 (first arch)). Then we draw our second arch to 90 (which will become our axis). The final prescription will be: –3.50 – 2.50 × 90. We still have to factor in our working distance (additional -2D): –5.50 – 2.50 × 90.

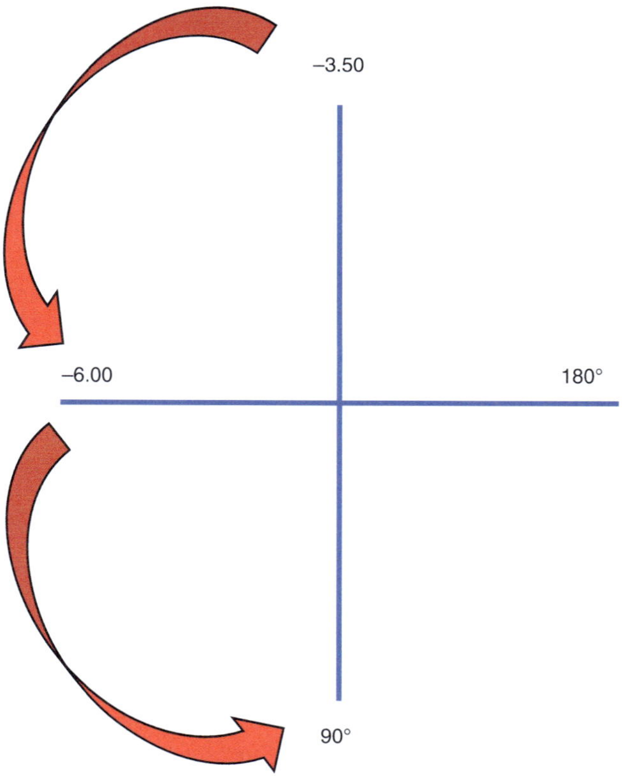

Fig. 37 Power cross and double arches method for practice question #2

We can do the same exercise using –6.00 as our "starting sphere lens". Using the double arches method, we would get a plus cylinder prescription of –6.00 + 2.50 × 180. We still have to factor in our working distance (additional -2D): –8.00 + 2.50 × 180.

If we have done our math/drawings correctly, the final prescription should be the same regardless of our chosen method.

3. Answer: We can again use either method. Let us do this question using only SC notation (we will do the next one only using a power cross).

$$\textit{SC Notation}: +5.50 \times 135 \text{ and } +2.00 \times 45$$

$$+5.50 \times 135 = \text{plano} + 5.50 \times 135 = +5.50 - 5.50 \times 45$$

$$+2.00 \times 45 = \text{plano} + 2.00 \times 45 = +2.00 - 2.00 \times 135$$

Suppose we chose the two "lenses" currently listed in the 45-degree notation:

$$+5.50 - 5.50 \times 45$$
$$\text{Plano} + 2.00 \times 45$$
$$\overline{\qquad\qquad}$$
$$+5.50 - 3.50 \times 45$$

Factor in working distance (67 cm), so additional –1.5D: +4.00 – 3.50 × 45.

Suppose instead we chose the two "lenses" currently listed in the 135-degree notation:

$$+2.00 - 2.00 \times 135$$
$$\text{Plano} + 5.50 \times 135$$
$$\overline{\qquad\qquad}$$
$$+2.00 + 3.50 \times 135$$

Factor in working distance (67 cm), so additional –1.5D: +0.50 + 3.50 × 135.

Note that if we have done our math correctly, either final prescription should yield the other final prescription if we flip between plus or minus cylinder notation.[15]

4. Answer: We can use power cross notation to solve this problem.

We know that the +1.00D lens is exerting its power at the 150-degree meridian; the –5.00D lens is exerting its power at the 60-degree meridian. We can draw a power cross that establishes this relationship and then use the Double Arches Method (Fig. 38).

[15] If you are feeling adventurous, you can try to solve this question using power crosses and should get the same answer.

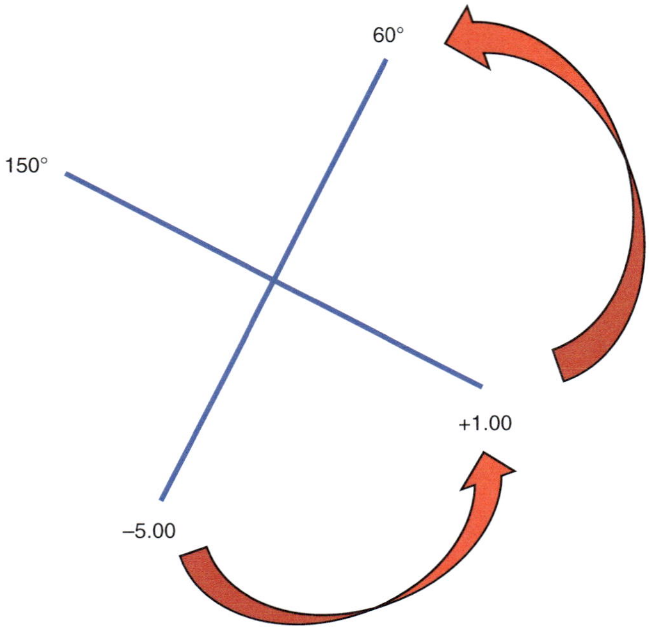

Fig. 38 Power cross and double arches method for practice question #4

Our prescription from the power cross is: −5.00 + 6.00 × 60. Alternatively, we could use +1.00 as our starting lens, and we would then get: +1.00–6.00 × 150.

Now factor in the additional −1.5D sphere for the working distance: −6.50 + 6.00 × 60. For minus cylinder: −0.50 – 6.00 × 150. Again, this is a lot of cylinder so make sure we are not missing a corneal ectasia!

5. Answer: For each of these prescriptions, we can use the Telephone Method after converting to the opposite cylinder notation:
   (a) −2.50 + 1.50 × 90 = −1.00 – 1.50 × 180
   (b) −6.00 + 2.00 × 180 = −4.00 – 2.00 × 90
   (c) −10.00 + 3.50 × 45 = −6.50 – 3.50 × 135
   (d) +4.25–2.75 × 20 = +1.50 + 2.75 × 110

   Now we can use the telephone method by connecting the sphere and axis of each prescription and setting these are our four positions of the power cross.

   The resulting power crosses can be seen in Fig. 39.

   We can check our work using the DAM for each power cross and make sure that we can get back the original prescriptions.
6. Answer: We should notice there is a 3D difference between the two meridians (60 and 150). The 60-degree meridian is the steep meridian ("big brother"). The 150-degree meridian is the flat meridian ("little brother").

   In order to help the little brother, we will need to place +3D of cylinder in the 60-degree meridian (axis meridian) so that it acts at the 150-degree meridian (power meridian): +3.00 × 60.

   In order to maintain a spherical equivalent of plano, we will have to add −1.50D sphere. The final prescription will be: −1.50 + 3.00 × 60.
7. Answer: We should notice a 2.50D difference between the two meridians (115 and 25). The 25-degree meridian is the steep meridian ("big brother"). The 115-degree meridian is the flat meridian ("little brother").

   In order to help the little brother, we will need to place +2.50D in the 25-degree meridian (axis meridian) so that it acts at the 115-degree meridian (power meridian): +2.50 × 25.

   In order to maintain a spherical equivalent of −2.50, we will need to add −3.75D sphere to the final prescription, yielding: −3.75 + 2.50 × 25.
8. Answer: This question requires us to put together several topics we have learned thus far. Our knowledge of power crosses will help us arrive at the correct answer.

   First, we know that the lens focuses light at 20 cm at 60°. This means there must be +5D of power (100/20 = +5D) placed in the 60° meridian (axis meridian) which is exerting its effect at the 150° meridian (power meridian), which in turn forms a line at 60°. When we draw the power cross, the +5.00D should be linked to the 150°.

   Next, we also know that the lens focuses light at 33 cm at 150°. This means there must be +3D of power (100/33 = +3D) placed in the 150° meridian (axis meridian) which is exerting its effect at the 60° meridian (power meridian), which in turn forms a line at 150°. When we draw the power cross, the +3.00D should be linked to the 60° (Fig. 40).

   The circle of least confusion (COLC) is the average of these two powers: 3 + 5 = 8; 8/2 = +4D. The focal length distance for +4D is 25 cm. Therefore, the COLC will be located at 25 cm.

   For the second part of the question, we can use the above information to draw the power cross (Fig. 41).

   If we choose +3.00 as our starting lens, then when we draw our first arch to the +5.00, we must add +2.00 (which will be our cylinder). Then we can draw our second arch over to the 60, which will be our axis. The power of the unknown spherocylindrical lens is: +3.00 + 2.00 × 60 (or minus cylinder: +5.00–2.00 × 150).

   Alternatively, we could have used SC notation based on the question stem with the following "starting lenses": +5.00 × 60 and + 3.00 × 150. We should get the same answer.
9. Answer: To make our lives a bit easier, we need to get both lenses with the same axis notation, regardless of whether it is in minus or plus cylinder notation. We can go ahead and change the OS lens to 180-degree notation so that we can convert it to minus cylinder:

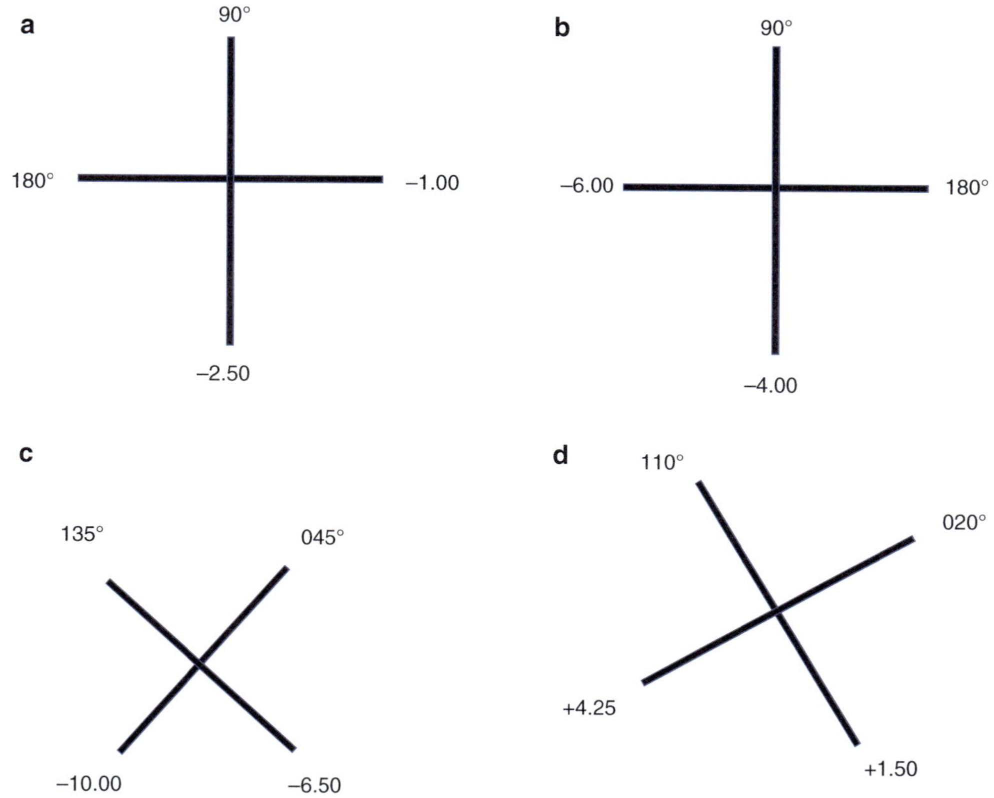

Fig. 39 Power crosses for practice question #5. Panels A-D correspond to the answers for Practice Question 5, A-D

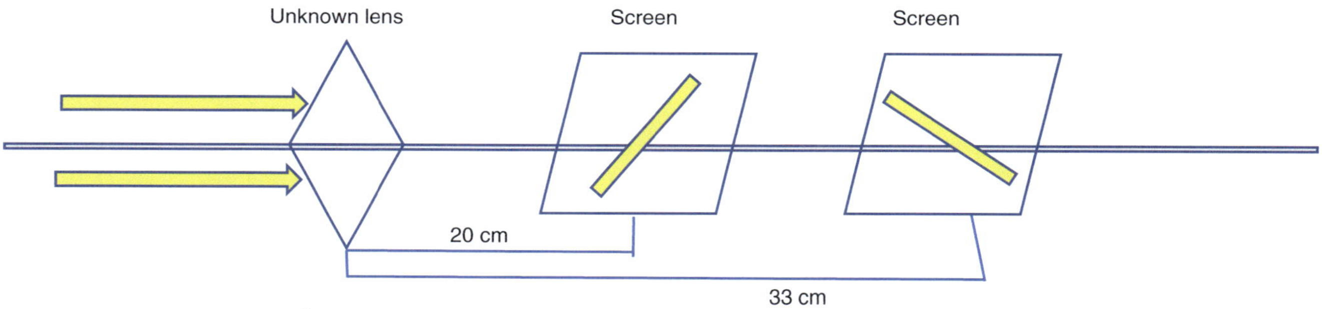

Fig. 40 Diagram for incoming light passing through a spherocylindrical lens of unknown power casting a line at 60° on a screen placed at 20 cm right of the lens and an additional line at 150° on a screen placed 33 cm right of the lens

$$\text{OS}: +2.50 + 2.50 \times 90 = +5.00 - 2.00 \times 180$$

For both eyes, we have cylinder power placed in the 180-degree (axis) meridian that is acting at the 90-degree (power) meridian (i.e., when the patient is looking up and down). When the patient is looking from side to side, only the +4.00D is having an effect in the right eye, and only the +5.00D is having an effect in the left eye.

We can draw this change in the pupillary distance and its prismatic effect in horizontal gaze (top panel of Fig. 42). In the top panel, we can see that if the patient's PD was actually 60 mm, the patient would be looking through the optical center of the lenses, and there would be no prismatic effect to consider. However, since the patient's PD is actually 70 mm, the patient will end up looking *temporal* to the optical centers of the glasses (bottom panel of Fig. 42). A base-in effect (additive) will be induced, and Prentice's Rule can be used to quantify the deviation.

As the patient is looking temporally to the optical center of the lenses in both eyes, there will be an induced BI prismatic effect. The prismatic effect is additive since both eyes are shifted nasally (i.e., in opposite directions). We now have to apply Prentice's Rule as follows:

$$\text{OD}: P = hD = (0.5)(4) = 2\,\text{PD BI}$$

$$\text{OS}: P = hD = (0.5)(5) = 2.5\,\text{PD BI}$$

Therefore, the net prismatic effect will be 4.5 PD BI.

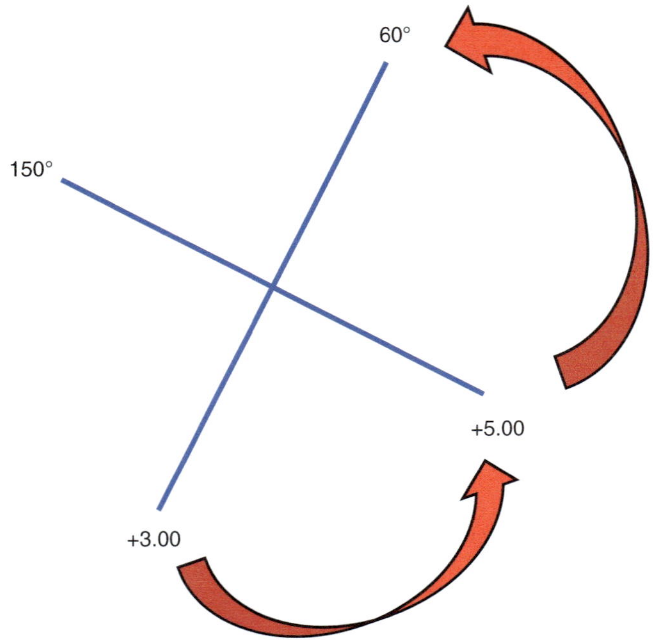

Fig. 41 Power cross and DAM for unknown spherocylindrical lens for practice question #8

10. Answer: We can again start this problem by getting both lenses with the same axis notation:

$$\text{OS}: +2.50 + 2.50 \times 90 = +5.00 - 2.00 \times 180$$

For both eyes, we have cylinder power that is placed in the 180-degree (axis) meridian that is acting at the 90-degree (power) meridian (i.e., when the patient is looking up and down). When the patient is looking from side to side, the +4.00D affects the right eye, and +5.00D affects the left eye.

We can draw this change in the pupillary distance and its prismatic effect in horizontal gaze as follows (top panel of Fig. 43). In the top panel, we can see that if the patient's PD was actually 60 mm, then the patient would be looking through the optical center of the lenses, and there would be no prismatic effect to consider. However, since the patient's PD is actually 50 mm, the patient will end up looking *nasal* to the optical centers of the glasses (bottom panel of Fig. 43).

Since the patient is looking nasal to the optical center of the lenses in both eyes, there will be an induced BO prismatic effect. We now have to apply Prentice's Rule as follows:

$$\text{OD}: P = hD = (0.5)(4) = 2\,\text{PD BO}$$

$$\text{OS}: P = hD = (0.5)(5) = 2.5\ \text{PD BO}$$

Therefore, the net prismatic effect will be 4.5 PD BO.

11. Answer: For these types of problems, it always helps to convert the given prescription into the opposite axis notation to determine the total power in this gaze position. Since we have been given 90-degree axis notation (vertical gaze), we can convert it into 180-degree axis notation, which would require minus cylinder notation and give us information about the horizontal gaze.

$$-2.50 + 3.50 \times 90 = +1.50 - 3.50 \times 180$$

We can see that +3.50D of cylinder has been placed in the 90-degree (axis) meridian and will therefore exert an effect at the 180-degree (power) meridian only. Therefore, only the –2.50D will have an effect in pure vertical gaze from the optical center. To solve part a, we can show the prismatic effects of inferior gaze by re-drawing the spherocylindrical lenses as simple minus lenses, as shown in Fig. 44 (top panel).

In inferior gaze, the minus lenses will cause a base-down effect. Using Prentice's Rule, we can determine the prismatic effects as follows:

$$P = hD = (0.6) * (2.5) = 1.5\,\text{PD BD in both eyes.}$$

Since both eyes have shifted downwards equally (i.e., same direction and same magnitude), there is no induced diplopia. No prismatic correction is needed for part a.

However, for part b, the situation is slightly different. When the patient looks nasal to the optical center in both eyes (horizontal gaze), we can see that we must incorporate the cylinder power, and these lenses will actually function like plus lenses. Therefore, we can show the prismatic effects of nasal (horizontal) gaze by re-drawing the spherocylindrical lenses as simple plus lenses, as shown in Fig. 44 (bottom panel).

In nasal (horizontal) gaze, nasal gaze to the optical center of plus lenses in both eyes will cause a base-out prismatic effect. Using Prentice's Rule, we can determine the prismatic effects as follows:

$$P = hD = (1) * (1.5) = 1.5\text{PD BO in each eye.}$$

Since each eye moves in the opposite direction, the net prismatic effect will be additive: 1.0 PD BO +1.0 PD BO = 2 PD BO total.

In order to correct this deviation, 2 PD BI must be given to either the left or right eye (but not both).

12. Answer: We can again start by getting both of our prescriptions into the same axis notation. Since we are primarily dealing with inferior gaze, the 90-degree notation will be helpful since that will allow us to ignore the cylinder portion and focus only on the lens's spherical component.

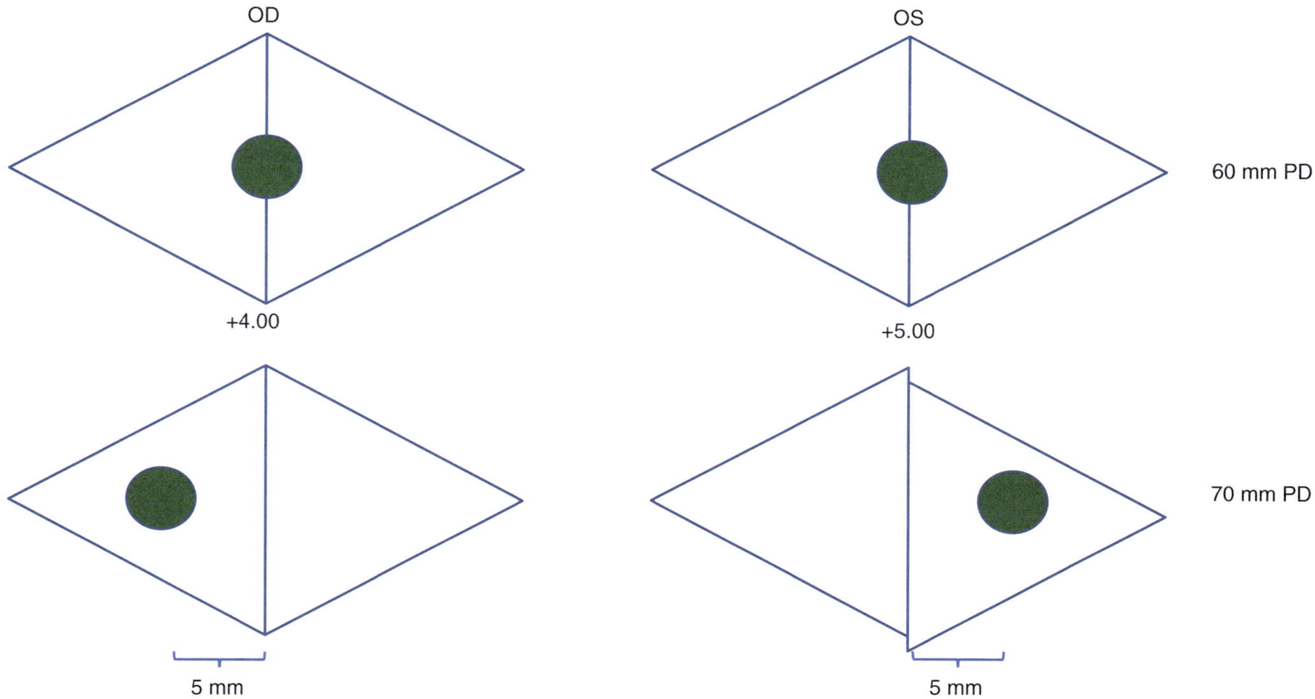

Fig. 42 When the patient looks through the optical center of the glasses, there is no prismatic effect. If the patient has a pupillary distance of 70 mm (instead of 60 mm), she will end up looking temporally to the optical center in both eyes. A base-in effect (additive) will be induced, and Prentice's Rule can be used to quantify the deviation

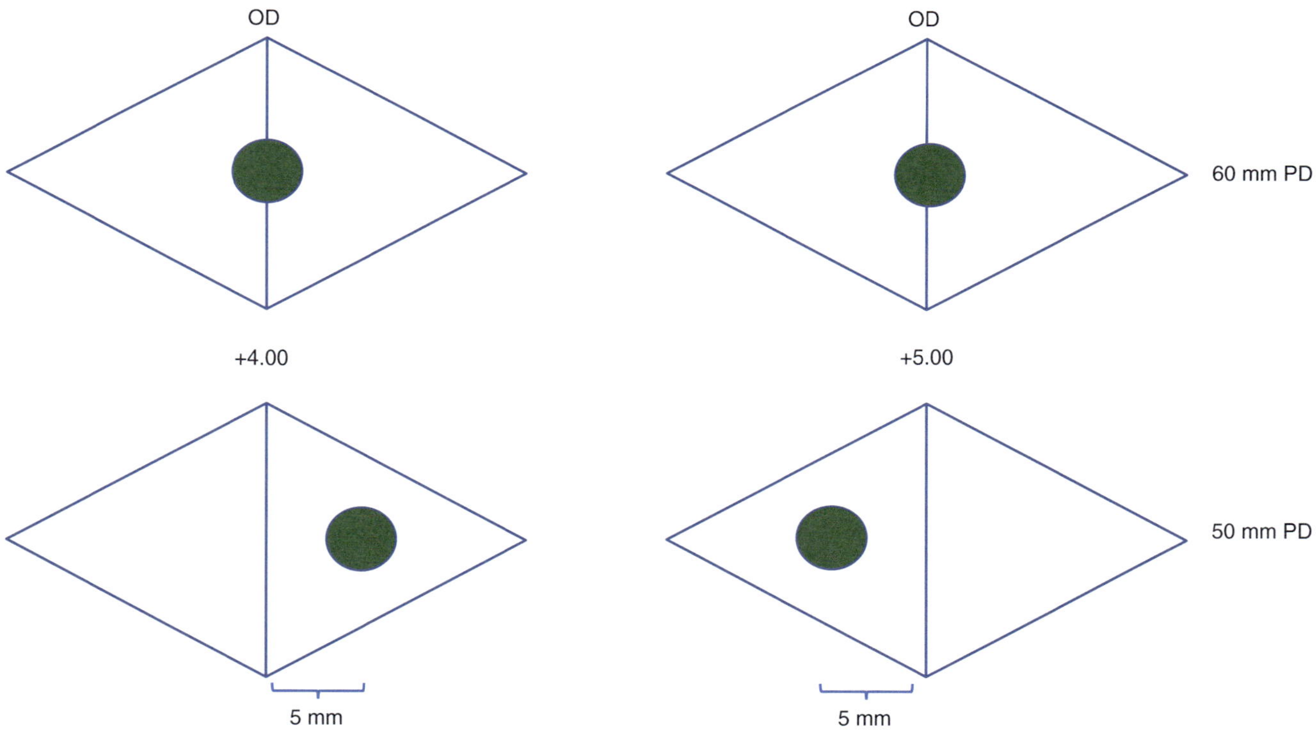

Fig. 43 When the patient looks through the optical center of the glasses, there is no prismatic effect. If the patient has a pupillary distance of 50 mm (instead of 60 mm), she will end up looking nasally to the optical center in both eyes. A base-out effect (additive) will be induced, and Prentice's Rule can be used to quantify the deviation

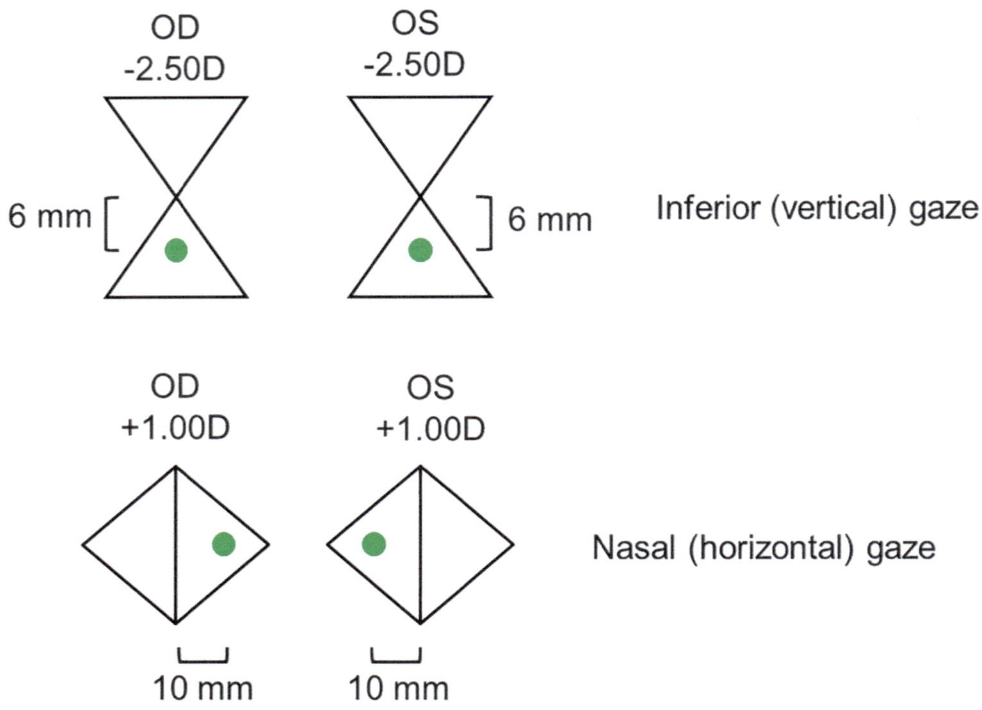

Fig. 44 Prismatic effects in vertical gaze (top panel) and horizontal gaze (bottom panel) when looking 6 mm inferior and 10 mm nasal to the optical center, respectively, of a −2.50 + 3.50 × 90 eyeglass prescription

$$\text{Preoperative refraction}: -4.00 + 2.00 \times 180 = -2.00 - 2.00 \times 90$$

$$\text{Postoperative refraction}: +2.00 + 2.00 \times 90$$

We can now redraw these lenses as shown in Fig. 45.

Now we can apply Prentice's Rule to the preoperative and postoperative lenses:

$$\text{Preoperative}: P = hD = (1)(2) = 2 \text{ PD BD}$$

$$\text{Postoperative}: P = hD = (1)(2) = 2 \text{ PD BU}$$

There is a net deviation of 4 PD BU when we compare the postoperative refraction to the preoperative refraction. In order to correct this deviation, we will need to dispense 4 PD BD in the postoperative glasses. We also need to go back and figure out what went wrong with the biometry measurements because we made a monocular myopic patient into a hyperopic patient![16]

13. Answer: This is yet another twist on asking the same concepts we have discussed thus far. If the vertical lines are focused sharply with the +3.00D lens, this means that a + 3.00 × 90 lens is needed; the lens is oriented in the 90-degree axis meridian, it exerts its power at the 180-degree power meridian, and an incoming light ray (in this case, the vertical lines of the Amsler grid) is focused at the axis meridian (90°). Similarly, if the horizontal lines are focused sharply with the +5.50D lens, this means that a + 5.50 × 180 lens is needed; the lens is oriented in the 180-degree axis meridian, it exerts its power at the 90-degree power meridian, and incoming light ray (in this case, the horizontal lines of the Amsler grid) is focused at the axis meridian (180°).

To summarize the above, we can draw a power cross showing that +3D is acting at the 180-degree meridian

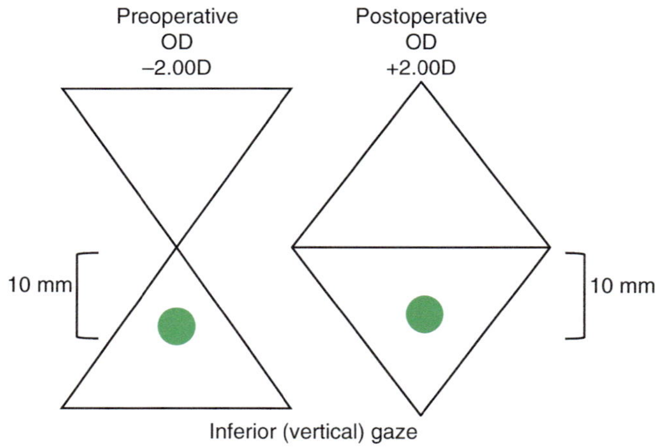

Fig. 45 Preoperative (left panel) and postoperative (right panel) prismatic effects induced in the reading position (10 mm inferior to the optical center)

[16] Causes for postoperative hyperopic surprise are discussed in chapter "Postoperative Optics for Cataract Surgery".

and a + 5.50D is acting at the 90-degree meridian. But the wrinkle to this problem is that we have to take into account the location of the Amsler grid at 50 cm. The patient will require +2D of accommodation to see the grid. The patient is 30 years old and should be able to generate this amount of accommodation on his own; however, because we have cyclopleged him, we are measuring this extra plus power that he actually does not need. In other words, we need to subtract 2D from each lens basically, and then generate our power cross (Fig. 46). Our power cross should connect +1.00 === 180 and + 3.50 === 90.

Using this power cross, we can determine the final prescription using the DAM : + 1.00 + 2.50 × 180 (or + 3.5 0 – 2.50 × 90).

14. Answer:
   (a) This one should be fairly easy by now: −4.00 + 1.00 × 90 = −3.00 – 1.00 × 180.
   (b) Using the Telephone Method, we can use our plus cylinder and minus cylinder notation to get our "PC Lenses": −4.00 === 90 and – 3.00 === 180. We can draw the power cross and check our work using the DAM (Fig. 47).
   (c) Our SC notation lenses should be the opposite of our PC components:
   −4.00 × 180 and – 3.00 × 90.
   We can check our work by using the SC method. We should get the original prescription.
   (d) The axis cross is drawn by setting the SC notation lenses as connected components and NOT using the DAM. In other words, our axis cross lenses are:
   −4.00 === 180 and – 3.00 === 90.
   Notice how these are *different* from our PC lenses. We can draw the axis cross, and following the arrows for the axis cross, we should be able to get back to our original prescription (Fig. 48).
   (e) Our expected streak refraction results will be as follows. From our SC notation lenses, we know that −4.00 STREAKS the 180 and – 3.00 STREAKS the 90. But these lenses have already had the working distance (50 cm = additional -2D sphere) incorporated into them. Thus, we must *add +2D sphere* to determine our streak results: -2.00D STREAKS the 180° and – 1.00D STREAKS the 90°. In other words, assuming a working distance of 50 cm, if we held the streak horizontally (and moved it up and down [vertically]), a −2D lens would neutralize the reflex. If we held the streak vertically, a −1D lens would neutralize the reflex.

15. Answer:
   (a) The circle of least confusion (COLC) will be formed halfway between the power of the above two lines. We can begin by using the information in the question stem.
   First, we know that the lens focuses light at 25 cm at 45°. This means there must be +4D power (100/25 = +4D) placed in the 45° (axis) meridian, which is exerting its effect at the 135° (power) meridian, which in turn forms a line at 45°. When

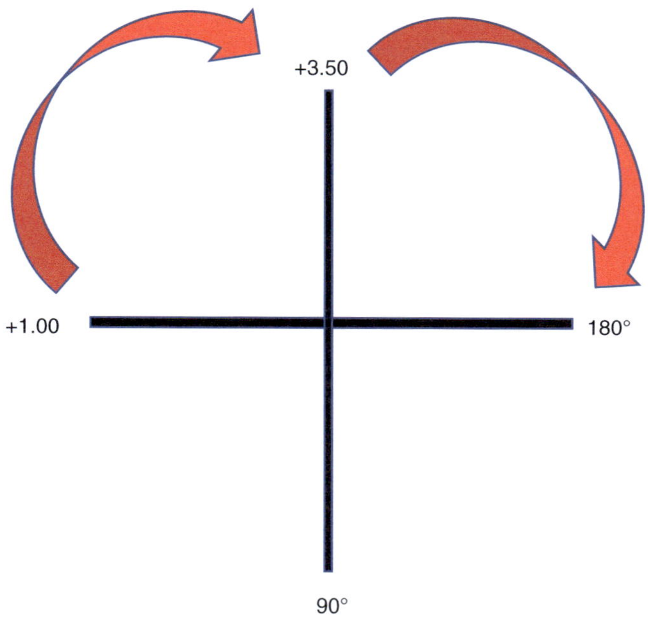

Fig. 46 Power cross for practice question #13

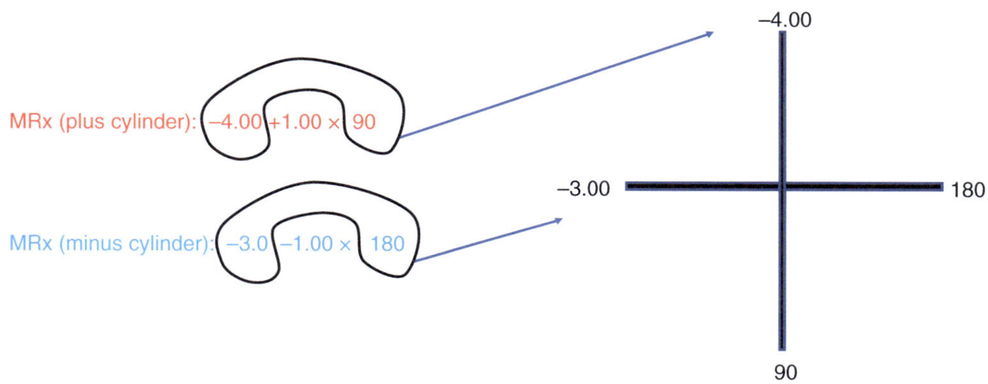

Fig. 47 Power cross for practice question #14

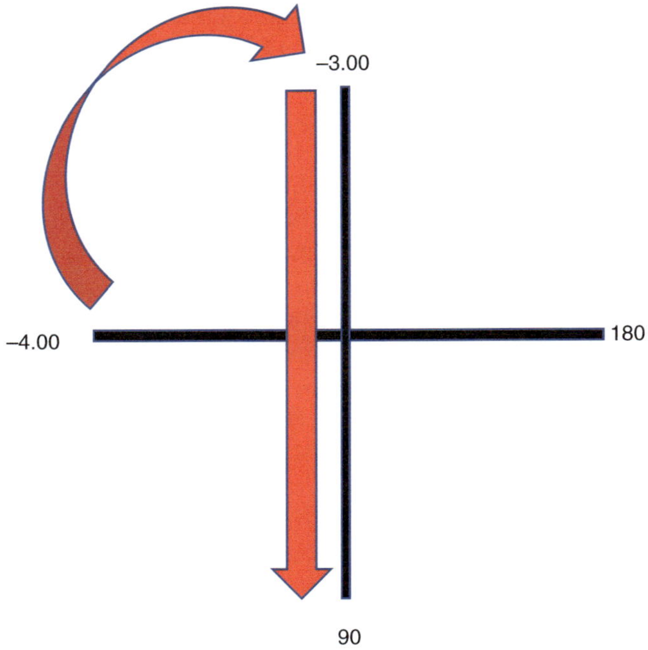

Fig. 48 Axis cross for eyeglass prescription: −4.00 + 1.00 × 90. Note how this differs from the power cross in Fig. 41. The double arches method *cannot* be used with the axis cross

we draw the power cross, the +4D should be linked to the 135°.

Next, we know that the lens focuses light at 67 cm at 135°. This means there must be +1.5D power (100/67 = +1.5D) placed in the 135° (axis) meridian, which is exerting its effect at the 45° (power) meridian which in turn forms a line at 135°. When we draw the power cross, the +1.5D should be linked to the 45°.

The COLC will be formed at the average power of these two powers: (4 + 1.5)/2 = 2.75D. The location of this will be 100/2.75D = 36.36 cm to the right of the lens (admittedly a difficult math number, which is why this is the last problem in the practice question set).

(b) From the previous solution, we can draw our power cross: +4.00 === 135 and + 1.50 === 45.

We can use the DAM to calculate the power of the unknown spherocylindrical lens: +1.50 + 2.50 × 45 (or +4.00 − 2.50 × 135).

Astigmatism

Daniel Wee

Objectives

- To understand the concept of astigmatism
- To differentiate between various types of astigmatism (corneal vs. lenticular astigmatism, refractive vs. ocular astigmatism, regular vs. irregular astigmatism)
- To classify various kinds of corneal astigmatism (with the rule, against the rule, and oblique) and apply this for clinical and surgical management of astigmatism
- To understand differences among simple, compound, and mixed astigmatisms
- To introduce the concept of pantoscopic tilt and astigmatism of oblique incidence, especially in clinical situations
- To review the concept and application of a Jackson cross cylinder
- To briefly discuss some additional advanced topics in clinical and surgical management of astigmatism

Introduction

This chapter is extremely useful for both exam and clinical purposes. All of us may have found ourselves explaining the concept of astigmatism to patients several times a day in the clinic. Some patients may be extremely concerned that they were told they have "an astigmatism"[1] and potentially vision-threatening consequences of this diagnosis! Other patients may be confused when they see their glass prescriptions look more like map coordinates with three different numbers.

Let us define astigmatism: linguistically, astigmatism is derived from "*a*" (Greek for "without") and "*stigme*" (Greek for "geometric point"). In other words, astigmatism refers to a refractive state in the eye wherein incoming light rays do not fall on the retina at a single point; instead, there is a set of two *focal lines* formed by these incoming light rays.[2] To review, in an emmetropic eye (without accommodation), incoming light rays should come together in love and harmony at a single point on the retina. When astigmatism is present, there is something evil and sinister happening so that these incoming light rays are broken into separate focal lines.

Why does this happen? Because there is no such thing as a perfectly round surface, the asymmetry present in the cornea and the crystalline lens will cause incoming light rays to be bent differently, depending on the portion of the cornea (or the crystalline lens) the light rays have passed through. Astigmatism is usually always present in conjunction with various amounts of spherical (myopic or hyperopic) refractive errors. Astigmatism has relevance in both clinical and surgical practice: we have to correct as many refractive errors as possible, including astigmatism, in order to give the patient his/her best possible vision. We discussed some of these introductory concepts in the previous chapter.

So, what is astigmatism? The short answer is that sometimes the cornea and/or the lens is shaped more like an American football than a soccer ball – voila, we have astigmatism.

The long answer: buckle up. We will cover that in this chapter in detail.

[1] Or, as some patients may call it, "stigmatism"

[2] You may wish to review the discussion in the previous chapter regarding conoid of sturm and the circle of least confusion (chapter "Spherocylindrical Lenses") that discusses these two focal lines formed by light rays passing through a spherocylindrical lens – in this case, that "lens" is the spherocylindrical cornea with astigmatism.

D. Wee (✉)
Center for Sight, Stockton, CA, USA

K. M. Riaz et al. (eds.), *Optics for the New Millennium*, https://doi.org/10.1007/978-3-030-95251-8_11

Types of Astigmatism

Astigmatism can be classified in several ways:

- Corneal vs. lenticular astigmatism
  - Corneal astigmatism itself can be subdivided in several ways, which we will discuss in the next section of this chapter.
- Refractive vs. ocular astigmatism
- Regular vs. irregular astigmatism
- Simple vs. compound astigmatism

Corneal vs. Lenticular Astigmatism

This classification is perhaps the easiest to understand. Simply put, we are describing how much astigmatism is due to the football shape of the cornea and how much astigmatism is due to the football shape of the lens. Every patient will have *some* amount of both corneal and lenticular astigmatism. For most patients, the amount of lenticular astigmatism may be quite minimal. Therefore, the refractive cylinder measured on manifest refraction may be very close to the corneal astigmatism measured on keratometry. For example, if a patient has keratometry readings of 44.50 × 45.50 at 90 (1D of corneal astigmatism), assuming zero lenticular astigmatism, a possible manifest refraction for this patient could be −2.00 + 1.00 × 90. In other words, we have to place +2D of cylinder *in* the 90-degree (axis) meridian in order to *act at* the 180-degree (power) meridian.[3] For this patient, all of the refractive astigmatism is coming from the football-shaped cornea.

However, as you may have gathered, this is not always the case. Just as the cornea can be shaped like a football, the lens can also have an ovoid shape. Lenticular astigmatism can therefore also play a significant role in the total amount of astigmatism present (ocular astigmatism) that may or may not show up in the refractive astigmatism (next section).

Lenticular astigmatism can be a funny creature that can have three faces (Fig. 1)

- Lenticular astigmatism can be so *minimal* that it has no/minimal effect on ocular astigmatism
- Lenticular astigmatism can *amplify corneal astigmatism*: if the directions of the "corneal football" and "lens football" are parallel to each other, then both astigmatisms will team up. For example, if manifest refraction showed 3D of refractive astigmatism but only 2D is present in keratometry readings, then it is very likely that the source of the additional 1D of refractive astigmatism is coming from lenticular astigmatism.
- Lenticular astigmatism can *neutralize corneal astigmatism*: if the directions of the "corneal football" and "lens football" are located 90° away from each other, then lenticular astigmatism may offset or neutralize corneal astigmatism. For example, if manifest refraction showed 1D of cylinder and 2D is present in keratometry readings, then it is very likely that there is 1D of lenticular astigmatism located 90° away that is neutralizing the corneal astigmatism.

Why is this important? Let us look at a few potential clinical examples:

Clinical example #1 Suppose you are going to do cataract surgery on a patient with a high amount of refractive astigmatism (as evidenced by his/her preoperative glasses) and you are deciding what type of intraocular lens (IOL) to place in that patient. Patient A has high corneal astigmatism and no lenticular astigmatism, while patient B has high lenticular astigmatism and no corneal astigmatism. Patient A may benefit from astigmatism correction at the time of cataract surgery (e.g., toric IOL or limbal relaxing incision). If this patient chooses no astigmatism correction at the time of surgery, it is crucial to explain to her that she will require cylindrical correction in the glasses because we will have unmasked the corneal astigmatism after surgery, even if she did not need cylindrical correction in the presurgical eyeglasses! Patient B will likely do well with a non-toric IOL and will likely do *worse* with a toric IOL. We will further discuss options for the surgical correction of astigmatism in Chaps. 26 and 27 "Preoperative Optics for Cataract Surgery", and What Is on the Menu: An Overview of Currently Available IOLs and Relevant Optics.

Clinical example #2 Suppose a 24-year-old patient presents to your office for her annual eye exam. She has worn glasses since age 10 but now inquires about wearing contact lenses. Her refraction in both eyes is −3.00D sphere (20/15). Keratometry readings are 43.50 × 44.75 at 90 (1.25D) in the right eye and 43.50 × 44.50 at 95 (1.5D) in the left eye. What type of contact lens would be the best option for this patient?

[3] See Chap. 10 "Spherocylindrical Lenses", for a review of this concept which is crucial to the rest of the discussion in this chapter.

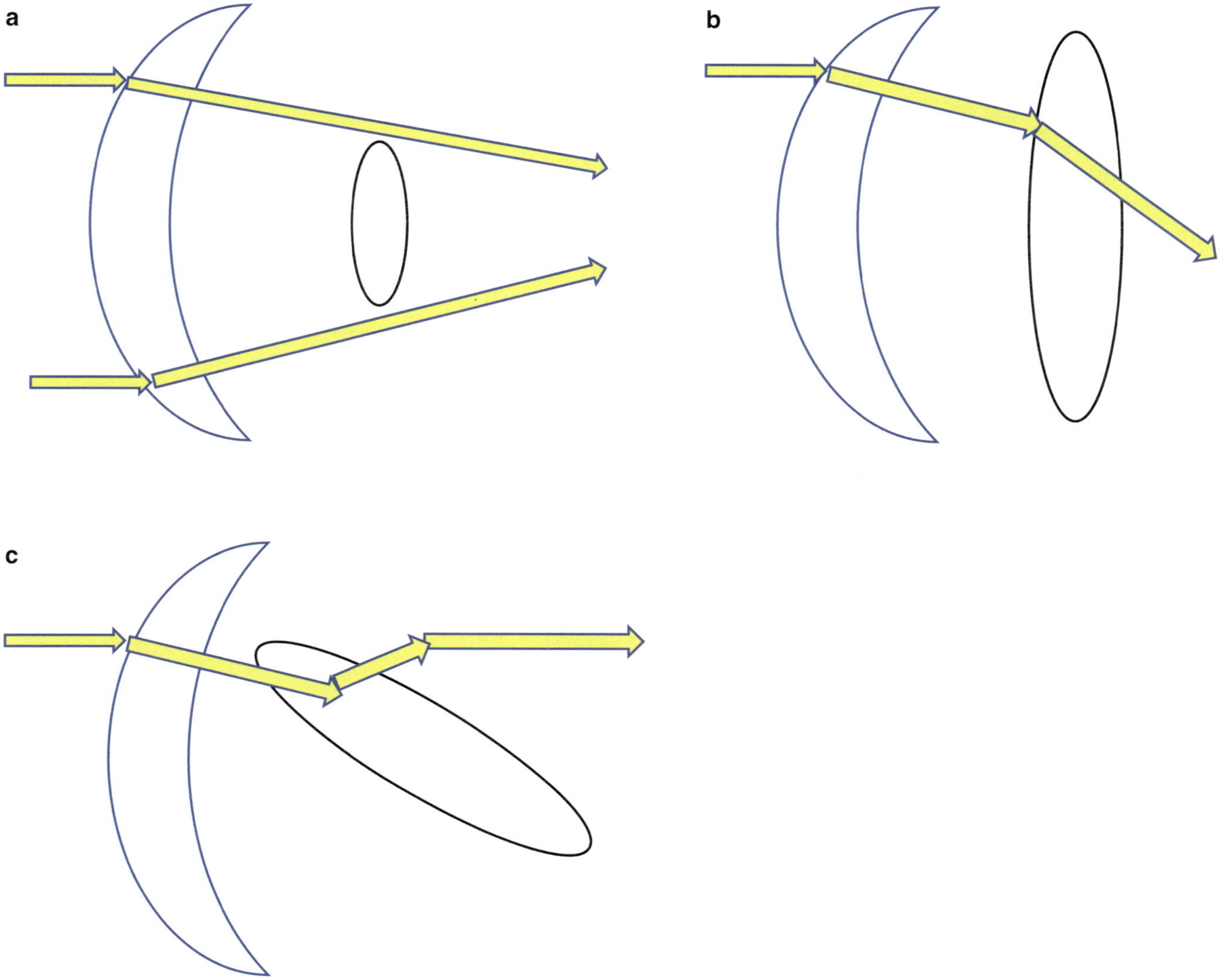

Fig. 1 There can be three varieties of lenticular astigmatism in relation to corneal astigmatism. Panel **a** shows minimal effect of lenticular astigmatism, drawn as a "small" lens that does not affect any incoming light ray. Panel **b** shows an eye wherein lenticular astigmatism is additive to corneal astigmatism, as shown by the effects of both the cornea and the lens (exaggerated) on an incoming light ray. Panel **c** shows an eye wherein lenticular astigmatism is located 90° away from corneal astigmatism and therefore has a neutralizing effect

This is an example of a patient that likely has the third type of lenticular astigmatism we discussed above. This is also known as *favorable lenticular astigmatism* because it is neutralizing (balancing) all of the corneal astigmatism; therefore, she only wears a spherical correction in both eyes and has excellent visual acuity. For this patient, she would probably do well with a *soft contact lens*. A *soft toric contact lens* is likely *not* necessary to correct this much astigmatism. Most importantly, a *hard contact lens* would be the *worst choice* because while it will neutralize the corneal astigmatism, it will unmask the lenticular astigmatism and paradoxically make the patient's vision worse! We will discuss more scenarios of clinical pearls for contact lens fitting in Chap. 20 "Contact Lenses in Clinical Practice".

Refractive vs. Ocular Astigmatism

In some ways, this may be semantics more than a true classification. Both are a combination of corneal and lenticular astigmatism and are often used interchangeably. *Refractive astigmatism* is the total astigmatism that can be detected during a manifest or streak refraction. Therefore, there is some dependency on the skill level of the examiner and the cooperation of the patient. For most clinical setting purposes, refractive astigmatism serves as a proxy for ocular astigmatism, and both are essentially equal. However, *ocular astigmatism* is the total astigmatism that is actually present in the eye and may only be detected on wave front aberrometry (see Chap. 14, "Physical Optics and Advanced Optical Principles"). It is a combination of corneal and lenticular astigmatism. Ocular astigmatism may or may not be equal in magnitude to the refractive astigmatism, but it has relevance for the purposes of laser refractive surgery, especially for wave front-guided and wave front-optimized ablations.

In the clinical setting, for example, a patient may have 1.5D of ocular astigmatism, but during manifest refraction, he may only require 1.25D of refractive astigmatism for 20/20 vision. For this patient, the "extra" 0.25D of ocular astigmatism is negligible and clinically irrelevant. However, on wave front measurement, the full 1.5D of astigmatism may be measured.

An additional type of astigmatism can be briefly mentioned here. Several terms have been used for this, but visuoperceptive astigmatism (VPA) may help describe the fact that a significant component in experienced vision involved tertiary neuroprocessing – in other words, outside the eyeball. Thus, in addition to refractive and ocular astigmatism, VPA refers to underlying neural processes that mediate retinal defocus and perceptual errors. VPA may neutralize or worsen ocular astigmatism. Don't worry too much about VPA, as it's beyond the scope of exams and clinical practice; we introduce it here only for completeness. VPA is an area of current and future study that may have greater clinical relevance in the future.

Regular vs. Irregular Astigmatism

If the astigmatism has the same orientation and is the same amount at every point in both the steep and flat meridians (which are 90° apart from each other), then we can say that the patient has *regular astigmatism* (Fig. 2). Regular astigmatism can usually be fully corrected with glasses and soft (including soft toric) contact lenses. *Irregular astigmatism* occurs when the astigmatism has variable orientation and amount in both meridians. The principal meridians may or may not be 90° away from each other: on retinoscopy or placido-disk-based keratometry, for example, an irregular streak reflex or irregular mires may be present, respectively. Irregular astigmatism usually requires imaging devices such as topographers and/or aberrometers to be quantified; in other words, irregular astigmatism is the summed total of higher-order aberrations (see Chap. 14 "Physical Optics and Advanced Optical Principles"). Irregular astigmatism usually *cannot* be fully corrected with glasses and may account for those annoying patients who objectively can see 20/20 but are incessantly complaining about their poor vision in your clinic. For these patients, a rigid gas permeable contact lens may correct most of the irregular astigmatism present. In recent years, topography-guided ablation has emerged as a potentially viable surgical option for treating irregular astigmatism.

Simple vs. Compound Astigmatism

As we stated above, refractive errors with astigmatism result in incoming light rays falling on the retina as vertical and horizontal focal lines. Depending on where exactly these lines fall on the retina (in front, directly upon, or behind), we can further classify refractive astigmatism into five subtypes. We will discuss this in greater detail in the section "Refractive Errors with Astigmatism: Simple vs. Compound Astigmatism" of this chapter.

Types of Corneal Astigmatism

Sutures and Corneal Astigmatism

A useful starting point for the discussion of corneal astigmatism (aka keratometric astigmatism) is to use an example that you may be familiar with, based on your experience in clinical and surgical settings. For example, if we place a single

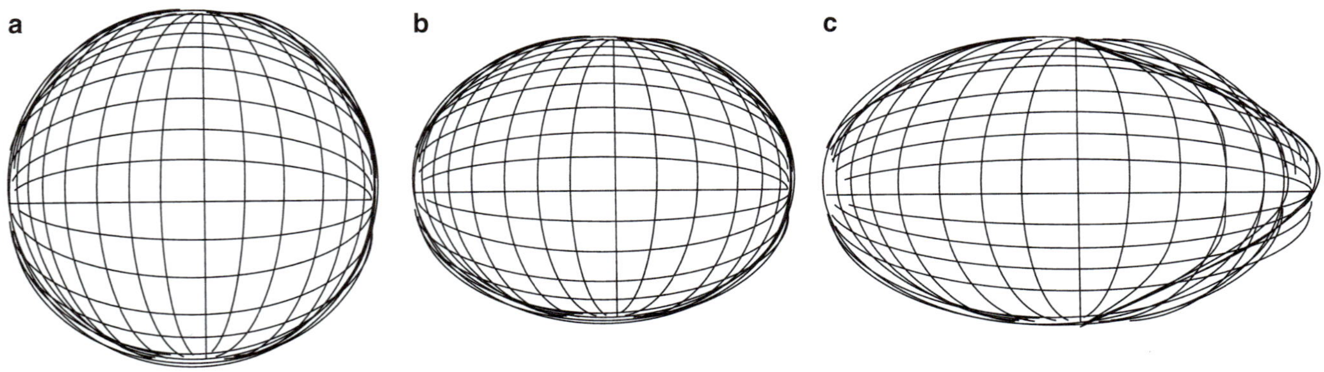

Fig. 2 Visual representation of no astigmatism (panel **a**), regular astigmatism (panel **b**), and irregular astigmatism (panel **c**). Note that in regular astigmatism (panel **b**), there is symmetry between long and short portions of the sphere. In irregular astigmatism (panel **c**), there is no symmetry between any portions of the sphere

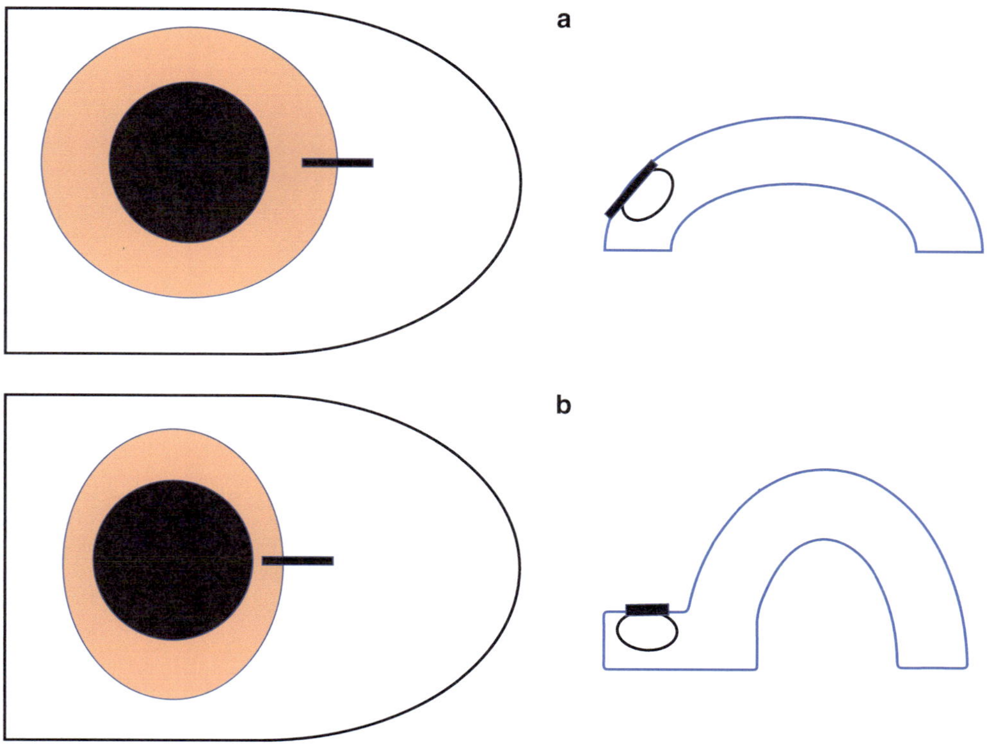

Fig. 3 Effects of a corneal suture on corneal astigmatism. In panel **a**, a properly tied suture will cause negligible change to the shape of the cornea and therefore will not affect the corneal astigmatism. If the suture is tied too tight (panel **b**), it will cause shortening of the 180-degree meridian and increased corneal astigmatism in this meridian. Keratometry readings will indicate the 180-degree meridian as the steep meridian, e.g., 44.00 × 47.00 at 180

suture to close a corneal incision made for cataract surgery of the left eye, we can see the effects of the suture on the corneal astigmatism (Fig. 3). If the suture is properly tied with equal tension, then its effects on the shape of the cornea (and therefore, corneal astigmatism) will be very minimal. However, if it is your first surgery and you are super cautious to make sure that this wound won't leak, you may end up tying it a bit too tight. When this happens (Fig. 3, panel b), we can see that the suture will cause *steepening* in the meridian of its placement and flattening of the meridian located 90° away.

Suppose that our main incision was a temporal clear corneal incision placed at the 0-degree meridian (since this is the left eye). Now that we tied our suture a bit too tight, we have induced steepening in this meridian. We would say that our steep meridian is at 0° (though 180° is preferred, in terms of the nomenclature and style points), and the flat meridian is at the 90-degree meridian. The corneal shape has become like a vertical football, as if the kicker is ready to kick a field goal (against-the-rule astigmatism). In the post-op period, keratometry readings may now read, for example, 44.00 × 47.00 at 180°, and the patient may require a manifest refraction of −1.50 + 3.00 × 180 to yield 20/20 vision (well, at least until you remove the suture).[4]

The suture example can be used as a reference to some nomenclature that we will use in following sections. The *steep meridian* is the shorter, "more protruding" meridian, the shorter side of the football. The *flat meridian* is the longer, "less protruding" meridian, the longer side of the football. This will be helpful to understand the next sections regarding the subtypes of corneal astigmatism.

[4]To review from our discussions in Chap. 10, this refraction is telling us that +3.00D cylinder has been placed in the 180-degree (axis) meridian in order to act at the 90-degree (power) meridian; it will "help" the 43D act like a 46D to equal the 180-degree meridian.

With-the-Rule (WTR) Astigmatism

With-the-rule (WTR) astigmatism refers to corneal astigmatism wherein the steep meridian of the cornea is at 90° (±20°): the range for WTR is 70–110°. We can imagine WTR astigmatism as a football placed down horizontally, as if the center is getting ready to snap it to the quarterback (Fig. 4). WTR astigmatism is most commonly seen in younger patients. Since the steep meridian is at 90°, the correcting cylinder (if using plus cylinder) has to be placed in the 90-degree (axis) meridian in order to act at the 180-degree (power) meridian. An example of an eyeglass prescription that may be used to correct WTR astigmatism would be −1.00 + 1.50 × 90.

A possibly useful (and silly) mnemonic to remember is that WTR astigmatism is more common in younger patients: "*w*ittle kids always go *w*ah-*w*ah-*w*ah."

Against-the-Rule (ATR) Astigmatism

Against-the-rule (ATR) astigmatism refers to corneal astigmatism wherein the steep meridian of the cornea is at 180° (±20°): the range for ATR is 160–200°. We can imagine ATR astigmatism as a football placed vertically (Fig. 4). ATR astigmatism is most commonly seen in older, adult patients. This is because of posterior corneal changes that occur gradually throughout life so that the net shift of cor-

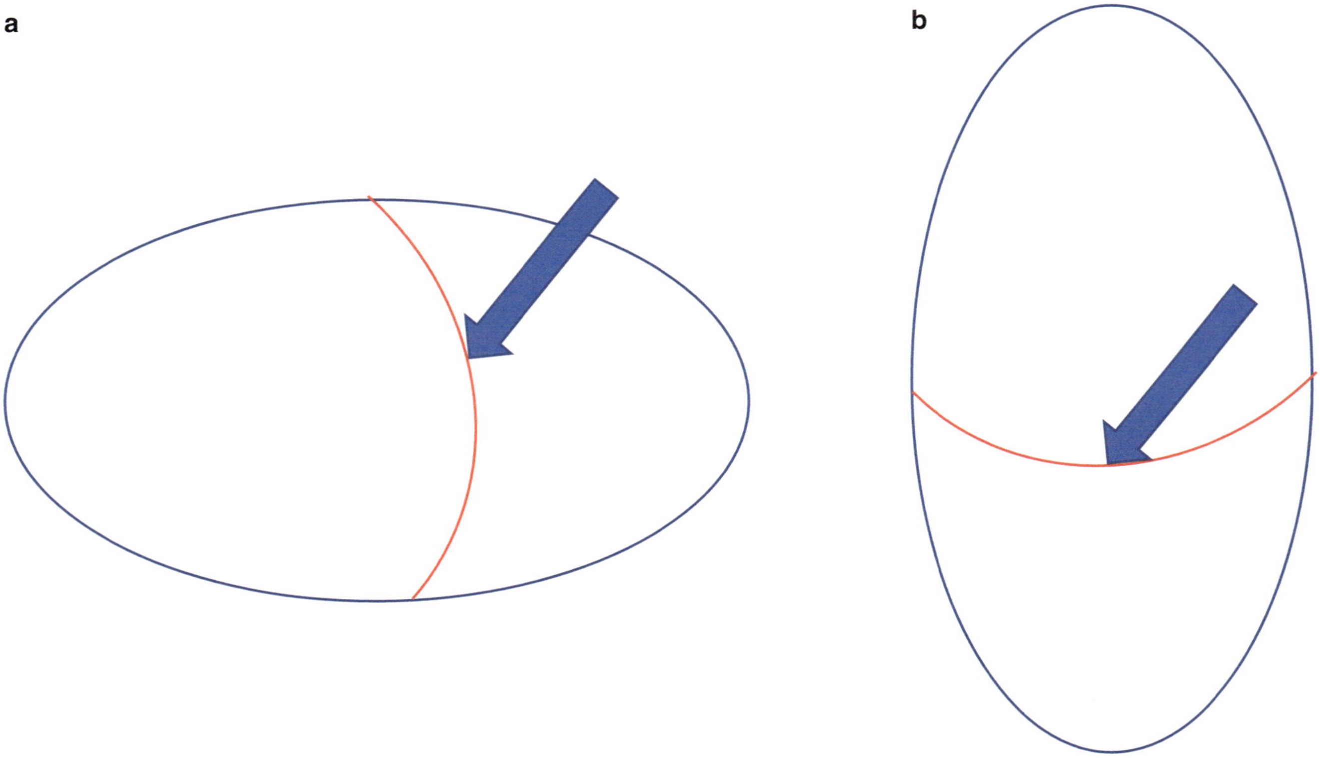

Fig. 4 Simplified representations of with-the-rule (WTR) and against-the-rule (ATR) corneal astigmatism. In WTR astigmatism (panel **a**), the steep meridian is located between 70° and 110° and can be visualized as a horizontally placed football. In ATR astigmatism (panel **b**), the steep meridian is located between 160° and 200° and can be visualized as a vertically placed football

neal astigmatism for many patients is from WTR to ATR.[5] Therefore, it is more likely to see ATR in older patients, though ATR may also be seen in younger patients. Since the steep meridian is at 180°, the correcting cylinder (if using plus cylinder) has to be placed in the 180-degree (axis) meridian in order to act at the 90-degree (power) meridian. An example of an eyeglass prescription that may be used to correct WTR astigmatism would be −1.00 + 1.50 × 180.

A possibly useful (and silly) mnemonic to remember this is "*a*ncient *a*dults will have *A*TR."

Oblique Astigmatism

Oblique astigmatism refers to corneal astigmatism that falls in between WTR and ATR astigmatism. In other words, the range for oblique astigmatism is 20–70° and 110–160°. Both WTR and ATR are typically better tolerated by adult patients as compared to oblique astigmatism.

Oblique astigmatism has significant relevance in clinical practice, especially in prescribing glasses and clinical/surgical management of oblique astigmatism. We will discuss this further in Chap. 21 "Clinical Problems with Optics and Refractive Manifestations".

A summary diagram showing WTR, ATR, and oblique astigmatism is in Fig. 5.

Refractive Errors with Astigmatism: Simple vs. Compound Astigmatism

As we have previously discussed, in an eye with refractive astigmatism, incoming light rays will not focus at a single point and instead will produce a set of focal lines. These two focal lines will basically give the eye two distinct focal points (Fig. 6). The five different types of refractive astigmatism can therefore be classified according to where these two focal points fall in relation to the retina – either in front of, directly upon, or behind the retina.

Note that both plus-cylinder and minus-cylinder notation can be used to determine the type of astigmatisms we will discuss below.

Simple Myopic Astigmatism

In simple myopic astigmatism, one focal point is anterior to the retina, and the other focal point is directly on the retina

[5] This will be of significant importance during our discussion of strategies and options for the surgical correction of astigmatism (Chap. 26 "Preoperative Optics for Cataract Surgery").

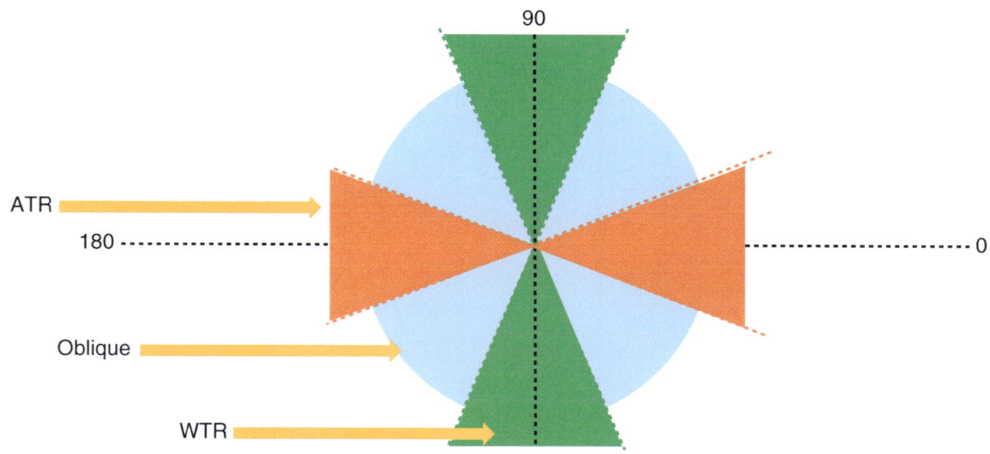

Fig. 5 Summary diagram of WTR (green), ATR (orange), and oblique astigmatism (blue) locations and ranges

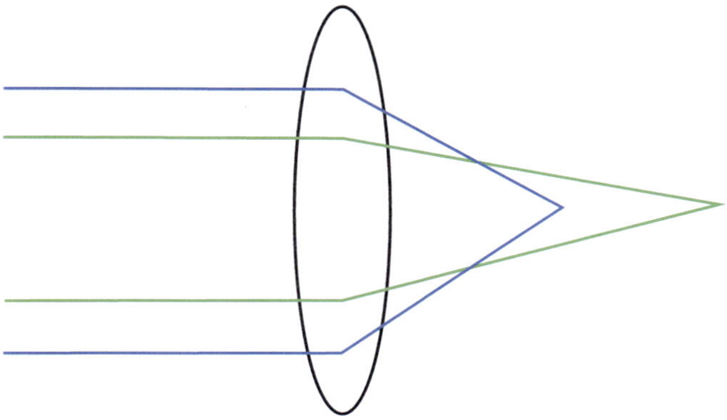

Fig. 6 Spherocylindrical lens with ray tracings coming to two separate focal points

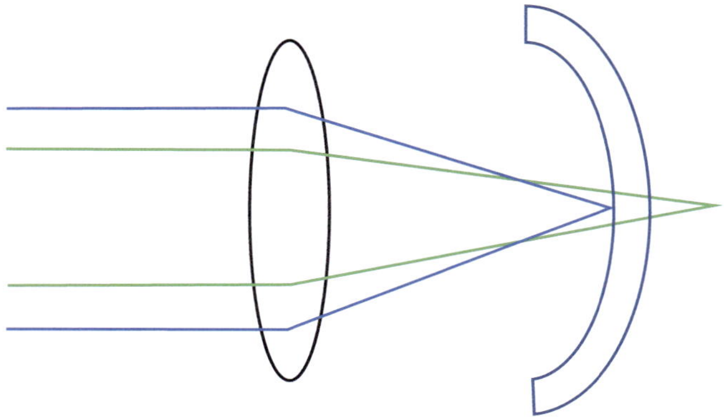

Fig. 8 Simple hyperopic astigmatism diagram showing two focal points: one posterior to the retina and one falling directly on the retina

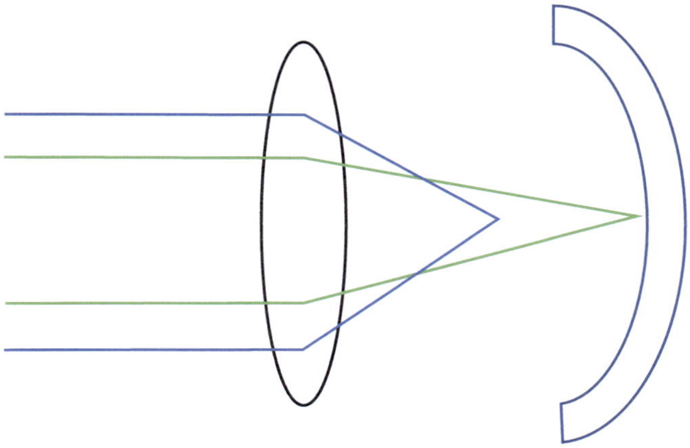

Fig. 7 Simple myopic astigmatism diagram showing two focal points: one anterior to the retina and one falling directly on the retina

(Fig. 7). Examples of manifest refractions that can be classified as simple myopic astigmatism include −2.00 + 2.00 × 90 and this should be: plano + 2.00 x 180.

When trying to determine if a prescription is simple myopic astigmatism, one method is to take the prescription and convert it to the opposite cylinder notation. If one of the resulting spheres is now plano and the other sphere is minus, then this is a simple myopic astigmatism prescription.

In the example above, note that the first prescription is the plus-cylinder notation of the second prescription. When converted to minus-cylinder notation, the sphere portion has become plano. Hence, this refraction is a correction for simple myopic astigmatism.

Simple Hyperopic Astigmatism

In simple hyperopic astigmatism, one focal point is posterior to the retina, and the other focal point is directly on the retina (Fig. 8). Examples of manifest refractions that can be classified as simple hyperopic astigmatism include plano +2.00 × 90 and +2.00–2.00 × 180.

In the two prescriptions above, notice that the first prescription is the plus-cylinder notation of the second prescription. Since the sphere portion of the first prescription is plano and the sphere portion of the second prescription is

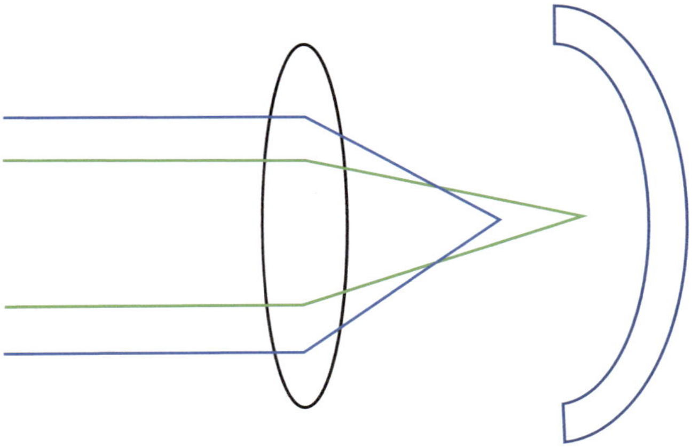

Fig. 9 Compound, myopic astigmatism diagram showing two focal points: both anterior to the retina

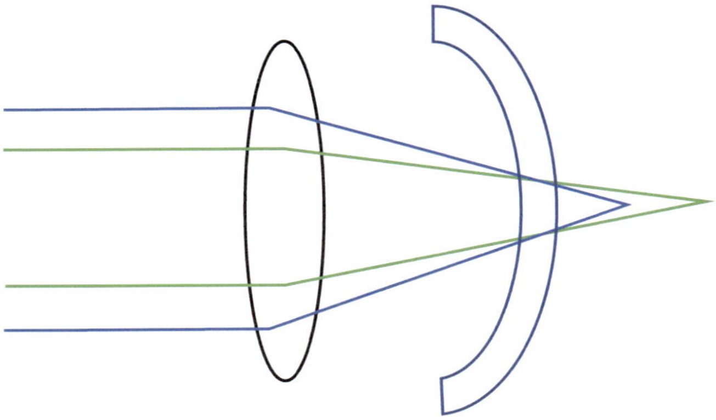

Fig. 10 Compound hyperopic astigmatism diagram showing two focal points: both posterior to the retina

+2.00D sphere, this is a simple hyperopic astigmatism prescription.

Compound Myopic Astigmatism

In compound myopic astigmatism, both focal points are anterior to the retina but in two different locations (Fig. 9). Examples of manifest refractions that can be classified as compound myopic astigmatism include −4.00 + 2.00 × 90; −2.00 – 2.00 × 180.

For example, if we consider the first prescription (−4.00 + 2.00 × 90) and convert it to minus-cylinder notation (−2.00–2.00 × 180), we note that both sphere components are minus sphere; therefore, this is a compound myopic astigmatism prescription.

Compound Hyperopic Astigmatism

In compound hyperopic astigmatism, both focal points are posterior to the retina but in two different locations (Fig. 10). Examples of manifest refractions that can be classified as compound hyperopic astigmatism include +2.00 + 2.00 × 90 and +4.00 – 2.00 × 180.

For example, if we take the first prescription (+2.00 + 2.00 × 90) and convert it to minus-cylinder notation (+4.00 – 2.00 × 180), we note that both sphere components are plus sphere; therefore, this is a compound hyperopic astigmatism prescription.

Mixed Astigmatism

Mixed astigmatism is a concept that may be confusing at first glance. In mixed astigmatism, one focal point is anterior to the retina, and one focal point is posterior to the retina (Fig. 11). What is confusing about the refraction is that simply looking at the sphere may make you think that it is a myopic or hyperopic prescription, but when you convert to minus-cylinder notation, you may get an opposite-signed sphere.

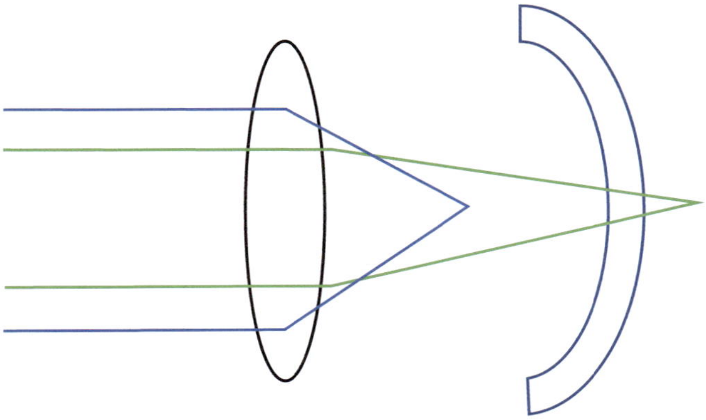

Fig. 11 Mixed astigmatism diagram showing two focal points: one anterior to the retina and one posterior to the retina

Examples of manifest refractions that can be classified as mixed astigmatism are as follows:

- −1.00 + 3.00 × 180 → convert to minus cylinder, +2.00 – 3.00 × 90; SE, +0.50
- −2.50 + 3.50 × 40 → convert to minus cylinder, +1.00–3.50 × 130; SE, −0.75
- +2.75 – 3.00 × 90 → convert to plus cylinder, −0.25 + 3.00 × 180; SE, +1.25

For each of these prescriptions, notice how sphere values change to an opposite-signed sphere value when we convert to the opposite cylinder notation.

As you may have sensed from examples given above, a commonly tested type of question may be "given the following refraction, what type of astigmatism does this patient have?" While we have solved some examples above, we will now present a systematic method to follow to ensure that you do not make an error in classification:

- Step 1. If the refraction is given in a plus (or minus) cylinder notation, write the opposite cylinder notation next to it (as we did above).
- Step 2. Look *only* at the spherical power of each notation. Ignore the cylinder and axis values:
  - *Both* spheres are *positive*: compound hyperopic astigmatism.
  - *One* sphere is *positive* and *one* is *plano*: simple hyperopic astigmatism.
  - *One* sphere is *positive* and *one* is *negative*: mixed astigmatism.
  - *One* sphere is *negative* and *one* is *plano*: simple myopic astigmatism.
  - *Both* spheres are *negative*: compound myopic astigmatism.

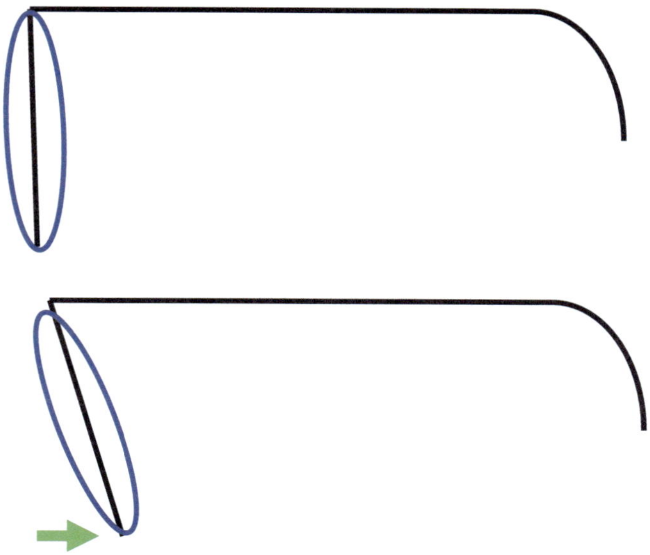

Fig. 12 Profile view of glasses sitting on a face demonstrating no tilt (top figure) and the preferred, typical pantoscopic tilt (bottom figure). Note that the typical amount of tilt is 7–8°; this has been exaggerated in the diagram for effect

Pantoscopic Tilt and Astigmatism of Oblique Incidence

Pantoscopic tilt (PT) is a confusing topic because, depending on which textbook you consult, it can refer to two similar yet slightly different concepts. We can begin our discussion using eyeglasses as an example.

If you look at a pair of single vision lens (SVL) glasses from the side, you will notice that the lenses are not exactly vertically aligned. They are usually constructed with an angle such that the lower edge of the lens is closer to the face/cheek, i.e., tilted along the horizontal (180-degree) axis (Fig. 12). This makes it easier for a person wearing SVL glasses to rotate his/her eyes from distance to near (and vice versa) without changing the vertex distance. The range of PT is 1–12°; the ideal tilt is 7–8° on the lower rim edge. This will place the optical center of the SVL glasses slightly below the center of the pupil (usually around 4 mm). As a general rule of thumb, the optical center should be dropped inferiorly about 0.5–1 mm for every 1–2° of PT in order to reduce the amount of induced power caused by normal PT. Bifocal and progressive glasses have varying amounts of PT as well.

A large degree of tilt, especially on high myopic prescriptions, will produce considerable amounts of nonuniform hyperopic shifts, along with peripheral astigmatism and coma in the visual field.[6] Therefore, the amount of PT is even more important for higher prescriptions.

Theoretically, *retroscopic tilt* (lower rim of the glasses tilted away from the cheek) also exists but is very rarely used.[7] One main drawback of retroscopic tilt is the high amount of induced refractive errors based on changes in gaze position, much more than those seen with PT. Additionally, *faceform tilt* (tilt along the vertical axis) is rarely used.

Pantoscopic Tilt: Tilting a Spherical Lens

Have you ever had a patient tell you that they see better when they tilt their lenses? This is especially common in myopic patients due to PT. In our previous discussions on lens effectivity (Chap. 6 "Lens Effectivity"), we discussed how moving the lens toward the eye and away from the eye can change the effective power of the lens. In this scenario, if we have a spherical lens but tilt the lens around its axis (either 90° or 180 axis), then we will see a resulting increase in lens power and induced cylindrical power in that axis. Since PT is typically used when describing glasses, the tilt will occur in the 180-degree axis. If you attempt to tilt around the 90-degree axis, you will probably end up breaking the glasses!

Why does tilting the lens help a patient, mathematically? This is where we can introduce the concept of *Martin's law of lens tilt*. This law helps us to calculate the power of a given spherical lens depending on how much you tilt it. Note: you will never ever be asked to calculate this on an exam because

[6]See Chap. 14, "Physical Optics and Advanced Optical Principles", for a more detailed discussion regarding coma and other higher-order aberrations.

[7]For those of you who simply must know, retroscopic tilt can be used for patients with unique facial anatomy, such as patients with low-set ears and protruding cheeks, or to maximize the amount of the frame's bridges touching the patient's nose.

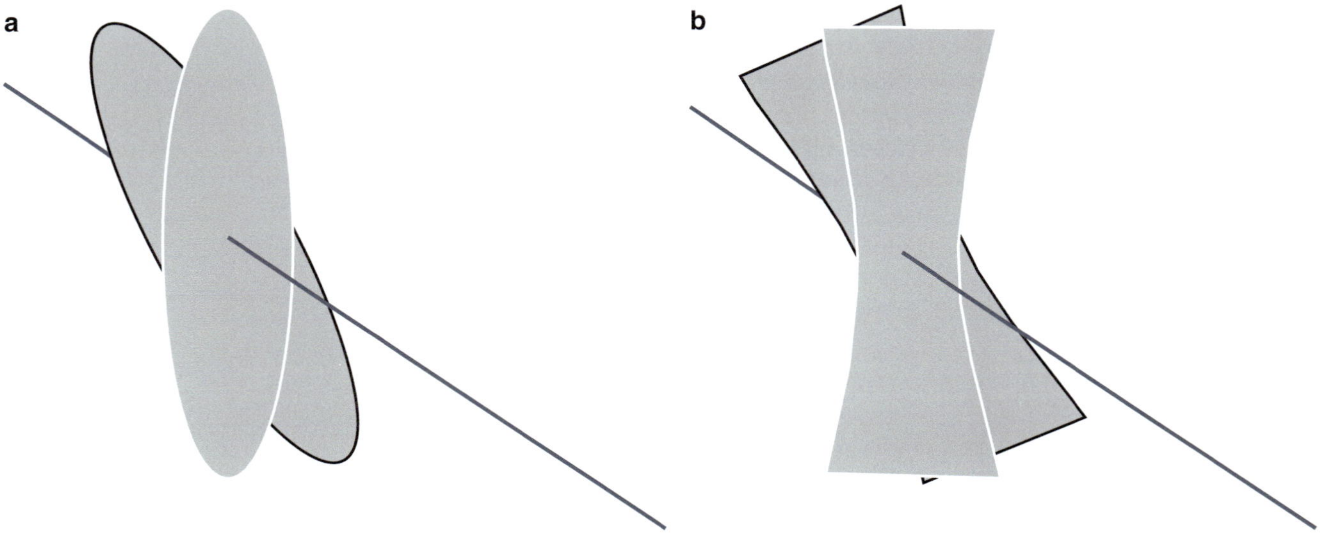

Fig. 13 Tilting a plus lens (panel **a**) induces additional plus cylinder in the axis of tilt, in this case axis 180; tilting a minus sphere lens (panel **b**) induces additional minus cylinder in the axis of tilt

the math will be incredibly difficult – if you can do this math in your head, then you are wasting your time in ophthalmology, and you should have been a Nobel laureate in mathematics instead!

We can see what all the fuss is about when it comes to Martin's law of lens tilt:

$$\text{PT new sphere} = \text{Sphere} \times \left[1 + \left((\sin a)^2 / 3\right)\right]$$

$$\text{PT new cylinder} = \text{New sphere} \times \left[(\tan a)^2\right]$$

Example #1 +15.00D glasses with 10° of tilt. Remember that most glasses are tilted about 180-degree axis:

- New sphere, 15 × [1 + ((sin 10 deg)^2/3)]:
  - Sin 10 = 0.17364 → (0.17364)^2 = 0.03015 → 0.03015/3 = 0.01005
  - 1 + 0.01005 = 1.01
  - 15 × 1.01 = 15.15 D sph
- New cylinder, 15.15 × [(tan 10 deg)^2]:
  - Tan 10 = 0.1763 → (0.1763)^2 = 0.031091
  - 15.15 × 0.031 = 0.47 D cyl

When tilted 10°, these glasses will function like +15.15 + 0.47 × 180.

Notice that these SVL plus glasses have *gained additional plus sphere and additional plus cylinder* in the direction of tilt.

Example #2 −15.00 D glasses with 10 degrees of tilt → −15.15 − 0.47 × 180

We can convert this to plus-cylinder notation, −15.62 + 0.47 × 90.

When tilted 10°, these glasses will give the myopic patient additional minus sphere power at the cost of some cylinder. This explains why an undercorrected myope will tilt his glasses – he is gaining some additional minus sphere power.

To summarize PT and Martin's law of lens tilt:

- Tilting a plus lens → extra plus sphere power and plus cylinder in the axis of tilt
- Tilting a minus lens → extra minus sphere and minus cylinder in the axis of tilt

Getting back to our clinical example, when a patient says they see better by tilting their glasses, they probably need stronger glasses, astigmatic correction, or both (Fig. 13).

Astigmatism of Oblique Incidence (AOOI)

Astigmatism of oblique incidence (AOOI) refers to oblique astigmatism that is induced astigmatism from light rays that are not on the principal axis. AOOI can be thought of as the "unwanted" astigmatism that happens when a patient looks through the lens at an angle away from the optical center (i.e., the peripheral portions of the lens). This type of astigmatism is dependent on the *shape* of the lens, specifically, the relationship between curves of the front surface and back surface. While PT assumes that the patient is still looking through the optical center when the entire lens tilts, AOOI can occur with and without PT, depending on where the patient is looking. As with many things with glasses, if only

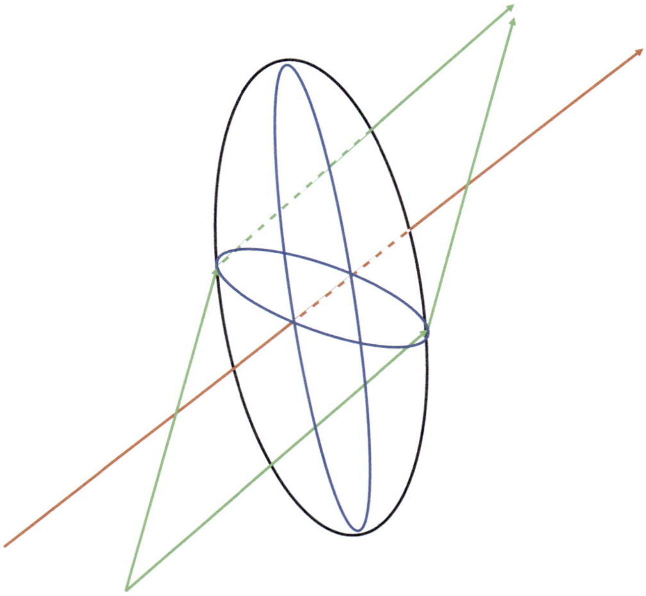

Fig. 14 Diagram of astigmatism of oblique incidence (AOOI) demonstrating a light source (green lines) off of the principal axis (red lines). AOOI may be caused by a spherical lens that has undergone unintended tilting

patients can be taught to strictly look through the optical center, then we would not have to worry about these issues!

When a patient looks through the optical center, spherical lenses induce spherical power, and spherocylindrical lenses induce both spherical and cylindrical power. However, if the light ray is off axis, the spherical lens also induces cylindrical power known as AOOI (Fig. 14).[8]

PT and AOOI usually occur together; it is difficult to have a situation where purely one of these is having an effect without accounting for the other. In fact, AOOI can further be broken down into AOOI caused by the cornea and AOOI caused by the lens; both of these AOOIs have opposite-signed astigmatism, which produces better image quality for the eye as a whole.[9]

We can conclude this section with a clinically relevant example. Suppose we have a patient with a history of pseudoexfoliation syndrome who underwent cataract surgery with placement of a + 20.00D IOL. His manifest refraction 1 month after surgery was plano (20/20). If this patient came in 3 months later complaining of blurry vision and we see on clinical exam that the IOL has tilted forward around the 180-degree axis (i.e., the superior part of the optic is now closer to the cornea, and the inferior part of the optic is now closer to the retina), then the IOL may no longer function as a + 20.00D IOL. Because it has tilted forward (similar to an eyeglass lens), it will gain some plus sphere and plus cylinder and thus may function as +21.00 + 2.00 × 180 due to PT (and resulting AOOI). The patient may present with a myopic astigmatism refractive error, such as −1.00 − 2.00 × 180, which converted to plus-cylinder notation that would be −3.00 + 2.00 × 90. Note that we used exaggerated whole numbers in this example to make the math easier for the sake of reinforcing the concept.

Jackson Cross Cylinders

Edward Jackson (d. 1942) first described the use of the Jackson cross cylinder lens (JCCL) to determine the *power* of astigmatism in 1887.[10] Then, in 1907, he described how the JCCL can be used to refine the *axis* of the correcting cylinder. The good Dr. Jackson was a pretty cool and accomplished guy: he established the first graduate course for ophthalmologists, suggested the formation of the instruction courses of the American Academy of Ophthalmology, and was the principal founder of the American Board of Ophthalmology.

A JCCL is simply a tool used to determine the axis and strength of astigmatism. It can look like a handheld tool or can be incorporated into the phoropter (Figs. 15 and 16).

A JCCL is basically two cylindrical lenses placed 90° away from each other. One cylinder is plano-convex and the other is plano-concave. A JCCL is made by grinding cylinder power on one surface and pairing it with a half-power sphere of the opposite sign on the other surface. In other words, the spherical equivalent of Jackson cross cylinders will always be zero because the cylinder power in a JCCL is double and of opposite power to the sphere. For example, commonly used JCCLs would include −0.25/+0.50 and −0.50/+1.00.

This may also make more (visual) sense if you imagine the JCCL as a power cross lens (Figs. 17 and 18).[11] In the first example, notice the power cross for a JCCL with −0.50/+1.00 power; in the second example, notice the power cross for a JCCL with −2.00/+4.00 power.

We can use the JCCL to help us answer three commonly encountered questions and scenarios:

Detecting refractive astigmatism If any refractive astigmatism is present, then using the JCCL to show the patient flip choices should reveal it because one flip choice should

[8]For those of you who wear glasses, especially higher-powered ones, you can try this by looking obliquely through your lenses in the periphery and trying to read a computer screen, for example. You will notice that the text is slightly blurry. It is much easier to turn your head and look at the screen directly (i.e., look through the optical center).

[9]Liu T, Thibos LN. Variation of axial and oblique astigmatism with accommodation across the visual field. J Vis. 2017 Mar 1;17(3):24

[10]Newell FW. Edward Jackson, MD – a historical perspective of his contributions to refraction and to ophthalmology. *Ophthalmology* 1988; 95: 555–58

[11]See Chap. 10, "Spherocylindrical Lenses", for a review of power crosses.

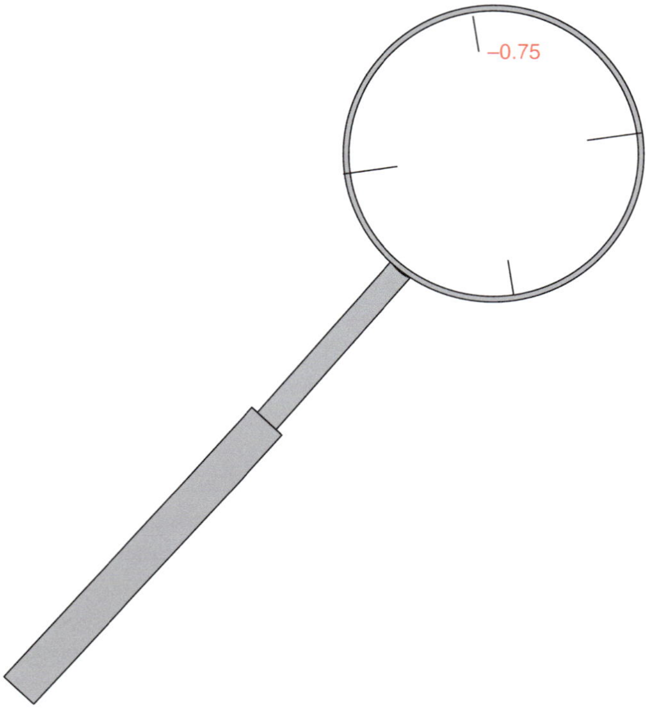

Fig. 15 Picture of a handheld Jackson cross cylinder lens

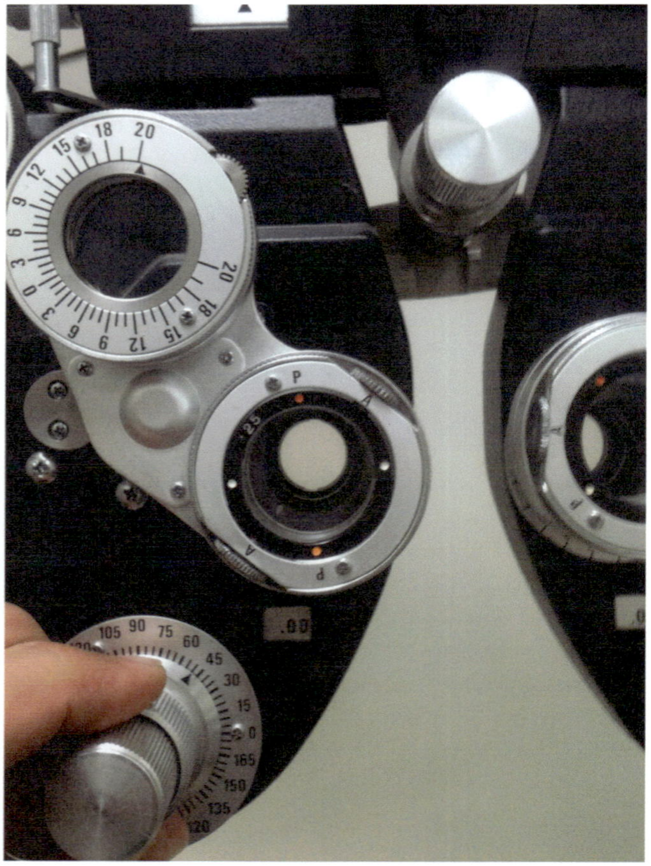

Fig. 16 Picture of a Jackson cross cylinder on the phoropter

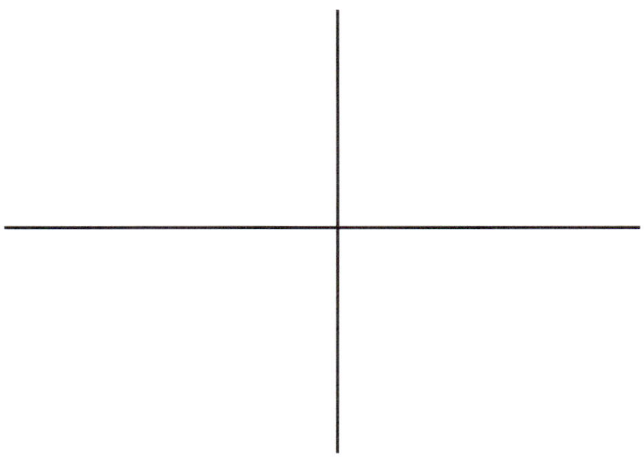

Fig. 17 Example 1 of power cross showing a Jackson cross cylinder lens with −0.50/+1.00 held in the 90-degree position

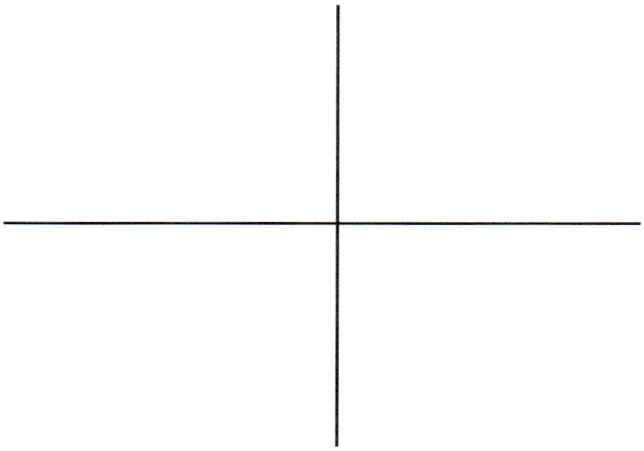

Fig. 18 Example 2 of power cross showing a Jackson cross cylinder with −2.00/+4.00 held in the 180-degree position

always produce less blur than the other choice. However, if we erroneously have placed the JCCL such that the JCCL axes are 45° away from the true axis of refractive astigmatism, then flip choices may be equally bad, and the patient may not report a preference for either choice. For example, if we place the JCCL in the 90°/180° position but the patient feels that both choices are equally lousy, then we may want to test at the 45°/135° position to attempt finding any refractive astigmatism.

What if the patient does not like any of the flip choices? If the patient does not like any of the flip choices, one or more of the following may be present: there is no significant refractive astigmatism; the axis of the refractive astigmatism is 45° away from where we are currently holding the JCCL;

the patient's vision is too lousy to appreciate any of the blur choices.

How much astigmatism can we refine using the JCCL? The cylinder power must be reduced if the clinician intentionally shifts the astigmatic axis, such as may be considered for a patient who has recently shifted from WTR to ATR, WTR to oblique, etc. In general, the smaller the amount of cylinder, the more degrees that can be refined. For example, if a patient only has 0.50D of refractive cylinder, then we can confidently refine 15–20° at a time. But if a patient has +2.50D of refractive cylinder, then we may only be able to refine 2–5° at a time. An analogy can be drawn from the more familiar example of toric IOLs: the greater the misalignment for a higher-powered toric IOL, the more effect it will have on under–/overcorrecting the patient's astigmatism.

Example

Which of the following is an example of a Jackson cross cylinder?

(a) −0.25 + 0.50 × 180
(b) −0.25 + 0.50 × 90
(c) −0.50 + 1.00 × 45
(d) −0.75 + 1.50 × 85
(e) All of the above

The answer is (e) all of the above. Notice that in each example, the opposite-signed cylinder is double the power of the sphere.

Advanced Topics in Astigmatism

We have thus far spent the bulk of this chapter talking about various types and classifications of astigmatism, including a discussion regarding WTR vs. ATR astigmatism.

One question that may seem philosophical but may have clinical relevance is *are there any advantages to retaining some astigmatism in the human eye?* In other words, since the human eye is imperfectly perfect, should we actively seek to neutralize all astigmatism and potentially miss out on some advantages that astigmatism provides, especially in the pseudophakic eye? While we may pat ourselves on the back after cataract surgery if a patient has no refractive astigmatism on manifest refraction, have we potentially missed out on certain advantages of mild amounts of WTR and/or ATR astigmatism?

As you may have gathered from the leading nature of the previous paragraphs' tone, there are theoretical and practical advantages to low amounts of astigmatism.

For example, low amounts (0.50–0.75D) of *WTR astigmatism* may be particularly advantageous in pseudophakic eyes.[12] Since there is more plus power at the 90-degree meridian, this will help bring in *vertical stroke letters at distance* (such as b, d, h, t, etc.) into better focus. There are more vertically stroked letters in English as compared to horizontally stroked letters. WTR astigmatism may also help with English language text because there is "less (vertical) space" between letters in a sentence as compared to the amount of space "between" sentences on a page. Furthermore, Javal's rule states that less cylinder correction is required to correct WTR astigmatism in glasses as compared to ATR; in other words, 1D of WTR keratometric astigmatism may only require 0.75D of refractive cylinder to correct it, as compared to 1D of ATR keratometric astigmatism.

Sawusch and Guyton demonstrated in an elegant model that the least amount of summated blur exists through the range of object distance 0.5–6 m that is −1.00 + 0.75 (SE, −0.63) with WTR astigmatism (as compared to ATR astigmatism) followed by −0.75 + 0.50 (SE, −0.50).[13] In other words, a postoperative pseudophakic refraction of −1.00 + 0.75 × 90 may be the "Goldilocks" prescription to give a good range of vision at the above range distances.

As for *ATR astigmatism*, the additional plus power at the 180-degree meridian helps to bring in *vertical stroke letters at near* into better focus; in other words, low amounts of ATR astigmatism may confer an advantage by improving the quality of a patient's reading vision after cataract surgery.[14] This may be particularly advantageous in patients with demands for excellent near vision, such as a jeweler or a coin collector.

Finally, in case we have not confused you enough, the benefits of WTR astigmatism for distance and ATR astigmatism for near work best for languages with vertical stroke letters. In considering languages with more horizontal strokes (Arabic, Hebrew, Hindi, etc.), the opposite may be true: low amounts of ATR astigmatism may help with distance text, and low amounts of WTR astigmatism may help with near reading vision.

[12]Morlet N, Minassian D, Dart J. Astigmatism and the analysis of its surgical correction. *Br J Ophthalmol*. 2002;86(12):1458–1459

[13]Sawusch MR, Guyton DL. Optimal astigmatism to enhance depth of focus after cataract surgery. *Ophthalmology*. 1991;98(7):1025–1029

[14]Trindade F, Oliveira A, Frasson M. Benefit of against-the-rule astigmatism to uncorrected near acuity. *J Cataract Refract Surg*. 1997;23(1):82–85

Practice Questions

1. What kind of astigmatism does a patient with this refraction have?
   Plano + 1.00 × 090:
   A. Compound hyperopic
   B. Simple hyperopic
   C. Mixed
   D. Simple myopic
   E. Compound myopic
2. What kind of astigmatism does a patient with this refraction have:
   −2.00 + 1.00 × 130
   A. Compound hyperopic
   B. Simple hyperopic
   C. Mixed
   D. Simple myopic
   E. Compound myopic
3. If a +2.00D sphere lens is tilted forward along its 180 axis, which of the following prescriptions *best* approximates the "new" power of this lens?
   A. +2.00 + 1.00 × 180
   B. +2.00 + 1.00 × 090
   C. +2.25 + 1.00 × 180
   D. +2.50 − 1.00 × 180
   E. +2.25 − 1.00 × 090
4. Which of the following statements is *true*?
   A. The anterior cornea may have with-the-rule (WTR) or against-the-rule (ATR) astigmatism; the posterior cornea usually has WTR astigmatism.
   B. A patient with keratometry readings of 44.00 × 47.00 at 90 has ATR keratometric astigmatism.
   C. A patient with keratometry readings of 44.00 × 45.00 at 180 may benefit from a temporal clear corneal incision at the time of cataract surgery.
   D. The posterior corneal astigmatism value will increase toward WTR astigmatism with age.
5. Keratometry readings of 44.00 × 46.00 at 90 are measured in a patient 6 weeks after cataract surgery. Which of the following statements is true (more than one answer choice may be correct)?
   A. If there is a tight suture placed in a temporal corneal incision, it should be removed at this time.
   B. The patient may require a manifest refraction of −1.25 + 2.00 × 180 to correct the refractive astigmatism.
   C. The patient may require a manifest refraction of −1.25 + 2.00 × 90 to correct the refractive astigmatism.
   D. If there is a tight suture placed in a superior corneal incision, it should be removed at this time.

Answers

1. Answer: B. Simple hyperopic astigmatism. First, we can write the refraction in both plus- and minus-cylinder notation:

   $$\text{Plano} + 1.00 \times 90$$
   $$+1.00 - 1.00 \times 180$$

   Since the sphere in one cylinder notation is plano and the other is plus, then this patient will have simple hyperopic astigmatism.
2. Answer: E. Compound myopic astigmatism. First, we can write the refraction in both plus- and minus-cylinder notation:

   $$-2.00 \ +1.00 \times 130$$
   $$-1.00 \ -1.00 \times 40$$

   Since sphere values in both cylinder notations are minus, then this patient has compound myopic astigmatism.
3. Answer: C. Remember that tilting a plus-powered spherical lens along its 180-degree axis will add some sphere and cylinder of that same power along the 180 axis. Note that we do not have to use Martin's law of lens tilt – we could, if we were so mathematically gifted and had access to a calculator. Instead, we can use the process of elimination. Since we know that the sphere power must increase with the tilt, we can safely eliminate A and B. Similarly, we know that the lens should gain plus-cylinder power. D and E are seemingly an increase in sphere power, but they also have an increase in minus cylinder so we can eliminate those as well. Only answer choice C gives us a value with increased plus-sphere and plus-cylinder powers.
4. Answer: C. The keratometry readings in choice C are indicative of ATR keratometric astigmatism; an incision at the steep meridian (temporal) may help to reduce this 1D of ATR astigmatism. While the anterior cornea may have WTR or ATR astigmatism, the posterior cornea nearly always has ATR astigmatism (choice A) that increases toward more ATR with age (choice D). The keratometry readings in choice B are examples of WTR keratometric astigmatism.
5. Answers: C and D. The keratometry readings indicated WTR astigmatism. A superior suture may be present at the 90-degree meridian and thus may be removed. Similarly, a manifest refraction of −1.25 + 2.00 × 90 indicates that +2D of cylinder placed in the 90-degree meridian will act at the 180-degree meridian (flat meridian) to help correct the keratometric astigmatism.

Glasses for Written Exams

G. Vike Vicente

Objectives

- To be able to list different types of bifocal segment options that may be tested on written exams
- Define image jump and image displacement
- Apply lessons from the previous chapter on prisms to understand how image jump and image displacement can be successfully managed

Introduction

Glass questions on written exams are infrequent. This topic is more relevant to oral boards and clinical practice; therefore, we will reserve the bulk of our discussion on glasses, including prescribing, dispensing, and troubleshooting glasses, for Chaps. 15 and 16 "Glasses in Clinical Practice" and "Construction of Glasses (Ophthalmologists as Opticians)".

We will focus our discussion in this chapter on a few key topics that tend to appear on written exams, such as questions regarding bifocals' advantages and disadvantages. Since these topics have some overlap and require an understanding of prisms (Chap. 2 "Prisms in Ophthalmic Optics"), we have placed this brief discussion on glasses here in the text. Topics regarding spherocylindrical lenses for distance vision were briefly covered in Chap. 10 "Spherocylindrical Lenses", but are also discussed in terms of clinical relevance in aforementioned Part II chapters.

We will begin by introducing various types of bifocal segments used in clinical practice and then discuss how Prentice's rule can help us understand (and differentiate) the two oft-confused (and dreaded!) topics of image jump and image displacement.

Bifocal Construction Types

Benjamin Franklin (yes, the kite guy, the hundred-dollar bill guy, and one of the first presidents of the United States... only one of those facts is incorrect) is credited with the first description of bifocals. Whether or not he actually *invented* bifocal spectacles is a matter of historical debate; however, he certainly played a key role in popularizing their usage in the United States. Shortly after the end of the Revolutionary War, the good Mr. Franklin wrote in a letter to his friend George Whatley about his happiness "…in the invention of double spectacles, which serving for distant objects as well as near ones, make my eyes as useful to me as ever they were."[1] We know that Franklin was likely a hyperope: therefore, his interest in and dependence on presbyopia-correcting glasses played a role in the popularity and further development of these glasses.[2]

Bifocals have changed considerably since Franklin's day. We can divide types of bifocals available based on how they are constructed (Figs. 1, 2, and 3):

Fused bifocal A craterlike depression known as a "countersink" (panel A) is made in the substance of the eyeglass lens to allow for a bifocal segment (made of a different material with a higher index of refraction, such as flint) to be joined (panel B) into the substance of the first lens. This added segment is then grounded (panel C) until it is level with the substance of the rest of this lens. Both round-top and flat-top bifocals can be made using fused construction designs. In these eyeglasses, the bifocal segment is attached to the front part (convex side) of the lens, allowing for any (minus) cylinder power to be placed into the back part (concave side) of the lens.

G. V. Vicente (✉)
Clinical Pediatrics and Ophthalmology Georgetown University Hospital, Washington, DC, USA

Eye Doctors of Washington, Chevy Chase, MD, USA
e-mail: vvicente@edow.com

[1] Taken from https://www.college-optometrists.org/the-college/museum/online-exhibitions/virtual-art-gallery/the-politician.html. Accessed March 31, 2020

[2] For American history fans, there is another famous story about how George Washington averted an insurrection by bringing out his reading glasses (see Chap. 9, "Accommodation and Presbyopia").

K. M. Riaz et al. (eds.), *Optics for the New Millennium*, https://doi.org/10.1007/978-3-030-95251-8_12

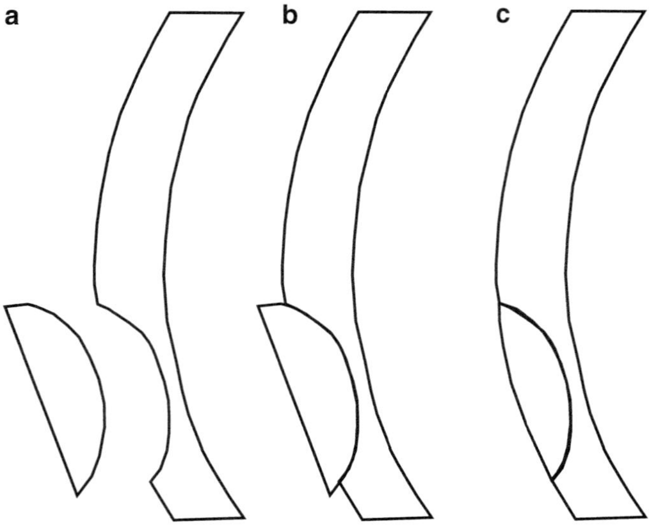

Fig. 1 Construction types of bifocals, fused bifocal

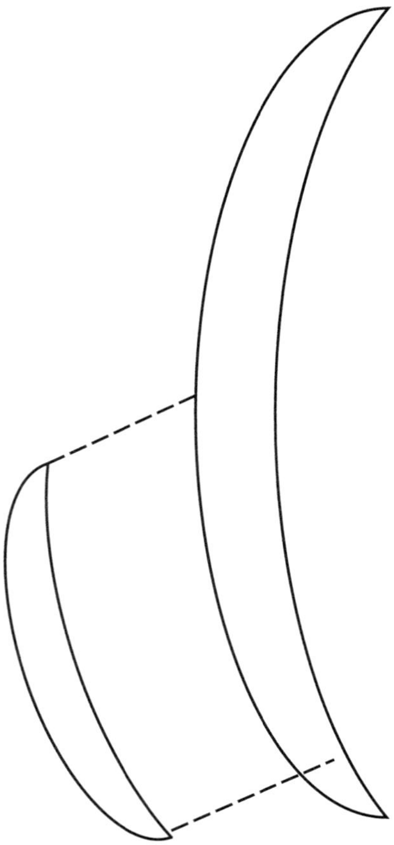

Fig. 2 Construction types of bifocals, cemented bifocal

Cemented bifocal The bifocal segment (usually of a different substance with a higher index of refraction) is attached to the surface of a single vision lens. The lower portion of the lens will have a greater thickness than the upper portion of the lens. This is the least commonly employed lens in clinical practice.

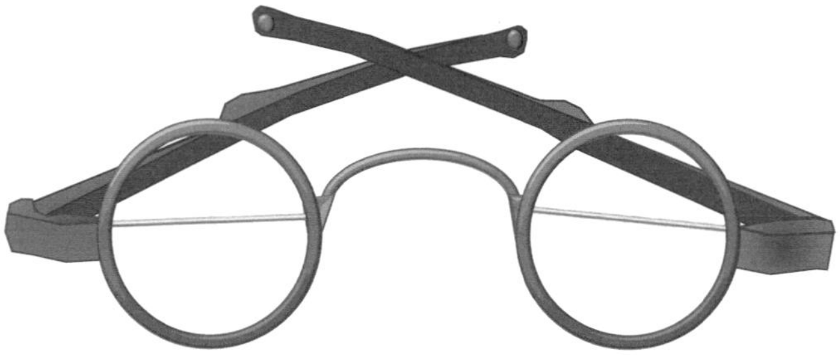

Fig. 3 Construction types of bifocals, a split-lens bifocal

Split-lens bifocal (aka executive style, aka "Ben-Franklin" bifocal) This is the granddaddy of them all. This bifocal involves two different lenses: the top segment (for distance) and the bottom segment (for near) are the combinations of two lenses (regardless of material) that have been cut in half and joined together in one frame. The optical center of the bifocal segment is at the *top* of the segment. Contrary to popular belief, these are not designed to read secret maps leading to ancient Masonic treasures.

Solid bifocal this is a one-piece bifocal made from a single piece of material. During construction, the lens surface is ground to create two different radii of curvature: the longer radius of curvature is used for the "distance" portion, and the shorter radius of curvature (having more plus power) is used for the "near" portion. A progressive lens (technically not a bifocal) is an example of a solid construction design.

Remember, a bifocal lens combines two lenses into a single lens. The small lens (the *segment*) is placed into the larger lens (the *carrier*). This next part is important: the total power when a patient looks through the bifocal segment is the *sum* of the carrier and the segment lens. For example, if a patient is wearing a lens in the right eye with the following power, OD = +1.50 + 0.50 × 90, +2.00D add, then the *total* power when the patient is reading will be +3.50 + 0.50 × 90. Note that the add power does not affect the cylinder power; it only affects the spherical component of the carrier lens.

As another example, suppose a patient wore a lens with the following power,

OD = −1.00 + 1.00 × 180, +2.50D add. The *total* reading power will be +1.50 + 1.00 × 180. So, this "minus" lens will function like a "plus" lens when the patient wants to read. This concept is important for the topics in this chapter and when solving exam questions (such as Prentice's rule-type problems) which involve the patient looking through glasses with bifocal segments with a given power.

Moving on from the construction types of bifocal lenses, we can shift our discussion to the four main designs of presbyopia-correcting glasses that we will encounter in clinical practice.

Bifocal Architecture Types

Round-Top Bifocal

The round-top bifocal is perhaps the easiest type of bifocal segment to understand (Fig. 4, panel a). It is basically a round lens placed into the carrier lens. It is common to remove the inferior portion of the round-top segment just below its optical center so that the optical center of the segment aligns with the inferior edge of the carrier. This lens is commonly used for hyperopic presbyopes – though there is a price to pay, as we will see in the next section!

Flat-Top Bifocal

We can imagine that the flat-top bifocal is basically a round-top segment whose head has been cut off (yikes!), which allows the optical center to be placed closer to the optical center of the carrier lens (Fig. 4, panel b). These are also referred to as "D" segments (since they look like a D) or a "straight top" bifocal segment. Flat tops are *excellent* options for myopes – as we will see in the next section!

Executive-Style Bifocal

As discussed previously, an executive-style bifocal (which has many names) is the combination of two lens halves that are joined together into a single frame (Fig. 4, panel c). This bifocal style, while cosmetically awkward (to some), offers excellent optical clarity because it not only distinctly separates the distance and near portions but also allows for sufficient "space" or "real estate" that the patient can use for distance and near vision. Ben Franklin certainly seems to know what he was doing!

Some patients may complain about the "visible" line in the executive bifocal, especially as this bifocal style makes

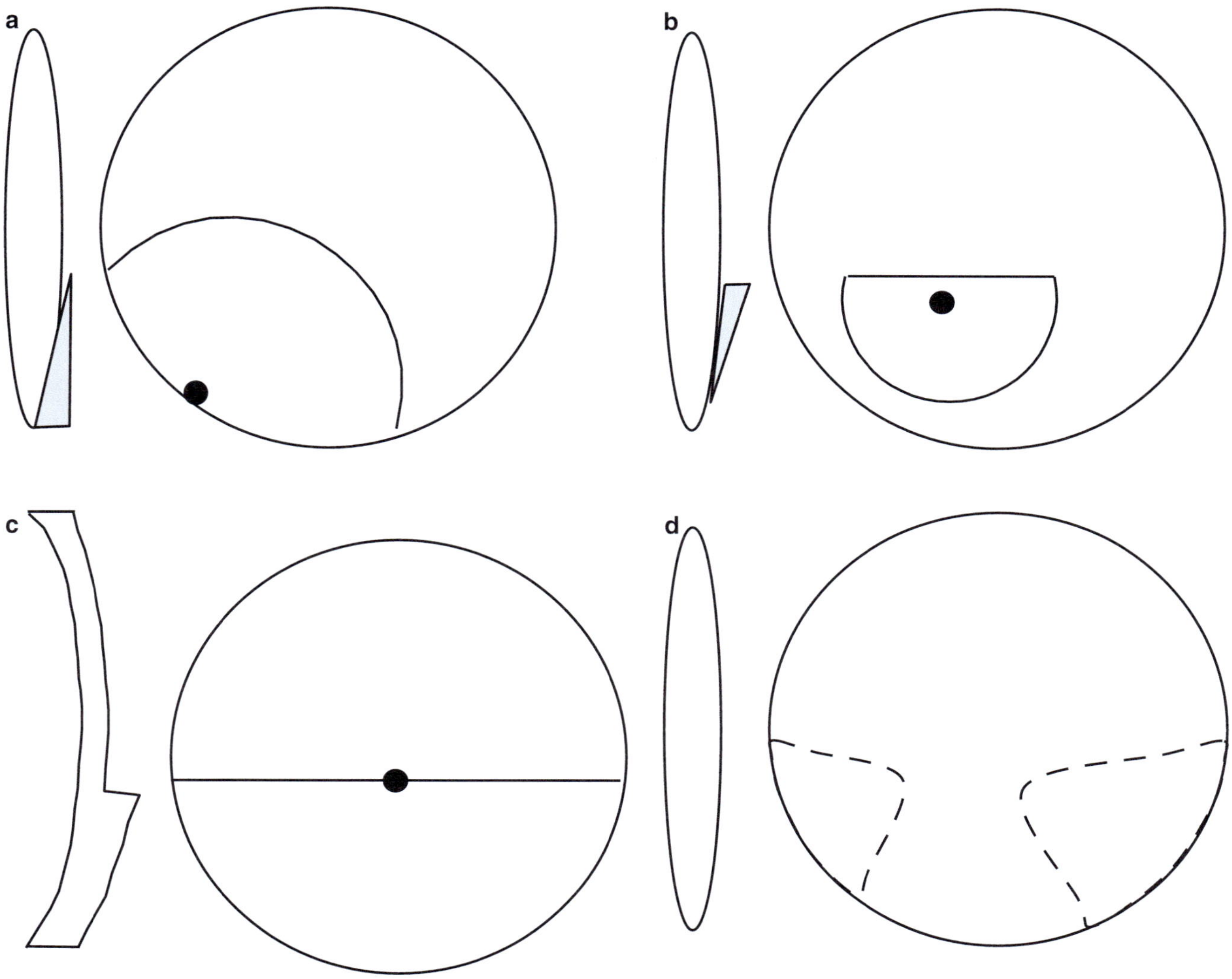

Fig. 4 Designs of commonly prescribed presbyopia-correcting glasses in clinical practice: round-top (panel **a**), flat-top (panel **b**), executive-style (panel **c**), and progressive add lenses (panel **d**)

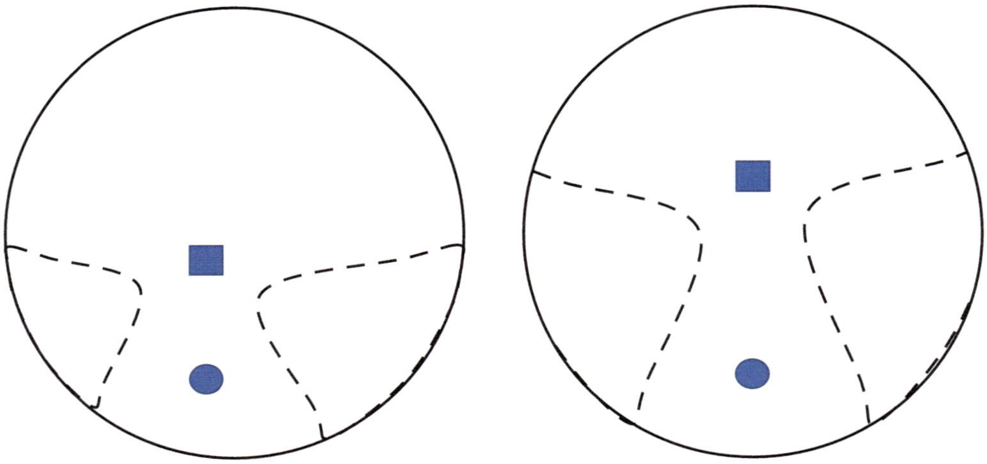

Fig. 5 A progressive addition lens (PAL) can be customized to give the patient a larger or smaller area for distance and near vision, depending on the patient's needs. In a "hard design" (left panel), the distance vision portion is larger, the near vision portion is smaller, and the peripheral distortions are more pronounced within the peripheral aberration zone. In a "soft design" (right panel), the PAL is designed to distribute the peripheral distortions over a larger peripheral zone

the lens considerably thicker, particularly in high-plus lenses. This "line" may be undesirable for cosmetic and social reasons. Furthermore, due to production techniques, some manufacturers may have an unwanted prism at the line or a blur zone slightly below it – this in turn may cause undesirable prismatic effects.

Progressive Lens

A progressive add lens (PAL) is not technically a bifocal because it does not contain distinctive or separate segments. We include it here because it is a useful extension of our previous discussions. PAL style glasses gradually change power between the top and bottom portions of the lens; they are the most commonly used presbyopia-correcting glasses in today's clinical practice. As a result of grinding techniques, a single lens can have multiple zones within the lens: distance, intermediate, and near within a vertical column field of vision (Fig. 4, panel d).

The optical lab can further customize pALs to give larger portions for distance or near vision, based on the patient's needs. The best vision with a PAL is achieved when the patient looks directly through the lens's middle "vertical column" (Fig. 5). Think of the vertical column as a "safe zone": inside it, the distance and reading optical centers are aligned, giving the patient the best possible vision for all distances. A "danger zone" of peripheral aberrations and distortions exists outside the safe zone. Therefore, all PALs involve a compromise between the amount of "safe zone" and "danger zone," given that increasing the size of the former will increase subjective distortions seen by the patient through the latter.

One option is to use a *hard design* PAL (Fig. 5, left panel): this design aims to maximize the distortion-free zones for distance and reading at the cost of smaller but much more severe peripheral distortion zones. Another option is to use a *soft design* PAL (Fig. 5, right panel). The distance and reading portions are slightly smaller in this design, but the larger peripheral zones allow for less severe peripheral distortions. In other words, we can think of hard design PALs as cramming a week of studying optics into a few days; those few days are tough (peripheral distortion zone), but other days involve no studying. The soft design PAL is like spreading out studying optics over many days so that the pain is less intense.[3]

PALs are constructed to have a progressive aspheric change in curvature throughout the lens, similar to an aspheric IOL design. This design has the advantage of improved vision quality when looking through the optimized central portions of the eyeglass (and IOL) but the disadvantage of the lens incurring unwanted aberrations when the patient looks to the side, similar to a decentration of an aspheric IOL.

PALs have other advantages as well:

- A PAL functions as a "multifocal" lens that provides a seamless progression of many lens powers for all viewing distances, especially intermediate vision, which is becoming increasingly necessary in the modern world for activities such as computer vision.
- Cosmetic advantages, as no "line" is present as in the three previous designs.
- "Optimal" power in the vertical center for all distances.
- Elimination of image jump *and* image displacement (see section "Prismatic Effects of Glasses").

[3] Authors maintain that studying optics every day is fun.

However, as with all things in life, there are disadvantages as well:

- Some patients may complain that the intermediate zone (which is usually relatively smaller than the distance and near portions) is insufficient for their visual needs, especially if they have high demands for intermediate vision.
- High hyperopes have a difficult time adjusting to PALs. Low hyperopes, emmetropes, and myopes tolerate PALs much better.
- Pupillary distance is extremely important when prescribing PALs. Since the patient has a narrow "safe zone" vertically, any error or change in pupillary distance may incur an unwanted journey into the "unsafe" peripheral aberration zone.
- Proper frame size (and eyeglass lens size) is essential. A small frame may have a lower amount of starting real estate for the optical lab to work within preparing the distance and near vision parts of the lens.

Prismatic Effects of Glasses

This subtopic is where our previous discussion regarding Prentice's rule will help us understand two concepts that are often challengingly frustrating to understand: *image jump* and *image displacement*.

Remember that when a patient shifts his/her gaze from the carrier (distance) lens into the segment portion of the lens, he/she is basically looking through a different lens power – recall our examples above. As a result, this new "reading power lens" will have not only its own power, but depending on how far away from the optical center a patient is looking through, prismatic effects will rear their ugly head.

Looking back at Fig. 4, we can see that the optical center for a round-top segment is the furthest away from the optical center of the distance lens, especially when compared to optical centers of a flat top and executive style. Appreciating this can help us understand why image jump and image displacement happen in the first place.

We only have to worry about image jump and image displacement problems when dealing with round-top and flat-top lenses. With executive style and PALs, we do not have to worry about image jump or image displacement.

Image Jump

Image jump happens when the eyes move from the carrier portion into the bifocal segment. As the patient moves his/her eyes downward to read through the bifocal, the image jumps upward from its anticipated location because of our "image goes to the apex" rule discussed previously. Think of the round top as a base down prism (Fig. 6): as soon as the patient looks through the segment, the (virtual) image will appear to jump upward toward the "apex of the prism," which can be frustrating. However, once the patient looks through and maintains focus through the segment, the image will stay in its place. Image jump is proportional to the power of the add segment: higher-power add segments will cause more image jump problems.

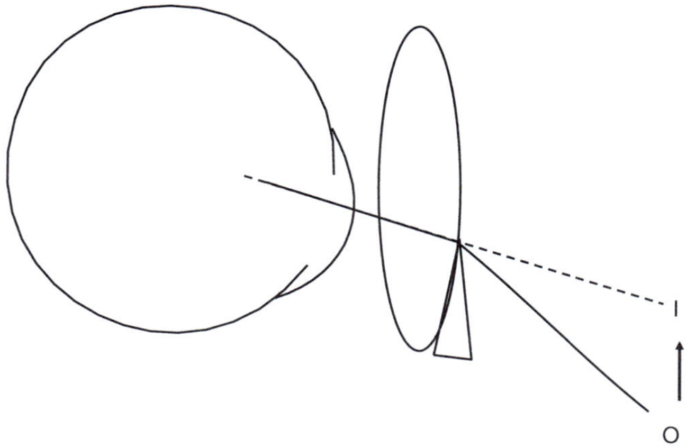

Fig. 6 Image jump is produced by the sudden introduction of prismatic power at the top of the bifocal (usually round-top) segment when the patient looks down to read. Image jump is momentarily bothersome: once the patient maintains focus through the bifocal segment, the image stays constant

Image jump is also proportional to the bifocal segment's optical center distance from the transition line. For example, the optical center of a *flat-top* segment is approximately 2–3 mm below the top of the segment; thus, these types of bifocals have fewer image jump issues.

The most important part of this entire discussion is what follows:

Round-top segments will *maximize image jump* (Fig. 7, panel a), regardless of whether they are given to myopes or hyperopes. We *definitely* want to avoid giving a round top to a myope (see section "Myopes vs. Hyperopes"). *Flat-top segments* (Fig. 7, panel b) have their optical center closer to the distance lens: therefore, there is *minimum image jump*. Executive-style segments have no image jump (Fig. 7, panel c).

Even though you can use your knowledge of image jump to impress people at cocktail parties and social gatherings, minimizing image displacement is much more crically, theoretically, at least on exams.[4] In real-world practice, this is quite different, as we will see in section "Myopes vs. Hyperopes".

[4]You may have gathered by now that none of the authors of this book have much of a social life because we are crazy enough to find things like image jump and image displacement interesting.

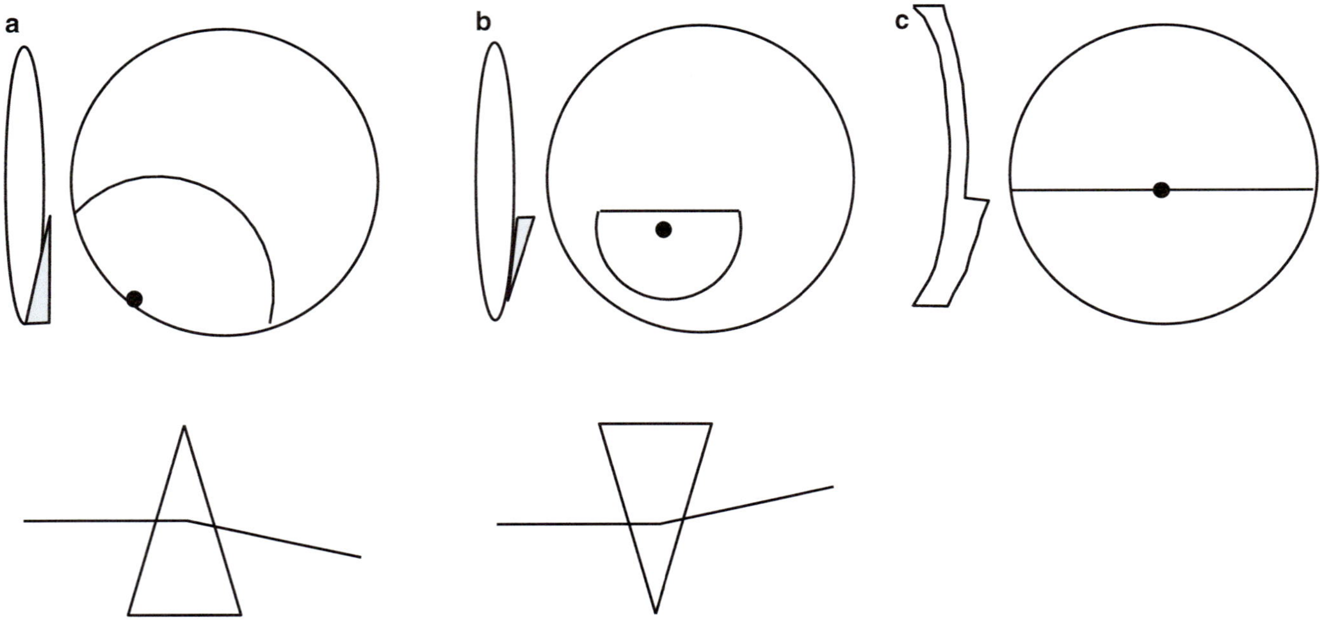

Fig. 7 A round-top segment will act like a base down prism, whereas a flat-top segment will act like a base-up prism. Therefore, image jump will be the worst for any patient who receives a round-top segment

Image Displacement

Image displacement occurs due to the *total prismatic power acting in the reading position*. In this scenario, the problem is not a momentary annoyance: it is persistently bothersome because you will want to look at a particular spot to read, but due to prismatic effects, the image will permanently be shifted elsewhere. The patient will have to constantly "search" for the image or look "off-center" to keep the image from moving around.

We can see what happens with image displacement if we have a hyperopic patient (Fig. 8) and a myopic patient (Fig. 9).

For a hyperopic patient, if we give her a round-top segment, notice that prismatic effects of looking off-center of the base up distance lens will be somewhat neutralized by prismatic effects of looking off-center of the base down bifocal segment (Fig. 8, panel a). In other words, the *round top* will neutralize some of the prismatic effects of the hyperopic distance lens and therefore *minimize image displacement*. If we instead gave her a flat-top segment (Fig. 8, panel b), notice that the base up effects of both the distance lens and the bifocal lens would be additive: this would worsen image displacement and, therefore, be a poor choice.

For a myopic patient, if we were to give him a round-top segment, notice that prismatic effects (base down) of both the distance and the reading lenses would be additive: this would worsen image displacement and, therefore, be a poor choice (Fig. 9, panel a). However, if we instead gave him a flat-top segment (Fig. 9, panel b), notice that the prismatic effects of the segment would somewhat neutralize prismatic effects of the distance lens. In other words, the *flat-top* segment will minimize *image displacement*.

Myopes vs. Hyperopes

Now that we have spent all this time discussing the optical principles of prismatic effects with bifocals, we can cut to the chase: *what kind of bifocal segment will work best for a given patient to minimize image jump and image displacement, both theoretically and in actual real-world practice*?

A simple solution is just to give everyone executive-style bifocals or PALs! This is perhaps one reason why PALs are so popular.

However, if we had to give a flat top or a round top, here is what we need to know:

We have previously discussed problems with both image jump and image displacement. Between the two problems, *image jump is the lesser evil*, and *image displacement is the greater evil*. Remember image jump is a momentary problem, but image displacement is a persistent problem. As a rule, we will always try to minimize both problems. However, if we had to pick our poison, we theoretically want to choose the option that *minimizes image displacement* (even if it maximizes jump).

How can you remember this? A silly mnemonic is as follows: suppose a criminal were to break into your home as you are studying for optics and tell you, "you can either jump up down a few times and I'll leave or you can be displaced

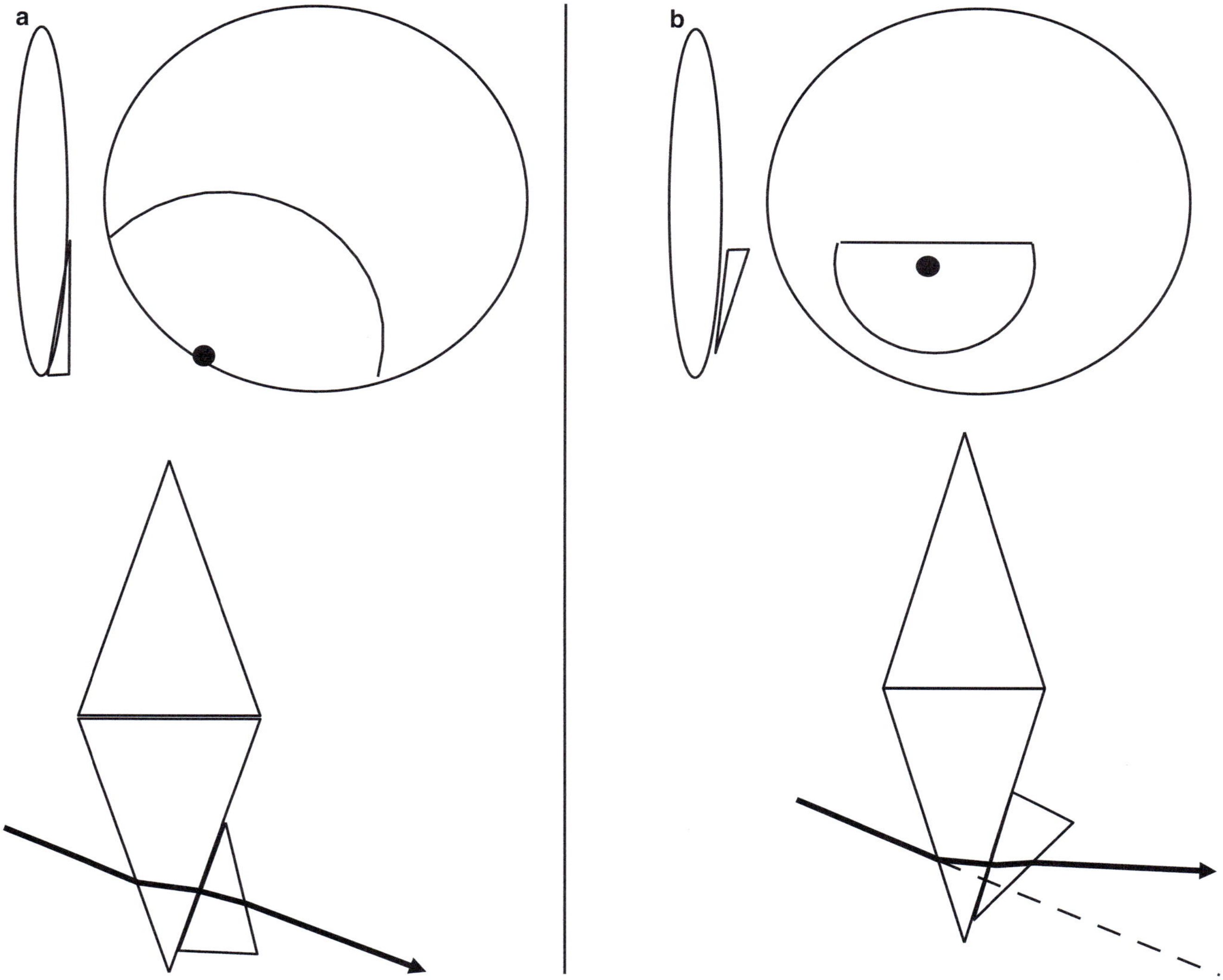

Fig. 8 A round top segment (panel **a**) will minimize image displacement for a hyperopic patient, but a flat top segment (panel **b**) will maximize image displacement

from your home forever – and no, you can't take your optics book with you." What will you choose? You will choose the jump option. Therefore, if you have to pick your poison, always choose to pay the price of accepting image jump to avoid image displacement.

For a *myope*, our solution is quite simple: we can *minimize both image jump and image displacement* by giving our myopic patient a *flat top* (Fig. 10). The visual mnemonic of a happy young myopic patient with his hipster flat-top haircut will help you remember that a myopic patient will benefit from a flat-top bifocal.[5]

For a *hyperope*, unfortunately, we theoretically *cannot solve both problems* – we are forced to pick between the two evils. Since we want to minimize image displacement, we are forced to pick the *round top*: as a result, we will *actually maximize image jump* for this patient, but at least we will *minimize image displacement* (Fig. 10). The visual mnemonic of a happy older hyperopic patient who is bald ("round-top haircut") will help you remember that a hyperopic patient will benefit from a round-top bifocal.

Another visual mnemonic is to think of the mouth of a stick figure's face. An uncorrected hyperope (Fig. 11) has a big upside-down U frowny face because everything is blurry up close and far away. That upside-down U frowny face looks like a round-top bifocal, which helps us remember: *hyperopes prefer round-top bifocals*. Similarly, in our visual mnemonic (Fig. 11), we can see that an uncorrected myope has a flat mouth, reminding us that he is neither happy nor sad: he is doing OK because he can see well at near but not at distance. This figure can help us remember that his "OK" (flat) mouth looks like a flat-top bifocal: *myopes prefer flat-top bifocals*.

[5]You can visually imagine Will Smith from *The Fresh Prince of Bel-Air* as a young myope with his flat-top hair cut benefiting from some flat-top bifocals.

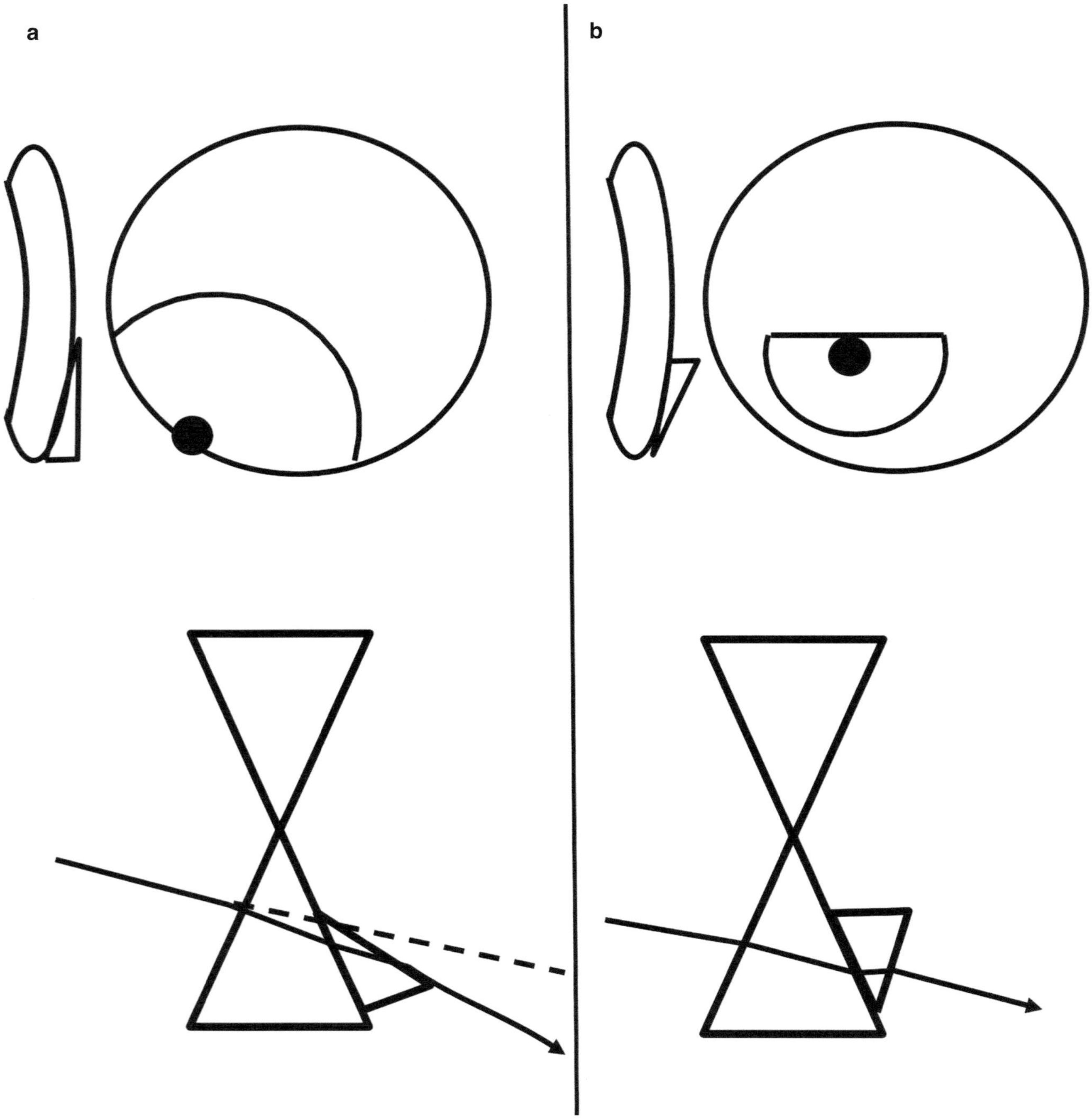

Fig. 9 For a myopic patient, a round-top segment (panel **a**) will maximize image displacement, but a flat-top segment (panel **b**) will minimize image displacement

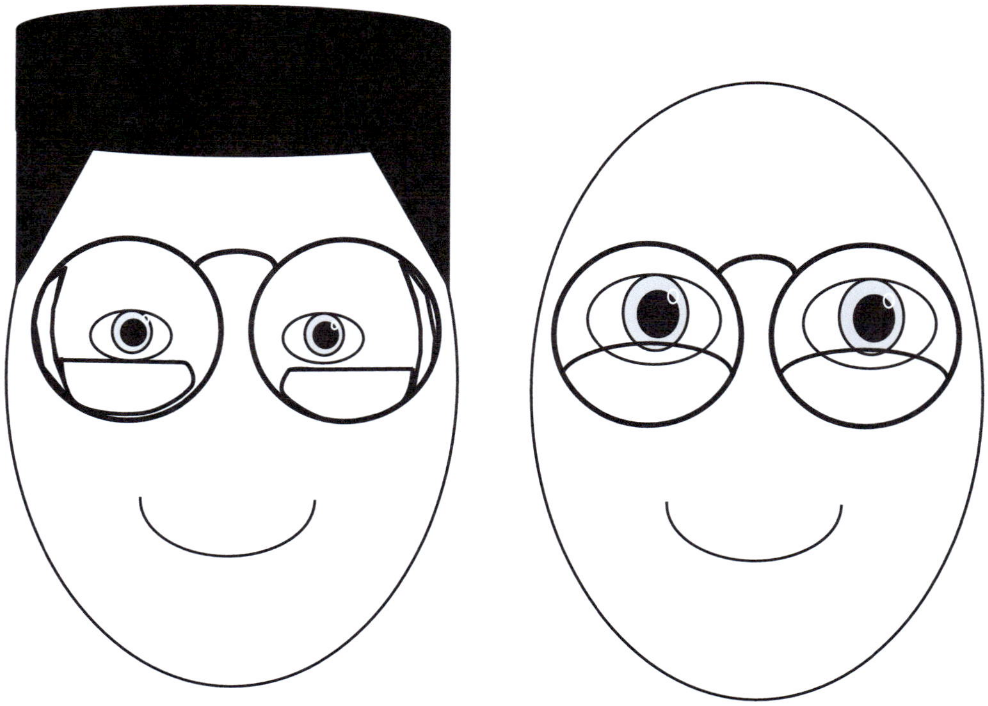

Fig. 10 Visual mnemonic of a happy myope with both a flat-top haircut and flat-top bifocals and a happy hyperope with a "round-top" haircut (bald) and round-top bifocals

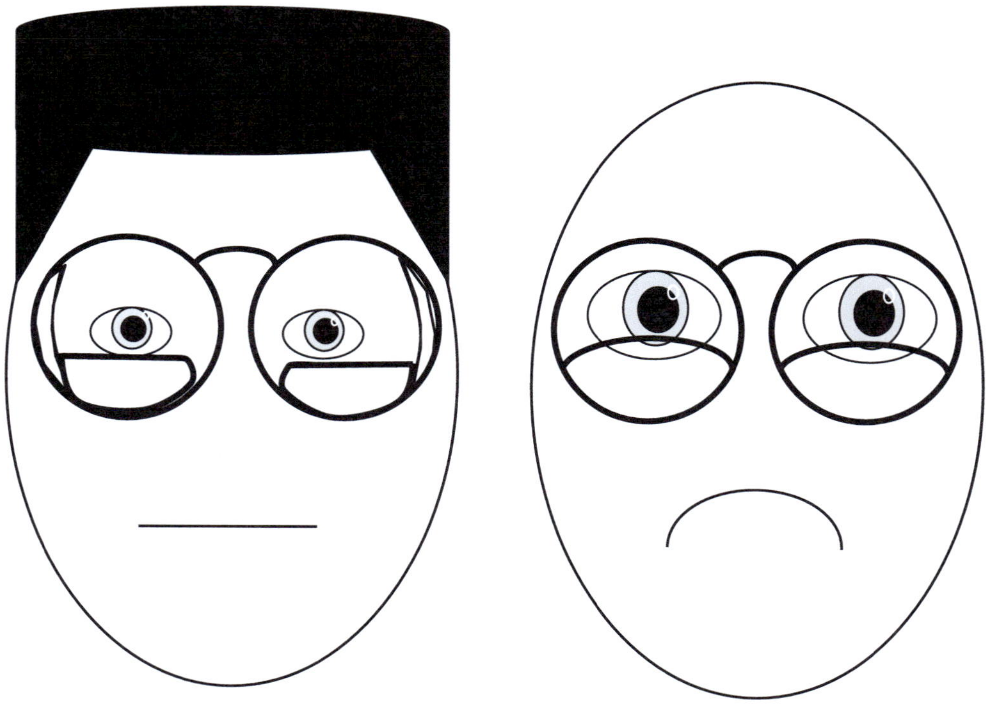

Fig. 11 Visual mnemonic of an even keel myope and an unhappy hyperope. The myope is even- keeled because he can see well up close but not far away; he prefers a flat-top bifocal The hyperope is unhappy because he cannot see well up close or far away; the frown helps you to remember that a hyperope benefits from a round top

Now for the plot twist, this previous discussion is classic teaching in ophthalmology textbooks of optics. However, this all may be a moot point when discussing real-world clinical and optical practice. While we previously stated that hyperopes should be given a round top to minimize image displacement (even at the cost of maximizing image jump), real-world applications are a bit more complicated.

On one hand, hyperopes that frequently switch between distance and near vision (e.g., a piano player, receptionist, barista, etc.) may be more bothered by image jump. On the other hand, hyperopes that do long periods of near work (e.g., a computer programmer, secretary, etc.) may be more bothered by image displacement. Therefore, the real-world dispensation of segment style may vary from patient to patient based on his/her needs.[6]

Another plot twist is in real-world optical practice, flat tops are often given to *both* myopes and hyperopes because they are cheaper to make, and the problem of image displacement is thankfully not as visually debilitating as it theoretically seems. Recent advancements in lens construction, such as "digital lenses" (laser-etched lenses), have further minimized previous generation image jump and displacement effects. The complete discussion of this point is beyond the scope of this text; interested readers should consult with an experienced optician and/or optical lab for more information regarding current manufacturing and construction standards.

Practice Questions

1. Which of the following statements regarding bifocals is *true*:
   A. In a fused bifocal, a countersink is used to place a bifocal segment made of a lower index of refraction than the substance of the first lens.
   B. In an executive-style bifocal, the center of the bifocal segment is at the top of the segment.
   C. In a round-top bifocal, the superior portion of the round-top segment is removed, and the segment is placed into the carrier lens.
   D. In a flat-top bifocal, the inferior portion of the round-top segment is removed, and the segment is placed into the carrier lens.
2. Which of the following statements regarding progressive add lenses (PALs) is *true*:
   A. In a hard design PAL, distortion zones are larger but have less severity of distortions within these peripheral zones.
   B. In a soft design PAL, distortion zones are smaller but have increased severity of distortions within these peripheral zones.
   C. PALs are constructed with a singular spherical design throughout the lens, in an effort to simulate the shape of the cornea.
   D. The intermediate zone in some PALs may not be sufficient, especially for computer vision.
   E. High hyperopes tolerate PALs much better than low hyperopes.
3. Which of the following statements regarding image jump and image displacement is *true*:
   A. Image displacement is more bothersome than image jump.
   B. Image displacement is a momentary shift in the perceived image when the patient looks from the distance portion into the near portion of the eyeglasses.
   C. Round-top segments will minimize image jump.
   D. Flat-top segments will maximize image jump.

[6]Again, this is why everyone should simply get a progressive add lens (PAL) to make our lives easier. However, a high hyperope may have problems with a PAL as well, so he/she may ultimately be happiest with an executive-style bifocal.

Answers

1. Answer: B. In a fused bifocal, the segment is made of a material with a *higher* index of refraction as compared to the substance of the "distance" lens. In a round-top bifocal, the *inferior* portion of the round-top segment is removed. In a flat-top bifocal, the *superior* portion of the round-top segment is removed.
2. Answer: D. In a "hard design" PAL, the distance vision portion is larger, the near vision portion is smaller, and the peripheral distortions are more pronounced within the peripheral aberration zone. In a "soft design" PAL, peripheral distortions are distributed over a larger peripheral zone. PALs are constructed with progressive curvature changes, similar to modern aspheric IOL designs. High hyperopes have the most challenging time adjusting to PALs compared to low hyperopes, emmetropes, and myopes.
3. Answer: A. While minimizing both image jump and image displacement is a worthy goal for eyeglass fitting, whenever possible, clinicians should minimize image displacement as it is much more bothersome than image jump. Image displacement occurs due to the total prismatic power in the reading position; therefore, it is not a momentary inconvenience to the patient. It permanently shifts the image away from the patient's desired or intended reading location. Round-top segments will always maximize image jump. Flat-top segments will minimize image jump.

Contact Lenses for Written Exams

G. Vike Vicente and Kamran M. Riaz

Objectives

- To learn how to fit, select, and calculate the power of a soft contact lens (SCL)
- To learn how to calculate the power of a rigid gas-permeable/hard contact lens (RGPCL)
- To understand the concept of the tear lens as it relates to RGPCL fitting
- To introduce concepts of soft toric contact lens (STCL) fitting
- To review principles of adjusting the fit of SCLs, RGPCLs, and STCLs pertaining to written exams

Introduction

You may have opened up this chapter and thought: *I am an ophthalmologist. I do eyeball surgery. I do not need to know anything about contact lenses!*

Well, that may be true for clinical practice as you may rely on your friendly neighborhood optometrist or contact lens specialist for the actual prescription and dispensation of contact lenses. However, there are some basics of contact lenses that every ophthalmologist should know. This chapter will primarily focus on how to solve contact lens problems that often appear on written exams. While we will discuss some clinically relevant information in this chapter, the bulk of information necessary for clinical prescription, dispensation, and adjustment of contact lenses will be discussed in greater detail in Chaps. 6 "Lens Effectivity", and 20 "Contact Lenses in Clinical Practice". Topics such as multifocal and scleral contact lenses will also be discussed in that chapter.

Note: topics related to contact lenses may appear on either written or oral exams. Therefore, whether you are preparing for written exams or oral exams, you may wish to read this chapter **and** the contact lens chapter in Part 2.

In this chapter, we will primarily focus on details about the power calculation of the given type of contact lens.

Soft Contact Lenses (SCLs)

Soft contact lenses (SCLs) are a good option for patients with mainly spherical refractive errors and low amounts of astigmatism (both refractive and keratometric). They are considered the "entry-level" contact lenses and likely comprise the majority of contact lens patients most ophthalmologists will encounter.

Most of the SCLs used in clinical practice today are silicone hydrogel lenses. These lenses have good oxygen permeability, come in various wear options (replacement schedules), and are usually well tolerated by most patients.

Features of Soft Contact Lenses

There are three features of a SCL that are important when solving exam problems (and even for clinical practice):

- Base curve (BC) – this is the posterior surface curvature of the SCL (in mm). A lower BC value corresponds to a *shorter* radius of curvature and, therefore, a steeper fit of the SCL. Conversely, a higher BC value corresponds to a *flatter* radius of curvature and, therefore, a flatter fit of the SCL.
- Diameter (DIA) – this is the edge-to-edge width of the contact lens. SCLs typically range from 13 to 15 mm in size. Increasing the DIA will lead to a steeper fit of the

G. V. Vicente (✉)
Clinical Pediatrics and Ophthalmology Georgetown University Hospital, Washington, DC, USA

Eye Doctors of Washington, Chevy Chase, MD, USA
e-mail: vvicente@edow.com

K. M. Riaz
Dean McGee Eye Institute, University of Oklahoma, Oklahoma City, OK, USA

K. M. Riaz et al. (eds.), *Optics for the New Millennium*, https://doi.org/10.1007/978-3-030-95251-8_13

SCL. Conversely, decreasing the DIA will lead to a flatter fit.

- Power of the SCL.

The fit of the SCL can be modified by adjusting either the BC or the DIA of the SCL. BC and DIA are inversely proportional to each other. For example, a SCL can be made *steeper* by either decreasing the BC or increasing the DIA.

Steps for Fitting Soft Contact Lenses

We can discuss a step-by-step (simplified) guide to fitting a SCL:

1. We first need to select the BC of the SCL. For a SCL, this is determined by obtaining keratometry readings and looking at the average K values:
   (a) If the average K is between 42.5 and 44.5D, use 8.6/8.7 BC SCL (flatter = longer radius of curvature).
   (b) If the average K is between 44.5 and 46.0D, use 8.3/8.4 BC (steeper = shorter radius of curvature).
   (c) This relationship explains why many manufacturers now use an 8.5 BC as a one-size-fits-all approach.
2. For written exam purposes, we can ignore the SCL "tear lens (TL)" (the tear film between the back surface of the SCL and the cornea) because it has minimal refractive power. The TL will have significance when we discuss RGPCLs.
3. Take the spherical equivalent (SE) of the patient's manifest refraction if the cylinder present is <1D. If ≥1D, then vertex correction must be done, as discussed in the next section. For higher amounts of cylinder, an RGPCL or soft toric contact lens will be necessary.
4. For sphere values below +4.00D/−4.00D, we can simply use the same eyeglass power as a starting power for the SCL.
5. For sphere values above +4.00D/−4.00D, adjust the SE value for vertex distance using a vertex table. These are available online or in handy reference charts in most offices. For example, suppose you calculated the SE as −8.50D with a vertex distance of 13 mm; a published vertex table chart will give the suggested power for the SCL as approximately −7.75D. Some online calculators will also do this step for you:
   (a) Otherwise, you may have to calculate the new power using the vertex distance formula:
      (i) Calculate the focal point of the given spectacle lens.
      (ii) Use the vertex distance to find the distance to the far point of the patient.
      (iii) Take the reciprocal of that distance in meters to find the power of the contact lens needed. See Chap. 6 "Lens Effectivity", for a review of calculations involved and the examples that follow:
         1. For **myopes,** you will have to *add the vertex distance* to the focal point.
         2. For **hyperopes,** you will have to *subtract the vertex distance* from the focal point.
6. Place the SCL on the patient's cornea *without fluorescein* and assess its fit. An optimum SCL fit will be comfortable for the patient and have good centration on the cornea with approximately 1.0 mm overlapping of the limbus in all directions and 0.25–0.5 mm movement with each blink in primary gaze:
   (a) If the SCL fits as described above, congratulations, you are done. Make sure to collect your SCL fitting fee.
   (b) However, if the SCL is either *too flat (loose)* or *too steep (tight)*, then proceed to step 7.
7. To adjust the fit, we can change either the BC or the DIA:
   (a) In order to **steepen the lens**, *increase the diameter* or *decrease the base curve.*
   (b) In order to **flatten the lens**, decrease the diameter or *increase the base curve.*
   (c) Mnemonic – "call SID if you have a flat tire." If the lens is flat, we have to steepen it. In order to **s**teepen a SCL, you can **i**ncrease the **d**iameter. You can figure out the other three relationships if you can remember that nugget.[1]
8. Perform an over-refraction as necessary.

Sample Problems

Sample Problem #1 What should the power of a *SCL* be if the patient's spectacle lens is +12.5D with a vertex distance of 13 mm?

Answer. For the contact or glasses to work, we must remember that the focal point of either lens must match the far point of the eye (Fig. 1). To calculate the far point of the eye, we can take the reciprocal of the spectacle lens, 100/12.5 = 8 cm or 80 mm behind the eye (to the right of the

[1]It is important to only use the SID mnemonic when the lens is flat. Do not use the SID mnemonic if the lens is steep. Remember that the "s" stands for "to steepen."

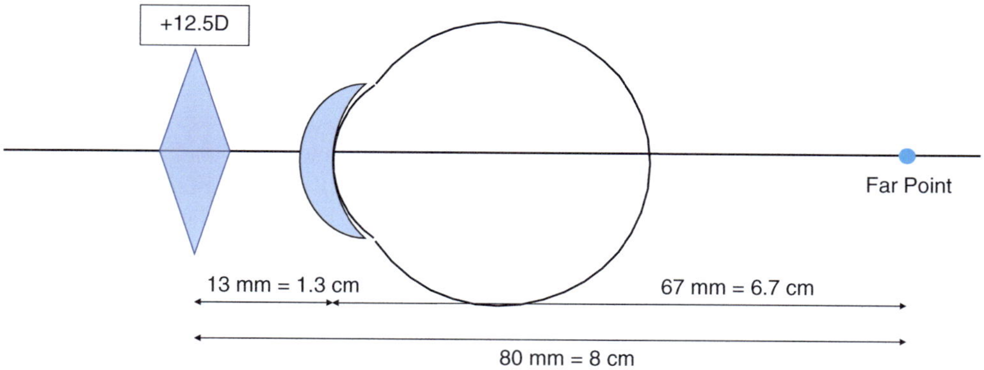

Fig. 1 Graphical representation for calculating a SCL needed for a patient wearing +12.5D spectacles with vertex distance 13 mm. When the patient is wearing glasses, the focal point of the glasses matches the far point of the eye. In calculating the power of the required SCL, we must determine the SCL power such that the focal point of the SCL similarly matches the far point of the eye

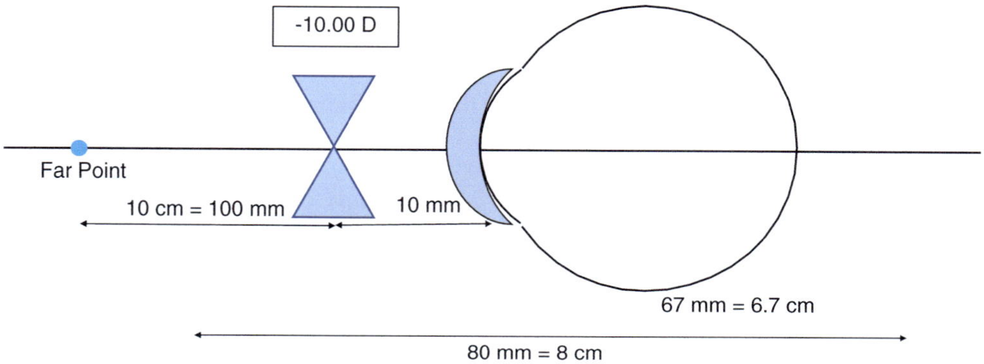

Fig. 2 Graphical representation for calculating a SCL needed for a patient wearing −10.00D spectacles with a vertex distance of 10 mm. When the patient is wearing glasses, the focal point of the glasses matches the far point of the eye. In calculating the power of the required SCL, we must determine the SCL power such that the focal point of the SCL similarly matches the far point of the eye

eye). This is both the focal point of the +12.5D lens *and* the far point of the (hyperopic) eye.

When we move the correcting lens onto the cornea (i.e., a SCL), we have to subtract the vertex distance.[2] Remember, we are going from glasses to contact lenses in a hyperope, so we must *subtract* the vertex distance, 80 mm − 13 mm = 67 mm (6.7 cm). Now we need to calculate the power of the "lens" with this new focal point, 100/6.7 (or 1/0.67) = +15D.

Thus, a + 15D contact lens on the cornea will focus light onto the far point of the eye, just as a + 12.5D lens that is 13 mm further away (vertex distance).

Sample Problem #2 What should the power of a *SCL* be if the patient's spectacle lens is −10.0D with a vertex distance of 10 mm?

Answer. For myopic patients, calculations are slightly different (Fig. 2). Since this is a myope, the far point will be in front (to the left) of the spectacles. We can again start by calculating the far point of the spectacle lens, 100/−10 = 10 cm to the left of the spectacle lens.

Since we are going from glasses to contact lenses in a myope, we must *add* the vertex distance, 10 cm + 1 cm = 11 cm. The power of the SCL therefore would be 100/11 = −9D.

Note: these questions may also be given in reverse for written exams. In other words, you may be given the SCL power and asked to calculate the spectacle lens power.

It may also be helpful to remember that when we go from spectacles to contacts in myopes, the contact lens power will be a "lower myopic correction power"; in hyperopes, the power of the contact will be a "higher hyperopic correction power." Thus, a − 6.00 myope will likely wear a − 5.50D SCL; a + 6.00 hyperope will likely wear a + 6.50D SCL.

Sample Problem #3 A patient complains that his SCL keeps falling out. You look at the box and notice the following numbers:

[2]See Chap. 6, "Lens Effectivity".

8.6 / 13.5 / –4.50

Which of the following adjustments would *most likely* help this patient?

(a) 8.4/13.0/−4.50
(b) 8.4/13.5/−4.50
(c) 8.6/13.5/−4.75
(d) 8.8/14.0/−4.50.

Answer. If the SCL keeps falling out, the SCL is likely *too loose (too flat)*. Since we have a flat tire, we can call on our friend "SID" to remind us that we can either increase the diameter or decrease the BC. Choice D allows us to increase the diameter, but it also increases the BC, so this can be eliminated. Choice C involves no change to either the BC or the diameter and involves increasing the power of the SCL; that won't help us, so this choice can also be eliminated. Choice A allows us to decrease the BC, but it also involves decreasing the diameter, so this can also be eliminated. This leaves us with choice B, decreasing the BC only, while keeping the diameter and the power of the SCL unchanged.

Note: in the above questions, the option to change the contact lens diameter was presented. In real-world clinical practice, however, most manufacturers have a fixed diameter of the contact lens (e.g., between 13.8 and 14.6 mm), while offering several different BC options. Therefore, we are limited to either increasing or decreasing the base curve when we want to flatten or steepen the SCL, respectively, in everyday practice.

Rigid Gas-Permeable Contact Lenses (RGPCLs) or Hard Contact Lenses

Solving this type of problem is a rite of passage for written exams. We can start by discussing the concept of the tear lens and what role it plays in our discussion of RGPCLs.

The Tear Lens in RGPCL Problems

The tear lens (TL) refers to the tear layer created between the posterior surface of the RGPCL and the anterior surface of the cornea. Since we ideally want the center of the posterior surface of the RGPCL *not to* touch the central cornea, this will create a "vault" of the RGPCL over the cornea. This silly little TL has (sometimes) significant power that must be accounted for when deciding on the power of the final RGPCL.

This concept gets slightly confusing for many students: in general, **the power of the TL is + 0.25D for every 0.05-mm difference** between the BC of the RGPCL and the BC of the central corneal curvature. What does this mean exactly? It means that if we take keratometry measurements of the cornea, we have to convert them to BC measurements. We will look at the two base curves that correspond to the flat and steep corneal meridians and pick the flatter of these two base curves; we will pick a contact lens with a BC that is slightly *steeper* than the flatter corneal base curve. Why do we do this? We do this to create some vaulting between the cornea and the RGPCL. Diopter-to-base curve tables are published references that can easily be found online and in most offices. It is improbable that you would be expected to convert between diopters and base curves for test purposes because the math involved is much too challenging to solve without a calculator. It is far more likely that the diopter value and the corresponding base curve value will be given to you in an exam situation.[3]

For example, suppose that a patient's keratometry readings are 42.50 (BC, 7.95 mm) x 45.00 (BC, 7.50 mm) @ 100. Our flatter *K* value is 42.50D (BC 7.95 mm), so we will want to fit a contact lens with a BC that is slightly steeper than this flatter *K*. Suppose we decide to fit this patient with an RGPCL that has a BC 7.85 (corresponding to 43.00D). Our chosen BC is 7.95 − 7.85 = 0.10 mm steeper than the flattest *K* value. Therefore, since every 0.05-mm difference between the BC of the RGPCL and the BC of the cornea will create a +0.25D TL, a 0.10-mm difference will create a + 0.50D TL.

Now that we have created a messy situation with this silly TL, we need to call in another friend. Our second friend for contact lens fitting is "SAM," which reminds us that if you fit **s**teeper than the flattest *K*, you have to **a**dd **m**inus.[4] Technically, this is actually the "SAM-FAP" rule, but fitting flatter than the flattest *K* (and therefore adding plus) is reserved for special situations, such as orthokeratology and extreme keratoconus, which is beyond the scope of what we need to know for exams. To summarize, we need to know that since we typically fit steeper than the flattest *K*, we will have to "add minus" to overcome the effects of the TL.[5]

Calculating and Fitting RGPCLs

We can discuss a step-by-step (simplified) guide to calculating and fitting RGPCLs:

[3]For the sake of completeness, the formula to convert between diopters and base curves is as follows: 337.5/diopters = BC (in millimeters).

[4]As an added reminder, you can imagine a friend named "Sam" who is always yelling at you to "add minus!"

[5]This is a simplification of clinical practice for purposes of ophthalmology trainees. Contact lens specialists typically choose a base curve corresponding to a "mid-K" value between the two keratometry values for a "steeper-than-flattest K and flatter-than-steepest K" fitting strategy. The full discussion of this topic is beyond the scope of this text.

1. Obtain a manifest refraction and keratometry readings (this should be given to you on an exam).
2. Start by thinking like an optometrist: convert the manifest refraction to *minus cylinder* and adjust for zero vertex distance.[6] We can discard the cylinder (and axis) and use this new sphere value as a starting point for the intended RGPCL.
3. Now we can look at the *K* readings and convert them to BC values, usually using a BC conversion table:
   (a) In general, we will want to pick a steeper BC (lower) than the flattest K value to allow for some apical clearance.
   (b) On written exams, BC values corresponding to keratometry values will usually be given to you.
   (c) If no BC values are given, we can choose to fit 0.1 mm steeper than the flattest *K* (corresponding to +0.50D TL power).
4. If we fit steeper than the flattest *K*, the RGPCL will vault over the cornea, and the TL will have a convex lens shape. Hence, the TL will have plus power that we have to additionally neutralize when determining the power of the RGPCL. Therefore, we can call upon "SAM" as a reminder to "add minus" power to the sphere value obtained in step 2.
5. Now we can use the power of the TL (step 4) and the power of the sphere (step 2) and add them together to determine the final RGPCL power.
6. We must assess the fit of the RPGCL at the slit lamp *with fluorescein staining*. This technique will be further discussed in chapter "Lens Effectivity", Contact Lenses in Clinical Practice.
7. Perform an over-refraction as necessary.

Example #1 A patient has a refraction of +11.50 + 1.00 × 50 with a vertex distance of 13 mm. Keratometry readings are 44.25 × 45.25 at 50, corresponding to BC of 7.63 and 7.46, respectively. If the BC chosen is 7.55 (44.75D), what is the power of the RGPCL needed for this patient?

Answer. This problem seems to have a lot of math, and we may be tempted to simply skip it on an exam. We can simplify it step-by-step using the method above. First, we already have the manifest refraction and the keratometry values. Next, we can think like an optometrist: let us convert the manifest refraction into minus-cylinder notation, +11.50 + 1.00 × 50 = +12.50 − 1.00 × 140. Now we can use the +12.50 and adjust for the 13-mm vertex distance. Note that these are the same numbers we used in Fig. 1. From this previous example, we have already determined that the power of the contact lens will be +15.00D. Now we can look at the *K* reading (and a BC conversion table if needed): they have been helpful enough to tell us that the flattest BC is 7.65 and the BC of the RGPCL is 7.55. Basically, we have a 0.10-mm difference in base curves, so we know that our TL will have +0.50D power.

However, *unlike the SCL example*, our job is not done by simply prescribing the +15.00D into a RGPCL. We still have to deal with our old enemy, the dastardly TL.[7] Remember, this fellow has a power of +0.50D, so we have to call in our old friend "SAM" to help us out: SAM tells us we have to "add minus" (add −0.50) to neutralize the TL.

Therefore, the final power of the RPGCL is +15.00 + (−0.50) = +14.50D.

Soft Toric Contact Lenses (STCLs)

Calculating the Power of STCLs

We can discuss a step-by-step (simplified) guide to fitting STCLs. We should know that STCLs share some features of SCLs but also have additional steps necessary in the fitting process:

1. We first need to select the base curve (BC) of the STCL. For a STCL, this is determined by looking at keratometry readings and looking at average *K* values, similar to our discussion with SCLs.
2. For our next step, we will again think like an optometrist: convert the manifest refraction to minus cylinder just like we did with RGPCL. However, we have to use all three values for the power of the STCL:
   (a) Adjust the sphere value based on vertex distance as needed for higher sphere powers.
3. Select the STCL based on the BC value and the vertex adjusted minus-cylinder refraction value:
   (a) For example, if a patient had −3.00 + 2.00 × 90, we will use −1.00 − 2.00 × 180 as the power of the STCL.
4. Place this STCL on the patient's eye and check the fit at the slit lamp (*without fluorescein*) to ensure that the centering mark sits at the 6 o'clock position (as discussed above). Wait at least 5–10 min to allow the STCL to settle before assessing the axis and rotation:
   (a) If the centering mark is **not** at the 6 o'clock position, then the *axis* of the prescription needs to be adjusted (see next section).

[6] Refer to Chap. 6, "Lens Effectivity", and the previous examples in this chapter on how to adjust for zero vertex distance.

[7] While, in this case, we have facetiously referred to the tear lens as an "enemy" (because of the calculation adjustment that we have to make), remember that the tear lens is actually our friend because it is mainly responsible for correcting the corneal astigmatism.

5. Perform an over-refraction to finalize the sphere and cylinder power if necessary.
6. The fit should be similar to the previous discussions regarding optimum fit for a SCL. Adjust the BC or DIA of the STCL if it appears to be too tight or too loose.

Assessing the Fit of STCLs

Soft toric contact lenses (STCLs) share many similar features as SCLs. One key difference is that STCLs have a "line(s)," a "ballast," or a "black dot" that helps the examiner assess whether the STCL is appropriately positioned or not. Note that the patient cannot see this mark: only you as the examiner can see it when examining a patient wearing STCLs at the slit lamp. Depending on the manufacturer, the "mark" may be simply one mark; a combination of three marks at 6 o'clock; a combination of three marks at 3, 6, or 9 o'clock positions; or even a combination of two marks at 6 o'clock and 12 o'clock positions.

If the STCL has been fit properly, the dot/mark/line should be sitting nicely at the 6 o'clock position, *regardless of the axis of cylinder correction*. Note that the mark on a STCL is unlike the marks on a toric IOL wherein we have to ensure that the marks on the latter are aligned with the steep meridian on the cornea intraoperatively. For the STCL, regardless the axis meridian of the correcting cylinder, the mark should be at the 6 o'clock position. If this centering mark is not exactly at the 6 o'clock position, we have to adjust the **axis** of the STCL. Do not change the sphere or the cylinder based on the mark alone!

At this point, if the mark is not at 6 o'clock, we have to call in our third friend in contact lens fitting, "LARS" (We seem to have some weird friends in the contact lens-fitting world!). The "LARS" rule tells us that if the mark has rotated to the **left**, we need to **add** to the axis; if the mark rotated to the **right**, we must **subtract** from the axis (Fig. 3). As a general rule, one clock hour of rotation equals 30 degrees.

Suppose we fit a patient with a STCL in Fig. 3, panel B, with −4.25 − 2.25 × 90. In applying the "LARS" rule, we can see that the STCL has rotated to the left by approximately one clock hour. Therefore, we have to **add** to the axis by 30 degrees. The new STCL should be −4.25 − 2.25 × 120.

Now suppose we fit a patient with a STCL in Fig. 3, panel C, with −4.25 − 2.25 × 90.

In applying the "LARS" rule, we can see that the STCL has rotated to the right by approximately one clock hour. Therefore, we have to **subtract** from the axis by 30 degrees. The new STCL should be −4.25 − 2.25 × 60.

Curveball question: What if the STCL has rotated 1.5 clock hours. Then we have to adjust by 45 degrees (i.e., the average of 30 and 60 degrees, which would correspond to 1 and 2 clock hours, respectively). If the STCL rotates 2 clock hours, we have to adjust by 60 degrees, etc. However, any excessive rotations should make us recheck the refraction and consider alternative CL options.

As a final note to the above STCL questions, while these examples have been presented for "test" purposes, in clinical practice, there is rarely a STCL that is stable if it has more than 10–15-degree rotation. In other words, if the STCL has rotated more than 10–15 degrees, it may be a "steep/flat" issue (i.e., a BC issue) rather than the wrong axis. If the STCL is moving "too much," the BC should be checked as a decrease in BC may fix the problem rather than adjusting the axis.

Additional Resources Additional information is available for free online at www.gpli.info, including a contact lens-fitting pocket guide.

Practice Questions

1. A patient would like to try a soft contact lens (SCL). Manifest refraction is −8.00 + 1.00 × 90 with vertex distance of 12 mm. Keratometry readings are 44.0 × 45.00 at 85.

   What *K* value(s) would you use to determine the BC? What power would you use for the final SCL?

   A. *K* = 45.0D, PWR = −7.50D
   B. *K* = 44.5D, PWR = −7.00D
   C. *K* = 44.5D, PWR = −7.75D
   D. *K* = 44.0D, PWR = −7.00D

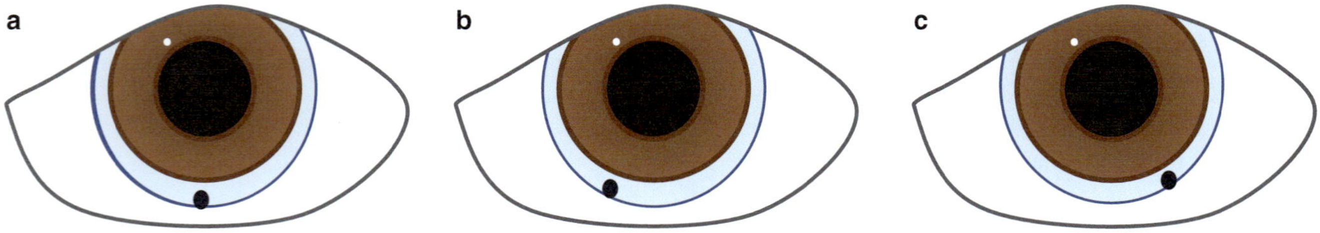

Fig. 3 The LARS rule for soft toric contact lenses (STCLs). If the STCL has been fit correctly (panel A), the centering mark will be seen at the 6 o'clock position, regardless of the axis of correction. In panel B, the resting mark has rotated to the left of the 6 o'clock position; therefore, we have to add to the axis of the STCL. In panel C, the resting mark has rotated to the right of the 6 o'clock position; therefore, we have to subtract from the axis of the STCL

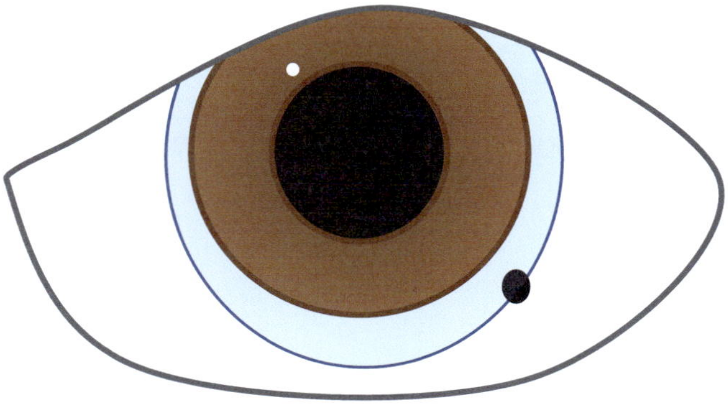

Fig. 4 Rotation of STCL corresponding to practice question #4

2. A patient presents to your office after recently receiving new SCLs from another provider 3 weeks ago. He complains that his eyes start to hurt within a few hours of wearing SCLs. Slit-lamp examination reveals significant pannus in both eyes with several prominent areas of corneal neovascularization near the limbus. You look at the box and note the following numbers, 8.5/13.0/−4.00. Which of the following adjustments would be most helpful for this patient?
   A. 8.5/13.0/−4.25
   B. 8.7/14.0/−4.00
   C. 8.7/13.0/−4.00
   D. 8.3/12.8/−4.00
3. Suppose a patient needs a RGPCL. Her manifest refraction is +10.0 + 1.0 × 180 with vertex distance of 13 mm. Keratometry readings are 40.0D x 41.0D at 180.

   Which *K* would you base your BC on and what power would you use for contact lens prescription?
   A. *K* = 40.0D, PWR = +12.5D
   B. *K* = 40.5D, PWR = +12.5D
   C. *K* = 40.0D, PWR = +9.75D
   D. *K* = 41.0D, PWR = +13.0D
4. Suppose you fitted a patient for a soft toric contact lens (STCL). If the power chosen was −5.50 – 1.75 × 150 and the following pattern was noted on slit-lamp assessment, what would the new power of the STCL be (Fig. 4)?
   A. −5.50 – 1.75 × 105
   B. – 5.50 – 1.75 × 15
   C. −5.50 – 1.75 × 60
   D. −5.50 – 1.75 × 120

Answers

1. Answer: B. For the BC determination for SCL, we can simply take the average of *K* values: (44 + 45)/2 = 44.5D.

   For the power calculation, first determine the spherical equivalent −8.0 + ½(+1.0) = −7.5D. Then we have to use vertex distance calculations to determine the power for zero vertex distance. The focal point of these spectacles is 100/7.5D = 13 cm; since the patient is a myope, we know that the far point of this patient is 13 cm to the left of the spectacle lens. Now we have to adjust for the vertex distance (12 mm or 1.2 cm):

   Far point = (13 cm + 1.2 cm) = 14.2 cm to the left of the cornea. The power of the SCL is the reciprocal, 100/14.2 = −7D. (Watch the decimal places!) A – 7.00D contact will have the same focal point as a – 7.5D spectacle lens at 13 mm.
2. Answer: C. The SCL is **too tight**. We have to flatten the SCL by either increasing the BC (to more than 8.5) or decreasing the diameter (to be less than 13.0). Choice D seems to allow us to decrease the diameter, but it also decreases the BC, so this will not be helpful. Choice A can safely be eliminated since the only change is to the power of SCL, so that will not be very helpful either. Both B and C increase the BC, but B also increases the diameter (which will steepen the SCL). Therefore, C is more likely to help this patient with a tight fitting SCL.
3. Answer: A. For the BC determination in RGP with low astigmatism, choose the lowest *K*, in this case 40.0D. To create a tear lens with +0.50D power, we will want to fit a half-diopter steeper than the flattest K. Thankfully, they have not given us any other BC values here, so we can dictate what *K* values we are going to use.

   For the power calculation, convert the manifest refraction into the minus cylinder: +10.00 + 1.00 × 180, minus cylinder: +11.00 – 1.00 × 90. We can eliminate the cylinder and axis value and use this "new" sphere to calculate the power of the lens if the vertex distance = 0. The focal point of this "new" sphere is 100/11 = 9 cm or 90 mm behind the eye. We are told that the vertex distance is 13 mm. Since the patient is a hyperope, the far point of the eye will be behind the eye (to the right of the lens and the eye). We can adjust for the vertex distance by subtracting it from the focal point to find the far point:

   9 cm – 1.3 cm = 7.7 cm Now we can find the focal length of this new far point, 100/7.7 = +13.0.

   Finally, we have to "add minus" due to the tear film effect, +13.0 – 0.5D = +12.5D.
4. Answer: A. The figure shows that the centering mark has rotated by approximately 1.5 clock hours to the right. We can use the "LARS" rule to remind us that a STCL that rotates to the **right** needs to be adjusted by subtracting from its axis. A 1.5-clock hour rotation would correspond to 45 degrees. Therefore, 150 – 45 = 105 degrees. Note that choice B would be wrong because it would be adding 45 degrees instead of subtracting. Choice C is way off because it involves changing the axis by 90 degrees. Choice D could be considered, but it does not make enough of an adjustment since it is only

30 degrees (1 clock hour) instead of the needed 45 degrees. Again, for real-world clinical purposes, if this lens has rotated 45 degrees, we may need to assess the BC before adjusting the axis. This example has been given mainly for test purposes.

Acknowledgments Authors would like to thank Rachel M. Caywood, OD, FAAO, Dean McGee Eye Institute, University of Oklahoma, for her assistance in the writing of this chapter.

Physical Optics and Advanced Optical Principles

G. Vike Vicente and Kamran M. Riaz

Objectives

- To introduce other theories of light, including wave theory, particle theory, and quantum electrodynamics.
- To understand key topics within Physical Optics, including interference, coherence, polarization, scattering, and diffraction.
- To review various devices and technology commonly used in ophthalmology utilizing these concepts.
- To understand how lower-order aberrations (LOAs) and higher-order aberrations (HOAs) affect both objective and subjective visual acuity.
- To discuss the effect of spherical aberration in the clinical and surgical setting.
- To understand key principles of spectral sensitivity and visual pigments.
- To understand how lasers used in clinical practice exert their effects through principles of photocoagulation, photodisruption, plasma-induced ablation, photoablation, and photoactivation.

Introduction to Physical Optics

Note to the reader: we think this is one of the coolest and most interesting chapters in ophthalmic optics. Though it may have the least relevance for exams, many of the topics discussed in this chapter have significant relevance to the current challenges and the next frontiers of ophthalmology, especially in cataract and refractive surgery. Our knowledge as a profession regarding some of these topics remains limited; thankfully, people much more intelligent than the authors are actively performing research in this arena. More answers will likely be discovered in the near future (and in the next version of this book).

As ophthalmologists, we are masters of the sensory perception of light, and to master it, we must understand it.

Theories of Light

Is light a ray, a wave, or a particle? Well, the answer is all of the above – and more. Light cannot make up its mind, so it can behave and be described as all three things, often simultaneous and interchangeably. Thus far, we have primarily (and artificially) conceptualized light as *rays* that travel in straight lines during our discussions of topics in most of Section I. However, saying that light travels in rays is like saying ophthalmologists only do cataract surgery – it fails to encompass so many other things we do, especially our subspeciality colleagues. Therefore, when it comes to light, Geometric Optics (light traveling in rays) only partially explains the nature of light. In this chapter, we will explore some of these other theories.

Wave Theory of Light

The first additional theory we can discuss is the *wave theory of light*. In this model, we can also think of light as propagating and expanding in three-dimensional space as a wave with both wavelength and frequency.[1] Waves can interact with one another by summation or cancellation, and they can even bend around corners (see *interference* and *diffraction* sections later in this chapter, which is best understood when imagining light as waves). Imagine you are relaxing after your board exams sitting on a dock, and you see a ripple on the surface of a pond. Ripples are only visibly happening in two-dimensional space (on the surface of the water), but in reality, ripples are happening vertically (underneath the surface of the water) as well (Fig. 1).

[1]We can visualize this in a two-dimensional space as water waves moving in a straight line toward the beach.

G. V. Vicente
Clinical Pediatrics and Ophthalmology Georgetown University Hospital, Washington, DC, USA

Eye Doctors of Washington, Chevy Chase, MD, USA

K. M. Riaz (✉)
Dean McGee Eye Institute, University of Oklahoma, Oklahoma City, OK, USA

K. M. Riaz et al. (eds.), *Optics for the New Millennium*, https://doi.org/10.1007/978-3-030-95251-8_14

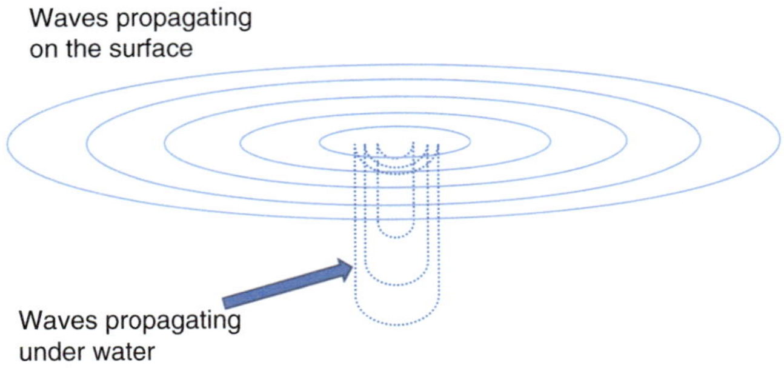

Fig. 1 Ripples on the surface of a pond seemingly extend only in a two-dimensional space on the water's surface. However, vertical ripples extend underneath the surface of the water, which serves as a foundational analogy to understanding how light can travel in waves

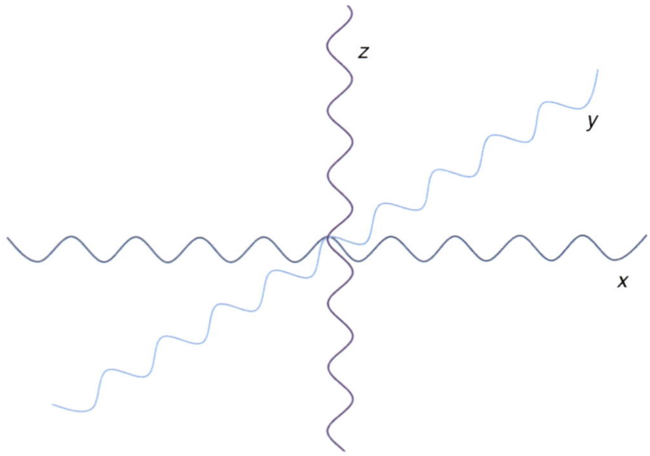

Fig. 2 Light can travel as waves in multiple directions. Here, we can visualize light as waves that travel in the x, y, and z directions for simplicity

When we extend this to light, we can see that light will travel as a wave in all three dimensions (x, y, and z directions). We will refrain from discussing whether light permeates the fourth through tenth dimensions because it is unlikely to ever be tested on an exam, even as an experimental question (Fig. 2).

Under the Wave Theory of Light, we can now imagine that light emanating from a light source will travel as waves in multiple directions (Fig. 3).

At this point, you might be wondering if we lied to you all along during Geometric Optics by saying that light can travel as rays in straight lines previously, and now we are telling you that light travels in waves. We can find our "rays" within the waves as follows: if we draw a line connecting points that are tangential (at 90 degrees) to each curve, we can see our familiar friend, the ray of light, hiding and hanging out within the waves (Fig. 4). We did not lie to you, good sir/madam, because if light could not be a ray, space villains in a galaxy far, far away could not have death rays!

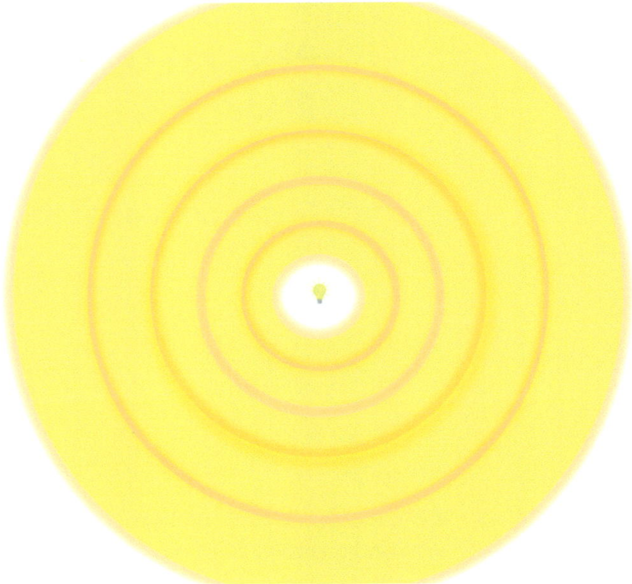

Fig. 3 We can visualize the Wave Theory of Light by imagining light as waves traveling in all directions emanating from a light source

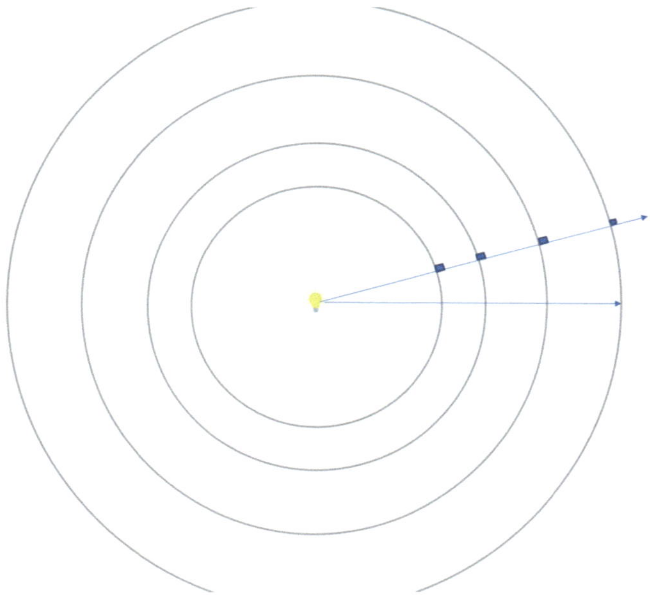

Fig. 4 If a line is drawn connecting all the tangential points to each wave emanating from our light source, we can find our familiar ray of light

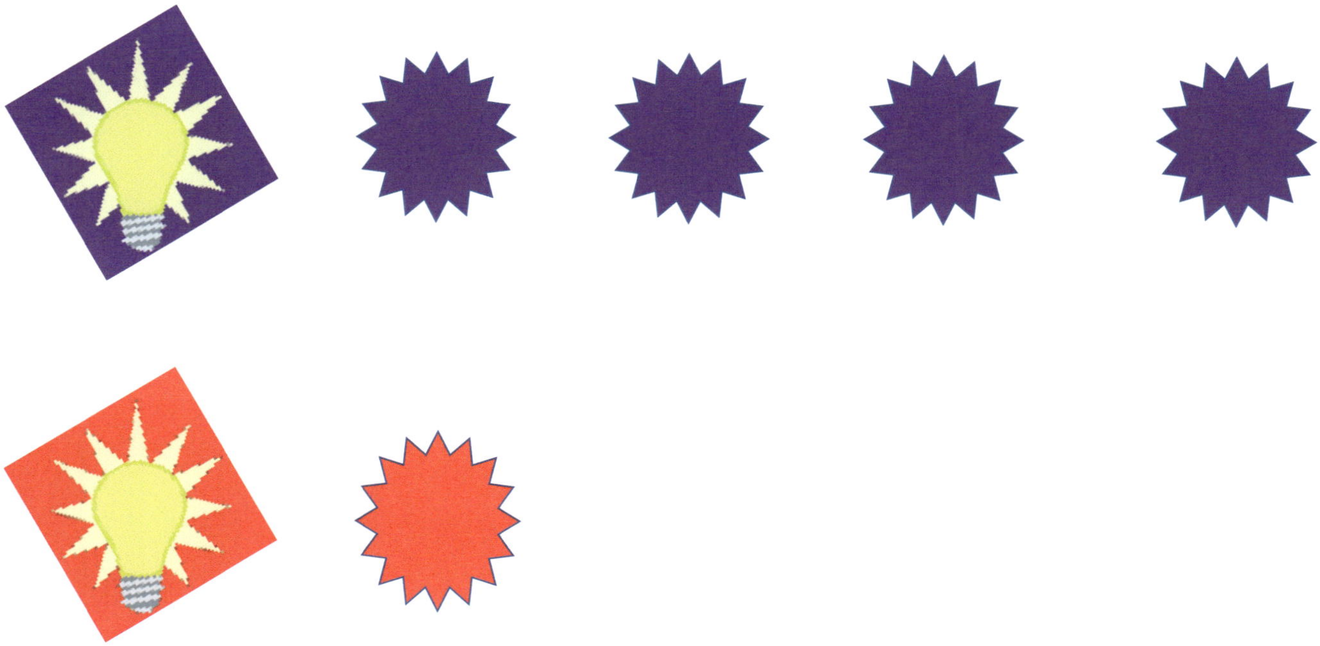

Fig. 5 Light particles emanating from a light source are termed photons. The higher the frequency of the light source, the more energy within the photons

Particle Theory of Light

The second theory is the *particle theory of light*, wherein we can think of light as a particle (photon) to help us understand how it can carry energy.[2] A photon is a discrete packet of light energy; imagine a BB pellet of light filled with energy. Light with a higher frequency (e.g., the purple spectrum of light) will have more energy than light with a lower frequency (e.g., the red spectrum of light, Fig. 5). We take advantage of this conceptualization of light as photons in developing and applying lasers in ophthalmology. Due to time travel paradoxes, we will avoid discussing photon torpedoes until the twenty-fourth century.

Quantum Electrodynamics (QED)

Just as there is *one ring to rule them all*, the theory of *quantum electrodynamics (QED)* is currently the one theory that unifies all other theories. While you may want to consult other texts for a more detailed explanation of this theory, we can simplify it: electrons and photons are like hormonally amplified young people using a social dating app – they are constantly hooking up and breaking up. Electrons (matter) pick up photons (light) for a while and then leave them for another photon, who are only too happy to connect with another electron.

For example, when we discussed refraction in Geometric Optics, we stated that an incoming light ray will bend toward the surface normal and emerge on the other side. In the QED theory, an incoming light particle (photon) hooks up with an electron in the medium and travels a little bit, and then a new photon is emitted to the adjacent electron. This hookup-breakup routine continues until, eventually, a photon is emitted at the back surface of the refractive medium as the "refracted ray of light." Interestingly enough, the incoming photon is not the same photon that emerges from the medium.

We have included QED mainly for the sake of introducing the topic. For the rest of this chapter, we will primarily use the Wave Theory and Particle Theory to explain some of the following concepts.

Interference

Using the Wave Theory of Light, we can imagine two waves meeting and forming a larger wave or two waves meeting and canceling each other out. Both of these are examples of **interference**.

Suppose that we had a point source of light that passed through a barrier with two openings (Fig. 6).[3] We can see that two different "routes" are open for light waves to pass through the first barrier before reaching the final screen.

[2]Historically, Newton termed this particle as a corpuscle of light until Einstein came along and named these individual packets of energy as photons, giving rise to the quantum theory of light. We are intentionally skipping some of the quantum theory of light principles because it involves conceptualizing light as both a wave and a particle. It is somewhat a confusing theory because one is never really sure when to use the "wave" part of light or the "particle" part of light, so we are going to skip it in this text.

[3]This is our simplified way of explaining Young's famous "double-slit" experiment.

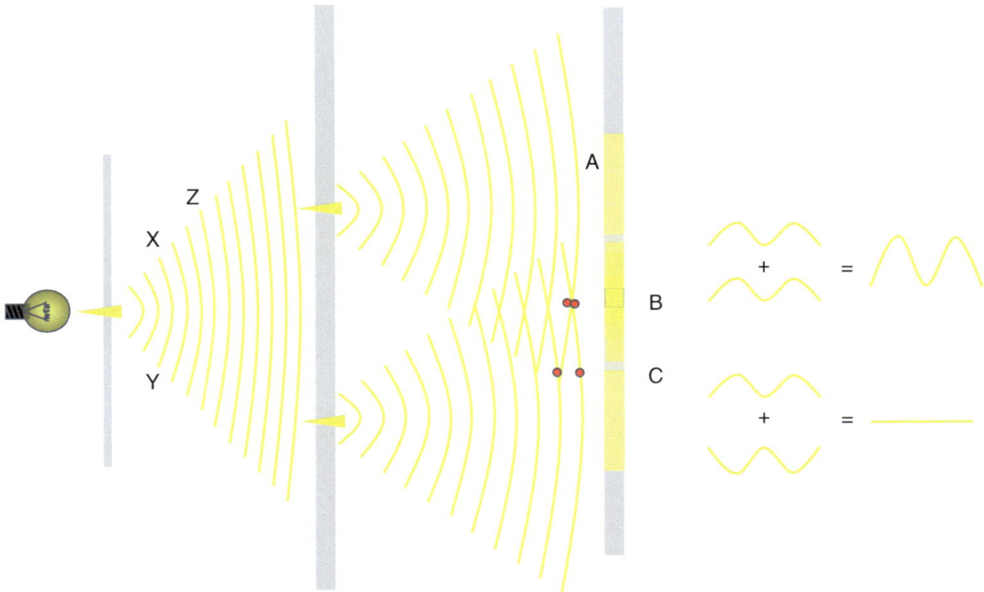

Fig. 6 A light source passing through a barrier with two separate openings will demonstrate both constructive interference (point B) and destructive interference (point C)

There are now three different "flavors" of light waves on the final screen. As seen at point A, the first kind is light waves that pass through the superior opening and never encounter any light waves that have passed through the inferior opening. These loner waves will have the same intensity as the original light source. The second kind of light wave can be seen at point B. This location is where light waves from the superior opening and inferior opening have teamed up together in love and harmony ("in phase") to create a more intensive light pattern – this is known as *constructive interference*. Finally, the third kind of light wave is seen at point C. At this point, light waves from the superior opening and inferior opening have some deep beef and simply refuse to join forces. This now creates a less intensive light pattern than either point A or B, known as *destructive interference*. You can demonstrate this to yourself if you have access to monochromatic light, a barrier with two openings, and plenty of time to spend on a boring weekend afternoon.

Therefore, the Wave Theory of Light is useful because it helps to explain how light waves can produce different intensity patterns. If we only assumed that light traveled as rays and ran those rays through the same barrier-opening setup, we can see that our diagram will artificially (and falsely) show that the resulting light pattern will be of equal intensity at all points on the final screen (Fig. 7).

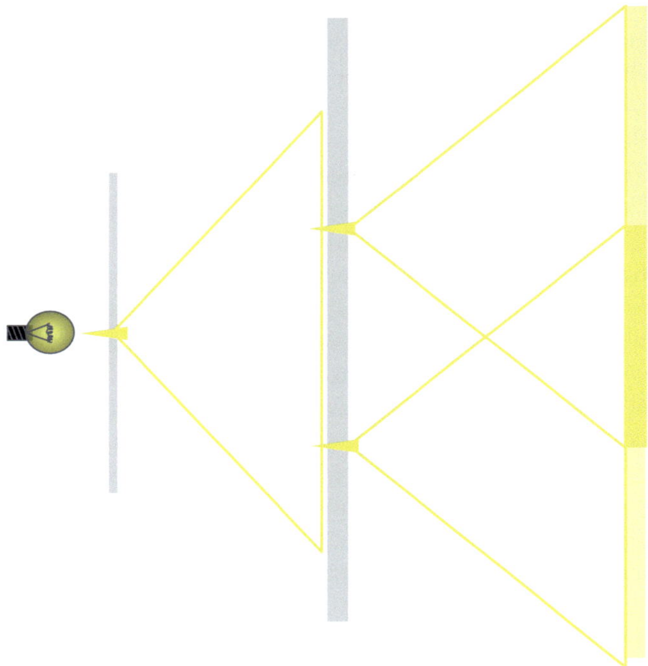

Fig. 7 If we only assume that light travels in rays, the resulting pattern will (falsely) have equal intensity on the final screen

Fluorescein angiography is a good example of a commonly used diagnostic tool in ophthalmology that takes advantage of this property of interference (Fig. 8). When fluorescein dye is injected into a patient's arm, nearly 70–75% will remain bound to serum albumin, and the remaining 25% that enters the circulation will quickly reach the retinal blood supply. When the camera is first clicked, white light emerging from the camera will pass through a blue interference filter, primarily allowing the blue wavelengths of light (465–490 nm) to enter the eye. When the fluorescein molecule is excited by the incoming blue light, the molecule will, in turn, emit a yellow-green wavelength (530 nm) of light out of the eye.[4] This returning "green" light, in addition to other wavelengths of light "emitted" from the eye, now reaches the camera a second time, where a green interference filter will block all other wavelengths of light and only allow yellow-green light to be focused onto the film or a digital camera.

[4] Here again, electrons and photons are "hooking up and breaking up".

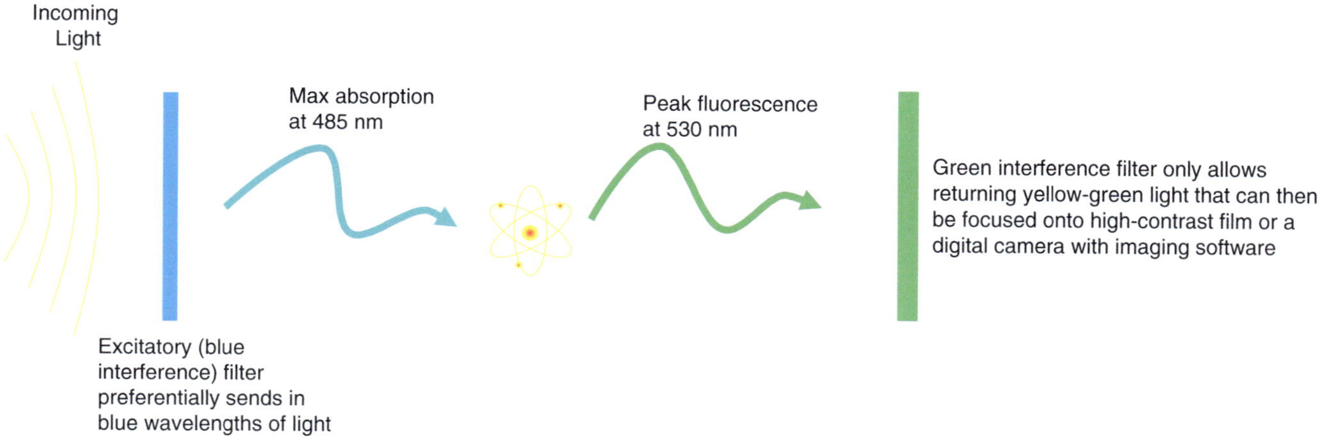

Fig. 8 The principle of interference is seen with both incoming and outgoing light during fluorescein angiography. White light goes through a blue filter into the eye, and this blue light is absorbed by the fluorescein molecule, which in turn emits green light that "returns" back to the camera. A green filter on the camera allows only the green light to reenter the camera

At this point, some of you may think to yourself: "I hate optics. I will not order any fluorescein angiograms so that I don't have to deal with this interference nonsense. I can get all the information I need about the retina from OCTs." Well, you may want to brace yourself for the next section.

Coherence

Coherence describes the ability of light waves or two parts of the same light wave to produce interference. If someone were to ask you to use "coherence" and "interference" in a coherent sentence, you can puff your chest boldly and declare: "if two light waves can produce an interference pattern, then they are coherent."

Types of Coherence

For completeness, Fig. 6 displays the two types of coherence. *Temporal coherence* is seen with points X and Z. These points are on two waves separated by time. If we waited for a few milliseconds, point X would be at the location of point Z (though Z would have moved on) and be the same size/magnitude as point Z. Temporal coherence is the basis for time-domain optical coherence tomography (TD-OCT) imaging.

Spatial coherence occurs within the same wave of light. Two different points on the same wave of light equidistant from the center are considered to have spatial coherence. For example, in Fig. 6, points X and Y have spatial coherence. Spatial coherence is the basis for spectral-domain optical coherence tomography (SD-OCT) imaging.

Examples of Coherence in Clinical Practice

At this point, one may wonder: *is any of this actually used in ophthalmology?*

You may have already guessed the answer, but yes, they are relevant and used frequently. Coherence and interference are used in various clinical applications, such as OCT, antireflective coatings, and modern optical biometry devices.

Optical Coherence Tomography

One area of considerable relevance is optical coherence tomography (OCT) – the word coherence has been hiding in the "OCT" phrase that you use in the clinic all the time and you may or may not have even realized it.

OCT uses **low-coherence interferometry**: long-wavelength, near-infrared light is used to penetrate into the scattering medium without damaging any tissue. An optical beam is directed at the tissue of interest (cornea, retina, etc.). The device's measuring instruments collect a small portion of this light that reflects from sub-surface features. Interferometry is then used to collect light directly reflected from surfaces of interest (and reject most photons that have scattered multiple times that cause "background noise").

In *time-domain OCT* (*TD-OCT*), if we can time gate the echo train of backscatter from the tissue of interest, we can generate an image by varying the path length of the reference arm in time (the reference mirror is translated longitudinally). By scanning the mirror in the reference arm, a reflectivity profile (A-scan) of the sample can be obtained. The device's software then amalgamates multiple A-scans to generate a cross-sectional tomography image (B-scan). Approximately *400 A-scans per second* can be generated using six radial slices oriented 30 degrees apart, yielding an accuracy down to the level of 10–15 microns.[5] Basically, we are comparing information about point X and point Z from Fig. 6.

[5]Yaqoob Z, Wu J, Yang C. Spectral domain optical coherence tomography: a better OCT imaging strategy. *BioTechniques*; 2005 Dec; 39: S6–13

With *Fourier-domain OCT (FD-OCT)*, interference components are collected simultaneously without using a reference mirror to measure the target tissue. FD-OCT significantly improves acquisition speed without compromising image quality. There are two subtypes of FD-OCT: *spectral-domain OCT* (SD-OCT) and *swept-source OCT* (SS-OCT). In both subtypes, a sensor within the device analyzes the beam intensity generated by the interference of the reference arm beam and the measuring arm beam – this includes constructive, destructive, and partially constructive interference.

SD-OCT systems use a spectrometer and high-speed line scan camera to analyze the reflected light; the SD-OCT mirror is static. Clinically important information can be gathered by distributing returning light waves (according to different optical frequencies) onto a detector stripe. This allows information from the full depth scan to be acquired within a single exposure. SD-OCT takes approximately *20,000–40,000 scans per second* to continuously image a 6-mm area of interest, yielding an accuracy down to the level of approximately three microns. Basically, we can obtain information about point X and point Y from Fig. 6 (and all points in between) to generate our scan. Since SD-OCT devices utilize lower-wavelength light sources (approximately 820–880 nm) with higher A-scans, they provide images with excellent resolution compared to TD-OCT devices, although with limited tissue penetration (decreased depth).

With SS-OCT, the longer-wavelength (1300-nm)-dependent reflected light is measured with a single detector. This narrow band light source is then rapidly tuned over a large optical bandwidth. The wavelength is rapidly swept within the laser, allowing for the use of a point detector. Due to its ultrafast scanning system, greater depth range, and less sensitivity to motion, SS-OCT allows for *several million A-scans per second* using high-speed swept-source technology. Thus, SS-OCT offers deeper tissue penetration (similar to TD-OCT devices) and improved image details (improving upon SD-OCT devices). Of clinical relevance, SS-OCT technology is used in the IOLMaster 700 (Carl Zeiss Meditec, Jena, Germany), a recently introduced biometry device.

If we thought OCT devices only dealt with coherence, we are in for a surprise: we also have to deal with our good old friend, refraction, which distorts the acquired image. Recall that the OCT signal has to pass through different media (air, cornea, aqueous, crystalline lens, and vitreous) with a wide range of refractive indices. Therefore, the acquired image has to compensate for these refractive effects by applying several previously discussed optics principles, such as Snell's law, power of a refracting surface, and power of lenses in different media.

Antireflective Coatings

When light reaches a lens, some of the light will refract through, and some of the light will be reflected (away) from the lens. However, if we could add a very thin, semi-transparent material of approximately one-fourth wavelength thickness of the incoming light to the lens, we would have created a second reflected wave out of phase with the first reflected wave and caused destructive interference. The two waves would cancel each other out, and very little light would be reflected (Fig. 8). The filter's troughs and peaks would look similar to the incoming ray. More importantly, the filter's peaks and troughs would neutralize the outgoing reflected ray's troughs and peaks, respectively (Fig. 9).

Antireflective coatings are especially useful for high-index lenses (e.g., some of the newer Crizal®-type materials) since the higher index of refraction also means there is more reflection of incoming light.

How do opticians or optical labs apply antireflective coatings to lenses? Well, the best thing to do is to visit an actual lab and see for yourself – seriously, it is pretty incredible some of the things that can be done with modern technology and newer materials. As mentioned above, antireflective coatings are customarily chosen to be approximately one-fourth the wavelength of incoming light. Given that yellow light (580 nm) is the average wavelength visible to the human eye, most antireflective coatings are chosen to be approximately 145-nm thick. In order to form this extremely thin coating, optical labs will allow vaporized particles to slowly condense on the lens surface until it forms a layer of approximately 145 nm.

Optical Biometry Devices

Optical biometry devices are interferometers: they use coherence and interference to more accurately image the eye (Fig. 10). A laser light source sends highly coherent light toward a beam splitter; this splits half the incoming ray toward the eye (red line) and the other half toward movable mirrors (blue line). The reflected light, both from the eye and the mirrors, is directed toward a photosensor which determines the intensity of the reflected light by measuring both the constructive and the destructive interference of the reflected light (i.e., both red and blue rays in the diagram).

The red ray will be affected by ocular structures (due to the change in refractive index [RI] of each structure); constructive interference will occur when these "returning" red rays of light arrive at the same time as reflected blue rays. Mirrors can be moved to coincide with spikes of interest, such as the anterior corneal surface, posterior corneal surface, etc. The distance between spikes is known as the optical path length (OPL) of the cornea, aqueous, etc. The length

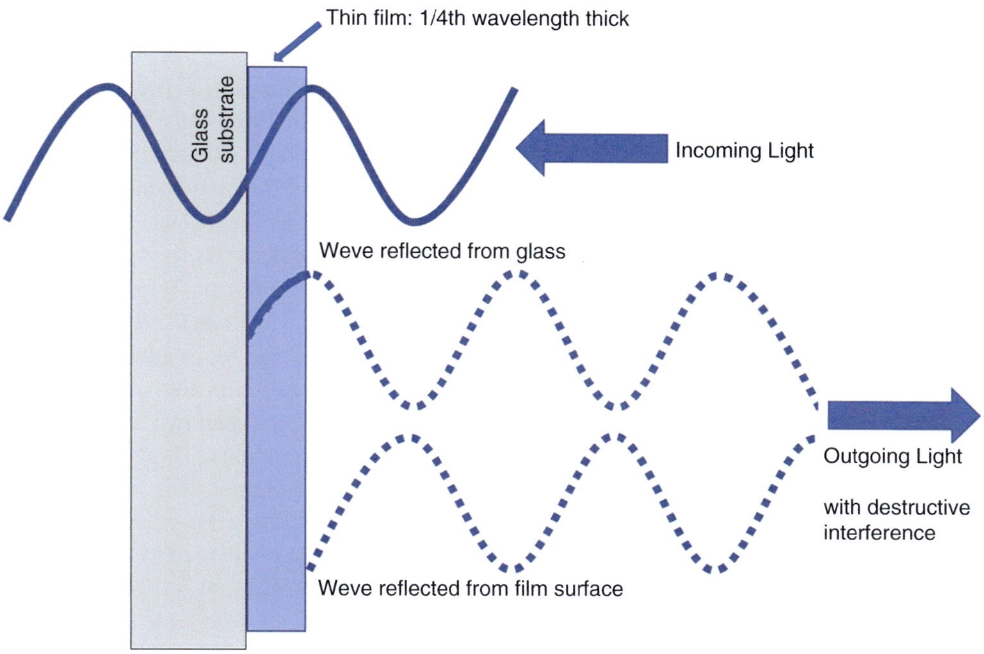

Fig. 9 Destructive interference can be used to a favorable advantage in the construction of antireflective coatings. Some of the incoming light (solid blue wave) will pass through the glass substrate (gray rectangle), whereas some will be reflected from the surface of the thin film (blue rectangle). The two waves will experience destructive interference and will not be seen by the observer

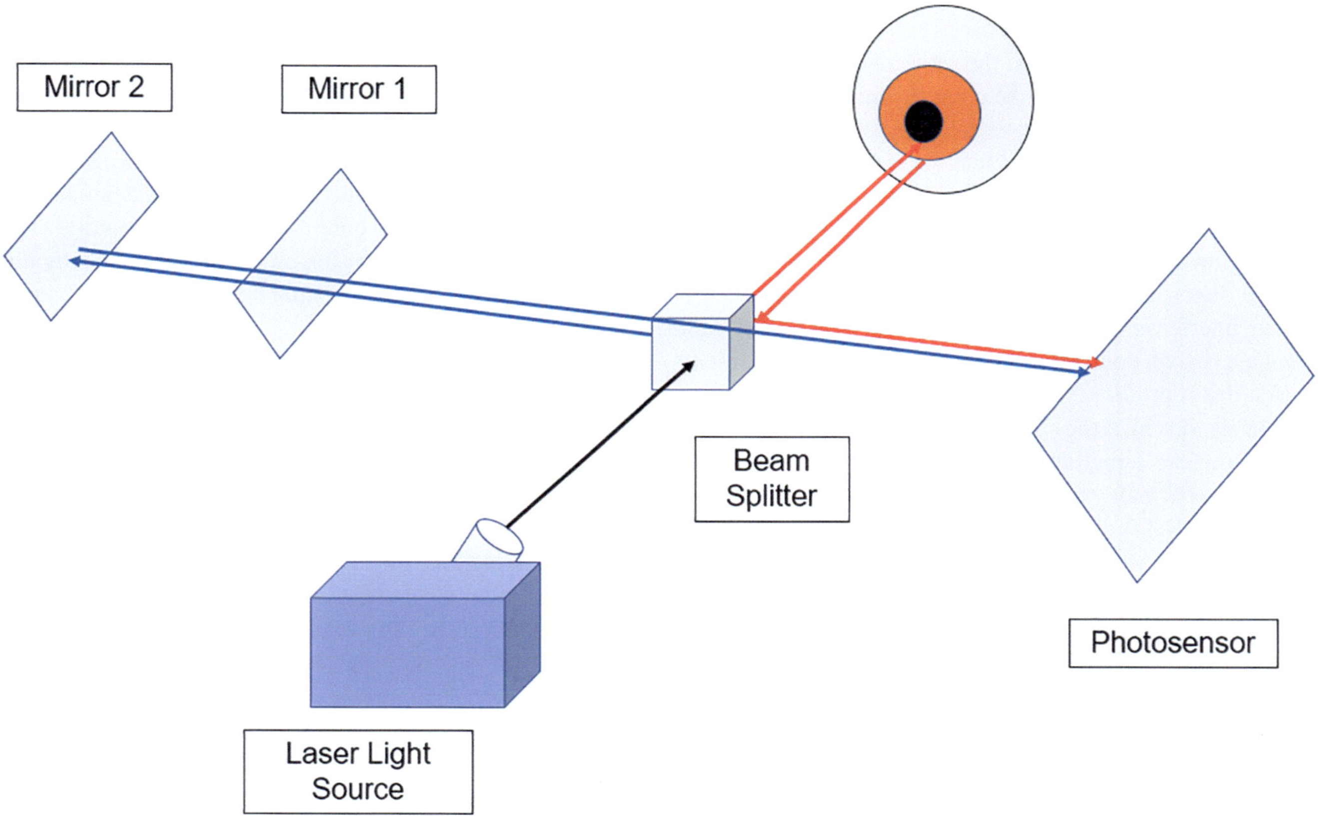

Fig. 10 A commonly used setup for interferometry

of each segment in the eye can be determined by a simple measurement of OPL/RI; unfortunately, since we do not know the "true" RI of each ocular structure, we have to either come up with one for the entire eye (e.g., 1.3375 as used by many biometry devices in the United States, or 1.332 as used in many European countries) or devise one for each segment of the eye – this is known as "sum of segments (SOS)," which is a more accurate way to measure axial length. SOS axial length differs from the traditional axial length, especially in very short and very long eyes. Traditional axial length tends to "underestimate" the length of short eyes and "overestimate" the length of long eyes, leading to myopic and hyperopic surprises, respectively, especially when using older-generation IOL calculation formulas.

In getting back to our interferometer example, if both the red and blue rays have the same OPL, then constructive interference occurs; if the OPL is <1, then the peak of one wave will destructively interfere with the trough of another wave. The key principle is that we want to see some alternating patterns of interference; by using low-coherence light (instead of white light, which is incoherent), we can create favorable interference patterns that the photosensor can measure.

Partial coherence interferometry (PCI) and optical low-coherence reflectometry (OLCR) are two of the most commonly used technologies in modern biometry devices, such as the IOLMaster 500 (Carl Zeiss Meditec, Jena, Germany) and the Lenstar (Haag-Streit, Switzerland), respectively.[6]

With PCI, a dual-beam setup is used: one beam to measure reflected light from the cornea and the second beam to measure reflected light from the retina. A mirror is used to increase the path length of the corneal signal. When the corneal and retinal signals are equal, interference is detected. Then using the index of refraction for the entire eye (usually n=1.3375), the entire axial length (AXL) can be measured. OLCR is a bit more complicated,[7] so we will instead focus on the low-coherence interferometry part: low-coherence light is directed into the eye, and reflected light is measured by an interferometer, which interprets this reflected light from every scan point as an interference pattern and presents it as a depth profile (A-scan). A cross section (B-scan) can also be generated at the same time.

PCI utilizes a multimodal (pulsed) laser diode (infrared laser light, 780 nm), whereas OLCR uses a superluminescent (continuous light) diode (820 nm). Because of the "partial" portion of PCI, every measurement signal will create secondary (smaller) peaks on either side of the "measured" peak; in other words, the software may falsely measure one of the smaller peaks, such as in the case of a pseudophakic patient, which may lead to an incorrectly measured axial length. Since OLCR uses continuous, low-coherence light, a full A-scan can be obtained, including axial length, lens thickness, corneal thickness, etc.

[6]See Chap. 26, Preoperative Optics for Cataract Surgery, for a more detailed clinical discussion of these two devices, including the most recently introduced swept-source OCT (SS-OCT) optical biometry device (IOLMaster 700, Carl Zeiss Meditec, Jena, Germany).

[7]An internal reference path is used to measure the patient's eye by using a rotating glass cube system to change the optical path length in the reference arm.

Polarization

Polarization (not the political kind) of light is a term used to describe light waves in which vibrations occur in a single plane. Polarization happens whenever light waves are transmitted, reflected, refracted, or scattered. This is another quite complex topic, and interested readers may wish to consult other texts for more information. We will primarily focus on *linearly polarized* light.[8]

Polarization has many uses outside of ophthalmology. For example, in addition to its influence on photography, polarization is also used to create 3D movies, which are nothing more than two movies filmed from slightly different camera locations. The two "films" are 90 degrees away from each other and then broadcast at the same time through two projectors; 3D glasses are basically two lenses with two different polarized filters – usually, one is vertical, and the other is horizontal – that allow us to visualize "both films" that are then fused by our brains to give a perception of three-dimensionality. A recent area of interest is the use of polarization in polarization-sensitive OCT technology (PS-OCT), which can measure the polarization properties of ocular tissues and generate an OCT image by mathematical processing (Jones matrix OCT). Collagen fibers, in particular, exhibit high phase retardation and birefringence, which can be used by PS-OCT devices to yield high-resolution images of the tissue of interest. The use of PS-OCT is an area to monitor in the future as it continues to develop rapidly.

We will focus our discussion on the four most commonly encountered types of polarization before discussing some examples.

Types of Polarization

Transmission

Most "naturally" occurring light sources, such as a candle or the sun, will emit light that travels in multiple directions with vibrations in multiple planes (unpolarized light). However, if a polarized filter is placed in front of an unpolarized light source, the filter will filter out (i.e., "block") one-half of the vibrations that pass through the filter. For simplicity, we can assume that all polarization is vertical or horizontal (Fig. 11).

Imagine that the polarized filter is like a bouncer at a nightclub that only lets in the light waves that meet the club's criteria for admission. A vertical filter will only allow in vertical waves, and a horizontal filter will only allow in horizontal waves. Suppose light passes through a vertically polarized filter. All the horizontally oriented waves will be excluded,

[8]There are other "flavors" of polarization, such as circularly polarized light and elliptically polarized light. Chocolate-chip cookie dough is unfortunately not an available flavor.

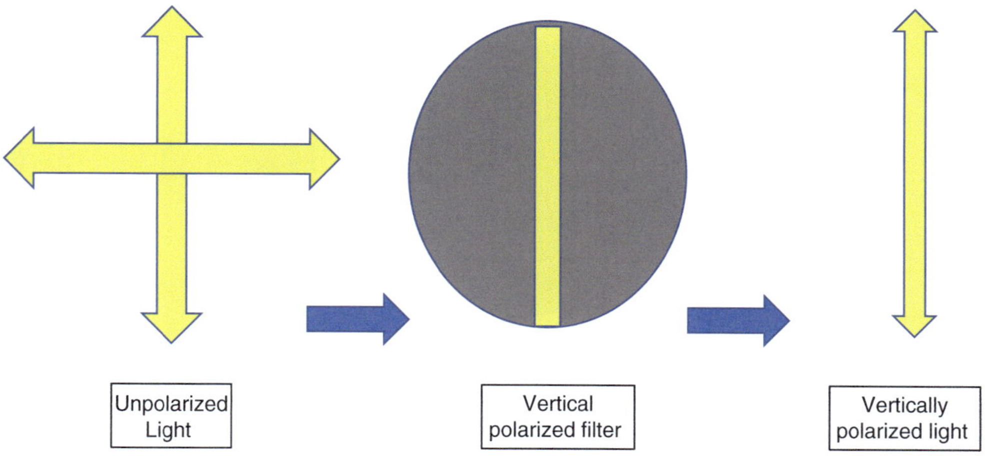

Fig. 11 Light waves emanating from a light source will have polarization in all directions (shown only as vertical and horizontal in the figure). If a polarized filter is placed in front of unpolarized light, only light waves that are oriented in the direction of the filter will be transmitted on the other side. A vertical filter will only allow vertically oriented light waves to pass through

and only the vertically oriented light waves will pass through and be transmitted on the other side.

Reflection

When unpolarized light approaches nonmetallic surfaces (such as asphalt, sand, etc.) and undergoes multidirectional reflection, reflected waves will also undergo partial polarization: some of the reflected waves will be polarized, and some of the waves will be unpolarized. The amount of polarization that happens depends on the angle of incidence of the light waves.[9] Nonmetallic surfaces will reflect a large concentration of waves parallel to the reflecting surface. This reflection causes glare off the surface of a lake, for example, that further blocks our fisherman (from Chap. 1, "Geometric Optics") from being able to find his fish underwater.[10] For simplification, we can divide polarization of reflected light into *horizontal* and *other* (e.g., *vertical*, etc.) types. When we consider a surface, such as the fisherman and the lake, much of this reflected light is horizontally polarized. Therefore, a pair of sunglasses with *vertical filters* will help our fisherman the most; we will discuss this example in greater detail in the next section.

Refraction

We have previously defined refraction as incoming light (rays or waves) bending as they pass from one medium into another. We can build upon this understanding by adding that the refracted beam will acquire some degree of polarization, usually *perpendicular to the surface*. A famous example often used in undergraduate physics classrooms is that of the Iceland Spar double-refracting crystal. If an object is viewed by looking through this crystal, two images that have resulted from the double refraction of light may be seen. A polarized filter may be used to block one of the images and enhance the other image. The observation of double refraction was a foundation to the eventual Wave Theory of Light.

As an interesting bit of history, Vikings may have been lovers of optics too: they may have used this special crystal as a "sunstone" to identify the sun's location on cloudy days for navigational purposes. Due to the amount of polarization of sunlight at the Arctic Circle, the crystal's "double index of refraction" can be used to separate incoming light waves based on the amount of polarization. In other words, on a cloudy day, an ancient Viking optics nerd could move the crystal along a cloudy sky to find the sun indirectly by observing a yellow entoptic pattern, similar to, of all things, Haidinger's brush, an example we will discuss in greater detail below.[11] We have no information on whether the good Wilhelm Karl von Haidinger (an Austrian physicist) was descended from Vikings.

Scattering

When light waves encounter atoms within a material, they will cause additional electromagnetic vibrations within the medium that subsequently cause a series of absorption and re-emission of light within the medium.[12] This is known as *scattering*. We will discuss scattering further in the next section, but for now, we should understand that scattered light also has significant directional polarization. For example, the polarization of scattered light is seen on a clear day with blue skies as glare in the skies. Photography in these conditions requires a polarizing filter to reduce the glare and increase the "blueness" of the photographed sky. These polarizers can be rotated to achieve desired contrast effects under various lighting conditions.

[9]This is known as the Brewster angle, using the formula, wherein n_t and n_i are refractive indices of the transmitted and incident mediums, respectively. Basically, at this angle, all of the reflected light is polarized (linear polarization).

[10]Remember he must throw his spear *in front* of the fish.

[11]See also Chap. 26, Preoperative Optics for Cataract Surgery, for additional information.

[12]The same electron-photon hooking up and breaking up

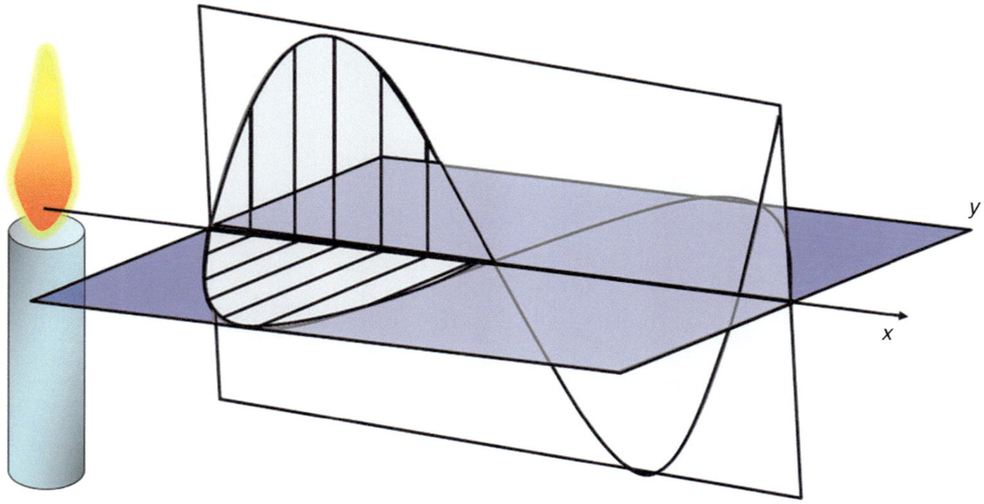

Fig. 12 Polarized light waves can be simplified as traveling along the horizontal (x) or the vertical (y) axis

Examples of Polarization

Within ophthalmology, three common clinical scenarios are worth mentioning about polarization. Multiple types of polarization are present in these examples, but we will try to highlight the main type(s) of polarization to reinforce the previous discussion.

Polarized Sunglasses

Recall our fisherman (it seems we shall never be rid of this fellow) who was having difficulty finding fish under the water's surface. After we have educated him in Chap. 1 "Geometric Optics", suppose he now complains about the glare caused by the polarization of reflection (multidirectional polarization):

Fisherman:	"Doc, can you give me some really dark sunglasses that I can use in case I ever get trapped on an island and have to spear fish again?"
Ophthalmology resident:	"Sure, here you go. And don't plan any more vacations because you are not very good at fishing if you get trapped on an island again."
Fisherman (puts on the dark glasses):	"But doc, I can't see anything."

At this point, the ophthalmology resident may be tempted to call in a psychiatry consult. Instead, we should realize that we can offer this patient a special lens that can significantly reduce glare without making lenses too dark. We can take a step back and remember how polarized light travels: even though polarization happens in all directions, for the sake of simplicity, we will limit polarization to either the horizontal (x) or the vertical (y) axis (Fig. 12).

What if we could create a filter to block off light traveling along the vertical (y) axis? If we place a horizontal filter in front of the light source, all the vertically oriented light waves will be blocked by the filter, and only the horizontally oriented waves will pass through (Fig. 13A). An observer standing at point A will see a diminished amount of light (dimmer light intensity) since the first (horizontal) filter has blocked half the light.

Now suppose that we placed a vertically oriented filter as a second filter in this system. This second filter will block out all horizontally polarized light waves, as shown in Fig. 13B. As there are a negligible amount of vertical light waves remaining at this point, an observer at point B will not be able to see any light waves from the candle.

Now, back to our fisherman. Instead of giving him intensely dark glasses, we can instead offer him *polarized sunglasses* with a **vertical filter** that will *block out all horizontally polarized light waves* and only allow in vertically oriented light. This construction works since most light reflected from roads, bodies of water, and windshields will be polarized along the horizontal plane. Therefore, a vertical filter will block out these horizontally polarized light waves and reduce his glare and sensitivity in bright light conditions.

Crossed Polarizers and Polarized Microscopy

We can also take advantage of polarization in the ophthalmic pathology lab, for example, when trying to visualize substances that demonstrate birefringence, such as amyloid seen in lattice corneal dystrophy. Birefringence is a unique optical property wherein a material can have a different refractive index depending on the polarization and direction of incoming light.[13] In other words, such materials can demonstrate a "double refraction" of light in a transparent material.

[13] Remember the Iceland spar crystal discussed previously?

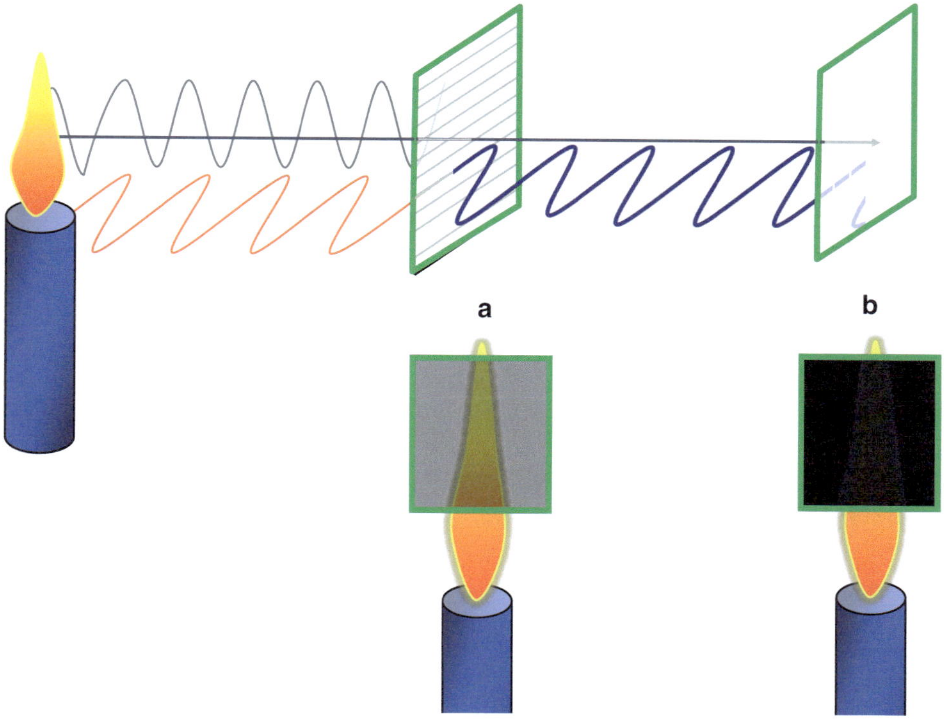

Fig. 13 A horizontal filter will block all vertically oriented light waves. An observer at point A will perceive this as a dimmer light source. A second filter (vertical filter) placed at point B will block all horizontally oriented light waves. An observer at point B will not perceive any light waves from the initial light source

Anisotropy refers to a non-equal, non-uniform distribution of properties within a material. Depending on which direction the material is analyzed, the observed properties of the material can be quite different. When light enters the true optical axis of anisotropic materials such as amyloid, all the light will pass through at a single speed. However, if light enters in a direction away from the true optical axis of that material, then it will undergo double refraction or birefringence.

Crossed polarizers can be useful in microscopy. A birefringent substance placed between both filters will refract light, causing some of the light to no longer be on the horizontal plane (Fig. 14). This shifts the "horizontal" light to a slightly different position, allowing it to pass through the second (vertical filter).

When amyloid is stained with Congo red, it is said to demonstrate "apple-green birefringence" in polarized light. You've probably memorized that fact from other texts, including the Marilyn Monroe mnemonic for corneal dystrophies, abnormality, and relevant stains. But what does that mean exactly? The birefringence of Congo red varies with wavelength of incoming light waves and includes both negative birefringence (blue light) and positive birefringence (yellow light). When mixed together, this will produce green light. When the polarizer and analyzer are uncrossed, birefringence effects are removed, and instead dichroic effects appear, changing the observed light from green to red. This asymmetry of effects – the birefringent "green" light and dichroic "red" light – can be used by pathologists to confirm the presence of amyloid.

Polarized light microscopes contain two polarizers: one positioned before the specimen and one positioned after the specimen (as shown in Fig. 14). As light passes through the microscope, the plane-polarized light will interact with a birefringent specimen to create two individual wave components oriented perpendicularly to each other. These light components are then recombined through *constructive and destructive interference* as they pass through the analyzer. Polarized light microscopy takes advantage of this contrast to improve the quality of images of birefringent materials. So even you, ophthalmic pathologists, cannot escape optics!.

The retinal nerve fiber layer (RNFL) is also highly birefringent: incident light undergoes polarization as it passes through the RNFL. Scanning laser polarimetry takes advantage of this polarization to measure the RNFL thickness. Interestingly enough, the cornea also polarizes some of the incident light, so there is a mechanism in the device that compensates for the corneal polarization effects. So even you, glaucoma specialists, cannot escape optics!.

Haidinger's Brush

This topic is another "rite of passage" type of question that may come up infrequently. See also Chap. 26, "Preoperative Optics for Cataract Surgery" for more information about this topic. Haidinger's Brush refers to a technique wherein the examiner can use a lens (such as a lens from a pair of polarized sunglasses) to rotate polarized light in front of a blue-white background to create an entoptic phenomenon that the patient may perceive as a yellow light. The "spinning" nature of the yellow light creates a "brush" (rotating yellow and

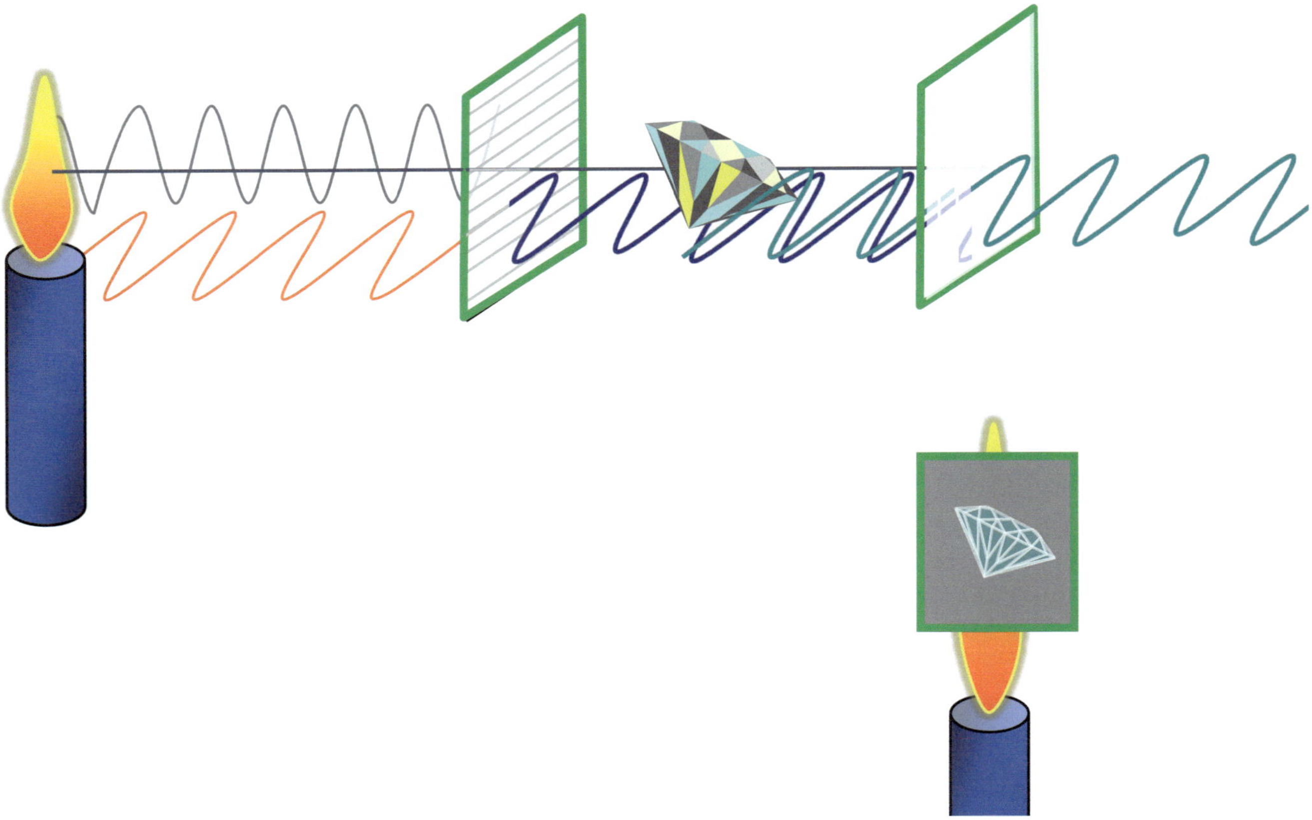

Fig. 14 Cross polarizers can be used to visualize a material of interest by highlighting its anisotropic optical qualities

blue patterns perpendicular to each other) that can be better described as a propeller-like phenomenon that the patient can visualize as the brush is centered on the fovea.[14]

The perception of the "brush" of yellow light is thought to be due to the *dichroism of xanthophyll pigment* in the macula as some pigment molecules are arranged circularly. Because the fovea is not flat, some nerves will run *orthogonal* to the central fovea, while other nerves will run *parallel*. This arrangement creates different areas of the fovea that are sensitive to two different degrees of polarization.

The classic use of Haidinger's Brush is to assess vision potential in a patient with dense cataracts. If the patient can see the "brush," this implies that macular function is present, and the patient has good vision potential with cataract surgery. Of course, other instruments such as pinhole acuity and potential acuity meter (PAM) may be easier to use for clinical testing purposes.

This test has two other uses that we can comment upon briefly. First, it may also test for and break eccentric fixation (EF) in strabismus patients. In order to confirm the presence of EF, the brush can be presented to a suspect patient. If a patient has EF, the brush will appear away from the fixation point since the brush will fall on the foveal center (Fig. 15, panel B). The brush phenomenon can also be used to break EF, as during therapy, the patient may point to the brush instead of the eccentric fixation point (Fig. 15, panel C). Eventually, the goal would be to get the patient to be able to superimpose the brush with the fixation point.

Finally, Haidinger's Brush may also be used to diagnose macular degeneration in older patients, similar to an Amsler grid. If a patient has macular degeneration, the brush pattern would be incomplete or disrupted, raising the suspicion of clinically significant macular degeneration.

Basically, no ophthalmologist can ever escape optics (insert evil maniacal laugh).

Scattering

When light interacts with particles similar in size to its wavelength, it can scatter ("spread out") in all directions. Technically, scattering is due to electron effects on photons of light, primarily occurring during reflection and refraction; we observe these fascinating interactions as the visible appearance of colors.

There are several types of scattering worth reviewing, as discussed below.

[14]Note: the "brush" used to describe this entoptic phenomenon can be a misleading term since it more closely resembles a propeller. Nevertheless, since Haidinger described it as a brush, we will maintain the nomenclature, but it may be easier to understand this as a propeller shape instead.

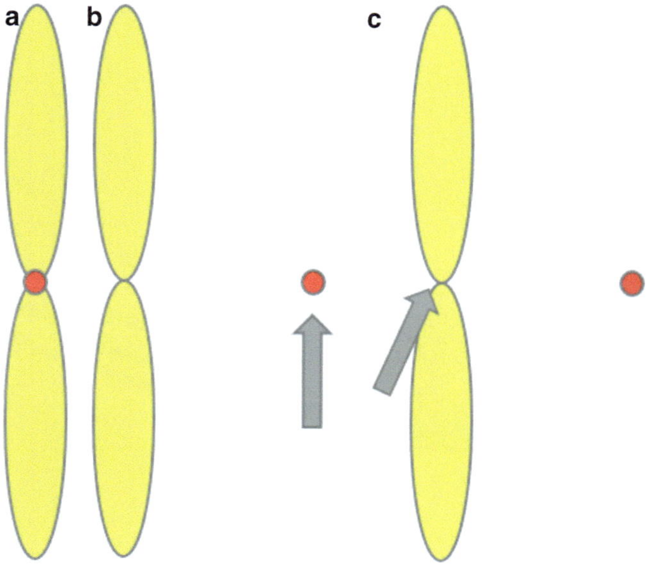

Fig. 15 Haidinger's Brush may be used to screen for and break eccentric fixation (EF). A patient without EF will have overlap of the fixation point (FP, red circle) and the Haidinger's brush (HB, yellow propeller) (panel A). A patient with EF will have an FP that will be either nasal or temporal to the HB. Screening for EF (panel B) will be positive if a patient points to the FP (arrow) instead of the HB since the HB is falling on the macula. With therapy to break EF, a patient may learn to eventually point to the HB (arrow) instead of the FP (panel C)

Selective Scattering (Rayleigh Scattering)

This type of scattering occurs when incoming light waves interact with *microscopic particles* (smaller than the incoming wavelength of light). For example, because air molecules are extremely small in size, they are more effective at scattering shorter wavelengths of light (blue and violet) than longer wavelengths (red and orange).

This type of scattering also helps us answer the proverbial rite of passage question: "Why is the sky blue at noon and red-orange at sunset?"

Before light from the sun reaches Earth's surface, it interacts with the molecules in our atmosphere (Fig. 16). Since air molecules are small in size, they are good at scattering shorter wavelengths of light; as a result, blue light is scattered approximately 16 times more than red light. Since sunlight includes all colors of the rainbow, violet and blue wavelengths will scatter more and appear to come not just from the sun but from all over the sky. There is the highest amount of blue light scattering at noontime because longer wavelengths (red) continue on a straight path without being scattered toward an observer's eyes. The red wavelengths of light are obviously still present, but there is so much scattering of blue light happening at this time that it is "blocking" the red light from being visible. At sunset, we can think of the blue light as having "finished scattering" so now we can observe longer wavelengths of light (red/orange) at this time.

If you are incredibly bored on a weekend, you can see Rayleigh scattering without having to take a trip up to the clouds. You can use a glass bowl filled with water and sprinkle in a few drops of milk. Using a flashlight as a proxy for the sun at noontime, if you shine it from straight above, you will see a blue tinge to the bowl; if you shine it from the side of the bowl (mimicking a sunrise/sunset), you will see a red tinge to the bowl.

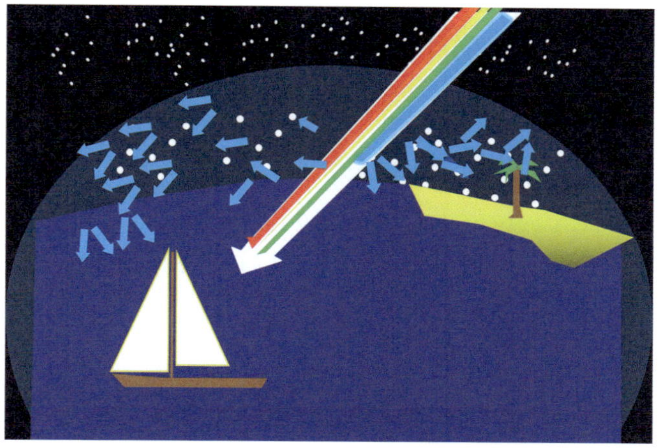

Fig. 16 The sky appears to be blue at noontime due to effects of Rayleigh scattering

Fun fact: due to the lack of an atmosphere on the moon, if we looked up at the "sky" from the moon's surface, it would appear black because no scattering occurs due to the lack of atmosphere. Similarly, if we were on the surface of Mars, the sky would appear pink-red due to the unique combination of particles in Mars' atmosphere that cause selective scattering of the red wavelengths.

Tyndall Effect

Technically, this is not a "pure" form of scattering, but we can group it here because it is a similar concept. The Tyndall effect is restricted to scattering that happens because of particles present in a suspension that make the incoming light beam "visible." Again, we can recall that shorter wavelengths are reflected more due to scattering while longer wavelengths are transmitted. We can see two routinely encountered clinical applications of the Tyndall effect:

- Visualization of cell and flare in the anterior chamber – light waves get scattered by white/red blood cells and proteins in the aqueous humor, allowing the examiner to assess the amount of flare present. The next time you get scolded for incorrectly grading the cell and flare in a patient, take solace that at least you know the Tyndall Effect and now must focus on using it clinically.
- Visualization of blue-green iris – There is less melanin and collagen present in patients with blue/green eyes in the iris stroma. As a result, incoming light waves will undergo "backscattering" toward the observer. As a result, the observer will see shorter wavelengths (blue) much more prominently as longer wavelengths will get absorbed

by the pigment epithelium. There is a higher melanin concentration in the iris stroma in patients with brown eyes. As a result, a higher percentage of light waves will get absorbed and not "backscatter" to the observer, giving the appearance of "brown" eyes.

Mie Scattering

This type of scattering occurs due to particles that are the *same size* as the incoming wavelength of light. Another way of thinking about this type of scattering is that it deals more with *forward scattering* as compared to backward scattering. For example, water droplets in clouds will cause scattering of incoming light waves, giving a white cloud's classic appearance.

Clinically, Mie scattering is relevant both before and after cataract surgery. For example, lens changes (e.g., cortical spoking), and associated Mie scattering can be seen as the "whiteness" of the cataract on clinical exam. For the patient, because this incoming light is getting scattered by cortical spokes, there is loss of objective visual acuity and increased subjective complaints such as increased glare. After cataract surgery, Mie scattering helps to explain some of the degradation of visual quality that occurs due to subsurface nanoglistenings (SSNGs) that may occur postoperatively on particular acrylic intraocular lenses. Light scatter from off-axis light that strikes SSNGs causes forward scattering (rather than the previously discussed backscattering). The **Strehl ratio** is used to define the height of a point spread function compared to an ideal diffraction-limited system for *on-axis* (as compared to *off-axis*) light. A higher Strehl ratio is desirable, as this means that there is less Mie scattering. IOLs with low Strehl ratios (secondary to SSNGs) are more likely to cause subjective degradation of visual acuity, leading to the classic "20/unhappy" patient. While tempting, a YAG capsulotomy will not improve visual quality in these situations as the cause for decreased visual acuity lies in the IOL itself, not in the posterior capsule.

Geometric Scattering

Geometric scattering occurs when incoming light encounters much larger particles than the incoming light waves. A commonly seen example is a rainbow (or maybe even, wow, a double rainbow!) because when light encounters water molecules (which are larger than incoming light waves), scattering that happens during refraction and reflection accounts for the breakdown of incoming light into colors of the rainbow.

Diffraction

We briefly introduced the concept of diffraction in Chap. 1, Geometric Optics, but will explore it further here. When light waves encounter an opening or barrier in their path of movement, there is a subsequent change in direction as light waves seek alternative paths of movement. Seemingly, light appears to find a way to bend around corners – what is happening, as you might have guessed by now, is that incoming light photons are engaging in various shenanigans with electrons at the edge of the material.

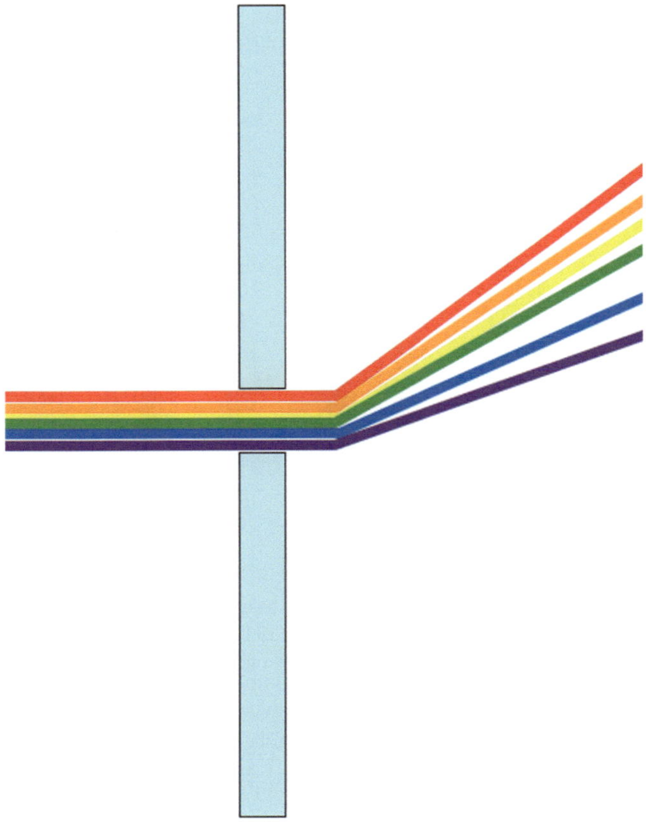

Fig. 17 Diffraction can be seen when a light wave passes through an aperture. Longer wavelengths (red) will undergo more diffraction than shorter wavelengths (blue)

This change in direction is known as **diffraction**. The *amount of diffraction increases* with *longer wavelengths (red)* and *decreases* with *shorter wavelengths (blue)* (Fig. 17). If the wavelength of waves is smaller than the obstacle, then no noticeable diffraction will occur. Note that *this is the opposite of refraction*, wherein shorter wavelengths (blue) are bent much more than longer wavelengths (red).

Diffraction will occur whenever light passes through an opening, such as the pupil. Recall that the *Airy disk phenomenon* describes the best-focused spot of light that a perfect lens with a circular aperture can make. When light passes through any aperture, diffraction will cause a pattern that looks like a target, a bright central region with a series of concentric rings of decreasing intensity (dimmer rings) around it. A larger aperture will create a smaller Airy disk pattern, whereas a smaller aperture will create a larger Airy disk pattern (Fig. 18).

Fig. 18 Diffraction increases as the aperture size decreases. The Airy disk pattern will be larger and have a noticeably brighter central region as it passes through a smaller aperture (as compared to a larger aperture)

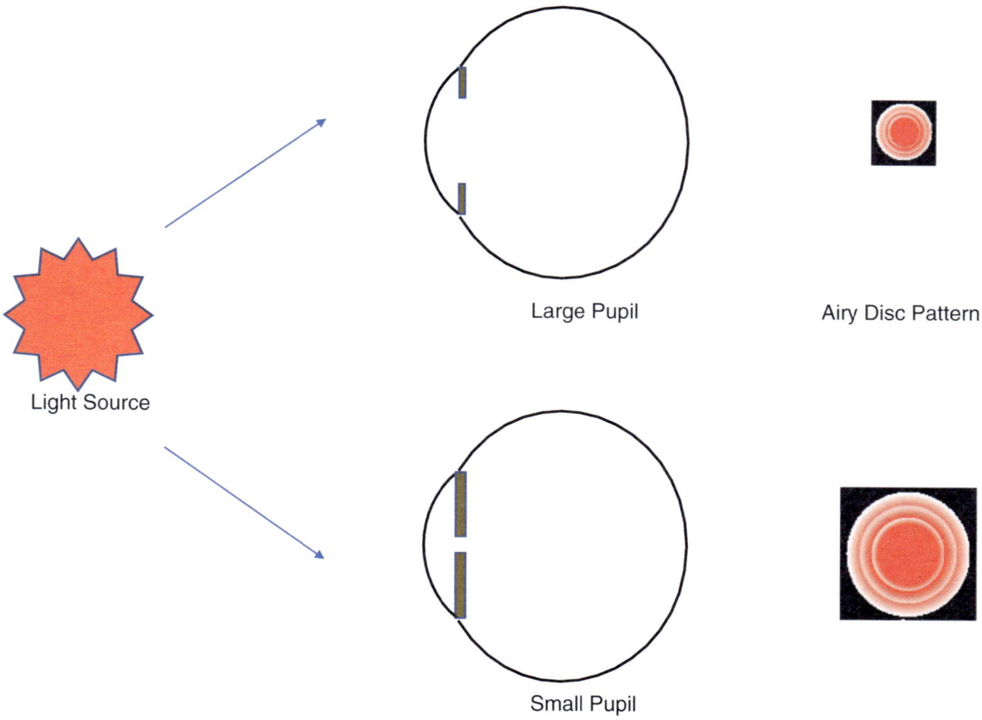

Furthermore, longer wavelengths (red) will create larger Airy disk patterns compared to shorter wavelengths. The size of the Airy disk (Θ_o) can be calculated using the equation[15]:

$$\Theta_o \approx 1.22 * (\lambda / D)$$

In this equation, λ is the wavelength, and D is the size of the circular aperture. Therefore, the *brightest Airy disk pattern* will be produced by *longer wavelengths of light* that pass through a *very small aperture*. As Airy disk patterns from different points of an object of interest are formed, they may begin to overlap, causing constructive interference to reduce contrast and eventually becoming indistinguishable from each other.

For example, if we consider light that passes through the pupil (a circular aperture), light at the edge of the pupil will get diffracted much more than light at the center of the pupil. If we make the pupil smaller, we can increase the theoretical number of paraxial rays that can reach the fovea, but the final visual acuity will be limited by diffraction. If we make the pupil bigger, the final visual acuity will be limited by higher-order aberrations, predominantly spherical aberration (discussed in the next section). When the aperture is extremely small, recall that longer wavelengths (red) of light will get diffracted in a higher ratio than in a larger opening. Essentially, there must be a compromise in the size of the opening to maximize the number of paraxial rays that strike the retina while minimizing the deleterious effects of both diffraction and spherical aberration.

We can now discuss three common scenarios where the principle of diffraction may be evident.

Optical Corona

An optical corona (not the virus!) may be seen due to the diffraction of sunlight or moonlight by small water droplets in the atmosphere (similar to scattering) that creates a concentric pattern of rings around the object (e.g., moon) with a bright central area (aureole). The aureole may appear to have a circular rainbow appearance, with a blue-white center and red-brown peripheral edge – confirming our previous discussions about longer wavelengths of light undergoing more diffraction. A similar phenomenon known as "rainbow glory (morning glory)" may also be seen in the atmosphere. The glory is caused by multiple optical properties (such as internal refraction, wave tunneling, etc.), including diffraction. The next time you are on a plane during a daytime flight, you may be able to see the corona if the sun is above and behind the plane and you look down at the clouds – you can consider this if the in-flight movie selection is extremely boring.

Pinhole Testing

In clinical practice, we often employ the pinhole test to measure a patient's potential visual acuity. When the patient looks through this 1.2-mm hole, we have maximized the number of undeviated paraxial light rays that strike the retina

[15] This is a simplified form of the classic Airy disk diameter equation, $\Theta_o \approx 2.44\lambda*(f/D)$, previously given in Chap. 1, where D is the exit pupil diameter and *f is the focal length*. The classic equation requires more math so we can use the simplified one to illustrate learning points from the text.

while limiting negative effects of diffraction (perceived as blur by the subject). If we made the pinhole any smaller, then adverse effects of diffraction would outweigh the increased number of paraxial light rays. Therefore, we can say that at a 1.2-mm-sized opening, we have an increased *depth of focus* and limited negative effects of diffraction. Recall that pinhole testing can correct up to 3D of refractive error if due to corneal or lenticular pathology but may reduce the visual acuity if the refractive error is due to retinal pathology.

Diffractive Multifocal IOLs

Diffractive multifocal intraocular lenses (DMFIOLs) and all diffractive-optics advanced technology (presbyopia-correcting) IOLs, such as diffractive-optics extended depth of focus IOLs and trifocal IOLs, take advantage of diffraction to enhance near and intermediate vision. When light waves encounter microscopic steps (diffractive zones) on a DMFIOL optic, parts of the incoming light wave will slow down, change direction, and instead be directed toward distant and near focal points. The *height* of the step will determine which focal point the incoming light will be directed toward. If the step height is the *same wavelength* as the incoming light, all incoming light will be directed to the *near focal point*. If the step height is a *smaller fraction of the wavelength*, it will direct more light toward the *distance focal point*. Therefore, DMFIOLs use a combination of varying step heights to split incoming light towards the distance, intermediate, or near focal points. We will discuss more about this technology in Chap. 27, "What's on the Menu: Overview of Currently Available IOLs"

Optical Aberrations

Note that throughout this section, we will flip between referring to light as rays and waves because some concepts are easily understood using Geometric Optics and other concepts using the Wave Theory of Light.

The human eye is an "imperfectly perfect" system. When a ray (or wave) of light goes into the eye, it will undergo distortion by the cornea and the crystalline lens; therefore, it cannot cannot be focused at a single point on the retina. Some of these distortions are actually quite helpful, as they may increase depth of focus and depth perception. Other distortions may degrade subjective visual acuity and can only be measured using special imaging devices. Several definitions are important to know before we continue our discussion.

Wavefronts and Aberrations

Light emanating from a real object will pass through an aperture (such as the pupil) and not focus in a perfect circle; instead, this light will form an irregularly shaped blob with some areas brighter than others. This "blob" is known as the **point spread function (PSF)**; in other words, the PSF describes the quality of the image: how light from a single point in the object will "spread" out as it forms the image. Therefore, every image we see is a combination of various PSFs from a given object that form the image.

Paraxial light rays will create relatively small PSFs; however, "peripheral" light rays will not focus stigmatically. These peripheral rays will cast large PSFs – it is these troublemaker light rays that cause most optical aberrations. However, nonparaxial light rays also contribute to image brightness and depth of focus.

A **wavefront** is a term used to describe the physical transmission or propagation of a ray of light. In other words, a wavefront is what happens to light as it gets affected by components of an optical system (such as the cornea and the crystalline lens). Wavefront analysis can be used to measure parallel light waves that enter the eye and undergo distortions creating **aberrations**. An aberration is a term used to describe distortions and deviations of light waves from an ideal wavefront pattern. Ideally, we would want the "shape" of the light going into the eye to equal the "shape" of the light that comes out of the eye, but this (almost) never happens because of aberrations.

We can use an analogy to reinforce this concept further: imagine that light rays emanating from an object toward the eye are like Black Friday shoppers departing from the same location and headed for the same store (the reference sphere of the eye) that is giving away 80″ high-definition TVs for the first ten shoppers. Some of these shoppers are faster than others; others are able to squeeze into the store through side doors, etc. The *geometric wavefront* is a snapshot of **where** all these shoppers are when the fastest shopper enters the store; the *wavefront aberration* of each shopper (light wave) is **the time** at which each subsequent shopper enters the store (reference sphere) as compared to the first shopper (who got the big TV).

A wavefront, therefore, captures light rays that pass through an optical system at a given time (this is known as isochronic, or equal-time, surface). In an ideal optical system, every point of light from an object would come into focus at the same location on the retina. We could place an artificial sphere (known as the reference sphere) anywhere in the optical system to show the uniformity of light. However, as discussed above when introducing the PSF, this is not the case: light is unruly, and incoming light, like Black Friday shoppers, does not pass through the optical system in a single-file, orderly fashion. The wavefront is more useful because it shows where all the "behaving" and "not-behaving" light (aka aberrations) is at a given point in time when compared to the reference sphere. Therefore, the wavefront is an irregularly shaped smooth surface that shows these aberrations.

We can divide our discussion of optical aberrations into two main categories: lower-order aberrations (LOAs) and higher-order aberrations (HOAs). A combination of LOAs and HOAs is usually present in any given eye, and these can be further subclassified into distinct entities. We can use a *Zernike polynomial* (a mathematical equation) to describe and visualize wavefront aberrations (usually arranged in a hierarchical pyramid shape). The more significant aberrations are visually represented at the base of the pyramid, and the less significant aberrations are at the peak of the pyramid (Fig. 19). Zernike reconstruction involves using about 36 data points to generate a wavefront pattern. More recently, Fourier reconstruction is another strategy to analyze data from any shaped pupil and provides more information to treat irregularly shaped corneas using about 240 data points.

Even though over 65 total aberrations (up to the eighth order) have been identified, the human eye can only perceive distortion effects from optical aberrations only up to the fifth or sixth order. We will limit our discussion up to the fourth-order aberrations.

At this point, dear reader, you may be wondering why we care about all this terminology. This is one area of Ophthalmic Optics wherein significant recent developments have occurred. More will undoubtedly occur in the near future, especially regarding cataract and refractive surgery. For example, understanding a wavefront will help one appreciate the significance and differences between wavefront-guided and wavefront-optimized excimer laser ablation strategies. These topics will be discussed in greater detail in Chap. 30, Optics for Refractive Surgery.

We can measure aberrations using **aberrometry**. Aberrometry measures distortions that a wavefront of light undergoes as it passes through the cornea and the crystalline lens. The most common method of aberrometry, Hartmann-Shack aberrometry (HSA), involves using a device (aberrometer) that can send a monochromatic beam of light into the eye (Fig. 20). After this light passes through the cornea and the lens, it will reach the retina and be reflected back toward the aberrometer. This reflected light from different

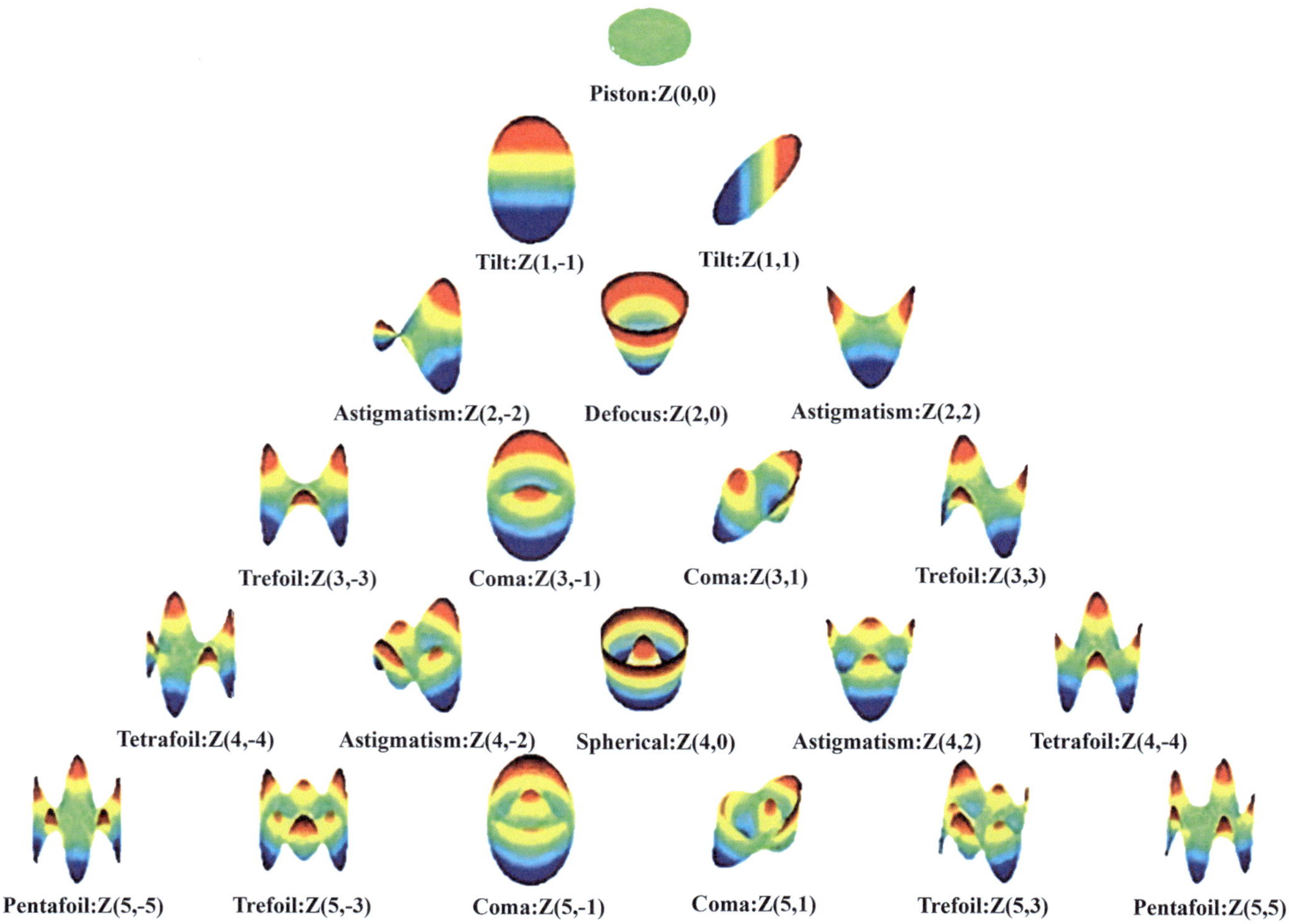

Fig. 19 Classification of lower-order aberrations (LOAs) and higher-order aberrations (HOAs). LOAs are located toward the top of the pyramid, and HOAs are located toward the base of the pyramid. LOAs can be corrected with manifest refraction. HOAs can only be measured by wavefront aberrometry

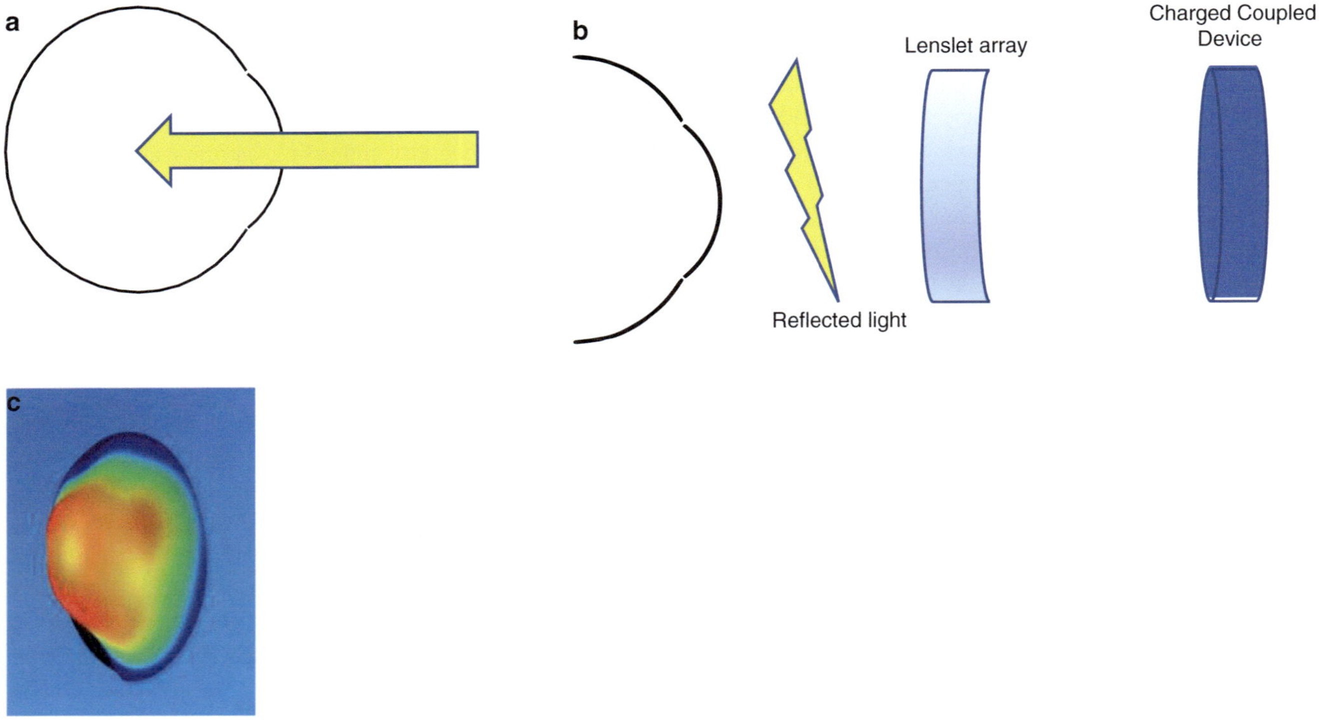

Fig. 20 Aberrometry involves generating a wavefront analysis of the eye's optical system to measure both lower-order aberrations (LOAs) and higher-order aberrations (HOAs). A monochromatic beam of light goes into the eye (panel A), which is reflected back toward a lenslet array in the aberrometer and then onto a charged coupled device (CCD) (panel B). These data are compared to data from an ideal optical pathway and used to map out LOAs and HOAs (panel C)

points of the optical path is captured by a lenslet array and then onto a charged coupled device (CCD). The computer in the aberrometer uses the CCD data and compares them to an ideal optical pathway; resulting differences (known as the optical path difference, or OPD) are then used to map out both LOAs and HOAs visually. In other words, we are looking at how the light sent into the eye differs from an ideal light path – these differences are LOAs and HOAs. One limitation of HSA is that because it measures reflected light, we can only measure "reverse" aberrations as a proxy for the "forward" aberrations happening to light waves going into the eye. A helpful analogy is to think that we are measuring the shadow of a tree to measure the height of the tree: the height of the shadow may vary depending on the sunlight (based on the time of day), so this method has some limitations in its accuracy.

While manifest refraction can describe the sphere and cylinder (LOA) present in the eye, it cannot measure HOAs in the total optical system as a wavefront aberrometry can. Aberrometry allows us to measure both refractive errors (such as myopia, hyperopia, and regular astigmatism) and the decreased vision quality due to HOAs. The term "aberropia" is a portmanteau that is rapidly gaining popularity for describing this combination of objective and subjective refractive errors.

Ray-tracing aberrometry (RTA) is another method of measuring optical aberrations that differs from Hartmann-Shack – in this method, ray tracing is used to measure "forward" light rays sent into the eye (rather than reflected) to calculate LOAs and HOAs. These aberrations can be quantified (in microns) and graphed visually to give the examiner an appreciation for the LOAs and HOAs present in the patient's eye. RTA can also simulate how a letter will appear to the patient and show PSF values and a refractive map at various points on the cornea.

Aberrometry (both HSA and RTA) has a variety of uses in clinical practice, including but not limited to pre-refractive surgery assessment of candidates for laser refractive surgery; assessment of LOA/HOA due to the cornea vs. the lens; pre-cataract surgery assessment of candidates for advanced technology intraocular lenses; and postsurgical assessment of unhappy patients after refractive and/or cataract surgery.

Lower-Order Aberrations

As discussed previously, lower-order aberrations (LOAs) are commonly encountered refractive errors seen in clinical practice, such as sphere and regular astigmatism (cylinder, including axis). These refractive errors can be easily detected on manifest refraction and can be adequately corrected with glasses and soft/toric contact lenses.

Higher-Order Aberrations

Higher-order aberrations (HOAs) cannot be measured during manifest refraction. HOAs may contribute up to 20% of a patient's subjective refractive error and can be a significant cause of the "20/unhappy" patients – these are patients that objectively may correct to ≥20/25, especially after cataract/refractive surgery, yet are bitterly unhappy with their vision. An inexperienced practitioner may be at a loss (or frustrated!) in dealing with these patients and addressing their complaints.

In the previous section, we discussed how optical aberrations occur due to the deviation of light as it passes through the eye. Patients will usually not report to the examiner: "I am experiencing a higher-order aberration." Instead, patients may describe HOAs as a combination of glare, halos, starbursts, and ghosting that contribute to subjective complaints of poor vision. Most HOAs comes from the anterior corneal surface and the lens; a small, clinically insignificant amount may come from the posterior corneal surface (and even the retina).

Risk factors for HOAs include but are not limited to, corneal disease (scars, Salzmann nodules, etc.), large pupil size, lenticular opacities, increased age, and post-refractive surgery, especially if done with conventional ablations (i.e., excluding wavefront-guided and wavefront-optimized ablations).

While there are many HOAs, we will focus our discussion on the three most important ones: spherical aberration, coma, and trefoil.

Spherical Aberration

Spherical aberration (SA) is the most important of the three HOAs that one must know about as it has significant implications on clinical and surgical practice.

When light rays pass through the cornea and the lens, they are not passing through spherical surfaces; in fact, they are passing through four refractive surfaces (anterior/posterior cornea and anterior/posterior crystalline lens). Recall that both the cornea and the lens are aspherical surfaces: there is different curvature at the periphery compared to the center. As a result, peripheral light rays are refracted (bent) more strongly than paraxial rays. They will thus come into focus slightly closer, that is, in front of the retina compared to their paraxial friends (Fig. 21).

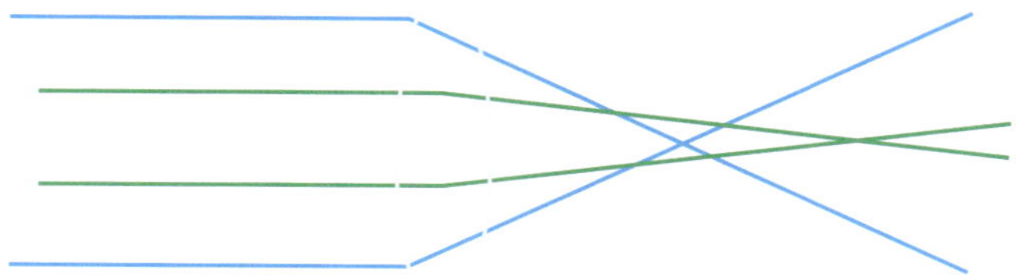

Fig. 21 Spherical aberration – peripheral light rays (blue) will be refracted more than paraxial light rays (green). Increased pupil size will increase the amount of spherical aberration noticed by the patient. A patient may report this as glare and halos, especially in mesopic and scotopic light conditions

Advantages and Disadvantages of Spherical Aberration

The most significant advantage of SA is that since incoming light rays land at different locations (either anterior to, directly on, or even slightly posterior to the retina), SA confers increased *depth of field* and helps with *stereo-depth perception*. Thus, having a small amount of "Goldilocks" SA may confer some benefits.[16]

However, drawbacks of SA are many, including, but not limited to:

- Night myopia – More peripheral light rays will fall in front of the retina in an otherwise emmetropic patient because of increased pupil size in low light conditions. Such patients, especially those with light-colored irises, may experience up to −0.50D myopia and may require spectacle correction, especially in low-light conditions (such as long periods of driving on dimly lit roads at nighttime).[17]
- Point image halos and glare – in addition to the night myopia, patients may subjectively experience increased spherical aberration as glare and halos, significantly worse in low-light conditions.
- Decreased contrast sensitivity – this is perhaps the biggest reason why spherical IOLs (discussed below) are not commonly used in surgical practice today. Increased spherical aberration will inversely affect contrast sensitivity[18]; while the objective vision may still be good, the subjective visual quality in a patient without significant spherical aberration will be much higher than the subjective visual acuity in a patient with significant spherical aberration. Furthermore, a patient with pre-existing mild-moderate glaucoma who undergoes cataract surgery with

[16] For the sake of thoroughness, this last point is also controversial. Some experts argue that SA, by definition is an "aberration", and degrades the image. Whatever increased depth of focus conferred by SA is lost when focusing at near due to pupil constriction (which will eliminate peripheral rays and only allow in paraxial rays). It is beyond the scope of this text to settle this debate, and this point has been introduced as a footnote merely for the sake of presenting a sampling of this debate. Interested readers are encouraged to consult other sources for more information.

[17] See Chap. 21, Clinical Problems with Optics and Refractive Manifestations, for more information on this topic.

[18] Piers PA, Manzanera S, Prieto PM, Gorceix N, Artal P. Use of adaptive optics to determine the optimal ocular spherical aberration. J Cataract Refract Surg. 2007 Oct;33(10):1721–6

a spherical IOL may test falsely worse on postoperative visual field testing due to the loss in contrast sensitivity.

On wavefront imaging, spherical aberration gives the shape of a grapefruit/orange squeezer device (Fig. 22). This image represents how peripheral light rays will come into focus before central light rays.

Patients may perceive spherical aberration as star-shaped glare or halos around point sources of light (Fig. 23).

Positive Vs. Negative Spherical Aberration

Positive spherical aberration means that more peripheral light rays are refracted and come into focus in front of the retina as compared to paraxial light rays, causing a myopic shift; this is

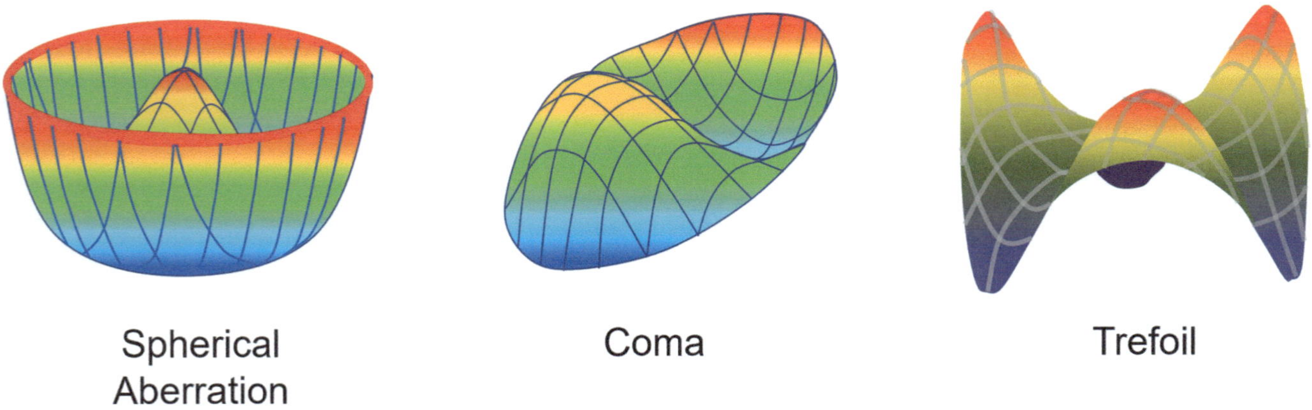

Fig. 22 Visual representation of the three most common higher-order aberrations: spherical aberration, coma, and trefoil

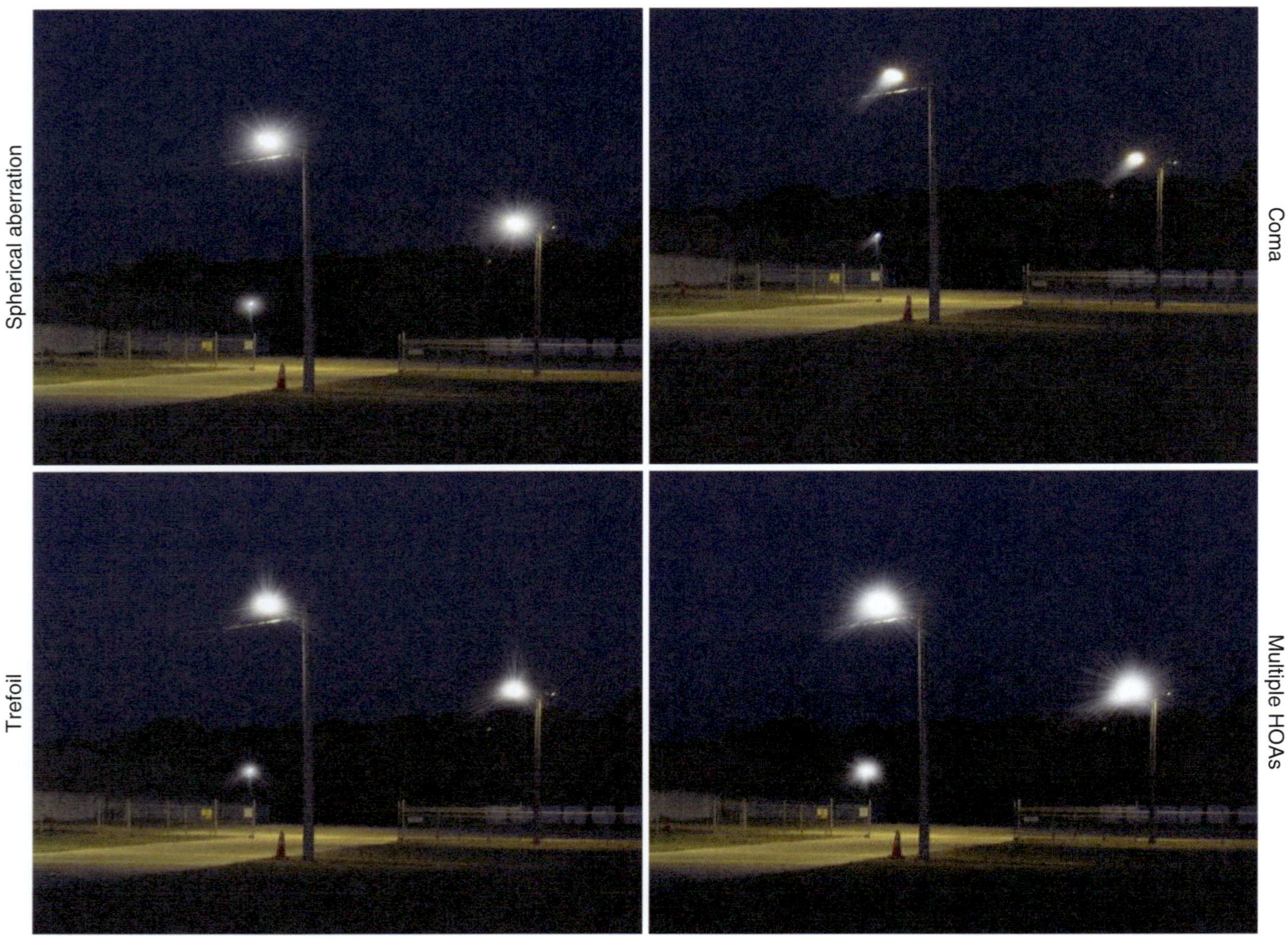

Fig. 23 Patient perception of spherical aberration, coma, and trefoil. Frequently, multiple HOAs are present, leading to a combination of visual distortions (image credit, https://lasikcomplications.com/hoa.htm)

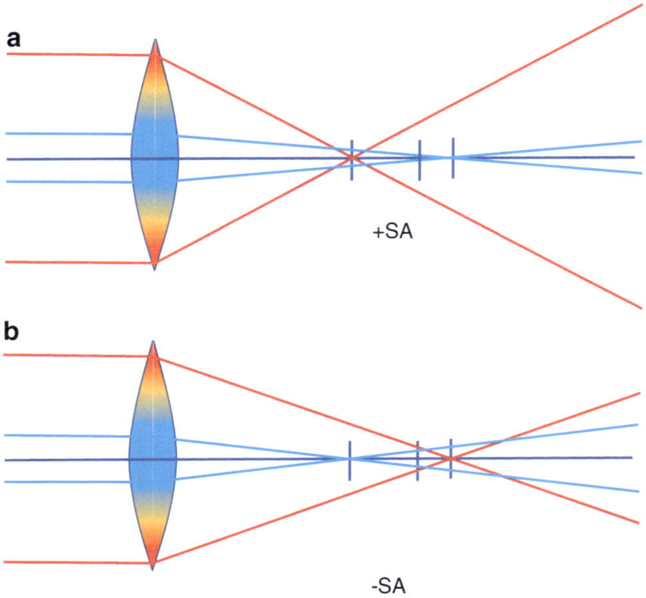

Fig. 24 Positive vs. negative spherical aberration. In positive spherical aberration (panel A), peripheral light rays (red) will focus anterior to paraxial rays (blue), as seen in myopic eyes. In negative spherical aberration (panel B), peripheral light rays (red) will focus posterior to paraxial rays (blue), as seen in hyperopic eyes

expressed in microns (Fig. 24). *Negative spherical aberration* is the opposite of the above and will cause a hyperopic shift in refraction. SA is very much dependent on pupil size: more positive SA is present in the eye when pupil size increases. Furthermore, refractive error may compensate for SA at larger pupil sizes but may introduce defocus at smaller pupil sizes. For example, a large pupil size (e.g., 6 mm may introduce +0.17 to +0.27 μm of SA) that may be neutralized with minimal myopia (-0.25 D) in pseudophakic patients. This may seem counterintuitive, but in such patients, the central part of the pupillary aperture is slightly hyperopic (relative to the peripheral pupil), balancing mild myopia. Nonetheless, minimizing SA will always yield the best quality of vision. Finally, to further complicate this (confusing) discussion, some authors have proposed that a small amount of negative SA in pseudophakic patients may be desirable as this may increase near vision - in such patients, there is more central power than peripheral, and activation of the synkinetic reflex (convergence, accommodation, and pupillary miosis) during near-vision tasks may make reading-distance letter clearer.

The cornea has positive SA, and the crystalline lens has negative SA. The net result is that *normal eyes* (especially *myopic eyes* much more than hyperopic eyes) usually contain a *low amount of positive SA*. The total SA is lowest in our teenage years, with nearly zero SA at age 19 as the positive SA of the cornea is nearly neutralized by the negative SA of the lens.[19]

This observation is admittedly a generalization because SA itself is not a static figure: not only does it change with age but it changes even with pupil size and accommodation. For example, low-light conditions that increase pupil size will increase positive SA; however, accommodation by the crystalline lens will induce additional negative SA power (approximately −0.05 μm per 1D accommodation). Thus, SA can range from slightly positive (e.g., when focusing at a distance target in low-light conditions) to slightly negative (e.g., when focusing on a near target in bright-light conditions). The mean net value for spherical aberration in an average population is approximately +0.27–0.36 μm (SD = 0.31).[20]

Recently, SA has gained attention in topics such as myopia control. Some experts have suggested that intentionally increasing positive SA may help bring *even more* peripheral light rays anterior to the retina to reduce image focus posterior to the retina ("hyperopic defocus) and subsequently slow down axial length increase and myopia progression in young patients. This topic merits additional discussion, as we will see in Chap. 24, Myopia Control.

As we age, the net positive spherical aberration increases: we typically develop more positive SA in the cornea, but at the same time, as the crystalline lens undergoes cataract formation, its SA changes from negative to positive as well. This explains why some of the more popular aspheric IOLs have negative spherical aberration built into the IOL to "restore" some of the negative SA present in the natural lens.[21]

Corneal Vs. Lenticular Spherical Aberration

While it seems redundant, we will repeat this for emphasis: the cornea has positive SA, and the crystalline lens has negative SA. However, as the eye accommodates for near targets, the lenticular SA becomes even more negative; with sufficient accommodation, there is so much negative lenticular SA that it reverses the eye's SA from positive to negative. Some authorities propose that having negative SA in pseudophakic presbyopic patients may help with near tasks as the postoperative negative SA may help with reading vision.

Spherical Aberration and Laser Refractive Surgery

At this point, we can address a commonly asked question: *what happens to SA values of patients who undergo laser refractive surgery*? The answer is that it depends on *what kind* of laser refractive surgery was done:

[19]See (1) Guirao A, Gonzales C, Redondo M, et al. Average performance of the human eye as a function of age in the normal population. *Invest Ophthalmol & Vis Science*. 1999;40: 203–213; and (2) Glasser A, Campbell MCW. Presbyopia and the optical changes in the human crystalline lens with age. *Vision Res*. 1998;38: 209–229.

[20]Racial demographics of a given population may influence the average spherical aberration as race and ethnicity have shown to be factors positively correlated to spherical aberration. The full extent of this variation is beyond the scope of this text.

[21]See Chap. 27 What's on the Menu: An Overview of Currently Available IOLs and Relevant Optics, for more discussion on this topic.

- Patients who undergo **standard (i.e., not wavefront-guided or wavefront-optimized)** ablations for *myopia* will develop an oblate corneal pattern. In the early days of laser refractive surgery (LRS), nearly all the treatment was limited to the central cornea (usually a 6.5 mm optical zone), and the peripheral cornea was left untouched. Thus, the post-myopic LRS cornea would show *central flattening* with a relatively *steep untreated peripheral cornea*. These patients' postsurgical wavefronts will show a significant *increase* in positive SA, even more than prior to LRS. A typical wavefront pattern for these patients may demonstrate emmetropia centrally (green) with "annular myopia" in the periphery (red).[22]
- Patients who undergo **standard** ablations for *hyperopia* will develop a more prolate corneal pattern (steeper centrally). Nearly all the treatment is directed toward the peripheral cornea (to flatten it) and creates secondary central corneal steepening. These patients' postsurgical wavefronts will show a significant *decrease in SA* (they may even have net negative SA due to the crystalline lens' negative SA "overpowering" the weakly positive corneal SA), and the wavefront shape pattern may become inverted.

Increased positive SA after LRS may lead to an unhappy patient, especially in a patient with large scotopic pupil size or a patient who needs good distance vision in low-light conditions (such as a long-distance trucker, etc.). These patients may have increased (and sometimes unbearable) glare and halos due to increased SA after LRS.

Spherical Aberration and IOL Options

As we have discussed (almost nauseatingly!), one potential advantage of SA is the increased depth of focus: but does this advantage outweigh the previously mentioned disadvantages?

We will discuss spherical vs. aspheric IOLs in greater detail in Chap. 27, What's on the Menu: An Overview of Currently Available IOLs and Relevant Optics. For now, we can summarize spherical IOLs as basically cylinder slices of a sphere: they have the same power throughout the entire optic of the IOL and actually have some positive SA themselves. Thus, patients who receive spherical IOLs will have an increased positive SA after cataract surgery that will function as a poor man's presbyopia-correcting IOL. Patients will not only see well at distance, but the increased depth of focus may theoretically confer some additional near vision without the need for reading glasses.

So why do not we use spherical IOLs and use benefits of SA to our advantage? The problem is that this depth of focus itself is a "blurred" depth of focus; it is not as sharp or clear as a singularly focused spot of light. Remember SA is an "aberration," not an "improvement." Furthermore, pupillary constriction may eliminate potentially beneficial peripheral light rays when a pseudophakic patient wants to read. Finally, studies have shown that *negative* SA may be more beneficial to pseudophakic patients: when the patient focuses at near, the synkinetic reflex increases the plus power of the eye and makes near objects sharper when the pupil constricts.[23]

Suppose we had two identical twins who underwent cataract surgery. One twin was left with +0.2 µm SA, and the other had −0.2 µm SA. Both patients may have a halo from the SA, but the twin with negative SA may be slightly happier: when he wants to read, the pupil will constrict, and the negative SA means that he has more power in the center and can potentially read better. This comparison has clinical relevance before cataract surgery too: a phakic post-hyperopic LRS patient may be happier at age 60 as compared to a phakic post-myopic LRS patient because the former's negative SA may allow her to read at close better than the latter's positive SA.

To confuse you further, the previous paragraph can be argued with a counterpoint: other studies have shown that pseudophakic patients with mild myopia (approximately −0.25 to −0.50D myopia) may have better uncorrected vision (as measured by contrast sensitivity function and macular threshold studies) if they have some *positive* SA.[24] However, this assumes the patient is *not wearing* any prescription glasses. If the patient's myopia is corrected, zero SA will yield the best quality of vision. Thus, there may be some benefit in leaving behind a small amount of pseudophakic positive SA in a patient who is −0.50D in both eyes and receives monofocal IOLs. However, for patients who wish to wear glasses or receive presbyopia-correcting IOLs and desire the sharpest vision possible, the surgeon's goal should be to correct all the refractive error and leave the SA as close to zero as possible.

We hope that we have not overwhelmed you with this deluge of information. We should appreciate how incredibly complex this entire discussion is and how we are still scratching the surface in understanding this topic.

Spherical Aberration and Q-Value

At this juncture, we can introduce a somewhat abstruse concept that confuses many people, including practicing ophthalmologists: Q-value. It is important to note that corneal

[22]See Fig. 1 in Chap. 30, Optics for Refractive Surgery, for a topography image of a post-myopic LRS cornea.

[23]Piers PA, Manzanera S, Prieto PM, Gorceix N, Artal P. Use of adaptive optics to determine the optimal ocular spherical aberration. J Cataract Refract Surg. 2007 Oct;33(10):1721–6

[24]Holladay JT. "Spherical Aberration: The Next Frontier". Cataract and Refractive Surgery Today, November 2006. https://crstoday.com/articles/2006-nov/crst1106_18-php/. Accessed January 10, 2021

SA and Q-value are **not the same thing**. They are related, but they are also different. Whereas **SA** measures the effect of the optical system on incoming light and is **measured in microns (as a root-mean-square, RMS)**, the **Q-value** describes and measures *the shape* of the refractive surface of the eye – most notably, the Q-value **has no units**. Even though they are *not* the same thing, it is helpful to discuss them side-by-side.

We can think of the Q-value as a way to describe how corneal shape can help to neutralize SA. The Q-value gives us information about how much the cornea is flattened in the periphery compared to its center. A Q-value = 0 will indicate a perfectly spherical surface, which does not exist in nature. A negative Q-value helps to offset some of the corneal SA. Since we have stated that most corneas are prolate with positive SA values, most patients (especially myopic patients) will have corneas with $Q < 1$. As can be deduced, $Q > 1$ is typically seen in oblate corneas. The Q-value varies among ethnic populations, ranging from −0.20 to −0.27 overall.

We can reinforce this with an example. If we have two Q-values (e.g., one cornea with a Q-value of −0.45 and another with −0.25), we can say that the lower (more negative) Q-value will describe a more prolate cornea. The Q-value is further defined as the best-fit ellipsoid shape to describe an apical ratio of change. Therefore, different corneal curvatures can produce different amounts of SA but still have the same Q-value. In other words, Q-value gives us information about the *form* of the corneal shape, but the spherical aberration gives us information about the *function* of the corneal shape.

Studies have shown that there is no "perfect" Q-value: there is no relationship between the shape of the cornea and the eventual best-corrected visual acuity (BCVA). Similarly, other studies have shown that maintaining a constant Q-value before and after laser refractive surgery, has no significant outcomes on a patient's BCVA or even other measures of visual acuity, such as contrast sensitivity.[25]

Thus far, we have stated that the ideal refractive surface will have no imperfections (Q-value = 0). Since the cornea is imperfectly perfect, the average human cornea has a Q-value of ≈ −0.26. This is where things get confusing: to correct the corneal SA, we would actually need a − 0.52 Q-value.[26] Amazingly, the crystalline lens has a Q-value of −0.25, which, when combined with the corneal Q-value, results in the neutralization of most of this SA. When we remove the crystalline lens in cataract surgery, we are now left with additional positive SA. Hence, some IOL manufacturers add additional "negative" SA to their aspheric IOLs to neutralize the (positive) corneal SA and yield better quality postoperative BCVA.

The Q-value may also be combined with keratometry to back-calculate (approximately) the SA of a given surface. All that fancy math is beyond the scope of this text, but if we took the average Q-value (−0.26) and average keratometry measurements (44.00D), the calculated corneal SA is approximately +0.18 μm. If we simply measured the corneal SA, this is approximately +0.27 μm. Most currently-utilized aspheric IOLs have about −0.18 to −0.27-μm SA built into the IOL.

Coma

This HOA occurs due to rays that pass through one edge of the pupil coming into focus before or after rays at the opposite edge (180 degrees away) of the pupil. Coma leads to a variation in image magnification. Patients may also perceive this as a "comet-like tail" emanating from a point source of light in low-light conditions. This HOA is common in decentered corneas, such as keratoconus (vertical coma due to asymmetry between the inferior and the superior cornea), irregular penetrating keratoplasty, and decentered ablations. On wavefront imaging, coma gives the shape of a baseball cap (Fig. 22). This figure represents how light rays at one edge of the optical system will come into focus before light rays at the opposite edge – imagine that some Black Friday shoppers have entered through the one side of the department store, while shoppers on the other side are still stuck behind the closed doors.

The cornea and lens both have coma; as you might have guessed, they both have opposite-signed values of coma. This allows the eye to maintain a good quality of vision despite the "misalignment" of its optical elements – remember the human eye is imperfectly perfect.

Trefoil

This HOA occurs due to incoming light that gets "smeared" in three directions. For example, both corneal opacities (corneal scars, Salzmann nodules, and epithelial basement dystrophy) and lenticular opacities (vacuoles) can smear incoming light. Patients may perceive this as a "peace-sign/Mercedes-Benz®" symbol emanating from a point source of light in low-light conditions. On wavefront imaging, trefoil gives the shape of a "tricorne hat" or "three-person saddle" (Fig. 22). Imagine a Colonial American-style hat (kind of) or a saddle upon which three people are sitting but facing three different directions. (Sorry, we couldn't come up with anything more clever than this!).

Spectral Sensitivity and Visual Pigments

While many animals can perceive extreme ends of the electromagnetic (EM) spectrum (including ultraviolet and infrared), the human eye can only perceive a small portion of the

[25] Tuan KM, Chernyak D. Corneal asphericity and visual function after wavefront-guided LASIK. Optom Vis Sci. 2006 Aug;83(8):605–10

[26] Ironically enough, at Q-values lower than −0.50 are clues that the patient may have a corneal ectasia present; usually, these corneas have Q-values around −1 or less.

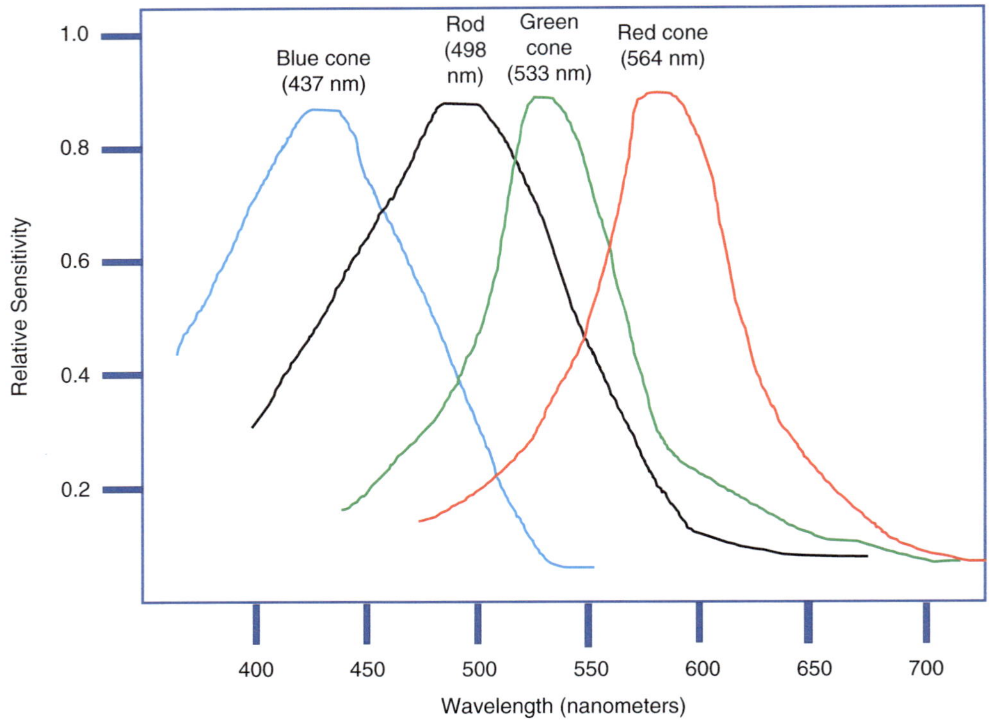

Fig. 25 Spectral sensitivity for rods and cones. Note that spectral sensitivities for each photoreceptor are curves. For example, a red cone will be stimulated by blue light (490 nm) but to a much lesser degree than a rod

EM spectrum from approximately 300–700 nm. The two main types of photoreceptor cells, rods and cones, have peak sensitivities to different portions of the EM spectrum. Note that these are curves: for example, at 500 nm, cones will still undergo some stimulation even though rods will undergo much more stimulation (Fig. 25).

Cones themselves can be further divided into three types, each with own peak range of sensitivity (Fig. 25):

- Red cones (560 nm) – technically peak at the yellow portion of the EM spectrum.
- Green cones (530 nm).
- Blue cones (420–40 nm) – technically peak at the violet portion of the EM spectrum.

The clinical relevance of these photoreceptors (and their respective peak sensitivities) can be seen in patients with color deficiency. Color deficiency is prevalent in the general population, affecting approximately 5–12% of male patients and 0.5% of female patients.[27] A *dichromat* is when a patient lacks one of the three cone systems. Dichromats can be further classified as follows:

- Protanopia (aka Daltonism) – these patients lack *red cones*. For these patients, red colors will have a black appearance.
- Deuteranopia – these patients lack *green cones*. For these patients, red and green colors will appear similar.
- Tritanopia – these patients lack *blue cones*. For these patients, blue objects will have a grayish appearance. Patients have an especially difficult time distinguishing darker shades of blue from black.

A silly (and possibly) useful mnemonic to remember these color deficiencies is as follows: "Protein (meat) is red; mountain deu is green; and the tritanic sank in the ocean (blue)" Red-green color vision defects are the most common forms of color vision deficiency.

We will discuss the diagnosis of color deficiency and deficits in Chap. 18, Visual Acuity Testing and Assessment, and the clinical management of these patients.

Lasers in Ophthalmology

You may be surprised to know that "LASER" stands for "light amplification by stimulated emission of radiation." We have been using "LASER" for so long that the acronym has become a word.

The physics of how lasers emit light is slightly complicated and beyond the scope of this particular text. We will give you a clue: it involves the same electrons and photons hooking up and breaking up. The interested reader is encouraged to consult other texts for this information.

For ophthalmologists, there are several properties of laser light are worth to memory:

- Laser light is *monochromatic*. All photons emitted by a laser have the same wavelength (color). As a result, there are negligible aberrations (spherical and chromatic) in laser light. Thus, the laser can be focused onto an extremely small spot down to the micron level.

[27] Source, https://ghr.nlm.nih.gov/condition/color-vision-deficiency#statistics. Accessed March 21, 2020

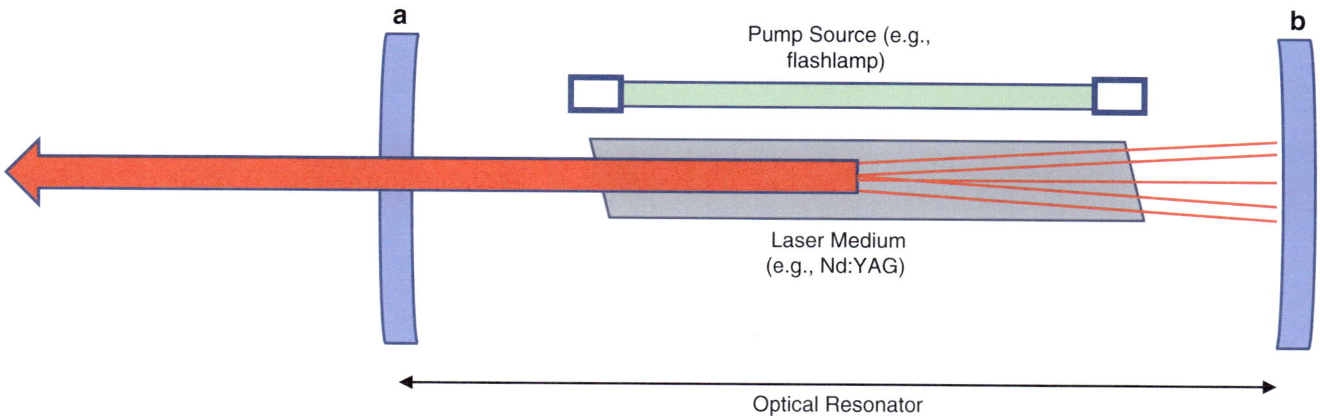

Fig. 26 A laser typically comprises three components: a pump source, gain medium, and optical resonator. As energy flows from the pump source into the gain medium, stimulated emission of photons occurs, leading to optical gain (amplification). Initially emitted photons will bounce hundreds to thousands of times between a highly reflective mirror (**b**) and a partially reflective mirror (**a**) before exiting the resonator toward the intended target

- Laser light is highly *coherent*. Photons emitted from a laser oscillate in the same direction simultaneously like a well-choreographed cheer routine (temporal coherence: "in phase"). As a result, laser light can produce an interference pattern – this causes the laser to "speckle" off irregular surfaces, such as ripples in a glass of water.
- Laser light is *highly directional* and can be polarized. This allows it to be emitted as an extremely narrow beam and targeted in a specific direction. This is very different from all other previous point sources of light that have negative vergence as light from these objects will emanate in all directions. In addition, even after its emission, laser light is *non-spreading* with minimal divergence per meter traveled. A laser beam will spread to less than 1-ft diameter at a distance from 1000 ft. from the laser; so even if a laser is sent from the earth to the moon (approximately 250,000 miles), it will only spread to cover an area of 2.5 miles on the surface of the moon (divergence angle = 5 rad). This minimal divergence allows a laser to deliver a large amount of energy to a small, targeted area even if it has to travel a considerable distance to reach it. Think of the Death Star (*Star Wars Episode IV: A New Hope*, 1977) and how a laser was able to destroy an entire planet from a far-off distance as the laser did not diverge much after being fired. Though we do not condone the destruction of Alderaan, we cannot fault the physics in the movie on this point - but don't get us started on the flawed physics of "laser" swords.
- Laser light can be *continuous* (such as an argon laser used for photocoagulation) or *pulsed* (such as a Nd/YAG laser). Pulsed lasers can be produced by two methods: *mode locking* and *Q-switching*. Again, we can skip some of the physics, but it is worthwhile to know that *mode locking* is the method used to create extremely short pulses, such as those used in femtosecond lasers (FSLs, 10^{-15} s).
- The power of a laser can be measured in watts or joules. A watt is 1 joule of energy delivered over 1 second. By decreasing the delivery time to less than a second (pulsing), we can significantly increase the power of the laser (i.e., increase the watts). For example, an FSL can deliver approximately 1 quadrillion watts!.[28]

A laser consists of three main components (Fig. 26):

- A pulsed power source to supply energy ("pump source") – This pump source provides energy to the system. Common pump sources include electrical discharges, chemical reactions, flashlamps, or light from another laser. For example, an Nd/YAG laser will usually use light from a xenon flashlamp or a diode laser; excimer lasers use a chemical reaction to provide energy. Lasers are *very inefficient* light sources: most of the energy used to power a laser is lost, and only a small amount of energy is emitted from the laser. Going back to our Death Star example, one Optics-nerd plot hole in the movie is that no explanation was given for where the energy was coming from to power the laser. We want answers.
- Gain medium ("laser medium") – the gain medium is the primary determining factor of the laser. Energy from the pump source flows into the gain medium to produce a population inversion, which is basically a complicated way of saying that most of the electrons in the medium are in higher-energy (excited) states than in lower-energy states. This will cause a spontaneous and stimulated emission of photons that will undergo optical gain (amplification) in the resonator. Examples of gain media include liquids, gasses (CO2, argon, krypton, and helium-neon),

[28]This author has often wondered what kind of pulsed technology and laser components were used by the Empire in the creation of the Death Star in order to deliver that much energy in such a short time that millions of voices suddenly cried out in terror and were suddenly silenced.

Table 1 Features of commonly used lasers in ophthalmology

Type of laser	Wavelength	Portion of electromagnetic spectrum
CO2	10,800 nm	Far infrared
Nd/YAG	1064 nm	Infrared
Krypton	677 nm	Red
Argon	488–514 nm	Blue-green
Excimer (Ar/Fl)	193 nm	Ultraviolet

and solids (such as crystals). Solid host materials, such as YAG (yttrium, aluminum, and garnet), are usually mixed with an impurity (neodymium).

- Optical resonator ("laser chamber") – the optical resonator is basically a chamber with two mirrors placed around the laser medium consisting of a highly reflective mirror and a partially reflective mirror. The light that has undergone stimulated emission will pass hundreds (or even thousands) of times between the two mirrors before exiting the partially reflective mirror toward the target of interest.

Uses of Lasers and Light Damage in Ophthalmology

We use many lasers in ophthalmology among various specialties that encompass a significant portion of the EM spectrum. A list of the most commonly used lasers is presented (Table 1).

It is worth nothing that FSLs have not been included in this list as they can be made from a variety of materials, such as Nd/glass and Nd/YAG, as the "base material." It is the *mode-locking* component that changes their destructively therapeutic abilities. Thus, while a typical Nd/YAG FSL uses a wavelength of 1053 nm (similar to the Nd/YAG laser, 1064 nm), the former can be used via plasma-induced ablation to "selectively destroy" target tissue, whereas the latter can be used via photodisruption to "forcefully destroy" tissue.[29] Thus, the FSL causes much lower collateral damage than the Nd/YAG laser – this allows us to use the FSL to create corneal flaps and incisions, which you *definitely* do not want to do with the Nd/YAG laser!

Ophthalmic lasers can affect tissue in five different ways:

1. **Photocoagulation** – photocoagulation involves lasers that use very short exposure times to produce highly powerful light energy absorbed by the tissue. This causes a *focal rise in temperature*, denaturation of proteins within tissues, and localized destruction (*scar formation*) of the tissue. Most of the laser energy is absorbed by **chromophores** (e.g., melanin, hemoglobin, xanthophyll, etc.) in tissues that convert the incoming light energy into heat and secondary destruction of surrounding tissue. These chromophores have to be activated by the appropriate type of incoming light. For example, argon blue-green (488–514 nm) and krypton yellow (568 nm) can be absorbed by hemoglobin. Xanthophyll preferentially absorbs 450–500 nm; thus, these wavelength lasers are used to treat macular disease. Finally, krypton red (647 nm) is *not* absorbed by hemoglobin, so it may be used in the presence of vitreous hemorrhage. Photocoagulation laser energy is usually measured in watts.
2. **Photodisruption** – photodisruption involves lasers that strike the target tissue and cause an acute *formation of plasma* (rapid ionization of molecules). This results in a shock wave and localized *mechanical disruption* of the target tissue. Because the laser does not need to be absorbed by the tissue (as in the case of photocoagulation), these lasers can be highly effective in removing and destroying semitransparent membranes. A typical example of this is the Nd/YAG laser; when we fire the laser, we can hear a mechanical "pop" sound. This force destroys the membranous scar tissue during a posterior capsulotomy and allows you to bill a 66821. Photodisruption laser energy is usually measured in joules.
3. **Plasma-induced ablation** – this type of laser damage can be considered a subset of photodisruption. Using a low-pulse energy laser with a short exposure time (e.g., femtosecond range), we can gently destroy tissue via plasma formation.[30] This creates a "wave" *of ablation*, as seen when creating a LASIK flap. Because of its transparency, the cornea can particularly be targeted for plasma-induced ablation with FSLs for precise surgical maneuvers, such as FSL-astigmatic keratotomy wounds and small incision lenticular extraction (SMILE). Similarly, the anterior lens capsule and nucleus can be surgically targeted using these principles for FSL-assisted cataract surgery.
4. **Photoablation** – photoablation involves *breaking covalent bonds* (carbon-carbon and carbon-nitrogen) in the target tissue such that it undergoes sublimation (conver-

[29]The Nd/YAG laser has a pulse duration in the nanosecond range (10^{-9} sec), whereas a FSL has a pulse duration in the femtosecond range (10^{-15} sec). Reducing the pulse duration will therefore reduce the amount of collateral damage caused by the FSL compared to the Nd/YAG laser – approximately 106 times less damage with the FSL.

[30]To be more specific, ionization (removing electrons from atoms and accelerating them) of atoms causes adjacent atoms to undergo ionization as well.

sion from solid to gas state).[31] These lasers create high-energy photons (range, 193–351 nm) that will be absorbed by all layers of the eye, including tears. The cornea should neither be too moist nor too dry during excimer laser surgery to avoid an undercorrection or overcorrection, respectively. Photoablation lasers are considered "cold" lasers since minimal heat/force is generated during the tissue destruction process.

5. **Photoactivation** – photoactivation lasers involve using laser energy with low energy and long exposure times to *convert a chemical from an inert form into an active form* to achieve a therapeutic effect. For example, verteporfin (used in photodynamic therapy) is activated by a low-power, long-duration (irradiance of 600 mW/cm2 over 83 sec) infrared laser (689 nm) and releases free radicals that initiate a series of inflammatory events and (subsequent) anti-inflammatory responses that induce regression of pathological neovascularization. Another example that has gained recent interest is corneal cross-linking for mild-moderate progressive keratoconus. In this procedure, riboflavin, a photosensitizer that can absorb light energy and then cause a chemical change in an adjacent molecule, is first applied to the de-epithelialized cornea (Dresden protocol). Ultraviolet-A (UV-A) light is then applied to the "riboflavin-marinated" cornea, generating reactive oxygen species, which induce the formation of covalent bonds between collagen molecules in the corneal stroma.

Light Damage, Accidental Laser Damage, and Laser Safety in Ophthalmology

As with anything in life, too much of something (or the wrong kind of something) can be dangerous. The intensity of incoming light (based on its wavelength) and length of exposure can damage sensitive ocular tissues, especially the retina, which has many *chromophores* that strongly absorb light, and can cause unwanted photochemical injury. The anterior segment of the eye serves as a protective shield for the retina. For example, the lens blocks UV-A light (310–400 nm) while the cornea blocks UV-B and UV-C (<310 nm), as well as infrared light. UV-A light is used in CXL because while it can penetrate the cornea, it is blocked by the crystalline lens and therefore causes no/minimal damage to the retina. However, long-term and repeated exposure to UV light can eventually break down this wall (similar to a nocturnal king who rode an ice dragon to break down a magical wall in the north of a fictional realm), leading to injuries such as photokeratitis and UV light-induced cataract ("glassblower's cataract"). As another example, aphakic patients can additionally suffer retinal injury due to the loss of UV-blocking properties of the crystalline lens. This is another reason why modern IOLs have UV-blocking or UV-filtering technology to protect the retina from light damage.[32]

Commercially available lasers include class II–IV lasers (Fig. 27). Accidental damage to ocular tissues can occur with any of these lasers. Laser injuries may cause various retinal changes, including ring-shaped hypopigmented lesions and pre-retinal/intraretinal hemorrhages. Late-term complications may occur, including epiretinal membrane (ERM), macular hole, choroidal neovascularization (CNV), and scars in the pigment epithelium. Although some pathologic damage may improve, permanent and irreversible changes such as chorioretinal scarring may be responsible for the delayed worsening of visual function after the initial improvement.

- Class I (class 1) – we can safely ignore these lasers as they are too puny to make a difference, and we will not waste any brain cells on them.
- Class II (class 2) and class IIIa (class 3R) – these lasers (e.g., laser pointer lasers) are considered to be safe for momentary viewing so long as the total power of the laser is $\leq$5 mW. In the USA, the FDA has imposed strict guidelines on the sale of laser pointers and only considers an output power of less than 5 mW safe.
- Class IIIb (class 3B) – these lasers typically have a power $\geq$ 5 mW and may be potentially damaging to the eye with any suprathreshold level of exposure (in less than one-quarter of a second). For example, a handheld laser pointer (with power $\geq$ 5 mW) or a military range finder (range 905–1550 nm) can cause significant and permanent retinal damage similar to solar retinopathy (Fig. 28).[33,34] Any laser class 3B (mnemonic, **think B for bad**) and above is damaging to the eye.
- Class IV (class 4) – this class encompasses most therapeutic lasers used in ophthalmology, including those previously discussed.

[31] This is why excimer lasers often have a vacuum fan near the laser that absorbs the sublimated corneal tissue during the ablation.

[32] As another example, older-generation surgical microscopes were known to cause light-induced retinal injury, especially with prolonged exposure in aphakic eyes or retinal procedures. Modern surgical microscopes contain additional UV filters that have reduced this risk. Nonetheless, if you are performing intraocular surgery and do not need the microscope light on the eye (e.g., the circulator nurse has to get additional viscoelastic, etc.), it is not a bad idea to move microscope light away from the eye to avoid potential retinal damage.

[33] Mainster MA, Timberlake GT, Warren KA, et al. Pointers on laser pointers. *Ophthalmology* 1997; 104:1213–14

[34] Roider J, Buesgen P, Hoerauf H, et al. Macular injury by a military range finder. *Retina* 1999; 19:531–35

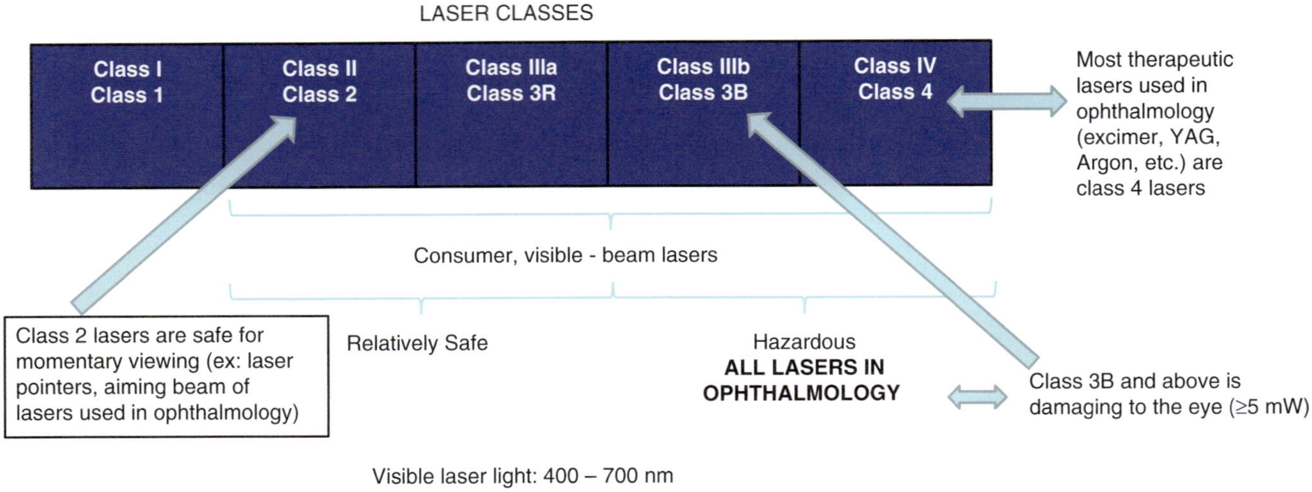

Fig. 27 Safety profile of commonly used lasers in ophthalmology

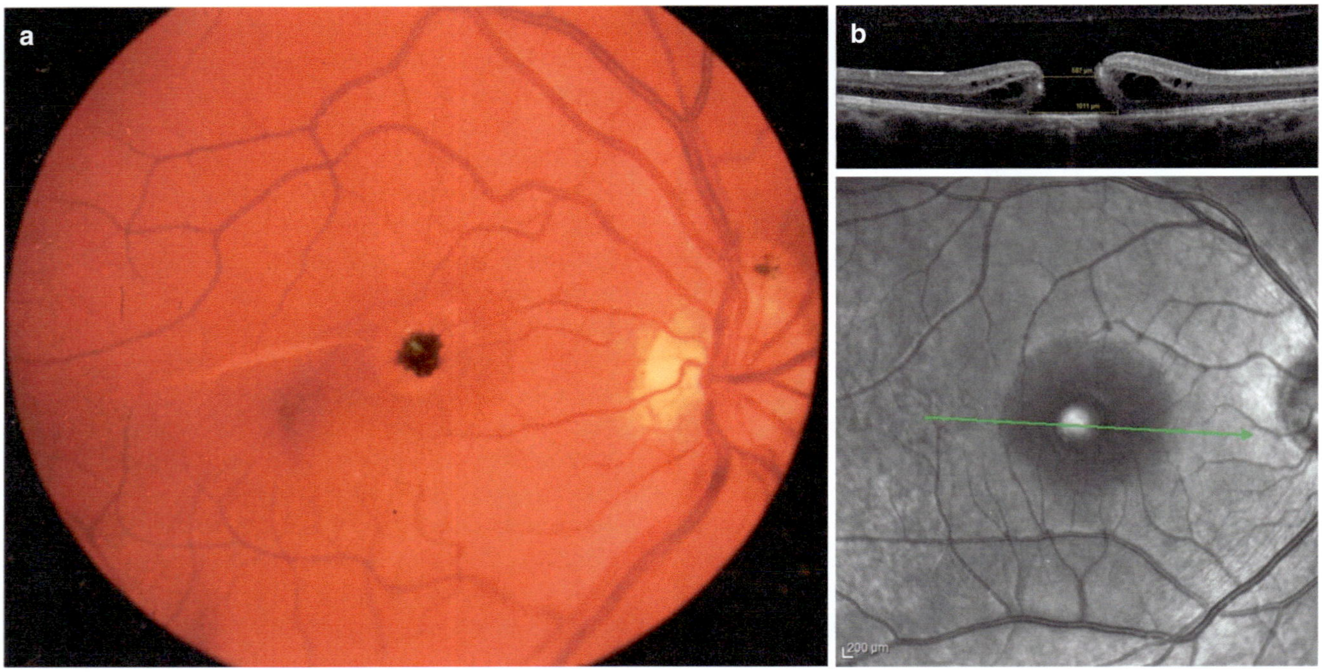

Fig. 28 Retinal damage due to accidental damage from lasers. Panel A shows accidental damage due to a military range finder laser. Panel B shows retinal damage in a child (visual acuity 20/100) due to a handheld laser pointer. (Courtesy of Dr. Yasha Modi, MD)

Since class 3R and 3B lasers can cause accidental eye damage, protective eyewear is highly recommended; for class 4 lasers, protective eyewear and other personal safety equipment are an absolute requirement.

In the USA, ANSI Z136 standard requires specification according to optical densities only and a nominal hazard zone (NHZ) to be determined by the laser safety officer of an institution.[35] Outside of the NHZ, diffuse viewing eyewear is allowed. In Europe, the standards are a bit more stringent as the power/energy density is also considered. There is no safe NHZ, and therefore laser safety glasses must protect against direct laser exposure.

Laser safety glasses usually involve materials with significant absorptive capabilities, such as polycarbonate or absorbing glass filters, to increase the optical density and decrease light transmittance. The color of the filter also matters: to protect against *ultraviolet/blue wavelengths*, a *yellow or orange filter* is commonly employed, whereas a *red filter* is used to protect against *green light*. In general, laser safety glasses should be ordered and customized based on the type of laser to be used.

[35] https://www.lasersafety.com/wp-content/uploads/2017/08/LaserSafetyGuide.pdf. Accessed March 22, 2020

Practice Questions

1. Which of the following is considered a cold laser?
   A. Excimer lasers 193 nm.
   B. Argon blue-green 488 nm.
   C. Krypton red 647 nm.
   D. Krypton yellow 568 nm.
2. How thick should an antireflective film be in relation to the wavelength you wish to block?
   A. ¼ wavelength
   B. ½ wavelength
   C. Same wavelength
   D. 2 X wavelength
3. If a patient had a vitreous hemorrhage which laser would best reach the choroid?
   A. Excimer lasers 193 nm.
   B. Argon blue-green 488 nm.
   C. Krypton red 647 nm.
   D. Krypton yellow 568 nm.
4. Which type of scattering causes the noontime sky to look blue?
   A. Mie scattering.
   B. Tyndall effect.
   C. Rayleigh scattering.
   D. Geometric scattering.
5. Which of the following statements about lasers is *true*?
   A. Laser light is highly divergent and therefore can deliver a large amount of energy to a large area.
   B. Laser light is monochromatic, polarized, and temporally coherent.
   C. Laser light can be diffusely spread out in multiple directions allowing for moderate amounts of energy to be delivered to multiple targets.
   D. Laser light is produced for an efficient use of input energy due to properties of the optical resonator.
6. Which of the following statements about coherence is *true*?
   A. Spatial coherence refers to two waves of light that come into focus at the same location at the target.
   B. Spatial coherence refers to two different points on the same wave of light that are equidistant from the center.
   C. Temporal coherence refers to two different points on the same wave of light that come into focus at the same time at the target location.
   D. Both temporal coherence and spatial coherence can be seen on the same given wave of light.
7. Which of the following optical principles is *correctly* paired with its technology?
   A. Polarization – antireflective coatings on lenses.
   B. Temporal coherence – fluorescein angiography.
   C. Polarization – Haidinger's brush.
   D. Diffraction – rainbow appearance.
8. Which of the following statements about scattering is *true*?
   A. Mie scattering is responsible for the degradation of visual acuity due to subsurface nanoglistenings (SSNGs).
   B. The Tyndall effect is best characterized by scattering of incoming sunlight due to atmospheric particles that bend blue wavelengths of light more than red wavelengths of light, leading to the appearance of a blue sky at noontime.
   C. Rayleigh scattering refers to particles in a suspension that create scattering of light, as seen by cell and flare in the anterior chamber.
   D. The Tyndall Effect states that because the melanin present absorbs more of the incoming light in a patient with a blue iris, the remaining blue wavelengths of light are visible to the observer.
9. Which of the following statements is *true*?
   A. Currently available multifocal intraocular lenses in the USA involve the use of refraction to split incoming light to distance and near focal points and increase unaided vision at all distances.
   B. The Airy disk is a description of the best focused spot of light that a lens with a circular aperture can make.
   C. Similar to spherical aberration, diffraction increases as the aperture size increases.
   D. Pinhole testing involves using a 2.4-mm hole to increase the depth of focus and decrease negative effects of diffraction to assess a patient's visual acuity potential.
10. Which of the following optical aberrations is an example of a higher-order aberration?
    A. Sphere.
    B. Cylinder.
    C. Piston.
    D. Coma.
11. Which of the following statements about spherical aberration is *true*?
    A. Spherical aberration in a myopic patient will decrease after conventional excimer laser ablation.
    B. Spherical aberration decreases the depth of focus and enhances contrast sensitivity.
    C. For most emmetropic patients, the net spherical aberration of the eye is a low amount of positive spherical aberration.
    D. Spherical aberration is worse during the daytime, especially on a bright sunny day.
12. Which of the following statements of the Q-value is *true*?
    A. The Q-value is a way to quantify combined corneal and lenticular spherical aberration and is measured in microns.
    B. A perfect spherical surface will have a Q-value of 1.

   C. The Q-value may be +1 or more in patients with corneal ectasias, such as keratoconus and post-refractive ectasia.
   D. A negative Q-value may help to offset some of the corneal spherical aberration.
13. Which of the following color deficiencies has been correctly paired with its pathology?
   A. Protanopia – lacking red cones.
   B. Deuteranopia – lacking blue cones.
   C. Tritanopia – lacking green cones.
   D. Vivanopia – lacking red cones.
14. Which of the following statements about aberrometry is *true*?
   A. Hartmann-Shack wavefront aberrometry involves the use of a lenslet array and a charged coupled device (CCD) to measure optical aberrations on light going into the optical system.
   B. Ray-tracing aberrometry measures reflected light emanating back from the retina from 240 points in the optical system.
   C. Spectacle glasses and contact lenses are not able to correct all the optical aberration measured by aberrometry.
   D. A Zernike polynomial can be used to describe wavefront aberrations in a pyramid shape with the most significant aberrations being visually represented at the top.
15. Which of the following types of laser light damage mechanisms has been *correctly* paired with its respective laser used in ophthalmic practice?
   A. Photoactivation – Nd/YAG laser.
   B. Photoablation – blue-green argon laser.
   C. Plasma-induced ablation – femtosecond laser.
   D. Photocoagulation – CO2 laser.
   E. Photodisruption – excimer laser.

Answers

1. Answer: A. Excimer lasers are considered "cold" lasers as there is no heat generated when breaking covalent bonds and converting solid tissue into a gas state (sublimation). This contrasts with lasers used in photocoagulation (choices B–D), wherein incoming light energy is absorbed by chromophores and converted into heat energy, causing tissue destruction and scar formation.
2. Answer: A. The antireflective film is a thin, semitransparent material of approximately one-fourth the wavelength of incoming light. This film creates a second reflected wave that interacts with the first reflected wave via destructive interference.
3. Answer: C. In the presence of vitreous hemorrhage, using a laser with a longer wavelength (i.e., a different color than the the vitreous hemorrhage) will allow the laser to penetrate the hemorrhage and the densely packed hemoglobin chromophore to reach the retinal tissue behind the hemorrhage for photocoagulation.
4. Answer: C. Rayleigh scattering occurs when incoming light waves interacts with particles smaller than themselves. The Tyndall effect (choice B) is not, strictly speaking, a form of scattering but instead refers to scattering due to particles in a suspension, such as protein or red blood cells in the aqueous humor in the anterior chamber. Mie scattering (choice C), also known as forward scattering, explains the appearance of white clouds; clinically, it accounts for glare caused by cortical spokes and subsurface nanoglistenings on IOLs. Geometric scattering (choice D) occurs when light encounters particles larger than the incoming wavelength of light, such as interaction with water droplets causing rainbow formation.
5. Answer: B. This is the summarized definition of a laser. Laser light is highly convergent (choice A) and demonstrates minimal spreading (choice C), even when directed to a target far away. Lasers are actually very inefficient sources of light as much of the input energy is lost in the "production" of the emitted laser (choice D).
6. Answer: B. This is the only correct definition listed. Temporal coherence refers to two similar spatial points on two separate waves separated by time in terms of when they come into focus. Spatial occurrence occurs within the same wave of light; it refers to two different points on the same wave of light equidistant from the center.
7. Answer: C. Polarization is used by the Haidinger's Brush technique to cause polarization of incoming light to preferentially stimulate orthogonal and non-orthogonal photoreceptors (relative to the fovea) to create an entoptic phenomenon and indicate gross macular function in the presence of a dense cataract. Destructive interference is used in antireflective coatings (choice A). Fluorescein angiography uses special interference filters (choice B) for incoming light (into the eye) and capturing outgoing light from the eye. Geometric scattering accounts for the appearance of rainbows as incoming light interacts with particles larger than themselves (choice D).
8. Answer: A. Mie scattering, or forward scattering, occurs when off-axis light strikes subsurface nanoglistenings on IOLs, causing a lowering of the Strehl ratio and degradation of visual acuity. See the explanation for question 4 for information regarding Rayleigh scattering and the Tyndall effect.
9. Answer: B. Multifocal IOLs (Choice A) use the property of *diffraction* to split incoming light into near and distance focal points. Diffraction is the inverse of spherical aberration; whereas the latter increases with larger aperture size (such as a pupil), diffraction decreases (choice C). Pinhole testing involves using a *1.2-mm* hole (choice D).

10. Answer: D. Sphere, cylinder, and piston (choices A–C) are examples of lower-order aberrations. Other important higher-order aberrations include spherical aberration and trefoil.
11. Answer: C. Spherical aberration (SA) will *increase* in a myopic patient after conventional laser refractive surgery. SA increases the depth of focus and worsens contrast sensitivity (choice B). SA worsens with a large pupil size (choice D).
12. Answer: D. The Q-value describes the asphericity (shape) of the corneal surface and has no units (choice A). A perfect spherical surface will have a Q-value = 0 (choice B); most patients will have a Q-value ranging from −0.20 to −0.27. The Q-value becomes increasingly negative in patients with keratoconus (choice C).
13. Answer: A. Deuteranopia means lacking green cones. Tritanopia means lacking blue cones. Vivanopia is a made-up term.
14. Answer: C. Hartmann-Shack wavefront aberrometry measures reflected light from the eye (choice A). Ray-tracing aberrometry measures light going into the eye (choice B). In a typical Zernike polynomial representation, the most significant aberrations are at the base of the pyramid (Choice D).
15. Answer: C. Femtosecond lasers use plasma-induced ablation to make fine cuts and cause changes to corneal tissue. The Nd/YAG laser uses *photodisruption*, which occurs when the laser strikes the target tissue and causes plasma formation via a rapid ionization of molecules within the tissue. This causes mechanical damage to the target tissue. The blue-green argon laser involves photocoagulation; in this process, incoming light energy from the laser causes denaturation of proteins in the target tissue and localized destruction (scar formation) within the tissue. The CO2 laser is a far-infrared laser that cut tissue via flash boiling water molecules within the target tissue, effectively sterilizing target tissue and sealing adjacent capillaries. The effectivity of the CO2 cutting depends on the target tissue's water content. This laser can also be used for periocular rejuvenation. Thermal effects of this laser cause dermal collagen to undergo neocollagenesis and tightening of adjacent facial skin. The excimer laser works via photoablation: through breaking covalent bonds, the laser causes sublimation of target tissue with minimal heat to surrounding tissues.

Part II

Optics for Oral Exams and Clinical Practice

Glasses in Clinical Practice

Kamran M. Riaz

Objectives

- To describe how to perform a subjective manifest refraction, cycloplegic refraction, and streak refraction.
- To appreciate the usefulness of the Duochrome test and the optical principles involved.
- To outline presbyopia-correcting options for glasses.
- To understand the unique challenges of prescribing, dispensing, and troubleshooting glasses in pediatric patients.

Introduction

Welcome to Part II! If you are reading this, we hope you have survived any or all written exams thus far and are ready to take on oral exams and learn something that has clinical relevance.

Some of you may believe that glasses are not the purview of ophthalmologists: you may only be partially incorrect in this assumption and belief. Nevertheless, even if prescribing and dispensing glasses are not a significant part of our clinical practice, we still need to understand some fundamental principles regarding glasses.

Remember: many times, in clinical practice, your best (or even only) solution may be to get your patient the best possible pair of glasses. And it is a bit more complicated than just sticking your patient in front of an autorefractor, accepting whatever prescription is generated, and sending your patient on his/her merry way. At least we think so; all of the authors have had numerous patients who have expressed immense gratitude when they simply receive a good pair of glasses that meets most of their visual needs, even in the presence of complex ocular pathology. Please do not underestimate the power of a good pair of glasses: it can be more life-changing than the most complex and impressive eye surgery and can help grow your practice in ways you cannot otherwise imagine.

Prescribing Glasses in Adults

Manifest Refraction

While discussing the full theory behind the how's and why's of clinical refraction is beyond the scope of this text, a review (and summary) of the important steps of subjective manifest refraction using a phoropter is important to commit to memory.

The standard refraction distance is 20 ft. (6 m)[1]; however, most ophthalmology clinic rooms are not this distance unless specifically designated as "research rooms". Using a shorter room distance, such as 10 ft., will cause the refraction to be *over-plussed* by approximately +0.25 to +0.50D (+0.33D exactly). The patient's **vertex distance** (distance between the back of the eyeglass lens and the patient's cornea) should also be measured. Usually, the vertex distance is 12–13 mm for most patients and does not need to be significantly adjusted for patients with refractive errors between −5.00D and + 5.00D. However, for patients with large refractive errors, the vertex distance should be carefully measured using a *distometer* (also known as a *vertexometer*).[2]

We can begin by positioning the patient correctly at the phoropter. Make sure that the patient's forehead is resting securely against the forehead rest, the pupils are centered through the openings, and the leveling bubble is centered. Check to make sure the lenses are free from smudges. Next, we can dial in a starting prescription from any (or a combination) of the following: streak refraction, autorefraction, or cur-

[1] See Chap. 29, "Postoperative Optics", for additional discussion regarding the relevance of exam room length in performing a refraction after cataract surgery.

[2] See Chap.17, "Optical Instruments", for more information regarding the distometer.

K. M. Riaz (✉)
Dean McGee Eye Institute, University of Oklahoma, Oklahoma City, OK, USA

K. M. Riaz et al. (eds.), *Optics for the New Millennium*, https://doi.org/10.1007/978-3-030-95251-8_15

rent wearing refraction. Those magical medications known as artificial tear drops to both eyes before refraction will make your life easier for patients with ocular surface disease. Start at the 20/60 line (assuming the patient has 20/20 vision potential). For patients with presbyopia, one eye should be occluded; for younger patients with intact accommodation, fogging the contralateral eye may be a preferable strategy, leading to less accommodation than occlusion.[3]

There are **four sequential refinements** that you should be able to list out (or summarize) in your own words. Please note that when you present choices in each of the following steps, allow your patient at least 2-3 seconds at each choice to have enough time to determine a difference. Moving too quickly between the choices may skew the refraction towards inaccurate results. Bolded words should definitely be committed to memory, and you may wish to use them as key concept words to develop your own checklist on how to perform a manifest refraction with the phoropter:

1. **Adjustment of sphere** – begin by dialing in **sphere with choices of +/− 0.50 D** apart and asking the patient to read each line down the chart. We can further refine this in 0.25D increments as needed. When giving the patient choices, you must remember there are actually *three choices, not two*: "is 1 better, is 2 better, or are they both the same?" If you forget to mention the third choice, some patients may become very frustrated as they may feel they have to choose between "1" and "2", when for them, "1 and 2" are equal for the two choices at a given reading line. The end point is where the patient reports the **clearest view** of the letter on the chart. Finally, we should always favor less minus between two sphere choices (especially in young adult myopic patients).
2. **Find the cylinder axis**:
   (a) Flip over the **Jackson cross cylinder (JCC)** such that white and red dots are on either side of the 90- or 180-degree axis ("straddle the axis") (Fig. 1).
   (b) Flip the JCC and ask the patient to **compare the first and second choices,** explaining that both choices will be a little blurry, and ask them to choose the "less blurry" choice.
   (c) Based on which JCC choice the patient prefers, rotate the axis in the direction of the white dot ("chasing the white rabbit") toward that choice in 10-degree changes.
   (d) Once the **patient prefers the red dot**, **shift the JCC back** in the original direction in 5-degree changes.
   (e) Repeat in smaller increment steps until the two choices are reported to be the same.
3. **Adjust the cylinder power**:
   (a) Rotate the JCC so that red or white dot is "on axis" with the axis determined in step 2 (Fig. 2).

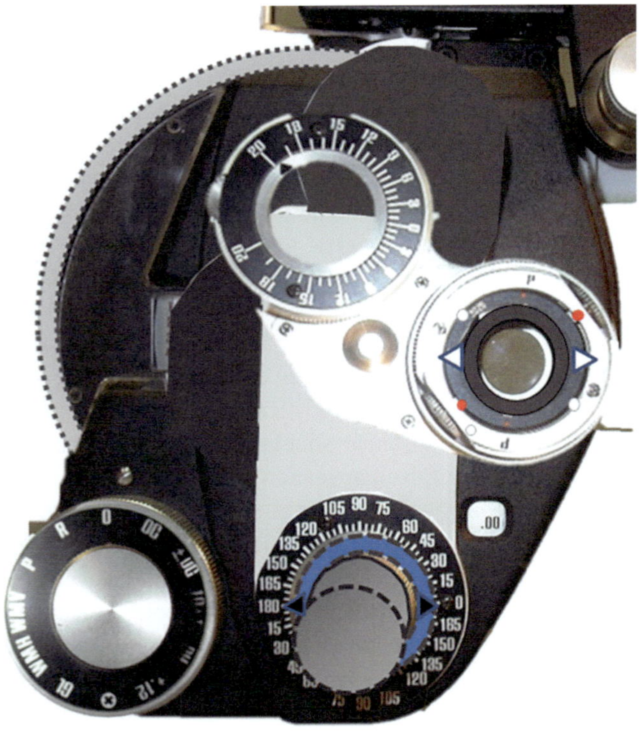

Fig. 1 Finding the cylinder axis – to fine-tune the axis, flip over the Jackson cross cylinder (JCC) so that the red and white dots straddle the "arrow" at either the 180-degree or 90-degree axis

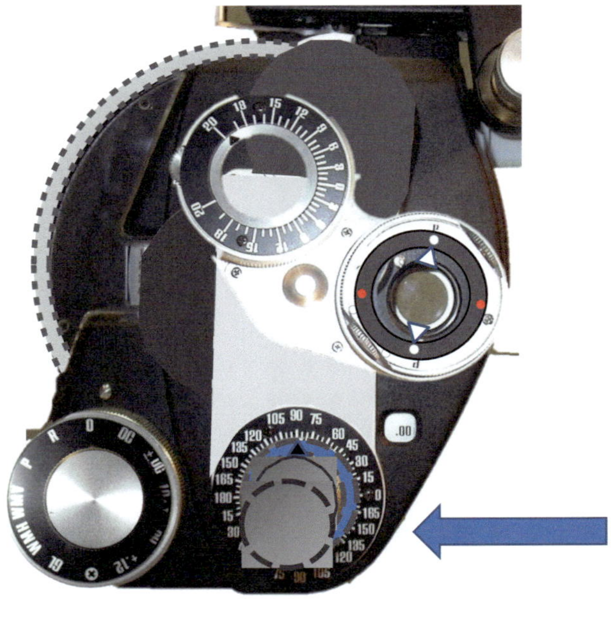

Fig. 2 Adjusting the cylinder power correction – to fine-tune the astigmatism power, rotate the JCC so that the red and white dots are on-axis. This will allow you to dial in cylinder power (blue arrow)

[3] Similarly, in patients with latent nystagmus, fogging is preferred over occlusion in order to determine the BCVA by refraction.

(b) Flip between red and white choices. If the patient reports that the **white dot choice letters are clearer**, then **add + 0.50D cylinder** power. If the patient reports that the red dot choice letters are clearer, add −0.50D cylinder power. This principle is true for plus- or minus-cylinder phoropters.
(c) For every +0.50D cylinder power added, **add − 0.25D sphere** to maintain the spherical equivalent and thus maintain the image on the retina.
(d) End when both red-white choices are the same, always favoring the lesser cylinder power.

4. **Final sphere adjustment**:
   (a) Remove the JCC. **Refine the sphere by 0.25D steps** until the patient reports the two choices to be the same. Again, always favor less minus ("push plus", especially in young adult myopic patients and pseudophakic patients with presbyopia-correcting intraocular lenses).

Congratulations, you have just refracted a patient. Make sure you remember to code CPT 92015 and collect any refraction fee(s) at this time.

Cycloplegic Refraction

Cycloplegic refraction (CRx) (also known as wet refraction) involves using anticholinergic agents to pupillary dilation and, more importantly, to paralyze the ciliary body and fully relax accommodation temporarily. Since the patient's eye cannot generate additional "plus" power (especially in younger myopic patients), a CRx can be helpful in many situations as follows:

- To help ensure we are not "over-minusing" a young myopic patient. In these patients, there may be several diopters of difference between the manifest refraction and the CRx. This is especially important for myopic patients presenting for laser vision correction.
- To diagnose other reasons why the objective dry manifest refraction does not provide the patient with good clarity and comfort in new glasses.
- To diagnose a patient with latent hyperopia (see Chap. 21 Clinical Problems with Optics/Refractive Manifestations).[4]
- To determine if another pathology is present in a patient with rapidly changing refractions in a short period of time.

[4]This is particularly relevant if the patient has an esotropia with an accommodative component, even as an adult.

Streak Refraction

Just as we previously discussed the significant steps for a manifest refraction, knowing the major steps for performing a streak refraction (and how to summarize them) is useful for both exams and clinical practice. The following scenarios are examples of when a streak refraction may be useful (or even necessary):

- Patients who cannot sit at or cooperate with a phoropter: physically disabled patients and pediatric patients, respectively.
- Malingering patient: the faker trying to get you to sign off on his unemployment benefits claiming he is blind may actually just need a −1D prescription. A streak refraction can objectively measure the true refractive error in these cases.
- A streak refraction can serve as a useful starting point before performing a manifest refraction in a patient with no previous history of wearing glasses.
- To determine if patients have irregular astigmatism present (such as corneal ectasia) based on the lack of an optimal streak or the presence of scissored reflex, this will warrant further imaging and evaluation by a cornea specialist.
- To determine if a patient has media opacities, such as oil-droplet cataract, lenticonus, etc., especially in the pediatric patient (in whom a prolonged slit-lamp exam may be difficult).

For detailed information on best performing a streak refraction, you may wish to consult other resource texts. For now, the bolded words in the checklist below should definitely be committed to memory, and you may wish to use them as key concept words to develop your own mini-speech on how to perform a streak refraction:

1. The patient should **fixate on a distant target**. Cycloplegia may be needed to relax accommodation, especially if performing a streak refraction in a pediatric patient.
2. Calculate your **working distance**. Usually, 67 cm (1.5D) or 50 cm (2D) are the standard distances. The working distance can vary: some people like to have their arm holding the lenses perfectly straight; others prefer a slight bend. You should have a colleague calculate your exact working distance once you find your "comfortable" arm position.
3. Starting with the patient's right eye, position the streak vertically and move it side to side to determine whether there is "against" or "with" motion (Fig. 3). Use the "SPAM" mnemonic (**s**ame motion, add **p**lus power; **a**gainst motion, add **m**inus power). The streak may need to be rotated in different meridians to find the one with the brightest reflex (Fig. 4).
4. Keep using SPAM until you have a **bright red reflex without any motion** that fills the pupil.

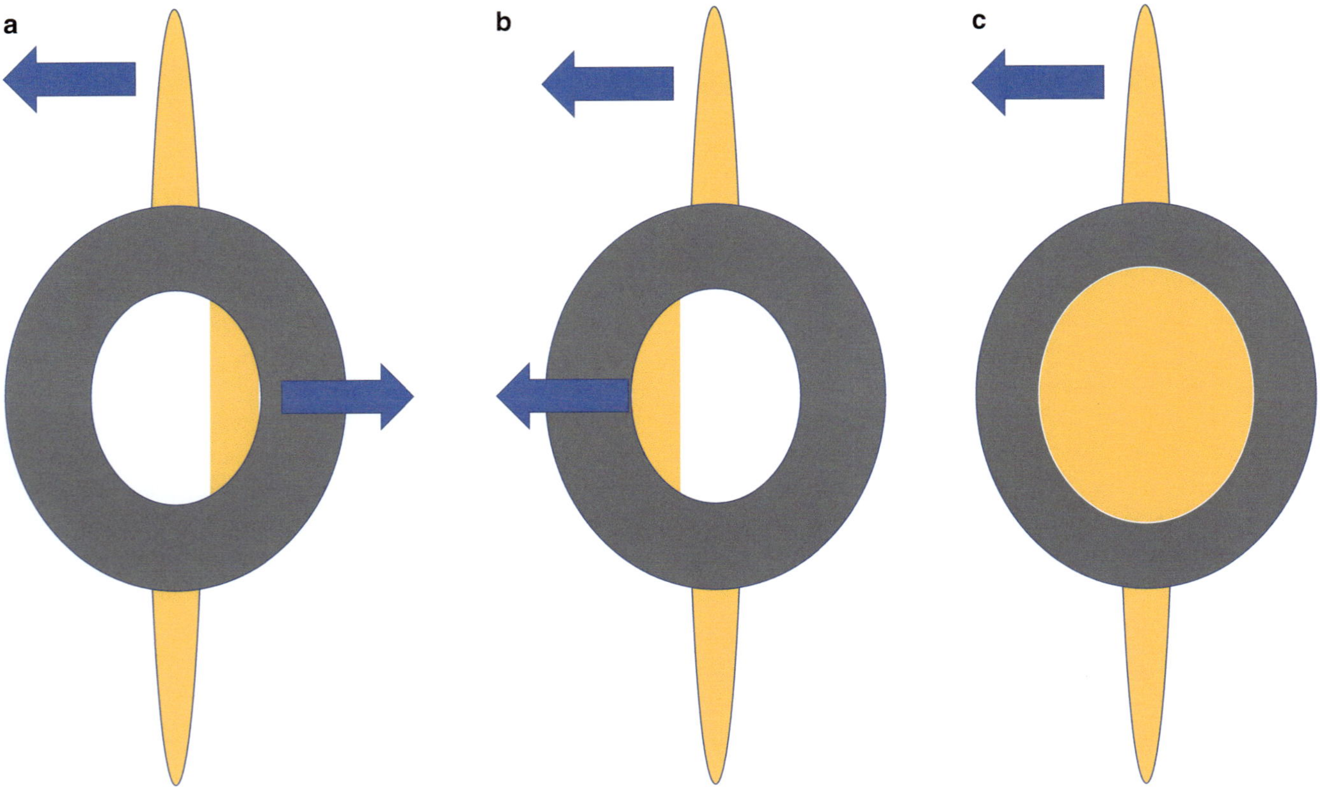

Fig. 3 Several possibilities may occur when moving the streak from side to side. If the streak demonstrates "against" motion (panel A), minus power needs to be added to the loose lens. If the streak demonstrates "with" motion (panel B), plus power needs to be added to the loose lens. The end result should be a neutral reflex that fills the entire lens (panel C)

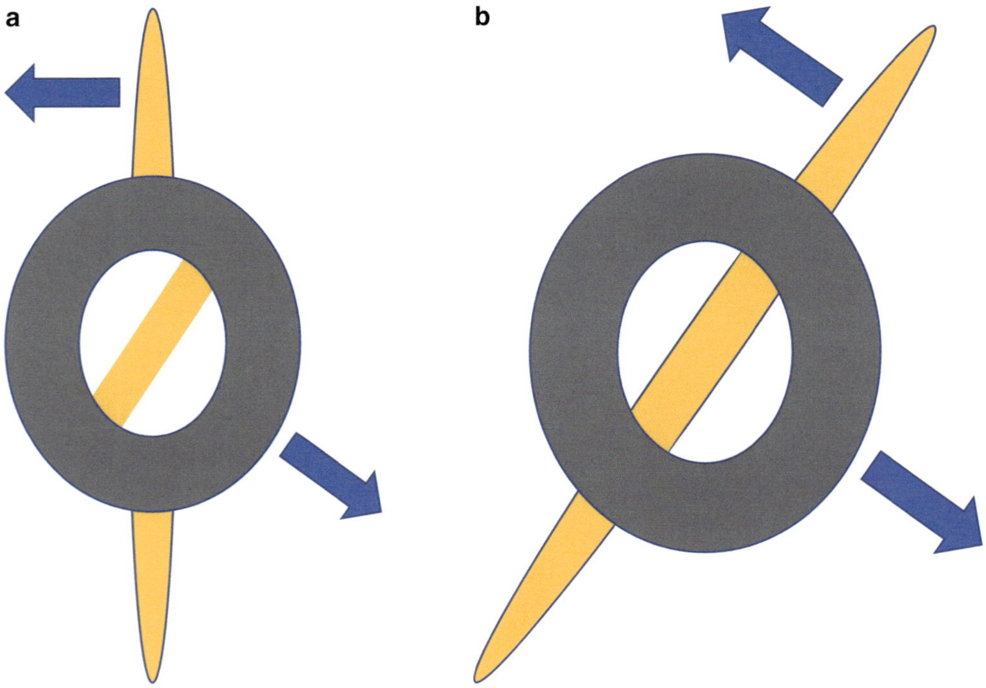

Fig. 4 If astigmatism is present, a streak held in the vertical position may not align with the reflex (panel A) and instead may show oblique motion. Rotating the streak ("on axis") may be necessary to neutralize the first meridian (panel B)

5. If the reflex has consistent width and brightness in all directions, there is no astigmatism – congratulations, you have an easy patient. However, there is usually some astigmatism to correct as well. So, we will have to rotate the streak 90 degrees away and **repeat steps 3–4 for the secondary meridian**.

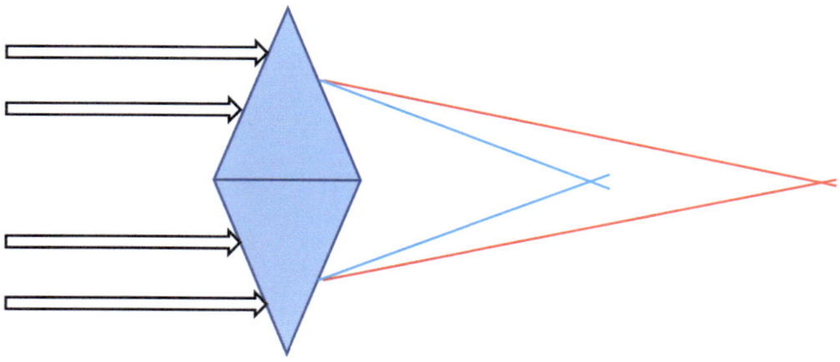

Fig. 5 An incoming ray of light will be bent according to individual colors that make up the ray of light. Blue rays will come into focus closer than red rays (intentional exaggeration shown for example purposes)

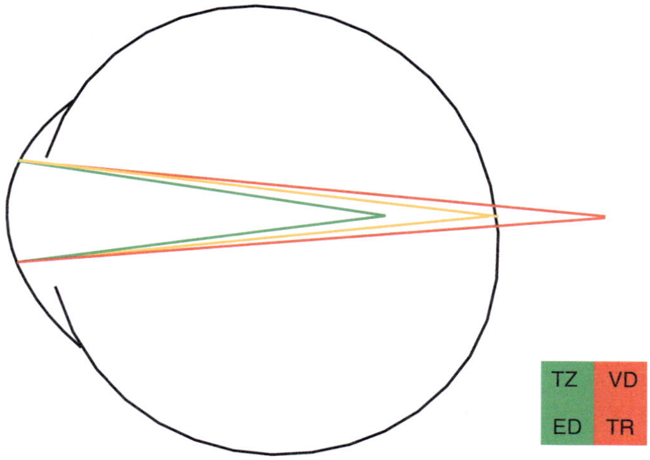

Fig. 6 In an ideal refraction, the yellow component of the incoming light will fall directly on the retina. Green components will land in the vitreous, and red components will land in the choroid (intentional exaggeration shown for example purposes)

6. **Repeat** steps 3–5 for the patient's **left eye**.
7. **Adjust for working distance** – remember you must **add additional −1.5D or −2D** of myopic sphere correction because of the working distance. For example, if -2D sphere (without any astigmatism) neutralizes the reflex and your working distance is 67 cm (1.5D), the final prescription will be −3.50D sphere.

Other Tests Used

Several other tests may be useful in selected cases to optimize manifest refraction.

Duochrome Test

Note to the reader: we will switch back and forth between referring to light as waves and rays in this section.

The duochrome test is one of the most important ancillary tests during a manifest refraction, especially when refracting a young myopic patient (even more so if said patient is presenting as a laser vision correction candidate). The test involves taking advantage of **chromatic aberration**. Remember that different wavelengths of light are bent differently by the eye's optical system: shorter wavelengths (blue) are bent more than longer wavelengths (red). In other words, the blue component of a light ray that passes through a plus lens will be bent much more than the red component; therefore, think that the blue will land in the vitreous and the red will land behind the retina in the choroid (Fig. 5). A helpful mnemonic is **bl**ue rays are **be**nt the most.

When we look at the eye, we can imagine that we will be able to get the "yellow component" of the light ray to fall on the retina in a perfect refraction scenario directly. Therefore, in this scenario, the green light components will be slightly in the vitreous, and the red components will be slightly in the choroid (Fig. 6).

The duochrome test takes advantage of chromatic aberration to ensure that we have not "over-minused" (or "under-minused") a patient. The test is performed as a final step after manifest refraction: after optimizing the refraction, *each eye is tested individually* by showing the patient the 20/20 (or 20/25) line with the "red-green" screen (one side of the screen is green, and the other side is red, as shown in Fig. 6). The patient should be fogged by adding about +0.50D sphere to their measured distance refraction; this will relax accommodation and (hopefully) will make the *red* letters bolder. It is important to let the patient know you will make it a little blurry on purpose. (If you forget to do this, they may point out your perceived incompetence.)

At this point, if the patient has been optimally refracted, he/she may report that red and green letters will appear equally clear. Congratulations, you are done. You can simply prescribe the glasses, charge the 92015, and move on.

However, if red and green letters are not equally clear, then the "**RAM-GAP**" mnemonic may be used to refine the refraction. This mnemonic reminds us that if the patient reports that red letters are clearer, the incoming light has been refracted "too much" and most of the light ray is falling in the vitreous. If we consider Fig. 7, we can see that if the red portion of the incoming light is on the retina, then yellow and green portions are in the vitreous. Therefore, if the **red is clearer**, we must **add minus ("RAM")** to the refraction. Similarly, if we consider Fig. 8 wherein the patient reports that **green is clearer**, the yellow and red portions are in the choroid; therefore, we have to **add plus ("GAP")** to the refraction.

Several questions are usually asked about the duochrome test, so pop quiz time, hotshot:

1. How much is the diopter difference between red and green components of light?

   Answer – approximately one diopter. The difference between red and blue is approximately 1.25 diopters.

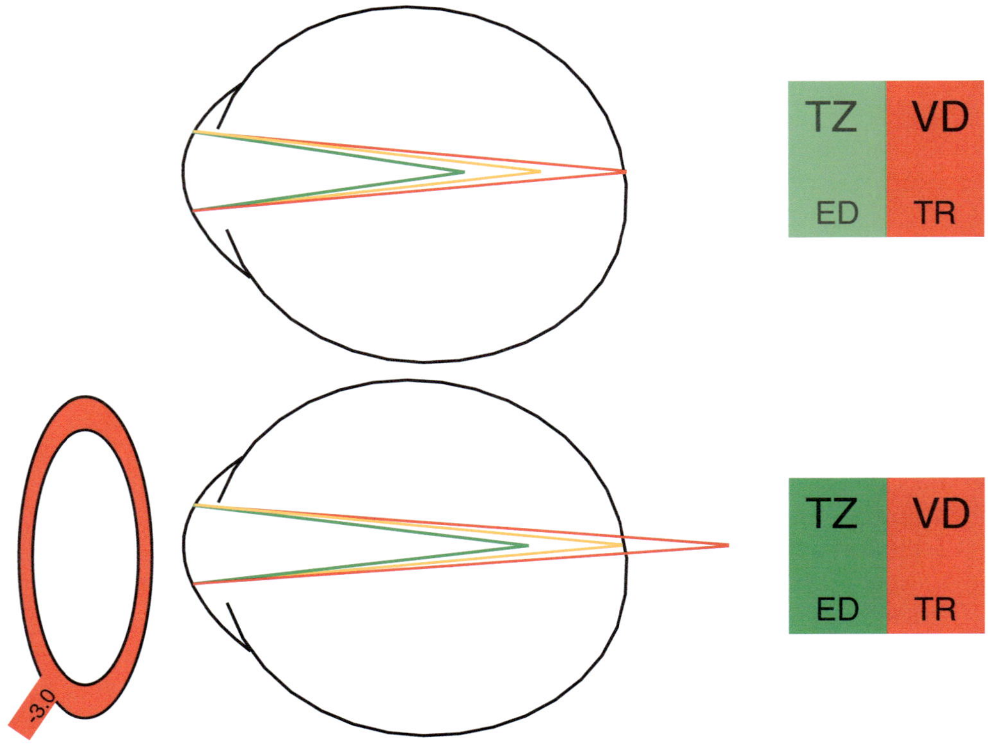

Fig. 7 Duochrome test. If the red is sharper, the patient needs more minus ("RAM")

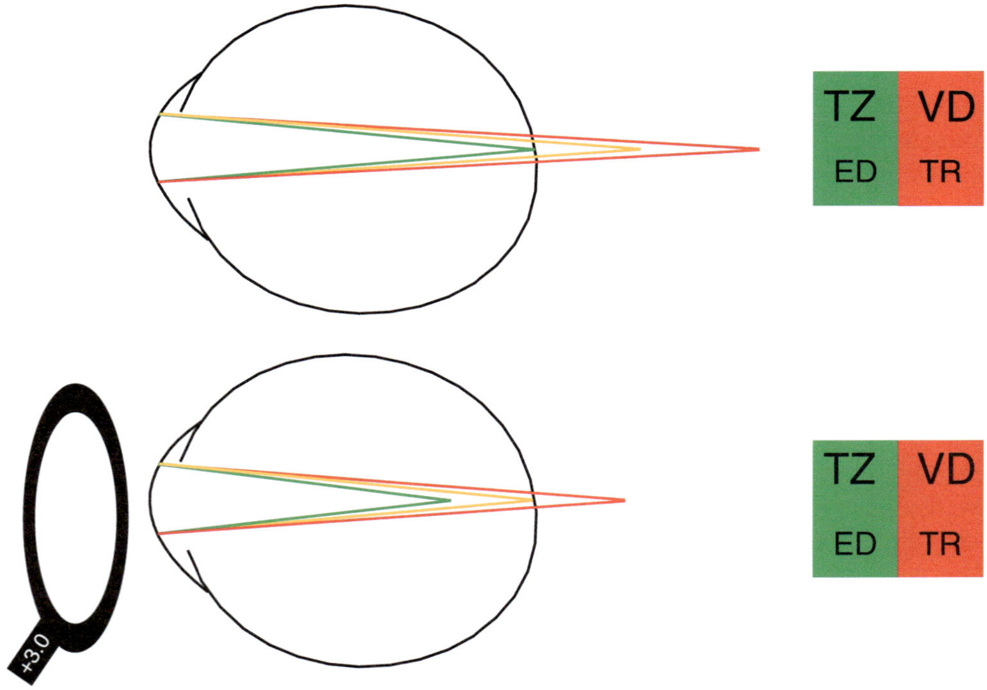

Fig. 8 Duochrome test. If the green is sharper, the patient needs more plus ("GAP")

2. **Should** this test be performed binocularly in routine patients?

   Answer – no, we just said above that this should be a monocular test, so don't be silly and perform it simultaneously with both eyes.[5]

3. Can this test be used on a patient whose best manifest refraction yields a vision of 20/50?

   Answer – no. This test should only be used on patients whose BCVA is $\geq$20/30 because it realistically can titrate about 0.50–0.75D. So, if a patient can only see 20/50,

[5]The duochrome test **can** be used binocularly to test binocular balance. This is **occasionally done** with a vertical prism to split screens and ensure equal accommodative relaxation between eyes since a young patient can still accommodate during monocular duochrome testing.

then the duochrome test will not be "as useful" since the difference is likely too small for the patient to appreciate.
4. Can a duochrome test be performed on a patient who is red-green color blind? Answer: Yes! Because the test involves the patient's ability to discern between wavelengths of light, it can be performed in patients with red-green color blindness. However, the patient may report that the "left" or "right" side of the chart is sharper, so the examiner will have to adjust accordingly.

Autorefraction and Wave Front Refraction

Objective autorefractor devices use low levels of infrared light to perform refraction. Because this technique does not involve visible light (as used in subjective manifest refraction), there is an error of approximately 0.75–1.00D between these two methods. Therefore, autorefractors are used as a screening tool or starting point to determine a patient's refraction and should *not* be used as a substitute for actual manifest refraction. However, there may be certain circumstances when an autorefractor may be more beneficial than a subjective refraction, such as in the presence of macular disease or lens opacity, to determine the refractive state of a patient's eye.

Depending on the type of autorefractor, several popular methods may be used to calculate the refraction of a patient's eye:

- Devices that use automated retinoscopy (dynamic sciascopy) are cost-efficient, integrate well with corneal topography, and rapidly generate a usable refraction (and information about aberrations). Examples of this technology include the Nidek OPD-Scan III (Nidek Technologies, Gamagori, Japan).
- The optometer principle can also be used in autorefractor devices.[6] The optometer involves using a standard lens of known power (and focal point) and using the patient's eye as an "unknown lens" to dial in power such that known lens and unknown lens focal points match. The power needed is used as a proxy for the eye's refractive power. Examples of this technology include the Nikon Auto Refractometer NR-1000 F (Nikon Corporation, Tokyo, Japan).
- The Scheiner disk principle involves using a lens with two small holes vertically oriented with a light source directed into the eye. The top hole is then covered, and depending on the refractive error, the top or the bottom spot of light disappears (for a myope and hyperope, respectively). The device can then measure the changes that occur when blocking both holes in 1–2 seconds to determine the refractive error present. Examples of this technology include the Nidek AR-2000 objective automatic refractor (Nidek Technologies, Gamagori, Japan).

As discussed in Chap. 14, Physical Optics, a wavefront refraction can be performed on inbound (ray-tracing devices) light and outbound (Hartmann-Shack) light from a patient's eye. These devices not only calculate the objective refractive error but can also give information about higher-order aberrations. Wave front autorefractors are commonly used for wave front-guided ablations in excimer laser refractive surgery.

Presbyopia Correction and Glasses

See the discussion on presbyopia in Chap. 12 "Glasses for Written Exams", for a detailed discussion regarding correction options with glasses.

In terms of how to determine the bifocal power, unfortunately, it's a bit more complicated than simply giving everybody a + 2.50 add and sending them on their way (even though that probably works in real life for ~90% of your patients).

Several methods can help us determine the needed bifocal add power:

1. Use an age approximated add power based on expected amplitudes of accommodation (AOA), such as Donder's table. Half of the AOA should be held in reserve to avoid asthenopia.[7] For example, a patient with 3 diopters of AOA should be given a + 1.5D add power. This will allow the patient to use half of their AOA.
2. Trial and error with different add powers in a trial frame – sometimes, you don't have to be elegant as long as you get the correct answer and don't break anything along the way.
3. Binocular plus build-up – put the patient in the phoropter with their full manifest refraction for distance. Hold a reading card at the patient's preferred distance (33–40 cm). Add +0.25D to each eye until the patient can read the lowest line on a near card. Note that this method essentially measures the AOA and may induce asthenopia if one were to prescribe only the minimum amount needed to read the J1+ line without cycloplegia.
4. Find the patient's near point by measuring the nearest point that a patient can maintain focus through their full distance correction. This maneuver can be facilitated by using a "Prince rule." This distance is divided into 100 to convert it to AOA. For example, if a patient wears −1.75D sphere OU and can see up to 33 cm with her glasses on,

[6] The optometer principle is also used in the lensmeter device. See Chap. 17 Optical Instruments and Machines, for more details.

[7] See Chap. 9 "Accommodation and Presbyopia", for more information on this topic.

then the AOA is 100/33 = 3D. Therefore, this patient will need +1.50D reading add in her glasses.

5. Fused cross cylinder test (Fig. 9) – place the patient in the phoropter and dial in his full distance correction. Move the Jacques blur point card (that tic-tac-toe-looking thing gathering dust in the corner of the exam lane) to the preferred reading distance. Next, dial in ±0.50 on the dial (not the JCC dial but rather the dial that we use for "open," "occlusion," etc.). Ask the patient: "are the horizontal lines darker?" If yes, keep adding plus power in both eyes until horizontal and vertical lines on the Jacques blur point card have equal intensity. This is the add power required.

Congratulations on wasting 15 min of your office time that you will never get back. You better bill that 92015 if you did option #5 from that list.

Prescribing Glasses in Kids

As in our previous discussions with adults, a combination of refraction strategies may be necessary for optimal refraction in pediatric patients, depending on age and (in)voluntary cooperation of the child (and the parent). We may have to schedule several appointments to optimize the refraction for a child. A more detailed discussion of this topic is presented in Chap. 23, Pediatric Optics.

The following section will focus on "considerations for pediatric patients," apart from the refraction issues discussed earlier in the chapter. In other words, we will discuss the "optician" stuff. Since every child is different, we have to consider a few additional considerations in this patient population.

Special Considerations for Glasses in Kids

The following is a list of factors that can increase success while dispensing glasses in pediatric patients:

- **Frame fit** – frame fit is equally important as a good refraction in pediatric patients. Remember that kids have a weird tendency (compared to your adult patients) to grow, especially before 10 years of age. For example, a child's head size is approximately 90% of adult size by age 10. Kids also have constantly evolving facial, nasal, and ear anatomy. Factors such as a flat nasal bridge should be considered in frame fit and size. Even if you have the world's most excellent refraction, if the frames are too big, too loose, too small, etc., the child won't wear them.

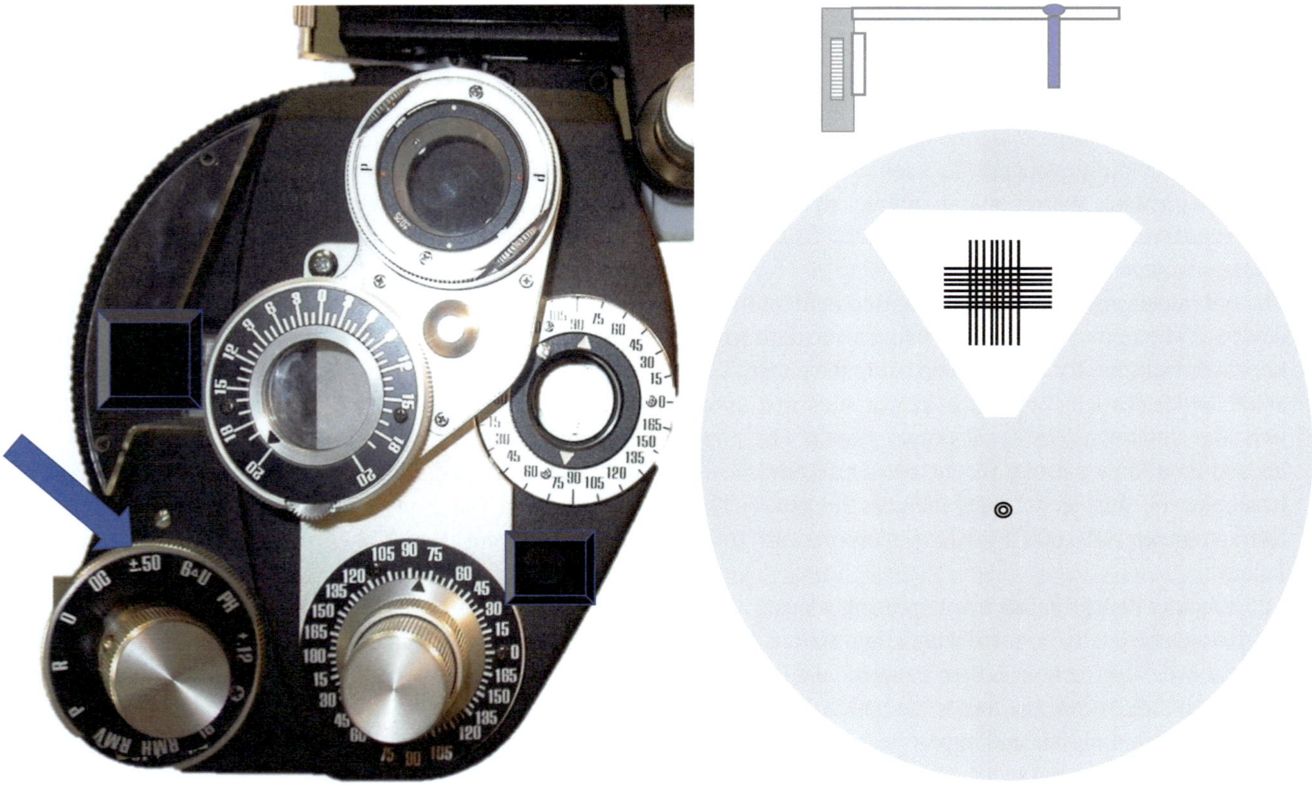

Fig. 9 The fused cross cylinder test. After setting the dial to the ±0.50 option (blue arrow) and giving the patient his/her full distance correction, the Jacques blur point card can be used to find the preferred reading distance. The patient is asked to look at horizontal and vertical lines (right panel). If the patient reports the horizontal lines are darker, the examiner dials in additional plus power until horizontal and vertical lines have equal intensity. The total amount of plus sphere dialed in during this process is the reading add required

For example, a head strap may be necessary if the child's nasal bridge is not large enough to support frames. A special "horseshoe addition" can be placed on the nasal bridge for added support.

- **Lens material** – shatterproof materials, such as polycarbonate, are preferred for lenses because of the higher risk of trauma in pediatric patients.
- **Cosmetic reasons** – children are fussy creatures with constantly changing tastes in preferences. A child may pick out blue frames because blue is his favorite color but then 3 months later change his mind that green is his favorite color. Aesthetic considerations for color, size, style, etc., may be prohibitive or motivating reasons for a child to wear (or not wear) prescribed glasses.
- **Psychosocial reasons** – other kids can be mean (some of you may still remember being bullied, or shame on you if you were the bully!). The child may not want to wear the glasses because she gets made fun of at school by her classmates. Similarly, a child may not want to wear her glasses because her parents picked out the frame, and she may feel that she did not have any control over choosing the frame color/style. Empowering the child to select his/her frames can be extremely effective in convincing the child to wear the glasses. Exploring these factors is crucial to ensure that the child will wear her glasses.
- **Family support** – unfortunately, we know that some parents can be... quite difficult. For example, some parents may not appreciate the need for their child to wear glasses and thus may not reinforce glasses wear. Other parents may be too overbearing regarding the child wearing the glasses. This scenario is where you may have to serve as a child psychiatrist and counsel the family to provide appropriate support for the child to wear his glasses as much as possible, especially if there is a risk for amblyopia. Unfortunately, there is no additional ophthalmology code (that we know of) that you can use to bill extra for your services as a life coach and therapist.
- **Reward approach** – sometimes, bribery is the best solution to life's problems. Kids respond to positive reinforcement, so especially with new glasses in pediatric patients, it may be necessary to have the parents "motivate" the child with candy, TV time, and other rewards to get junior to wear the new glasses.
- **Penalization approach** – at other times, if the carrot won't work, then the stick may need to be employed–not literally, of course! It may be necessary to provide negative reinforcement for some patients, for example, to "motivate" a pediatric patient with accommodative esotropia to wear glasses to prevent the development of amblyopia. Strategies such as eyeglass bands (to keep the glasses on) are relatively benign methods to provide negative reinforcement. More aggressive strategies may involve using arm splints or cycloplegia of the better-seeing eye in patients with amblyopia and hyperopia (such as with cyclopentolate).[8]
- **Cycloplegia** – while this may seem like the complete opposite of the previous sentence, there may be some situations where cycloplegia of the affected eye(s) is a highly appropriate and effective treatment. For example, if a child has a high hyperopic prescription and an accommodative ET, cycloplegia may help to relax accommodation and accept the full refraction in glasses. See Chap. 22, Optics for the Clinical and Surgical Management of Strabismus, for more details.

Practice Questions

1. Self-assessment – List all the steps of a manifest refraction in under one minute in your own words. Practice in front of a mirror or reciting this to a friend, colleague, and/or significant other. Apologize to this person and offer to buy them a coffee for their troubles.
2. Self-assessment – List all the steps of a streak refraction in under one minute in your own words. Practice in front of a mirror or reciting this to a friend, colleague, and/or significant other. Apologize to this person and offer to buy them a coffee for their troubles.
3. Which of the following statements regarding manifest refraction is *true*:
   A. A streak refraction is a useful method to determine the starting refraction point for a patient with aphakia.
   B. In performing a manifest refraction on a young myopic patient, it is preferable to occlude the non-tested eye.
   C. During the step of finding the axis using plus cylinder, if a patient reports the red dot is clearer, move the dial in that direction.
   D. When dialing in +0.50D cylinder, one should add −0.50D sphere to maintain the spherical equivalent.
4. Which of the following statements regarding the duochrome test is *true*?
   A. This test can be used in patients with BCVA of ≥20/50 to finalize the refraction.
   B. If a patient reports that green letters appear clearer, there may be unintentional overcorrection of the myopia present.
   C. Red-green color blind patients may need alternative methods of testing, such as a cycloplegic refraction, in lieu of the duochrome test.

[8]Note that older texts may discuss the use of phospholine iodide for this purpose. In modern practice, this has been essentially abandoned due to the high side effect risk profile, such as iris cysts, etc.

D. This test uses the principle of spherical aberration to titrate and finalize the refraction.

Answers

3. Answer: A. A streak refraction may be especially useful in patients with high refractive errors as a starting point, before placing the patient in the phoropter. In young myopic patients, fogging the non-tested eye may be a better method to hinder accommodation during the refraction rather than occlusion. When finding the axis using plus cylinder, if the patient reports the *white* dot is clearer, move the dial in that direction. If one dials in +0.50D cylinder, one should add −0.25D sphere to maintain spherical equivalent.
4. Answer: B. If green letters are clearer, it is likely that we have over-minused the patient, and we have to add plus power (using the "GAP" of the "RAM-GAP" mnemonic). This test can only be used in patients with BCVA of ≥20/40. Red-green color blind patients can effectively use the duochrome test, though they may need additional guidance on which "side" of the screen they should indicate is clearer. The duochrome test uses the principle of chromatic aberration.

Construction of Glasses (Ophthalmologists as Opticians)

Kamran M. Riaz

Objectives

- To describe the advantages and disadvantages of commonly used materials employed in the construction of glasses.
- To understand the role of lens coatings commonly used in glasses.
- To formulate an approach toward diagnosing and improving glasses and bifocals for the unhappy patient.
- To appreciate how patients' needs may require the construction of nontraditional or occupational glasses.
- To discuss the role of tints in glasses with consideration to patients' visual needs.

Introduction

Here's a closely guarded secret for our profession: besides being an ophthalmologist, you also need to know a little bit about what our optician friends do in the mystery tower known as the optical shop (or magical eyeglass-making laboratory). While we may never have to make glasses ourselves, it is helpful to know some of this information in order to appreciate better what our optician colleagues do, but also to know what kinds of options we can offer our patients who are unhappy with their glasses or are looking for custom-tailored glasses for their particular visual needs. Before you repeat that refraction for the third time, perhaps you may want to think about what could be wrong with the glasses' construction and design and what options you can discuss with your unhappy patient.

K. M. Riaz (✉)
Dean McGee Eye Institute, University of Oklahoma, Oklahoma City, OK, USA

Lens Materials

Commonly Used Materials

While many materials are used in the construction of lenses in glasses, there are several common ones worth discussing. These materials are usually a mixture of multiple base compounds put together in varying concentrations:

- **Crown glass (n = 1.5–1.6)** – this is the most frequently used material referred to as "glass" in eyeglasses. It is somewhat of a misnomer (as are all "glass" materials used in lenses) as it is actually a composite of silicone dioxide (sand, ~70%), Na20 (soda, ~15%), and calcium oxide (lime, 10–15%); the rest is a mystery like the colonel's 13 herbs and spices. Crown glass is a relatively durable surface resistant to scratches and cleans easily. Crown glass can be rendered stronger to resist shattering using various chemical and heat methods.
- **Flint glass (aka lead glass, n = 1.66)** – this material has a high index of refraction (compared to crown glass) and is commonly used as a bifocal segment for fused bifocals. It is a mixture of sand, soda, and lead oxide. These are less commonly used today as they are difficult to render impact resistant.
- **Barium glass (n = 1.58)** – this material consists mainly of barium oxide, sand, and other metallic oxides. It is commonly used for making bifocal segments for fused bifocals.
- **CR-39 (n = 1.498)** – a fun historical fact is CR-39 stands for "Columbia Resins 39"; during WWII, the company Columbia-Southern Chemical Corporation produced a variety of polymers, and the 39th polymer was found to be highly suitable for plastic eyeglass lenses. Today, CR-39 is among the most popularly used lens materials for most glasses due to several key features:
  - Weight – approximately 50% lighter than crown glass.

K. M. Riaz et al. (eds.), *Optics for the New Millennium*, https://doi.org/10.1007/978-3-030-95251-8_16

- Fogging – less likely to fog-up compared to glass lenses, especially with rapid temperature changes.
- Safety – if the lens breaks, it will break into larger pieces whose edges are not as sharp as broken glass edges.
- Impact resistance – CR-39 requires no additional treatment to enhance its natural strength as compared to "glass" lenses.
- Chromatic aberrations and reflections – less than "glass" lenses.

However, because CR-39 is "softer" than glass, it does tend to scratch easier, necessitating the addition of secondary scratch-resistant coatings.

- **Polycarbonate (n = 1.58)** – This material can be used to make a thinner and lighter lens than other materials. It is *extremely impact resistant*, making it a popular choice for safety glasses, children's glasses, sports glasses, and glasses for monocular patients. Polycarbonate is extremely sensitive to scratches and almost always requires a secondary scratch-resistant coating. However, polycarbonate has an extremely low Abbe value (see next section) that can cause significant subjective visual disturbances when the patient looks through the edge of the lens.
- **Trivex (n = 1.54)** – this is one of the lightest lens materials available. It offers the same clarity and excellent impact resistance as polycarbonate but has a higher (favorable) Abbe value and UV protection.
- **Hi-index glass (n = 1.7–1.8)** – This is a generic term for various glass materials popular for high-power lenses. Due to their high index of refraction (>1.70), the lens can be thinner and lighter, especially at the lens edge, making them desirable in highly myopic patients.

Abbe Value

In the previous section, we hinted at some of the pros/cons of each lens material. One particular property deserves its own section because of its high clinical relevance. The **Abbe value** (aka V-number) measures a given material's inherent dispersion properties. Recall our discussion on dispersion in Chap. 1 "Geometric Optics", dispersion refers to the change in the angle of refraction of *each individual color of light* that comprises a "white" light ray. In other words, dispersion tells us how much the incoming light breaks up into the many colors of the rainbow; we want colors to stick together like our favorite band and not break off and try to make it on their own.

Why should we care about this? We ideally want to use a lens material that has low dispersion. If a material has *low dispersion*, it will have a *low chromatic aberration* and therefore a *high Abbe value*. Conversely, if a material has *high dispersion*, it will have a *high chromatic aberration* and therefore a *low Abbe value*. The Abbe value of the human eye is 45–50; therefore, lens materials with lower Abbe values can affect the quality of a patient's vision by increasing the amount of chromatic aberration a patient experiences when looking at the edge of the lens. It is important to note that objectively, a patient's visual acuity should not be affected by the lens material. However, if you have a "20/unhappy" patient, you should consider these types of things.

Why else should we care about this? If a patient has eyeglasses constructed of a lens material with **low Abbe values** (classic example; polycarbonate lenses), then because of chromatic aberration effects, these patients may complain of a "rainbow glare" or "blue off to the side" when wearing their glasses, especially when he/she looks through the edge of the lens. This phenomenon is known as "off-axis blue glare" and is due to transverse chromatic aberration – as if just regular chromatic aberration isn't bad enough! Remember this is an "edge of the lens problem": there should be minimal/no subjective complaints when the patient is looking through the optical center of the lens.

Therefore, a desirable lens will have a *low* chromatic aberration and a *high* Abbe value. Ironically, some new "high-index" lenses have low Abbe values. Abbe values of commonly used lens materials are included in Table 1. We should emphasize that you should just understand trends in this figure and not waste time memorizing individual Abbe value numbers for a given lens material. Note the low Abbe values for polycarbonate and "high-index" lenses.

Is there any other reason to care about this? Acrylic is the most common material used in popularly implanted IOLs

Table 1 Abbe values for selected lens materials used in eyeglasses

Lens material	Type	Index of refraction	Abbe value
CR-39	Plastic	1.498	58
Crown glass	Glass	1.523	58
Trivex	Plastic – High index	1.530	45
1.7 glass	Glass – High index	1.701	40
1.8 glass	Glass – High index	1.802	35
High index plastic	Plastic – High index	1.658	32
Polycarbonate	Plastic – High index	1.586	30

today, which also have higher indices of refraction (ranging from 1.47 to 1.55) than older-generation IOLs, such as silicone IOL, that have much lower indices of refraction (ranging from 1.39 to 1.429). These acrylic IOLs also tend to have low Abbe values (therefore, higher chromatic aberration) and higher rates of postoperative dysphotopsia.[1]

Lens Coatings

Lens coatings can be used to enhance the properties of eyeglasses further. Some common types of lens coatings include the following:

1. Antireflection coatings (see Chap. 14 "Physical Optics and Advanced Optical Principles") – a clear, thin film (approximately one-fourth the wavelength of incoming light so that incident light is reflected out of phase, producing destructive interference of any additional reflected light) can be applied to the lens surface that reduces undesirable reflections. This coating secondarily increases the amount of light that enters the eye. These may be particularly advantageous in high-index and polycarbonate lenses.
2. Edge coatings – edge coatings are a popular choice for high minus lenses with thick edges at the periphery. A color coating can be applied to the lens edge that hides some of the lens edge thickness and reduces some undesirable lens edge aberrations and reflections.
3. Mirror coatings – using various materials (such as magnesium fluoride or titanium oxide), several layers of constructive interference can be added to the outer surface of the lens in order to create a "mirror effect" similar to a two-way mirror. This coating will decrease the amount of total light that enters the lens, and the patient may report a "gray-brown" tint when wearing them. These are especially popular for patients who desire high visual acuity in bright light settings, such as police officers and helicopter pilots.
4. Scratch-resistant coatings – as discussed in the previous section, "softer" lens materials such as plastic may benefit from a scratch-resistant coating. Many newer materials, such as high-index glass and Trivex, have inherent scratch-resistant coatings. These coatings may be particularly advantageous in patients (such as ophthalmologists!) who constantly rub their eyeglasses against surfaces (such as slit-lamp eyepieces and operating microscopes).
5. UV-resistant coatings (aka UV 400) – a coating used to cause destructive interference of incoming UV light (300–400 nm) can also be used on eyeglasses. Since the cornea can absorb UV light, overexposure can cause photokeratitis and accelerate the development of cataracts in patients with high sunlight exposure (both direct and indirect), such as skiers. A UV-resistant coating may be helpful for patients who work (or have fun) in high-UV light settings.

[1] See Chap. 29 for more information regarding dysphotopsias.

Troubleshooting Glasses

Imagine the following scenario: you have just spent an hour and a half with your favorite patient, I.M. Grumpyface, performing a meticulous refraction (including a duochrome test), discussing various presbyopia-correcting options, and answering his page of questions that he obtained from the internet "doing his own research" regarding lens materials and lens coatings. You finally give him his prescription and are relieved that he walks out of your office, hoping that he never returns (or becomes a patient of your crosstown competitor). Your staff gives you death stares because there are 20 patients still waiting.

Instead, he returns two weeks later, fuming mad and unhappy with his glasses.

Does this sound familiar? This is an all too common scenario, even for ophthalmologists. Let's explore how we can troubleshoot glasses for the unhappy patient before he writes a bad review online.

Diagnosing Problems with Glasses

The following checklist is a (somewhat) logical way to check why a patient may complain about his/her glasses:

1. Check the new glasses:
   (a) Place glasses in a lensmeter or another device and check if the glasses were made correctly (correct sphere, cylinder, and axis as the dispensed refraction).
   (b) Check the base curve of the new glasses with a Geneva lens clock and ensure that the new glasses have a similar base curve as the old glasses.[2] Patients often use the word "fishbowl" or "swimming sensation" to describe their dislike of a different base curve.

[2] See Chap. 17, Optical Instruments, for a detailed discussion regarding lens clocks.

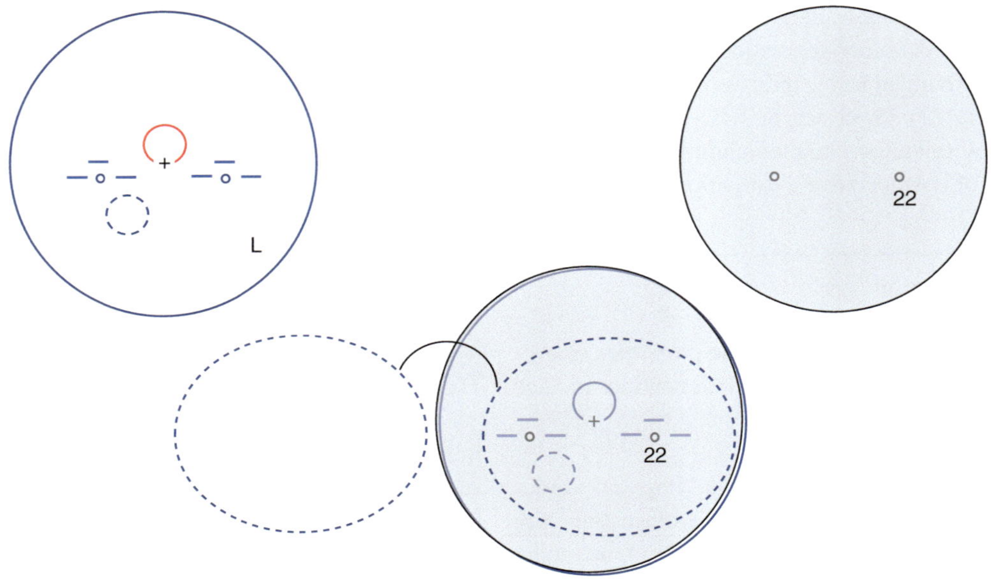

Fig. 1 Centration chart. *Top left* – a simplified centration chart, with the "+" sign indicating the optical center, the red circle indicating the area for best distance vision, and the dashed circle indicating where the pupillary center should be for reading at near. Horizontal bars additionally help to orient the lens. *Top right* – a progressive lens with +2.25 add prior to cutting. We can tell it is a *left eye* lens because the "22" watermark (short for +2.25) etching is located on the right side (temporal to the patient). *Bottom figure* – lens placed over the centration chart. This will help the optician know how to construct the lens for its final shape (dotted line)

   (c) Check the lens material to see if a different material (different index of refraction) or different/new coatings or tints are present.
   (d) Check the glasses to ensure that the *cylinder is ground on the back*. This teaching is somewhat a relic of older textbooks since most modern glasses, by convention, are made such that the cylinder is ground on the back surface of the lens.
   (e) Check to ensure that the cylinder power is placed in glasses in *minus cylinder* format. Again, this is a moot point for modern glasses because essentially, all glasses are constructed with this arrangement as it decreases meridional magnification and allows for bifocal segments to be placed on the front surface of the eyeglass lens.
2. Recheck the patient's refraction: perform a streak refraction or autorefraction and then recheck the manifest and cycloplegic refraction (especially for myopic patients):
   (a) Check vision with glasses on both at distance and at near.
   (b) Check the vision with glasses on both in dark and light settings.
   (c) If refractions match up, the patient may need additional time to adjust to the new prescription, especially if there has been a significant recent change in sphere, cylinder, or axis.[3]
3. Have the patient wear the glasses:
   (a) Check if the new glasses' frames are too big/too small for the patient's face; if the lenses are too thick/too thin; or if the patient has switched to a rimless frame, especially compared to the older glasses.
   (b) Check if the patient is looking through the optical center of the new glasses; otherwise, there may be an induced prismatic effect (Prentice's rule). This can be done by marking the pupil center with a dry-erase marker and finding the optical center with a lensmeter to ensure that they match.
   (c) Check the patient's pupillary distance (PD) and ensure that glasses were made such that the optical center aligns with the patient's PD. A centration chart (Fig. 1) may be helpful. Have the patient wear the new glasses and look at a distance target. Using a muscle light, ensure that the patient is looking through the optical center of the lenses (as confirmed with a lensmeter).
   (d) Check the fit of the frame, especially with pediatric patients:
      (i) Ensure that nose pads and nose bridge fit correctly. Look at the patient's facial anatomy and see if glasses are sliding down the nose or applying too much pressure to the nasal bridge.
      (ii) Ensure that the temples of the glasses are fitting snugly over the ears or check if the new frame has a different temple shape/size than the old glasses. Issues with glasses fitting at the ears may cause an unwanted tilt of the new glasses, leading to undesirable pantoscopic tilt issues.

[3]#ProTip – have the unhappy glass patient return when the next resident is on rotation.

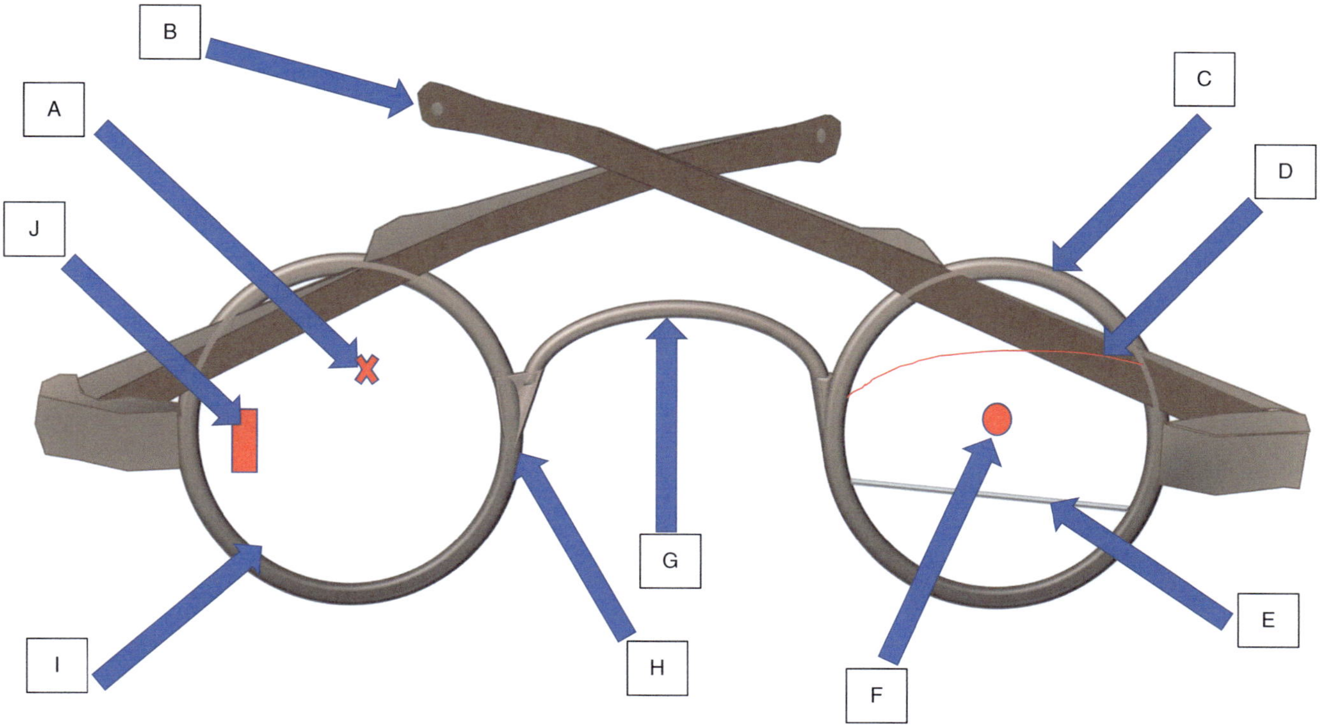

Fig. 2 Visual representation to spatially organize various problems in a pair of glasses. (**a**) Changes in the lens material (index of refraction and Abbe value issues); (**b**) problems with the temples causing pantoscopic tilt and fit issues; (**c**) problems with frames, such as too large/small, too thick/thin, and rimless frames; (**d**) changes in base curve, cylinder ground on the back of the lens, and changes in vertex distances; (**e**) problems with bifocals and progressive lenses; (**f**) problems with pupillary distance changes, optical center, and induced prismatic effects; (**g**) problems with the bridge of the nose and other facial anatomy; (**h**) problems with snug pads and other nasal anatomy; **i** problems at the edge of the lens, such as chromatic aberration, lens edge glare, etc.; and **j** problems with glare and lens coatings

(iii) Check if there is any facial anatomy (such as large brow, etc.) affecting the fit of the glasses or causing issues such as fogging.

(iv) Check to ensure there is no unwanted pantoscopic tilt or faceform issues that are affecting the patient's satisfaction with glasses.

(e) Check the vertex distance: using the distometer, make sure that the vertex distance of the new glasses is the same as the vertex distance of the old glasses.[4] This is especially important for higher prescriptions (both myopic and hyperopic), as discussed in Chap. 6 "Lens Effectivity".

(f) Ask the patient about glare and other subjective problems. These patients may benefit from a change or addition of coating(s).

(g) Ask the patient if he/she notices any subjective visual problems when looking at the edge of the lens. If so, there may be issues with the lens edge (such as a thick lens edge with high minus prescriptions, chromatic aberration with high index/polycarbonate materials, etc.).

4. Bifocals/progressives – see Chap. 12 "Glasses for Written Exams", for more details. There are several things worth mentioning here:
   (a) If this is the first time in bifocals or progressives (PAL), the patient may need additional time to adjust.
   (b) Check the type of bifocal/PAL given and see if there is a problem with image jump, image displacement, oblique astigmatism, etc.
   (c) Check the position of the bifocal segment, its relation to the optical center, vertex distance, and size in the context of the frame. For example, a patient who has switched to a smaller frame may now have a smaller (proportional) bifocal segment and may be unhappy with this "decreased real estate."
5. Other miscellaneous issues are as follows:
   (a) Scratches and defects.
   (b) Cost, frame colors, and cosmetic appearance. Patients are sometimes embarrassed to say they changed their minds about the frames, or perhaps they think they will not be charged for a different frame if they complain. Many street-smart opticians may ask, "do you think you would see better with a different frame?"

It may help to *visualize* all possible problems on a pair of glasses instead of memorizing a checklist (Fig. 2).

[4] See Chap. 17, Optical Instruments, for a discussion on the distometer and its clinical usage for vertex distance.

Slit-lamp examination of the patient may be helpful if the above checklist fails to reveal the problem. Specifically, we can consider the following (not an exhaustive list):

- Extraocular motility – new or decompensated phoria and convergence insufficiency.
- Eyelids – new ptosis may cause astigmatism; increased palpebral fissure height may exacerbate ocular surface dryness.
- Cornea – dry eye syndrome, epithelial irregularity, etc.
- Lens – lens opacity, posterior capsular opacification, etc.
- Retina – worsening of existing retinopathy (diabetes, AMD), ERM, etc.

Ancillary testing may also help detect the problem. While we can perform a million-dollar workup, tests that may be the most useful include corneal topography/tomography and ocular coherence tomography of the retina.

Fixing Problems with Glasses

Mr. I.M. Grumpyface is still unhappy with this exhaustive list of issues you have just rattled off. He is not impressed with your knowledge and instead wants to know how you can actually *fix* his glasses. The following is a list of options to fix glasses for the unhappy patient:

Always start by repeating the refraction and ensuring that it is accurate. Assuming it is, then we can do the following:

1. Remake the glasses, especially if the prescription has changed or the new glasses were made incorrectly:
   (a) Physical changes to the glasses may be necessary; for example, changing the vertex distance (usually closer to the cornea), changing the lens material (index of refraction; higher index of refraction will give a thinner lens but may increase aberrations), changing/adding a lens coating, etc.
   (b) Change the base curve back to the old pair of glasses; for high minus lenses, a flatter base curve may be used for the front of the lens.
   (c) Grind the cylinder on the back portion of the lenses: as discussed in the previous section, this is a relic of days past.
   (d) Plastic lenses are thinner and lighter than "glass" lenses.
2. Change the lens edge for high minus or high plus lenses, especially if there is an induced prismatic effect:
   (a) "Slab-off" – this is a favorite term for people to throw around in didactic conversations. What does it actually mean? Slab-off is done for high minus lenses with thick edges. Basically, we can **grind/thin out the lens edge** so it's not so thick anymore. If a patient has base-down prism effects in a high minus lens when looking down, we can slab-off the high minus lens to create a bit of a base-up effect.
   (b) "Reverse slab-off" – this is yet another favorite term for people to throw around in didactic conversations. It is basically the opposite of slab-off; therefore, we can do this to the more plus-power lens to give some base-down effect. In the optician world, **reverse slab-off is more commonly done** in practice because it is easier to do in the optical lab.
   (c) The lens edge may also be beveled or polished to improve glare and chromatic aberration issues.
3. Change the frame type – if anatomical considerations are the reason, switching to more ergonomically comfortable frames may solve the problem:
   (a) Larger frames (especially for high plus lenses) are usually better than smaller frames, especially if the unhappiness is due to problems at the edge of the lens (that is noticeable in the field of vision). By making frames larger, we can shift the problematic edge of the lens outside the patient's field of vision.
   (b) Somewhat paradoxically, for **highly myopic patients**, we can consider switching to a **smaller frame** to force the patient to look through the optical center and avoid looking around toward the edge of the lens. Smaller frames don't work well for high plus-power lenses.
   (c) Rimless/thin frames can be switched to thicker frames that can better hide the lens's edge, especially for high minus-power lenses.
   (d) Adjust the vertex distance as needed. We may not give much consideration to vertex distance for low power prescriptions, but this plays a significant role in high plus- and minus-power lenses.
4. Astigmatism issues are as follows:
   (a) Suppose there has been a significant recent change in the cylinder correction. We can attempt to decrease the cylinder power while sacrificing some visual acuity (~20/25–20/30) if the patient is not at risk for amblyopia.
   (b) Suppose there has been a recent change in the axis. We can try to rotate the cylinder closer to 90 degrees or 180 degrees to avoid diplopia and oblique astigmatism issues with the oblique cylinder. However, any change in cylinder axis in a patient 20–40 years of age should warrant a workup for possible corneal ectasia.
   (c) Some patients may need reassurance to get used to the change in cylinder amount and cylinder axis. For pediatric patients at risk for amblyopia, the full correction (including the axis) must be given; we can't play around and get all fancy due to the amblyopia risk.
5. Bifocal issues are as follows:
   (a) Image jump/displacement can be addressed accordingly if a round-top and/or flat-top has been given erroneously to a patient.
   (b) Switch the patient to an executive lens or PAL.

(c) Consider a trifocal pair of glasses for patients with high demands for intermediate vision who are willing to sacrifice "real estate" in their glasses.

(d) Prescribe separate glasses for distance and near vision. This solution is beneficial for patients with convergence insufficiency who need a base-in (BI) prism to avoid diplopia at near. These patients can have BI prism for the near glasses and no prism correction in distance glasses.

6. Prescribe separate glasses for distance and reading, night and day vision, and indoor and outdoor activities (e.g., changing tints or lens coatings). For example, suppose a patient needs glasses for night-time distance needs, such as long-distance driving or playing night-time sports. In that case, an additional pair of glasses with extra minus power may be considered to overcome potential problems with night myopia.[5]
7. Contact lenses, including monovision and multifocal contact lenses.
8. Refractive surgery may be considered as a last resort after all of the above options have been thoroughly discussed.

Problems with High Minus- and High Plus-Power Glasses and Potential Solutions

While some of the material in this section may be repetitive, it may be helpful to separately lump together problems that may occur with high minus- and high plus-power lenses for rapid review.

Problems with High Minus-Power Glasses

There are six high-yield problems to memorize that may occur with high minus-power glasses. A useful mnemonic is "BAG of MMC":

1. **B**arrel distortion – light rays that pass through the thicker edge of a high minus-power lens may cause the patient to experience a "barrel distortion" (see Chap. 1, "Geometric Optics"). Remember that real light rays are bent toward the base (edge of a minus lens), so central rays (passing through the thinner central portion of the lens) will seem to come in focus closer to the center as compared to the peripheral rays that will seem like they are "bent" toward the edge of the lens. We can also think of distortion as a disparity in linear magnification for paraxial light rays versus peripheral rays. The central light rays will be more minified than the peripheral light rays in myopic glasses. Therefore, the peripheral rays may appear "pushed out" towards the periphery.
2. **A**ppearance of glasses (thick lenses, especially at the edges).
3. **G**lare at the edge of lens – chromatic aberration.
4. **M**inification – recall that a myope is looking at the world through a reverse Galilean telescope (see Chap. 8, "Magnification and Telescopes"), so objects will appear smaller to her (as compared to an emmetrope).
5. **M**akes face smaller to others – recall that the temporal edge of a high minus-power lens is basically a base-out prism; therefore, virtual images will appear to be displaced toward the apex of the prism. For an observer looking at a patient wearing high minus lenses, the patient's temporal face/cheek may appear to be shifted ("smashed in") toward the nose. High minus lenses may create an undesirable cosmetic effect that the patient may be concerned about (Fig. 3).
6. **C**ost – to paraphrase a famous rapper from the 1990s, "More money, more problems." These lenses may require a significant financial investment from patients.

Ten things to consider in *improving high minus glasses* are as follows:

1. Perform a cycloplegic refraction and duochrome test to make sure the patient is not overminused.

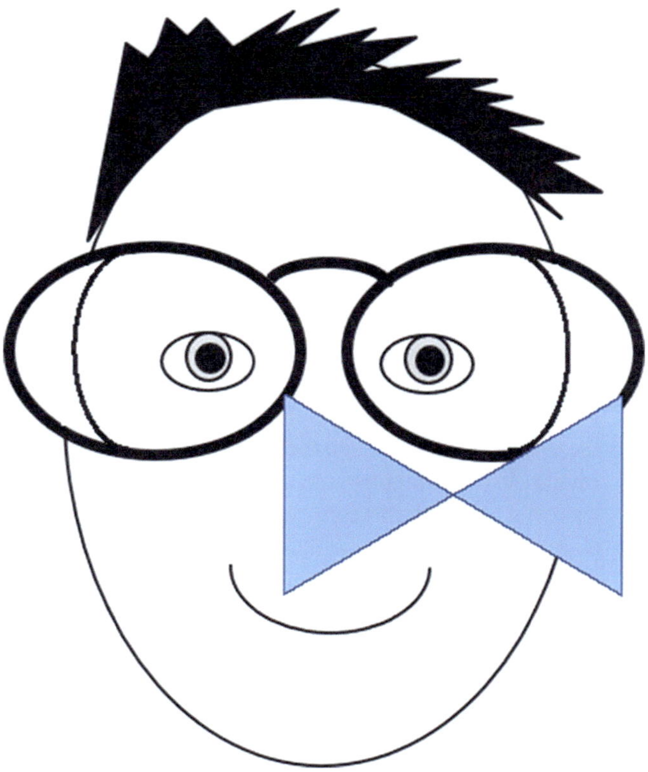

Fig. 3 An observer looking at a patient wearing high minus-power lenses may notice that the face appears to be shifted toward the nose ("smashed in" appearance) due to prismatic effects. Recall that the image of this patient's face is a virtual image to the observer; virtual images are shifted toward the apex of the prism

[5]See Chap. 21 Clinical Problems with Optics and Refractive Manifestations, for a more detailed discussion regarding causes and treatments of night myopia.

2. Smaller frames – these provide a smaller field of view but may force the patient to use the pure optical center of the lens and avoid looking toward the edge of the lens.
3. Larger frames – these push the edge of the lens out of the field of view. Yes, this is the opposite answer of the previous choice, but we discussed why both options might work in the preceding section.
4. Thicker frames – these may help to hide the edge of the lens better.
5. Polishing the edge of the lens – this may help with glare and chromatic aberration complaints.
6. Beveling/slab-off – this may help with prismatic effects encountered at the thick edge of a high minus-power lens.
7. Plastic (or lighter lens material) – this decreases the weight of the lens.
8. Flatter base curve for the front of lens.
9. Decrease the vertex distance.
10. Non-glasses options – contact lenses and refractive surgery. Again, for exam purposes, save this answer as the last option after you have thoroughly discussed the previous options.

Problems with High Plus-Power Glasses

There are ten high-yield problems to memorize that may occur with high plus-power glasses. We apologize, but we could not come up with a clever mnemonic to help you remember this:

1. Ring scotoma – secondary to prismatic effects. See below for a more detailed explanation.
2. Jack-in-the-box phenomenon – this goes hand in hand with ring scotoma. See below for a more detailed explanation.
3. Pincushion distortion – light rays that pass through the thinner edge of a high plus-power lens may cause the patient to experience a "pincushion distortion." Remember that real light rays are bent toward the base (in this case, the center of a high plus-power lens), so the central rays will reach the retina first. The peripheral rays will seem to focus much further away than the central rays – they will seem to be pulled away from the central visual axis. We can also think of distortion as a disparity in linear magnification for paraxial light rays vs. peripheral rays. In hyperopic glasses, central light rays will be more magnified, and peripheral rays will be less so, seemingly "pulled" out toward the periphery.
4. Spherical and chromatic aberration issues – due to optical effects at the edge of the lens.
5. Field of vision reduction – because of the four above issues, the edge of the lens is an optically problematic area for a hyperope. As a result, only the "center" of the lens is functional, so the patient may report a reduction in the field of vision.

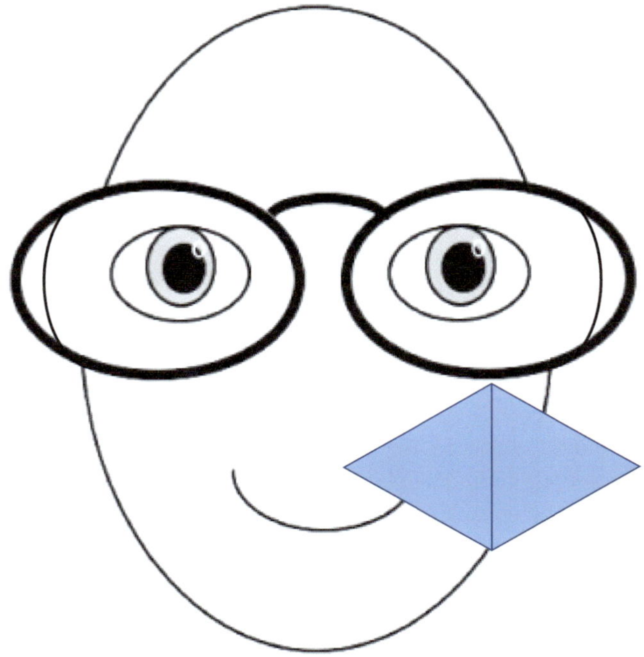

Fig. 4 An observer looking at a patient wearing high plus lenses may notice that the face appears to be shifted out toward the ear ("bug-eyed" appearance) due to prismatic effects. Recall that the image of this patient's face is a virtual image to the observer; virtual images are shifted toward the apex of the prism

6. Magnification – recall that a hyperope is looking at the world through a Galilean telescope, so objects will appear larger to her (as compared to an emmetrope).
7. Cosmetic considerations – recall that the temporal edge of a high plus lens is basically a base-in prism; therefore, virtual images appear to be displaced toward the apex of the prism (the patient's ear). For an observer looking at a patient wearing high plus lenses, the patient's temporal face/cheek may appear to be larger and shifted toward the ear ("bug-eyed appearance"). This may create an undesirable cosmetic effect (Fig. 4).
8. Increased convergence demands – when the patient wants to read, he will look through the nasal portion of the high plus lens, which creates an unwanted base-out prismatic effect. The patient will therefore have to converge more in order to compensate.
9. Weight of high plus glasses.
10. Cost. Again, more money, more problems.

It is helpful to discuss two problems mentioned above in a bit more detail. It is helpful to view these problems together as each helps explain the other.

Ring Scotoma (aka "Roving" Ring Scotoma) As discussed above, the edge of a high plus lens has base-in prismatic effects (for the patient). Real light rays are bent toward the base of a prism. As the power of the lens increases, there is increased refraction of incoming light rays towards the "base" of the two prisms that comprise the lens (known as angle alpha). Due to a large angle alpha, we can observe that light rays that hit the edge of the lens are bent so significantly toward the center of the lens (the base of the prism) that they never reach the retina, and thus the patient never "sees" them. Since the edge of the lens is shaped like a ring, this is perceived by the patient as a "ring scotoma." It is sometimes called a "roving ring scotoma" because the scotoma blocks objects of interest in the peripheral visual field, so the patient tries to look "around" it, but the scotoma also constantly moves; this can be very frustrating for the patient. This is why using a larger frame (such that the edge of the lens is outside the field of vision) may alleviate this problem.

Jack-in-the-Box (JITB) Phenomenon The JITB phenomenon is easy to understand in the context of the previous discussion on ring scotoma. Basically, when a patient wearing high plus-power lenses wants to look at an interesting object located in the peripheral visual field, he may move his eyes toward the object. As the eye moves toward the object, the image may momentarily land in the ring scotoma area and disappear; but then, as the patient continues to move his eye further, the image is no longer in the scotoma, so it appears in the visual field again. This sudden disappearance and reappearance of objects in the peripheral visual field is known as the JITB phenomenon. Like the childhood (or creepy!) toy, the object disappears and appears. JITB can be very frustrating for the patient, especially when considering peripheral vision needs for activities such as driving (e.g., seeing street signs, cars in parallel lanes, etc.). Again, this is why using a larger frame (such that the edge of the lens is outside the field of vision) may alleviate this problem.

Improving High Plus-Power Glasses As you may have sensed a theme in this entire textbook, it is no fun being a hyperope. There are a limited number of things we can do to improve high plus lenses:

1. Change frame design and size: as discussed previously, larger frames work exceptionally well for hyperopic patients because they can hide the edge of the lens, mainly to decrease problems such as ring scotoma and JITB. Unlike their myopic counterparts, using a smaller frame *will not* work well.
2. Change frame design: wraparound-style frames may also work because they may shift the edge of the frame out of the field of vision.
3. Switch to a high-index or lighter-weight material to decrease the weight. Usually, high plus-power lenses are heavier than their high minus-power lens counterparts.
4. Reverse slab-off: this can help with prismatic effects encountered at the edge of the lens.
5. Non-glasses options – contact lenses work extremely well in hyperopic patients, especially those with presbyopia, as they decrease the accommodative demand. Excimer laser refractive surgery has a lower rate of success in hyperopes than myopes. A secondary IOL may be an extremely effective option if a patient has hyperopia secondary to aphakia.

Custom Glasses

Mr. I.M. Grumpyface was so pleased with your abilities to troubleshoot and finally get him a pair of glasses that work. He has been telling everyone he knows about your skills, and your busy ophthalmology practice has now turned into a thriving optical shop. One of his referrals is Ms. Tara Daktyl, reportedly a "lady friend" of Mr. Grumpyface, looking for some custom glasses. She is a middle-aged female who is an electrician during the day and a concert pianist at night. Her hobbies include golfing, hunting, and fishing. She was told that you are the best in town and is eager for your advice on what kind(s) of glasses can help her visual needs.

Using Ms. Tara Daktyl as our starting point, we can discuss some options for "custom glasses" – creative, nontraditional ways to construct glasses with particular requirements for specific visual activities.

Nontraditional Bifocals (Occupational and Recreational Bifocals)

While we often assume that bifocals have to be made with a reading segment in the bottom portion of each lens, there are several options for nontraditional bifocals:

1. Glasses with bifocal segment(s) placed superiorly or superonasally. This option may be suitable for patients with occupational requirements (e.g., electricians, carpenters, car mechanics, etc.) for near work that involves looking upward (rather than downward for reading); these patients may therefore require near-vision correction when looking up rather than down. An add segment placed in the superior or superonasal portion of the lens (in one or both eyes) may help the patient with her near-vision needs when she is looking upward. Basically, these patients would have a "reverse bifocal" as the bottom portion would be for distance vision.
2. Glasses with a single bifocal segment placed inferiorly. This option may be viable for patients for activities requiring maximum field of vision for distance with a reduced bifocal area for quick, minimal near-vision needs. In other words, these patients may want a bifocal

segment for short periods of near vision, rather than prolonged periods of reading. For example, an avid presbyopic golfer (or a hunter) may only need to look at her scorecard momentarily to record her score; she may therefore want to maximize her distance vision during her recreational golf outings. Therefore, an add segment placed only in the inferonasal aspect of one lens (preferably the nondominant eye) will allow her to look down for quick near-vision needs while maximizing distance vision, especially in the dominant eye.

3. Bifocals with modified near segments. Some patients may need a bifocal for assistance with intermediate vision (such as a concert pianist or stock trader looking at computer screens) rather than near vision. Therefore, a modified bifocal can be made with the inferior add segment set for *one-half* the required reading add power. For Ms. Daktyl, if she wears +2.50D for near vision, we can construct her a pair of glasses when she plays the piano such that the bottom "add" is instead +1.25 (allowing her to look at sheet music), and the top portion of the glasses have the full distance vision correction (e.g., to look at the conductor). Such glasses may not be helpful for near-vision needs.

We have now given Ms. Daktyl three additional pairs of glasses for her various occupational and recreational needs. She is thrilled and purchases three $1200 frames to go with each prescription you have given her. At this rate, you may never need to see patients with actual pathology or do eye surgery ever again.

Other Modifications for Glasses

Like the gift that keeps giving, Mr. Grumpyface's referral patients keep coming in. A young man named Jed I. Knight (dressed in a brown, hooded robe) comes in asking for a pair(s) of glasses that will help with the following activities:

- Optimizing vision at dawn and dusk when he performs specific training exercises, such as handstands.
- Optimizing vision in low-light conditions as he navigates through an unknown swamp searching for a little green man.
- Optimizing vision while running back and forth between indoors and outdoors – because who knows?
- Reading a novel while sunbathing – it could happen?
- Optimizing vision while sailing on his yacht – yeah, we also don't know why he does this.

As you contemplate telling him to go elsewhere, he responds: "If you send me out, I shall become more powerful than you can possibly imagine."

His list of demands serves as a helpful starting point to introduce a few other things we can do for glasses: tints, gradients, and polarization.

Tints in Glasses

Tints in glasses are a somewhat controversial and evolving subject. The basic principle is to use tints (colors) in eyeglass lenses to preferentially block specific wavelengths of light to improve patients' subjective vision. For example, blocking shorter wavelengths (blue) may help reduce eyestrain and headaches in patients with extreme photosensitivity. It is known that blue wavelengths may additionally trigger special cells (intrinsically photosensitive retinal ganglion cells, IPRGCs) besides rods and cones that may be abnormally activated in patients with severe photophobia.[6] It has been shown that increased activation of IPRGCs may exacerbate photophobia. Among various tints, the FL-41 is a reddish-pink tint that has been used since the 1990s that has been shown to have usefulness in treating certain patient populations with photosensitivity and eyestrain.[7]

Historically, tints have been used to treat patients with various ophthalmic, neurological, psychological, and psychiatric diseases with varying degrees of success. More relevant to routine ophthalmic practice, removing a cataract (and the patient's intrinsic light filter) may be one reason why some patients report photophobia immediately after cataract surgery. Some authors have reported successful usage of tints in patients with ophthalmic diseases such as blepharospasm, achromatopsia, and cone dystrophies.

While a variety of options exist, there are several tint colors that we should be familiar with: FL-41, dark gray (smoke), brown (amber), and yellow. Dark gray and brown tints can be interchangeable for all intents and purposes:

- **FL-41 (boysenberry color) tints** – as previously mentioned, these tints block blue wavelengths of light and may be especially useful in patients with clinically significant photophobia and photosensitive neurological diseases (e.g., epilepsy, etc.).
- **Dark gray (smoke) tints** are meant for daytime wear in bright sunlight conditions. They may help to decrease brightness, especially from sunlight, without compromising color quality.
- **Brown (amber) tints** are meant for daytime wear on cloudy days or sunset/sunrise type of lighting conditions.
- **Yellow tints** are controversial as they are purported to enhance depth perception and visibility in low-light conditions – this is why they are a preferred color for safety glasses used in dim-light conditions, such as coal-mining safety glasses. However, they may filter out a large portion of blue wavelengths of light, subjectively giving patients

[6]Raabe J, Kini A, Lee AG. Optical lens tinting – a review of its functional mechanism, efficacy, and applications. *US Ophthalmic Review* 2019; 12: 85–87

[7]Wilkins AJ, Wilkinson P. A tint to reduce eye-strain from fluorescent lighting? Preliminary observations. *Ophthalmic Physiol Opt.* 1991;11:172–5

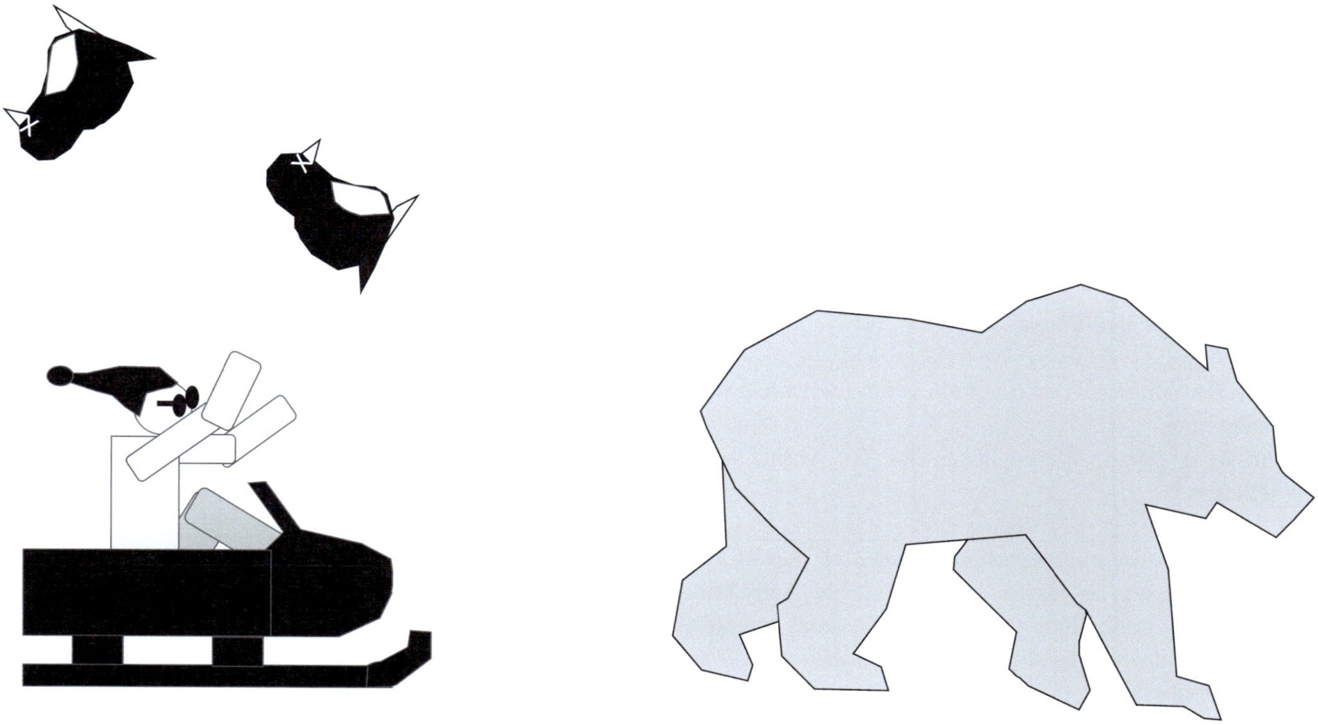

Fig. 5 Photochromic lenses are *not* recommended for outdoor activities in cold settings, such as snowmobiling, as the lenses may become too dark for the user and obscure vision. This is not good for penguins and polar bears encountered during such activities. Of note, no animals were hurt in the production of this book, and yes, we know polar bears and penguins would not be found in the same location

the impression of improved contrast vision in bright-light settings. Even more controversial, they are said to help "soothe strained eyes" from computer vision syndrome. However, research performed in simulated settings such as nighttime driving conditions has not demonstrated improved performance in subjects. At the time of this writing, there is no substantial evidence to suggest that yellow tints in standard glasses have anything more than a placebo or "cool-guy" fashion sense effect in patients.[8]

Photochromic lenses are a separate category of tints that can be lumped into this discussion. These lenses have molecules within the lens substance that automatically adjust the color based on light exposure; they can "transition" between darker tints outdoors and lighter/no tint indoors. A significant advantage of these lenses is that they allow a patient to use one pair of glasses for both indoor and outdoor needs. They also block nearly 100 percent of incoming UVA/UVB light. One disadvantage is that these lenses do not function as well as actual sunglasses outdoors; an actual pair of sunglasses may be optimal for prolonged outdoor activities. Another disadvantage is that these lenses may not work as well in bright environments with windows that block UV light (such as car windows) because windows may block some of the incoming light that stimulates the lens to change color – the photochromic tint may take several minutes to work. This delay may lead to frustration for the patient. As a final warning, lenses may become too dark in a cold outdoor setting, such as during skiing or snowmobiling (Fig. 5). A variety of photochromic tint options are commercially available.

Gradient Modification for Glasses

A gradient modification can be added to sunglasses such that the top of the lens is the darkest while the bottom of the lens has a very minimal tint (or even no tint). A gradient allows the patient to have the full benefit of sunglasses at the top of the glasses while allowing for better visibility in the lower portion of the lens. For example, this may be a valuable modification for patients who enjoy reading while sunbathing: the top portion of the glasses will provide sunlight protection and good distance vision, while the bottom portion of the lens has a minimal tint to provide greater visibility for near vision and reading.

Polarization for Sunglasses

We have previously discussed polarization filters in Chap. 14 "Physical Optics and Advanced Optical Principles". To review, vertically oriented polarization filters are commonly used in polarized sunglasses. A vertical filter will block most of the horizontally scattered light (such as incoming light off the surface of a lake) while allowing in vertically oriented light, making them an excellent choice for sunglasses used

[8]Hwang AD, Tuccar-Burak M, Peli E. Comparison of Pedestrian Detection With and Without Yellow-Lens Glasses During Simulated Night Driving With and Without Headlight Glare [published online ahead of print, 2019 Aug 1]. *JAMA Ophthalmol.* 2019;137(10):1147–1153

outdoors (e.g., when captaining a yacht on a bright sunny day).

Returning to our friend, Jed I. Knight, we can therefore prescribe the following tints, gradients, and other modifications:

- Prescribe brown (amber) tints for dawn/dusk activities.
- Prescribe yellow tints for his swamp (low-light condition) activities.
- Prescribe photochromic tints for his indoor-outdoor activities.
- Prescribe sunglasses with a gradient tint for reading while sunbathing.
- Prescribe polarized sunglasses for his yacht sailing activities.

After you write him prescriptions for each pair of these specialized glasses and as you begin to tally his hefty bill at checkout, you notice him waving his right hand and softly say: "These are not the dollars you are looking for." You don't remember much of what happened after that.

Glasses in Special Circumstances

We can conclude this chapter by discussing strategies for glasses for patients in special circumstances. Usually, this is addressed by a skilled optometrist or a low vision specialist in real life. While we may never actually have to do this in clinical practice, an understanding and appreciation for our colleagues' thought processes and strategies are worthwhile. Many vision pathologies may benefit from customized glasses, but there are also numerous ways to help a patient depending on the disease. A full review of all potential glasses options for every ophthalmic disease is beyond the scope of this text.

Consider three sample patients and different types of glasses that can benefit each.

Glasses for a Patient with Albinism There are several factors to consider for a patient with albinism: high incidence of refractive errors, astigmatism, nystagmus, and glare issues. Strategies for prescribing glasses to these patients include:

1. Due to these patients' photophobia/glare issues, *polarized sunglasses* for outdoors (along with headgear with a visor) can be extremely beneficial. Sunglasses may be accordingly *tinted* and/or have a *mirror coating*.
2. *Photochromic lenses with dark tint outdoors and light tint indoors* (as opposed to clear lenses indoors) may also be helpful for a single pair of glasses. Different tints may be helpful based on the activity, for example, light blue tints may be helpful for indoor lighting (school, workplace), whereas dark brown/smoke-gray tints may be helpful for outdoor activities.
3. Due to nystagmus issues, *contact lenses* may give better vision than glasses. Soft toric and rigid gas-permeable lenses may especially help neutralize moderate-severe corneal astigmatism.
4. *Handheld telescopes* may be useful for school-age patients (see Chap. 5 "Power of Lenses in Different Media", Chap. 19 "Low Vision and Vision Rehabilitation").
5. Other strategies to reduce glare include *screen tints* on computers and *yellow paper* (instead of white paper) for classroom work.
6. We must also remember that due to a limited BCVA, some patients with albinism will not appreciate the effect of glasses. A trial frame in the office is often helpful before finalizing the prescription.

Glasses for a Patient with Achromatopsia (aka "Rod Monochromatism") Recall that only the rods are functioning in these patients, and no cones are functioning. Rods are tolerant to red light because bright light will bleach out the rods. Therefore, using a *dark-red tint* on glasses will transmit red wavelengths of light, protect the rods, and allow the patient to utilize the rods' abilities for maximum vision.

As an added wrinkle, a subset of achromatopsia patients is blue-cone monochromats. In these patients, *both* the rods and blue cones are functioning. If we only used a red tint, we would lose out on the potential function of the healthy blue cones. Therefore, using a *magenta tint* will allow the patient to use both rods and blue cones to maximize vision potential.

Glasses for a Patient with Congenital Stationary Night Blindness (CSNB) CSNB refers to a group of nonprogressive retinal disorders characterized by an abnormal or absent function of the rod system; basically, *only* the cones are functioning. In these patients, using *yellow tint glasses* will maximize the peak sensitivity of yellow (560 nm) among red cones (which peak technically at the yellow portion of the electromagnetic spectrum; see Chap. 14 "Physical Optics and Advanced Optical Principles") and partially among green cones. Using a yellow tint/filter may interfere with color discrimination but maximize visual acuity potential in these patients.

Practice Questions

1. A 50-year-old patient (−4.00D myope) states she gets new headaches with her new single vision distance glasses when she uses them for driving and while she is binge-watching her favorite TV series.

You check the lenses and measure that both are −4.00 D sphere. You check her visual acuity with glasses at distance as 20/30 and at near as 20/60. A repeat refraction shows −4.00D sphere OU (20/20) in the phoropter. When you perform the duochrome test, she states that green letters are bolder than red with glasses on. Which of the following is the most likely cause of this patient's symptoms?
   A. The new frames have a shorter vertex distance.
   B. The new lenses have a different base curve.
   C. There is Jack-in-the-box (JITB) effect caused by the new frames.
   D. She is experiencing problems because of unmet accommodative needs in the new glasses; she should switch to a progressive or bifocal lens.
2. A 14-year-old patient presents with subjective complaints of poor vision after recently getting a new pair of glasses. He states: "It looks like I am looking through a fishbowl." On exam today, his vision is 20/20 with glass prescription +2.00 + 1.00 X 090 OU. Repeat manifest refraction is the same, yielding 20/20 corrected visual acuity OU. The patient is ortho without correction at both near and far. Which of the following is the most likely cause of this patient's symptoms?
   A. The patient likely has latent hyperopia and should have a cycloplegic refraction.
   B. The vertex distance may be too large and should be checked with a distometer.
   C. The patient is probably describing a ring scotoma given his hyperopic prescription.
   D. The problem is due to new lenses with a different base curve.
3. Which of the following statements is *true* regarding the construction of specialty glasses?
   A. A gradient modification is an effective substitute for polarized sunglasses for a patient who is an avid sailboater.
   B. FL-41 tints may be useful for patients with clinically significant photophobia.
   C. Most modern polarized sunglasses are made with horizontal filters in order to effectively block horizontally scattered light.
   D. A photochromic tint works equally well for outdoor activities and driving.
4. For each of the following complaints, indicate whether it is more likely to be reported by a patient wearing −10.00D OU glasses (A) or + 10.00D OU glasses (B):
   - Roving ring scotoma – ____.
   - Pincushion distortion – ____.
   - Minification of viewed objects – _____.
   - Barrel distortion – _____.
   - Magnification of viewed objects – _____.
   - Complaints of peripheral objects in the distance "suddenly" appearing – ______.
5. Which of the following statements is *true*?
   A. For a patient with a – 8.00D sphere prescription OU, a flatter base curve for the front of the lens may be helpful.
   B. Reverse slab-off means to grind or shave down edges of a high minus lens.
   C. Switching to a smaller frame is a very effective way to solve problems of a ring scotoma and Jack-in-the-box effect in patients with hyperopic prescriptions.
   D. Spherical and chromatic aberration effects are more likely at the center of a pair of glasses.

Answers

1. Answer: A. Results of the duochrome test indicate that the patient has been overminused ("green add plus" from the "RAM-GAP" mnemonic). However, the dilemma appears to be that glasses' power and repeat refraction are the same, yet the patient demonstrates signs of "extra" minus power. Due to lens effectivity, a minus-power lens will gain power if it is closer to the eye. In this scenario, it is likely that a shorter vertex (answer choice A) is causing the −4.00D lens to behave like a −5.00D lens (approximately). Restoring the old vertex distance should alleviate the problem. A different base curve (choice B) may cause problems such as a "swimming sensation," but would not cause a decrease in BCVA. The JITB effect (Choice C) is seen in patients with high plus-power glasses for objects in the distant peripheral field of vision, not with reading vision. Patients who are overminused may also experience problems with unmet needs of accommodation (choice D). However, the patient does not seem to be complaining about these issues in the question stem.
2. Answer: D. When a new base curve is introduced, the patient will often complain of a "fishbowl" effect (choice D). The remaining findings on the exam, including the lack of a tropia or phoria, further reinforce that the problem seems to be coming from the new glasses. Latent hyperopia (choice A) may cause blurred near vision and headaches, and usually manifests in patients after age 30. A longer vertex distance (choice B) would cause blurred distance vision. A ring scotoma (choice C) would be expected in high hyperopia and mainly with peripheral vision at distance.
3. Answer: B. The FL-41 tint (boysenberry color, answer choice B) preferentially blocks shorter wavelengths (blue) of light and may decrease activation of specialized cells (IPRGCs) that may be "overactivated" in patients with significant photophobia. A gradient modification (choice A) consists of a "dark tint" at the top of the lens with a

gradual decrease toward the bottom of the lens that has almost no tint at all. It can be useful for patients who enjoy activities such as outdoor reading in sunlight, as it provides some "sunglasses" like protection at the top of the lens while allowing for a relatively clear "inferior" reading portion. However, it does not offer the same benefits of a polarized pair of sunglasses that would more effectively block horizontally scattered light throughout the entirety of the lenses. Modern polarized sunglasses (choice C) contain vertically oriented filters that block horizontally scattered portions of incoming light, thereby allowing the vertically scattered (a minority portion of incoming light) to pass through the filter. A photochromic tint (choice D) may not work as well during driving as compared to outdoor activities. During outdoor activities, there is more "incoming light" to better activate the photochromic tint. The tints may not effectively or efficiently activate in a "dim-bright light" condition such as driving inside the car on a sunny day (due to light-blocking effects of the car roof, windshield, etc.).

4. Answer: The patient with −10.00D (pathological myope) is most likely to complain of a barrel distortion (B) and minification of viewed objects (B). The patient with +10.00D (high hyperope) is most likely to complain of a roving ring scotoma (A), pincushion distortion (A), magnification of viewed objects (A), and sudden appearance (A) of peripheral objects in the distance ("Jack-in-the-box" effect).
5. Answer: A. For high minus-power prescriptions, a flatter base curve for the front of the lens, as compared to the back of the lens, may improve subjective comfort and visual acuity. Slab-off (choice B) is a modification customarily done to high minus lenses: as these lenses have thick edges (compared to the thinner center), grinding/thinning out the edge of the lens may help alleviate problems at the lens periphery (prismatic effects) and lens edge (spherical/chromatic aberration). In modern optical practice, reverse slab-off is more frequently done: in this strategy, the edge of the plus lens is modified to give less base-down effect. In general, switching to a larger frame (especially one such that the edge of the lens is outside the patient's field of view) can be helpful for both myopic and hyperopic prescriptions. For the hyperope, a larger frame (choice C) can help minimize negative effects of ring scotoma and JITB effect. Spherical and chromatic aberrations (choice D) mainly occur at the peripheral edge of the lens.

Optical Instruments and Machines

G. Vike Vicente

Objectives

- To understand the optical principles involved in the development and usage of commonly encountered instruments in ophthalmic practice
- To know the components of the retinoscope and how to perform retinoscopy
- To know how to use the lensmeter to measure the power of single-vision, bifocal, and progressive glasses
- To review the various components of the phoropter
- To discuss advantages and disadvantages of trial frames
- To survey the optics involved in the construction and clinical usage of the direct and indirect ophthalmoscopes
- To review important components of the slit lamp, including correlation with previously discussed concepts, such as the telescope and prisms
- To discuss how to use the manual keratometer, as well as review advantages and disadvantages of this device
- To be able to assemble the optical instruments required by an eye care professional in a worst case/zombie apocalypse scenario

Introduction

We would like to start this chapter with a true anecdote about ophthalmic instruments. On the first day of his fellowship, one of the authors had the following conversation:

- Chairman – Please go measure the prism in this patient's glasses.
- New fellow – I'm sorry I do not know how.
- Chairman – You've never seen prism glasses before?
- New fellow- Oh! I've seen prism glasses before, but my residency program never taught us how to measure the prisms.
- Chairman – In three years, they never taught you? Shame on them!
- New fellow – Yes sir!
- Chairman – In three years, you never asked?

Since we have all these interesting ophthalmic gadgets in our clinics, we owe it to ourselves to understand what optical principles went into their development and implementation. Most importantly, we must learn how to use them properly.

Let's start the tour.

Retinoscope

Technical Components

A retinoscope is a portable, handheld instrument that allows the clinician to measure a patient's refractive error, detect regular/irregular astigmatism, assess the red reflex, and quickly screen for intraocular pathology (e.g., cataract, lenticular/retinal tumor, etc.)

Retinoscopy (a.k.a. skiascopy) is a technique wherein the retinoscope is used to objectively measure the refractive error present in a patient's eye(s). This is especially useful for pediatric, non-verbal, and physically handicapped patients who are unable to undergo subjective refraction at the phoropter. Retinoscopy may also be employed during an exam under anesthesia to assess refractive error in the operating room. A skilled retinoscopist may even be able to successfully refract patients with large spherical and cylindrical errors, such as patients with keratoconus, even when autorefractors and wavefront aberrometers fail! Retinoscopes produce a streak of light that reflects from the posterior fundus back through the eye toward the observer. By observing both the streak of light and the red reflex coming out of the eye simultaneously, the observer is able to determine both the

G. V. Vicente (✉)
Clinical Pediatrics and Ophthalmology Georgetown University Hospital, Washington, DC, USA

Eye Doctors of Washington, Chevy Chase, MD, USA
e-mail: vvicente@edow.com

K. M. Riaz et al. (eds.), *Optics for the New Millennium*, https://doi.org/10.1007/978-3-030-95251-8_17

patient's refractive error (myopic, hyperopia, and astigmatism) and accommodative ability.

The retinoscope is one of the oldest instruments still used in modern ophthalmic practice. This instrument was invented in the 1800s using candles to produce a spot of light. These spot retinoscopes have largely been replaced by **streak retinoscopes** so we will focus on the latter. Today, all retinoscopes have similar components (Fig. 1):

Several notes about the retinoscope are as follows:

- The crossed polarizing filter is helpful to cut down on reflections and allows retinoscopy to be performed closer to the axis of the correcting lens. It is rarely used in clinical practice but may be used in special situations, such as corneal ectasia, wherein the reflex may be skewed and may require an additional filter.
- The streak retinoscope may be converted into a spot retinoscope with a special bulb. Some practitioners may find a spot retinoscope to be easier to use for large vision screenings and assessing pediatric patients as this technique can help detect refractive error quickly without relying on patient fixation. In addition, a spot retinoscope may function as a poor man's keratometer/topographer and yield information about the tear film, corneal power, etc.
- The retinoscope sleeve can be moved up or down. Depending on the manufacturer of the retinoscope, "sleeve up" or "sleeve down" will correspond with a divergent light ("thick beam," a.k.a. "the fat guy") or a convergent light ("thin beam," a.k.a. "the thin guy") (Fig. 2). In general, we will want to use "the fat guy" to perform retinoscopy.[1]

If "the fat guy" (diverging light) is used 95% of the time, why do we need two sleeve settings? In other words, is there ever a time to use "the thin guy"? Yes, dear reader, using a narrow beam is advantageous in certain situations, such as determining the exact axis of astigmatism in the phoropter or trial frame (Fig. 3).

The sleeve can also rotate, making it easy to rotate the streak to check for astigmatic power at different degrees (Fig. 4).

Principles of Retinoscopy

In order to perform retinoscopy, we need to determine if the red reflex is filling the pupil ("neutralization"), moving in the same direction as the streak ("with motion"), or in the opposite direction as the streak ("against motion") (Fig. 5).

[1]The thick beam means that the emitted light rays are slightly divergent and the instrument acts as a plano mirror. The thin beam will focus the emitted light and the instrument acts with a concave mirror effect wherein the light rays cross and then diverge. Therefore, because this light has already crossed, performing retinoscopy with the thin beam means that the examined eye's reflexes will move in the opposite direction as compared to when using the thick beam. The thin beam may be helpful in certain situations, such as determining the astigmatic axis off the phoropter of trial frame.

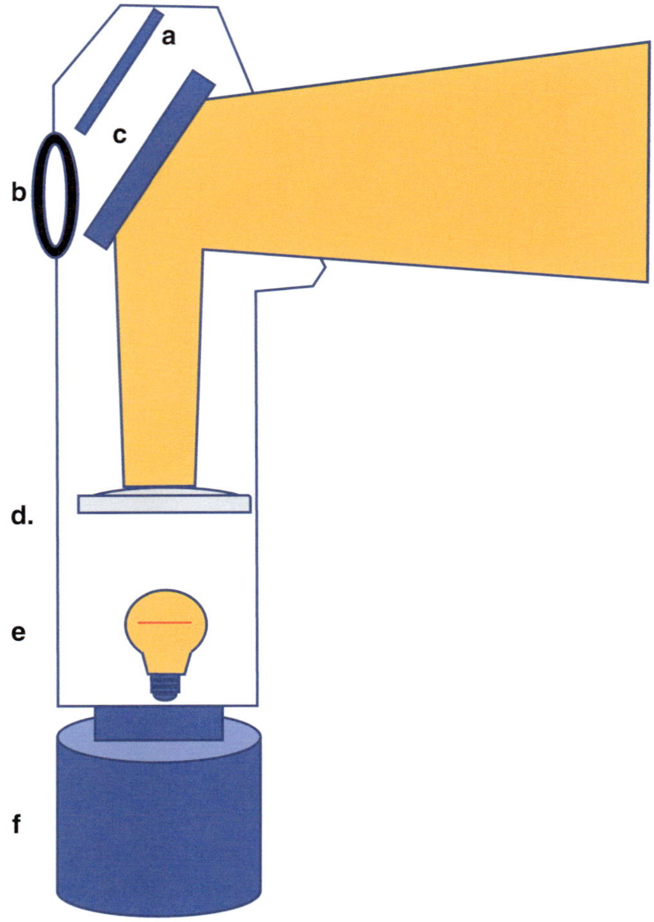

Fig. 1 Streak retinoscope components: (**a**) Crossed polarizing filter to reduce glare. (**b**) Examiner eyepiece. (**c**) Semitransparent mirror allows examiner's view to be coaxial to the streak. (**d**) (+) Condensing lens. (**e**) Linear filament bulb creates a linear streak of light. (**f**) Sleeve can rotate the filament and change the distance between the light and the lens making the light convergent or divergent

If the patient's far point is at the peephole, then the pupil will fill with a round red reflex as soon as the intercept reaches the pupil.

While doing retinoscopy. The observer should record his/her working distance from the patient. By convention, 66 cm is considered as the standard **working distance (WD)**; however, if you are taller or shorter, or prefer for your arm to be more extended or more flexed, your working distance may need to be adjusted accordingly. A fixed WD allows for a good view of the pupil and makes the math easier when determining the final prescription to be dispensed. In general, we can take the reciprocal of the WD and add **additional myopic sphere power** to the dispensed refraction. For example, if we set 66 cm as our WD, we would add an additional −1.5D sphere to the streak refraction; if we set 50 cm as our WD, we would add an additional −2D sphere to the streak refraction. Note: do not add any additional power to the cylinder or adjust the axis based on the working distance!

Here are some examples of streak refractions and dispensed refractions with an assumed WD of 66 cm:

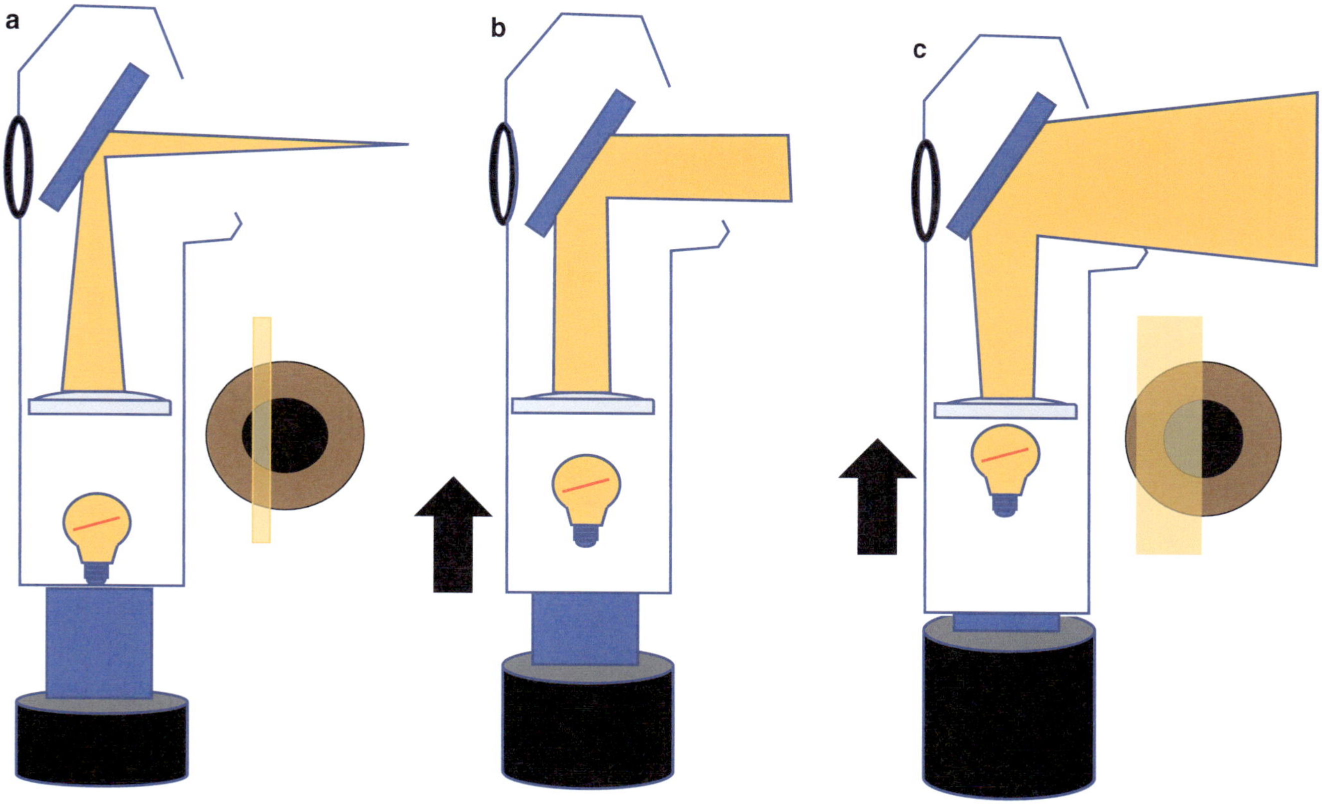

Fig. 2 Streak retinoscope sleeve settings. Never miss an opportunity to remember $U + D = V$. In panel A, the sleeve is down and the bulb is far from the lens. Thus, V (+) light will be converging and form a streak that is in focus at 33 cm. In Panel B, as the light moves closer to the lens, u becomes small, $U = D$ and $V = 0$. The light is at the focal point of the lens making the rays exit in parallel fashion. Panel C, the sleeve is up producing more diverging light, V (−). The light streak will be slightly out of focus

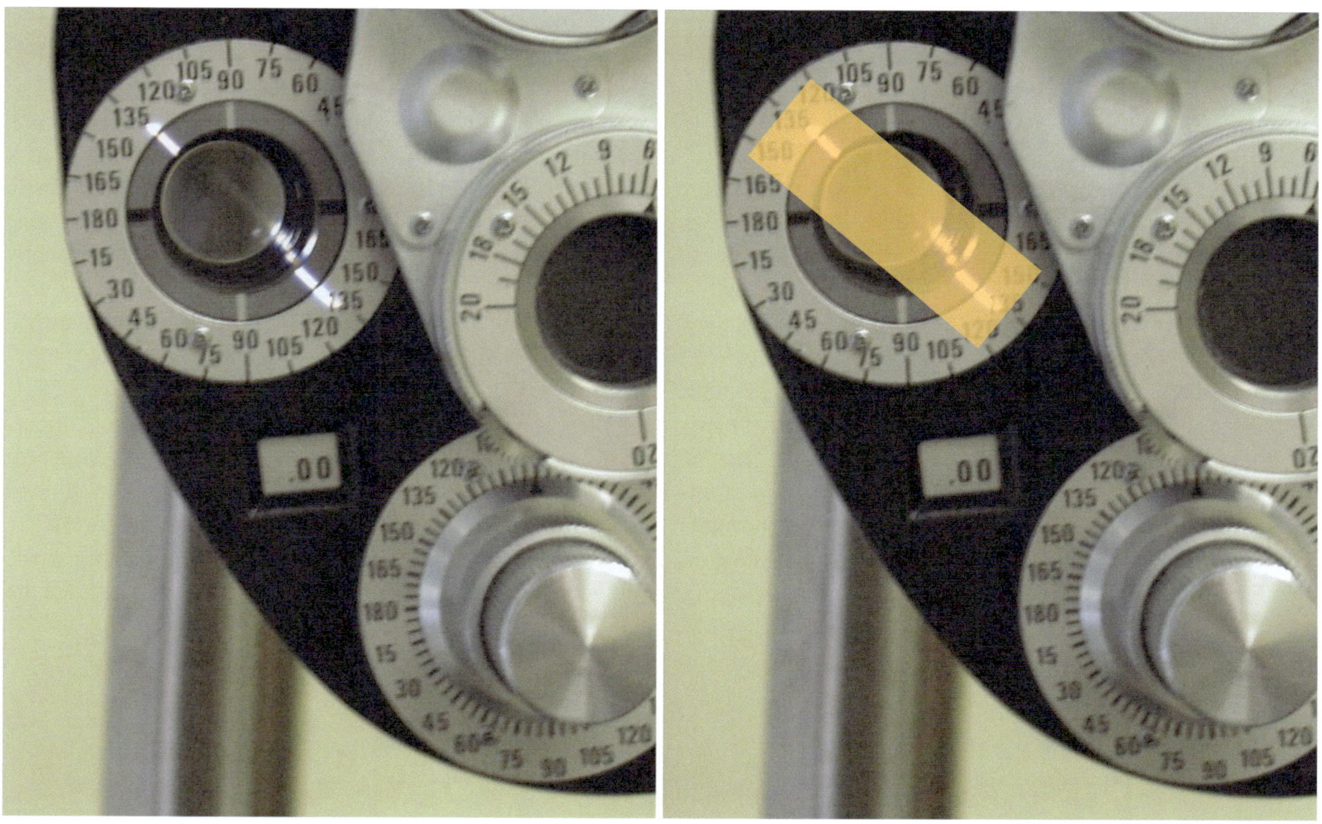

Fig. 3 A thin intercept "converging light" setting is used to better see where the oblique astigmatism is located. A wide intercept with diverging light would make it difficult to tell if the axis was 120, 135, or 150 degrees

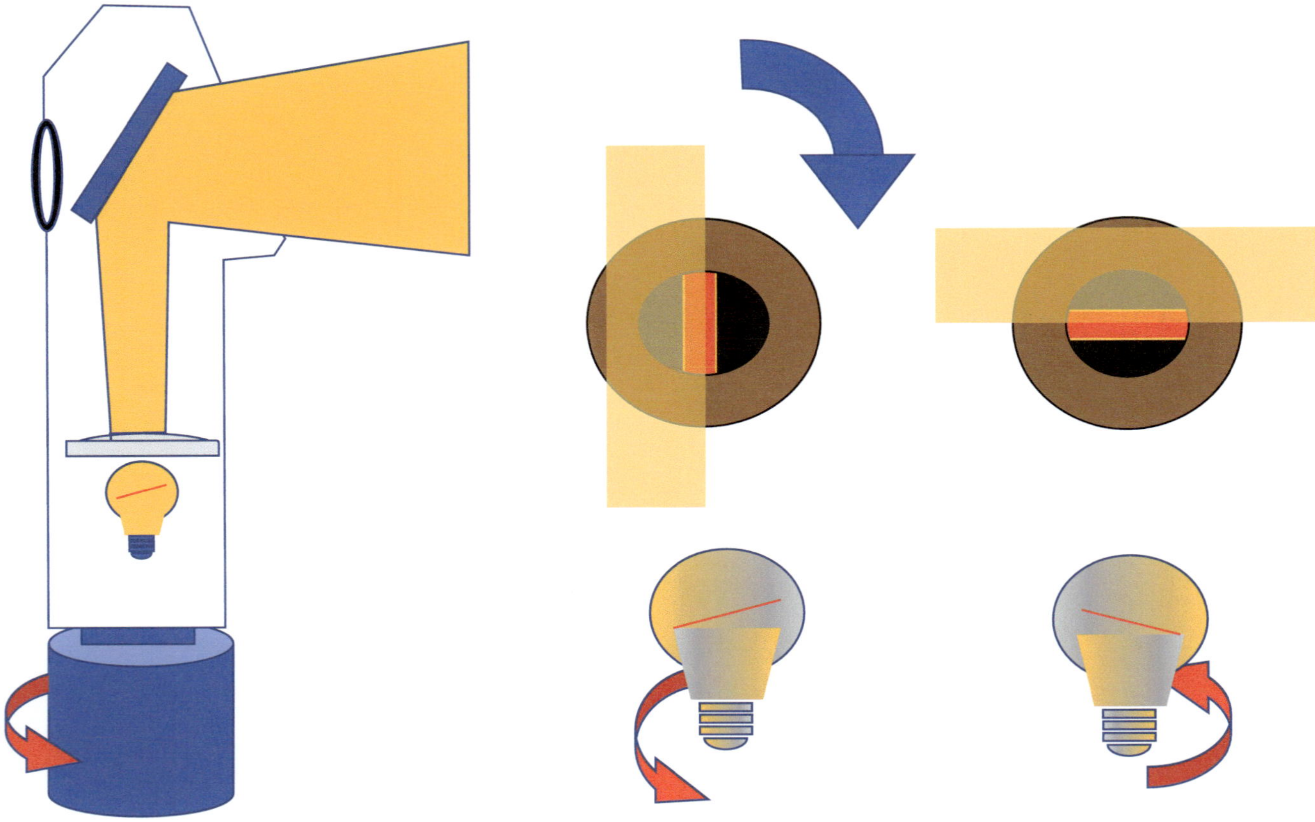

Fig. 4 By rotating the handle, the filament is rotated, which in turn rotates the streak vertical, horizontal, or oblique

Neutralization achieved with trial lens:	Final dispensed refraction:
−1.00 sphere	−2.50 sphere
−1.00 + 1.00 × 90	−2.50 + 1.00 × 90
Plano	1.50 sphere
Plano +2.50 × 90	−1.50 + 2.50 × 90
+3.0 sphere	+1.5 sphere

Suppose you are performing retinoscopy and you want to avoid having to adjust for the WD, there are two other options. The first option, which is only theoretically possible, is to perform retinoscopy from far away (beyond optical infinity). However, this has two main disadvantages: you would need a very strong light, and it would be hard to see a tiny pupil from far away.[2] The second and more practical option is to add a + 1.50D trial lens throughout the measurement and then remove it for the final prescription. The "*R*" setting in many phoropters places a + 1.50 D lens in your line of sight; you can then do retinoscopy adjusting the phoropter lenses until the pupil fills in. When neutralization is reached, then the "R" is removed and the "O" open setting is placed without the need to subtract any value from the readings on the phoropter.

[2]Socially distanced streak refraction may be quite difficult.

While we are discussing positioning, the examiner should sit in front of the patient but without blocking their view of the eye chart. Performing retinoscopy from too far to the side will cause false astigmatism to be observed.

It is also important to remember that because young patients can generate significant accommodation, it may falsely affect the retinoscopy.[3] Therefore, especially with pediatric patients, it is necessary to perform cycloplegic retinoscopy. Moreover, it is also easier to perform retinoscopy through a dilated (large) pupil than a small one. Older patients can be relied upon to simply fixate at a distant target, though a cycloplegic retinoscopy will always yield a "purer" result.

We have previously discussed that hyperopic patients have a far point behind the retina. When conceptualizing retinoscopy, it may be helpful to understand that the "mirror image" of this far point will be behind the examiner (Fig. 6). As the intercept comes down, it does not fill the pupil, so the red reflex forms a bar; the first red rays (A and B) to reach the

[3]Retinoscopy in this situation may be falsely myopic or hyperopic. It is not uncommon for an undilated pediatric patient to scope with +1.00D sphere at one moment, and then a few seconds later, scope with −4.00D sphere.

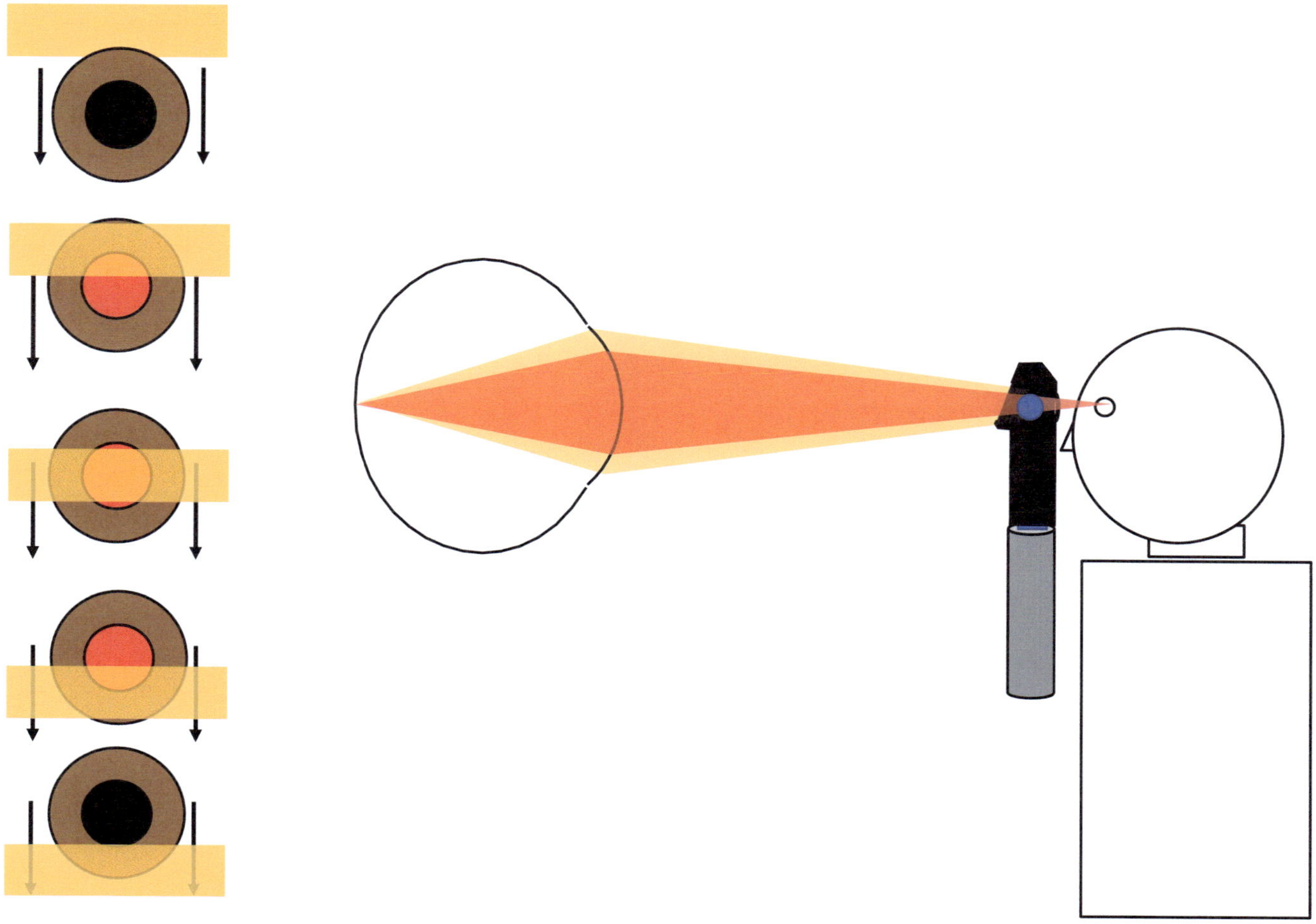

Fig. 5 With vs. against movement. When the far point (blue dot) is at the peephole, the patient's pupil will instantly fill with a red reflex as the yellow intercept comes down and reaches the pupil. This is known as neutralization

examiner's pupil come from the *top of the pupil* and move in the same direction as the intercept ("with motion").

When "**with motion**" is observed, **plus power lenses are added** with increasing power in order to bring the far point to the retinoscope peephole and achieve neutralization.

Patients who are nearsighted will have a far point between them and the examiner (Fig. 7). As the streak comes down and reaches the top of the patient's pupil, the first red rays (A and B) to reach the examiner will appear to be coming from the *inferior pupil*. The red reflex will move in the opposite direction ("against motion") as the intercept.

When "**against motion**" is observed, **minus power lenses are added** with increasing power in order to bring the far point to the retinoscope peephole and achieve neutralization.

A useful mnemonic to remember this is "SPAM": **S**ame ("with motion") requires **P**lus power, and **A**gainst motion requires **M**inus power. We can compare retinoscopy for hyperopes and myopes in the following two figures. Figure 8 depicts how adding minus lenses and plus lenses for myopic patients and hyperopic patients, respectively, will shift the far point to align with the examiner's peephole. Figure 9 shows the examiner's view of neutralization (top row), with motion (middle row), and against motion (bottom row).

This is a lot easier to understand with animation, but the editors decided against turning this textbook into a giant flip book. What happens when we neutralize the reflex on one axis but we see with motion at another axis? This means astigmatism is present. If you are working with plus cylinder, it is easier to first neutralize the most minus axis and then add plus power 90 degrees away until that reflex is neutralized as well. Let's look at a few examples:

Example #1 (Fig. 10): Suppose that when the streak is oriented horizontally (top left panel), neutralization is observed. When the streak is oriented vertically (top right panel), with motion is observed. Using the "SPAM" mnemonic, we know we must progressively add plus power in order to neutralize this reflex. We note that this reflex finally neutralizes with the addition of +4.00D (bottom panel). To determine the patient's required prescription, we can adjust for WD and dispense: $-1.50 + 4.00 \times 90$.

Example #2 (Fig. 11): Suppose that when the streak is oriented vertically (top right panel), neutralization is observed. When the streak is oriented horizontally (top left

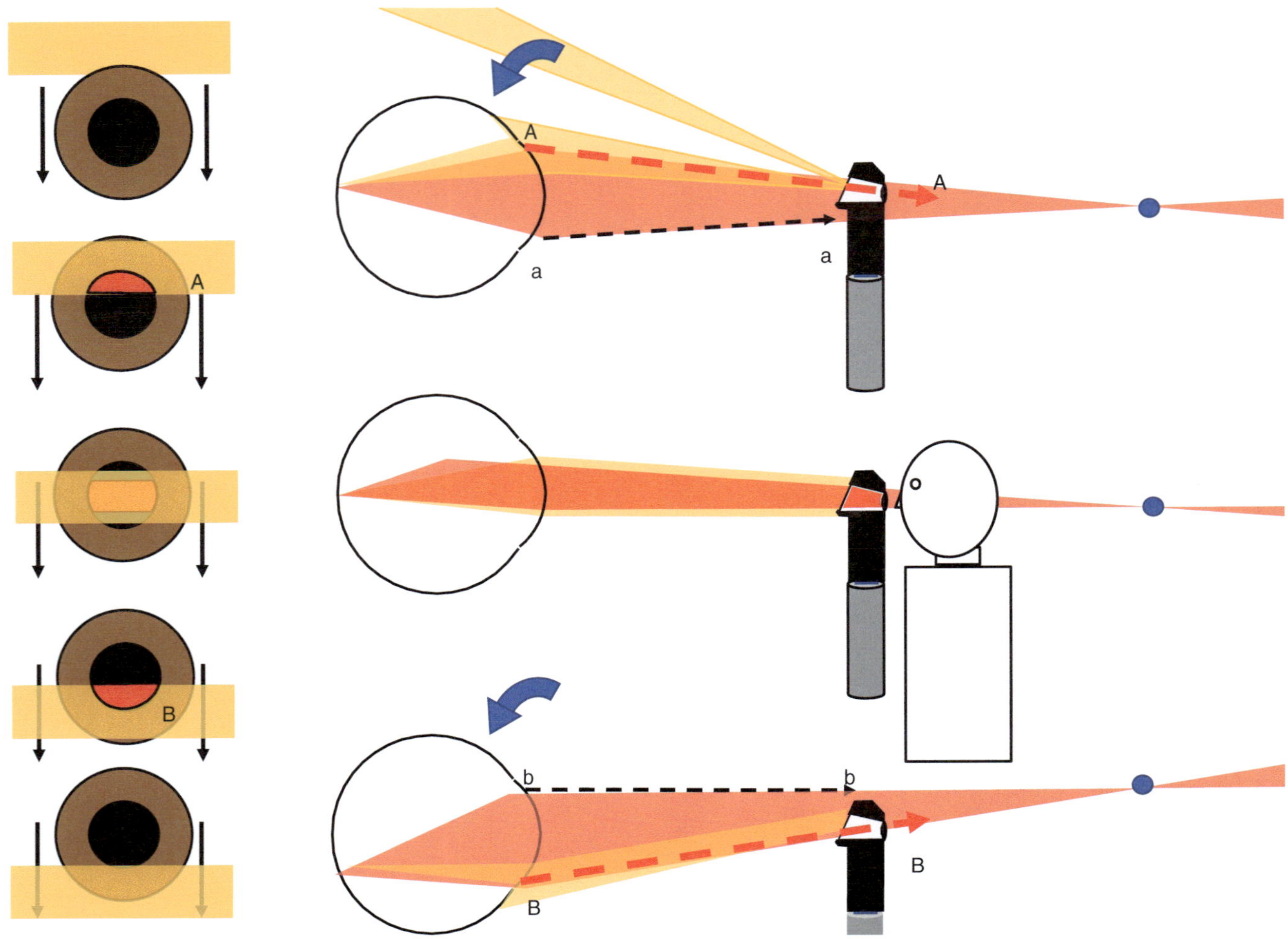

Fig. 6 With vs. against movement for hyperopes. When the far point (blue dot) is behind the observer, as in a hyperope, a red reflex will move in the same direction as the intercept. This is known as "with motion." Notice the red rays emanating from "A and B" enter the peephole and are visible. The black rays emanating from "a and b" do not enter the peephole and do not reach the observer

panel), with motion is observed. Using the "SPAM" mnemonic, we know that we must progressively add plus power in order to neutralize this reflex. We note that this reflex fully neutralizes with the addition of +4.00D (bottom panel). To determine the patient's required prescription, we can adjust for WD and dispense: −1.50 + 4.00 × 180. Note the key difference with this example compared with the previous one.

Example #3 (Fig. 12): In this scenario, neither meridian is successfully neutralized without additional lenses. Since we want to neutralize the against motion meridian first (top left panel), we will use the "SPAM" mnemonic to add progressively add minus lenses until the reflex is neutralized, in this example, with a − 1.50D lens (bottom left panel). We can then direct our attention to the vertical meridian that has with motion (top right panel) and progressively add plus lenses until the reflex is neutralized, in this example, with a + 4.00D lens (bottom right panel). We may be tempted to simply dispense −1.50 + 4.00 × 90, but we must remember to adjust for the WD. Therefore, the dispensed refraction should be −3.00 + 4.00 × 90.

Example #4 (Fig. 13): In this scenario, suppose we note that there is with motion in both the 90-degree and 180-degree meridians, but more so along the 90-degree meridian when the streak is moved left to right. In this case, the 180-degree is the "more minus" meridian (top left panel), so we can neutralize that with the addition of plus lenses until neutralization with +2.00 D sphere (bottom left panel). We can then direct our attention to the 90-degree meridian (top right panel) and progressively add plus lenses until neutralization with +4.00D cylinder (bottom right panel). After adjusting for WD, the dispensed refraction will be +0.50 + 4.00 × 90

Example #5 (Fig. 14): What happens if we have a patient with oblique astigmatism? In this case, we notice the reflex is neutralized with the streak held horizontally (top left panel). Suppose that when we hold the streak vertically, we notice with motion but with a tilted red reflex (top right panel). This indicates the location of the steep axis at approximately 70 degrees (oblique astigmatism). We will then progressively add plus lenses until neutralization with +4.00D cylinder to act at the 160-degree axis (bottom panel). After

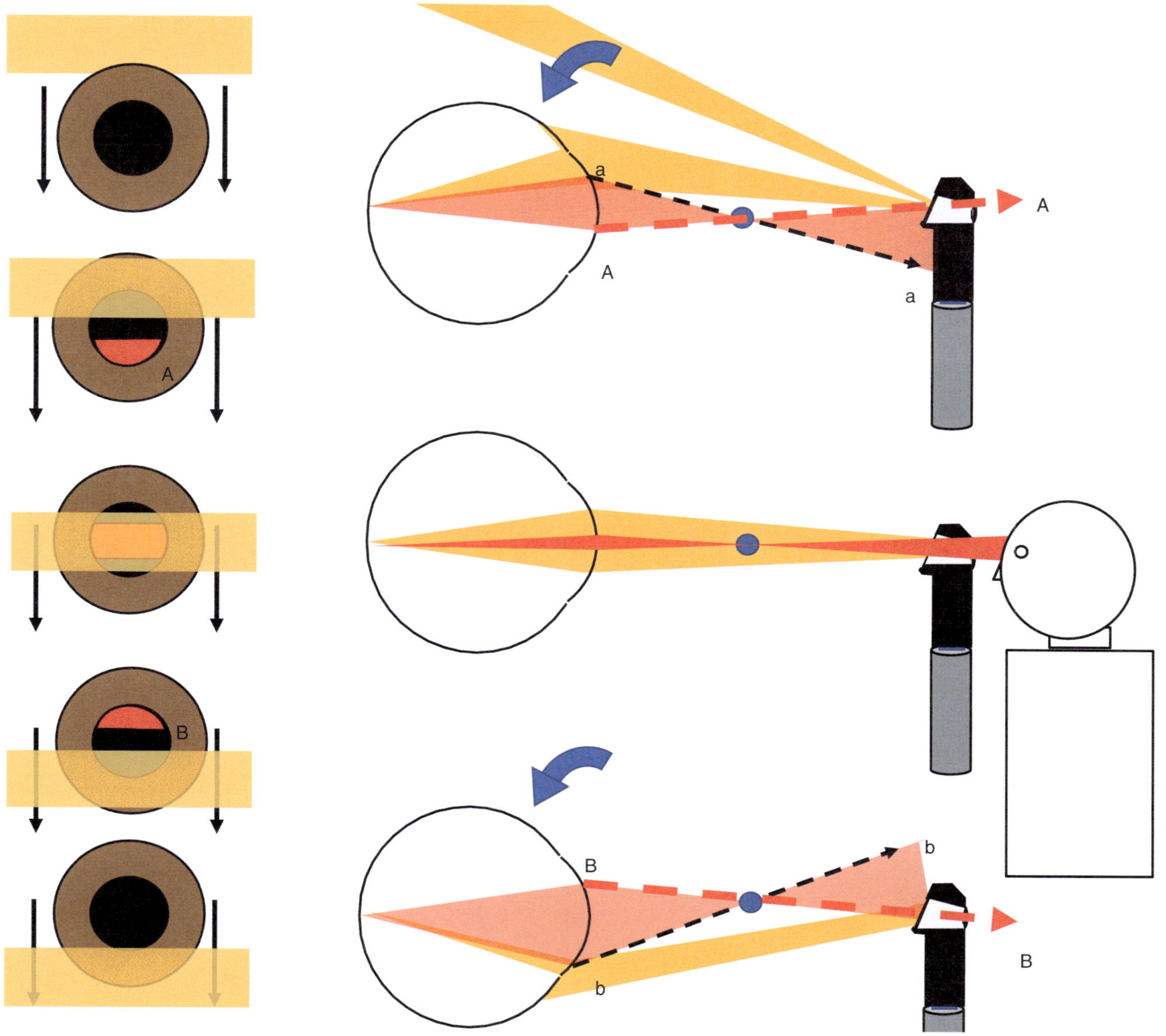

Fig. 7 With vs. against movement for myopes. When the far point (blue dot) is in front of the observer as in myopes, a red reflex will move in the opposite direction as the yellow intercept. This is known as "against movement." Notice the red rays emanating from "A and B" enter the peephole and are visible. The black rays emanating from "a and b" do not enter the peephole and do not reach the observer

adjusting for the WD, the dispensed refraction will be −1.50 + 4.00 × 70. Notice that this patient has mixed astigmatism, and corneal topography may be in order to assess for corneal ectasia!

There are two other types of retinoscopy findings that may be discussed here. **Skew phenomenon** occurs when the reflex is tilted because it is off axis with low cylinder powers. **Break phenomenon** is similar to skew but occurs with higher cylinder powers.

By now we can all agree retinoscopy is amazing: you can measure anything! Well, there are several challenges and noteworthy exceptions (Fig. 15):

- Keratoconus scissoring (Panel A): This can be an effective screening tool to warrant further investigation with topography, pachymetry, etc.
- Bull's eye motion (with motion in the middle, against motion in the periphery) (Panel B): In young patients with large pupils, we may notice a bull's eye pattern where the **central part** of the lens shows **with motion** and the peripheral part of the lens show **against motion** due to the peripheral rays converging more (i.e., our good friend spherical aberration). In this case, the examiner should focus on neutralizing the central reflex and ignore the peripheral reflex.

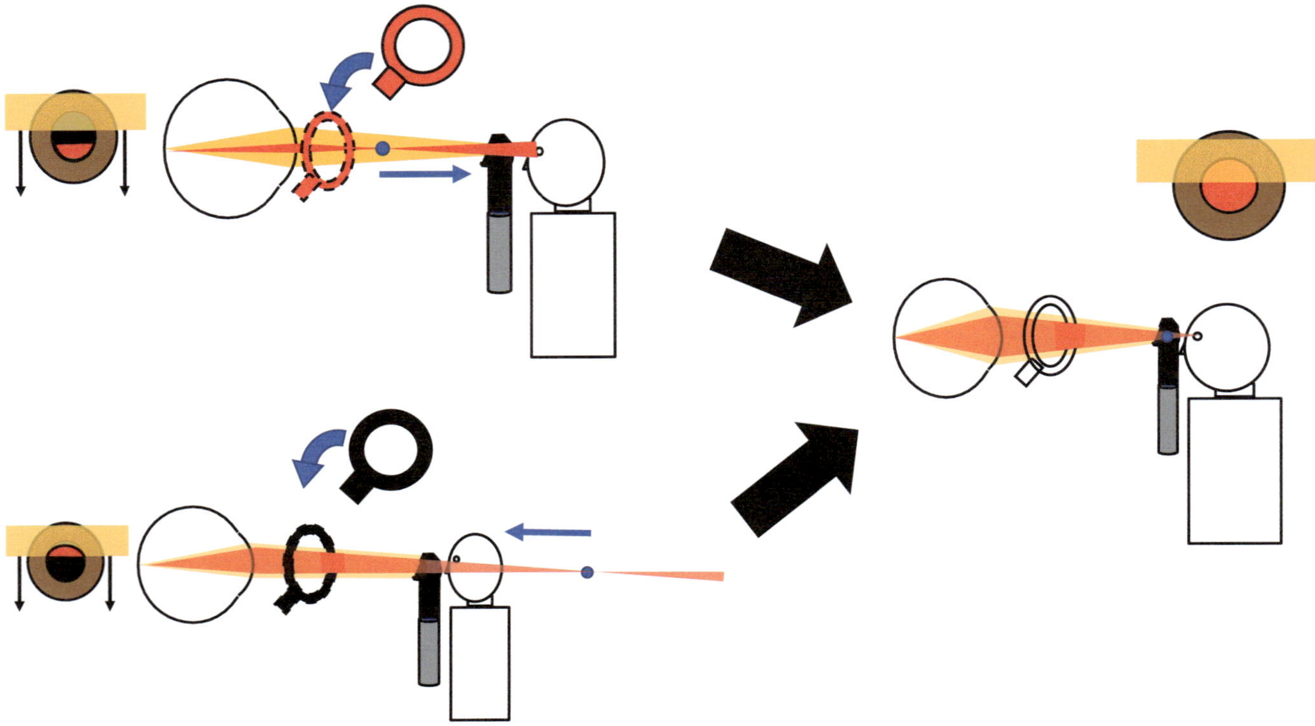

Fig. 8 For a myopic patient (top panel), the near point (blue dot) is between the observer and the patient. A minus (red) lens would add divergence to the red light coming from the eye and push the near point toward the peephole. For a hyperopic patient (bottom panel), a plus (black) lens will converge the red light and bring the far point onto the peephole

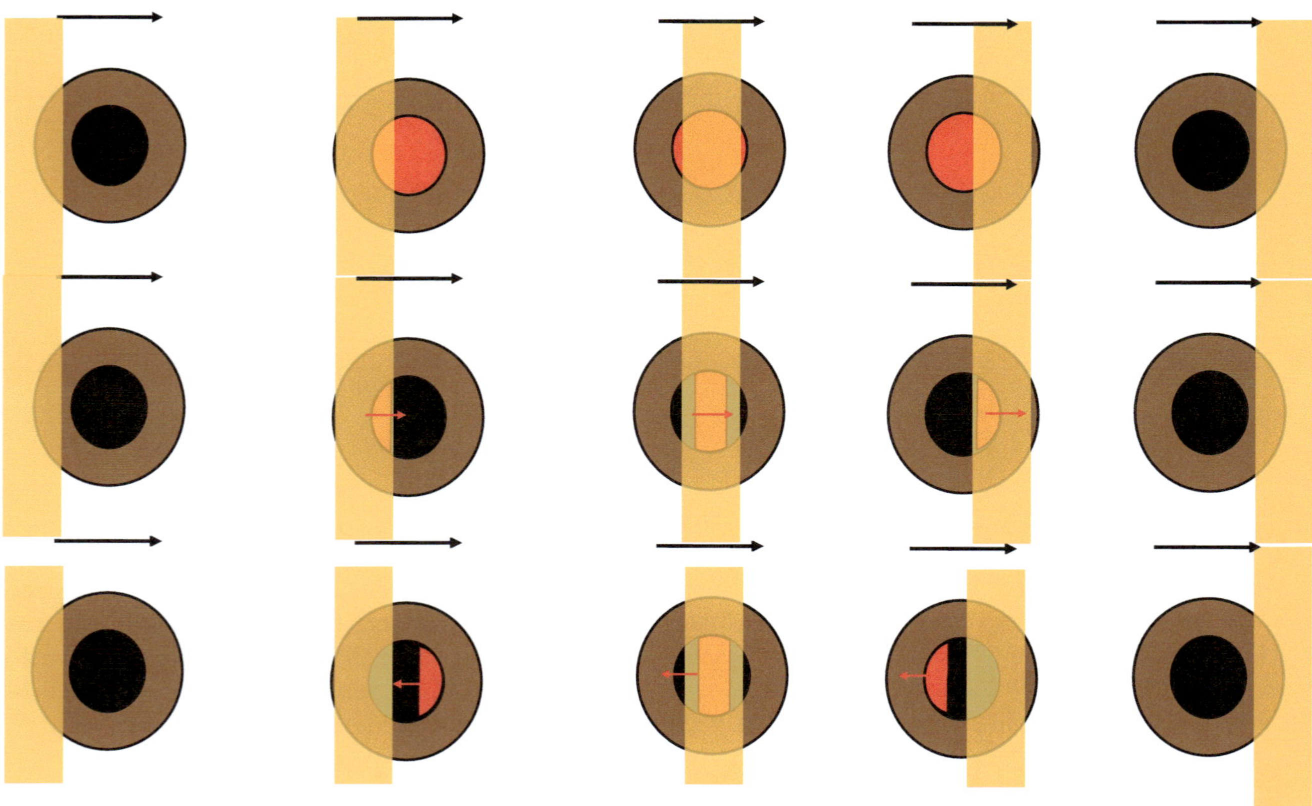

Fig. 9 Examiner's view of with vs. against movement (summary). Light intercept moves from left to right. Top row shows neutralization, middle row with motion, and bottom row against motion

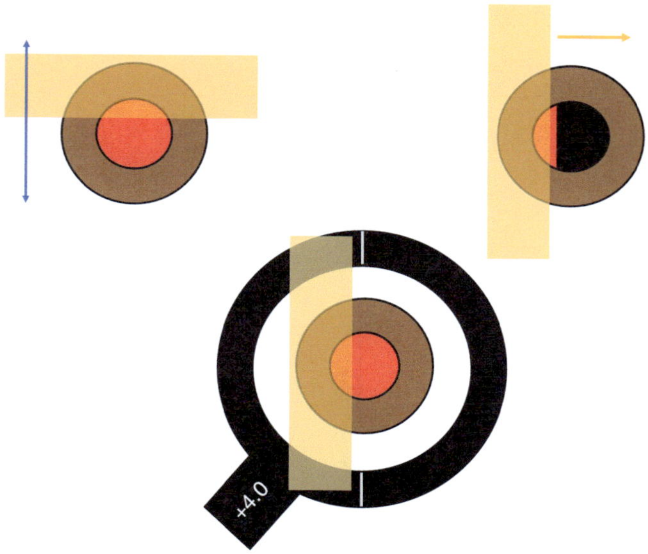

Fig. 10 Plus cylinder power placed in the 90-degree meridian is required to neutralize with motion observed (to act at the 180-degree axis). After adjusting the WD, the dispensed refraction will be −1.50 + 4.00 × 90

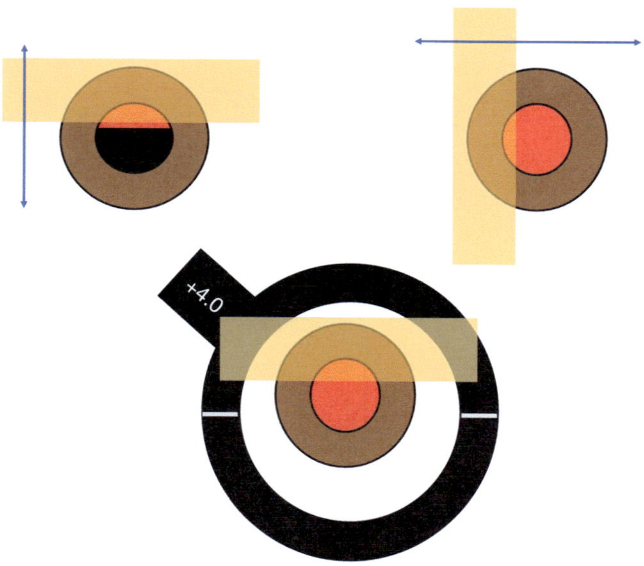

Fig. 11 Plus cylinder power placed in the 180-degree meridian is required to neutralize with motion observed (to act at the 90-degree axis). After adjusting the WD, the dispensed refraction will be −1.50 + 4.00 × 180

- Posterior capsular opacity (Panel C): Posterior lenticonus may also demonstrate this type of reflex.
- Lenticular/retinal opacity or extremely high refractive error (Panel D): A dull pink (or even white) reflex may be caused by nuclear sclerosis, high myopia, or high hypermetropia (e.g., −10 or +10 D, respectively).

In addition to the movement of the red reflex, three characteristics of the red reflex may be observed if retinoscopy is far from neutral:

- The **Speed** of the reflex will be slower (it might not even seem to move at times giving a false sense of filling the pupil).
- The **Brilliance** of the reflex will be lower.
- The **Width** of the reflex will be narrower.

We mentioned earlier that young patients should be dilated prior to retinoscopy. The one exception to this rule is if you are concerned the child may have an accommodative deficiency, which should be assessed in any child having reading difficulties. This can also occur in young patients (approximately 6–8 years of age) with Down syndrome or in any post-concussion patient. In these situations, **dynamic retinoscopy** may be more useful. A full discussion of this technique is beyond the scope of this book, but in brief, the examiner should have the child focus on an accommodative target (such as a sticker) at the peephole in an **undilated state**. If the examiner observes with motion, while the patient is trying to focus on the near target, then the patient may need additional plus power.

Summary: How to Perform a Streak Refraction

See Chap. 15 Glasses in Clinical Practice, for a seven-step, "to be memorized and summarized," method on how to perform a streak refraction.

Geneva Lens Clock

Dear reader: the Geneva lens clock (GLC) is not a steam punk doomsday device, but we're glad that crossed your mind. The GLC is an adapted spherometer that allows the observer to measure the curve of a spectacle lens and the location of the curve (front or back). If the lens material and its index of refraction are known, it can then also be used to determine the refractive power of that surface. A given GLC is constructed and calibrated to a specific index of refraction (and therefore a specific lens material) and can therefore only be used to assess that particular lens material. If the lens is made of some other material, the reading must be adjusted to correct for the difference in the refraction index. Different GLCs can be made based on the measured lens material.

The most commonly used index of refraction for GLCs is 1.53 (crown glass). Suppose we have a crown glass GLC,

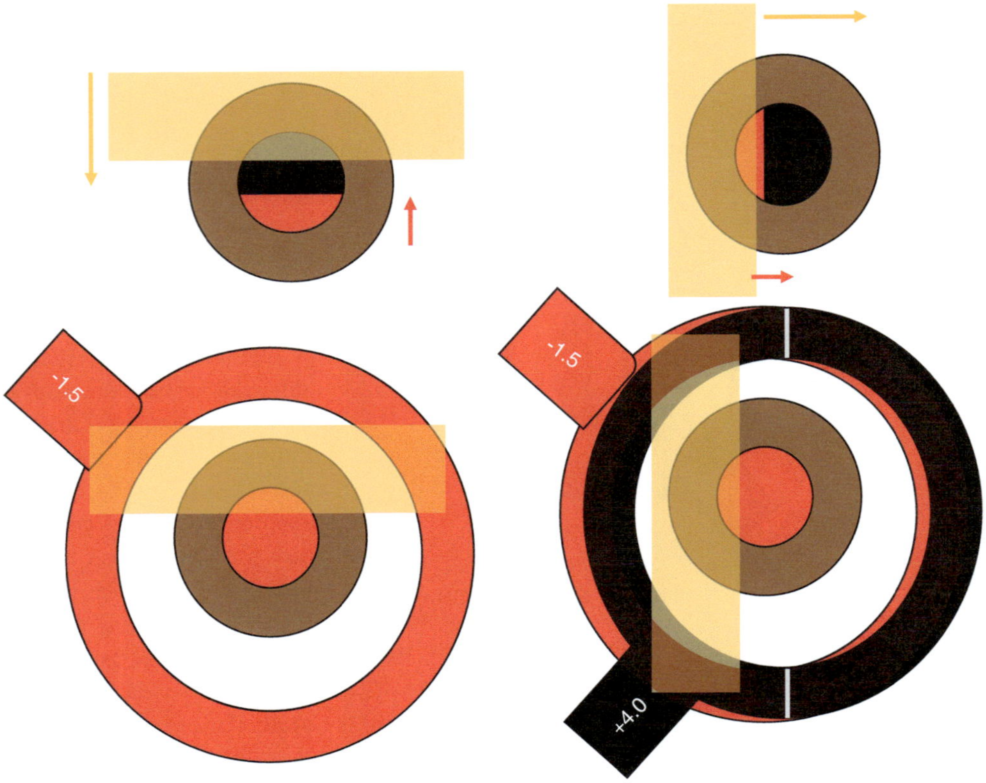

Fig. 12 A −1.5D sphere (red trial lens) is added to neutralize the against motion first (top left and bottom left panels). Then, a + 4.0D cylinder lens is used to neutralize with motion observed on the 90-degree meridian. After adjusting for WD, the dispensed refraction should be −3.00 + 4.00 × 90

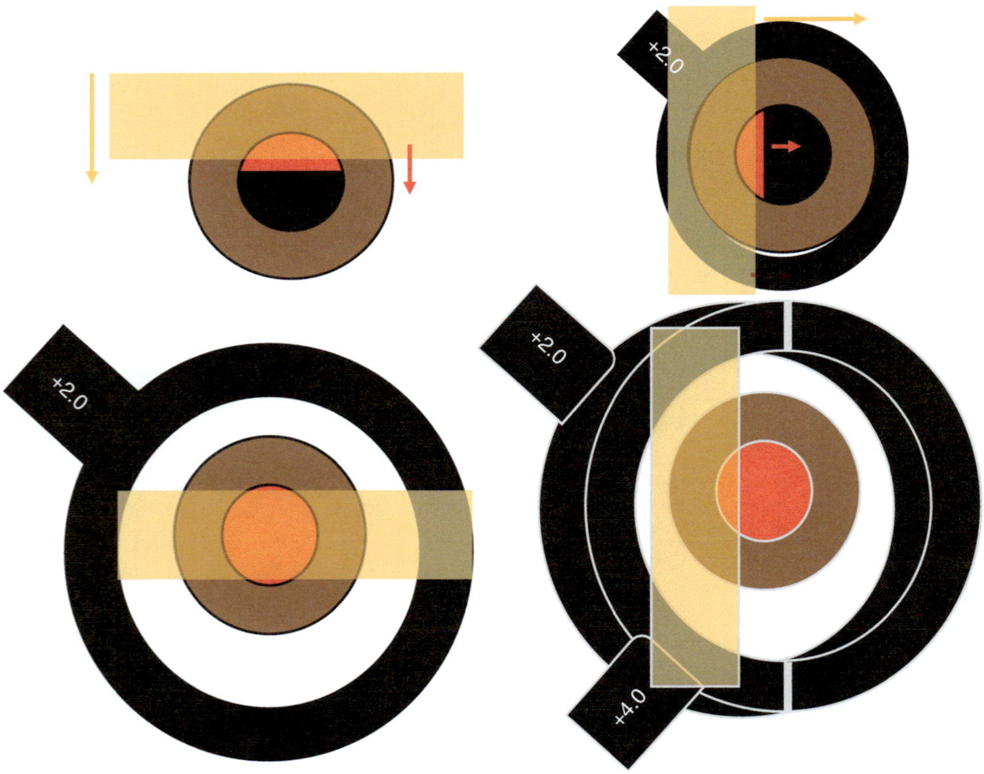

Fig. 13 When there is with motion in both meridians, begin with neutralization of the "more minus" meridian. Suppose there is more "with motion" along 90 degrees when the streak is moved left to right. A +2.00 D sphere lens neutralizes the 180-degree meridian, but there is still with motion along the 90-degree meridian. Thus, more plus cylinder (+4.00D) power is added to the 90-degree meridian until neutralization is noted. After adjusting for WD, the final dispensed refraction will be +0.50 + 4.00 × 90

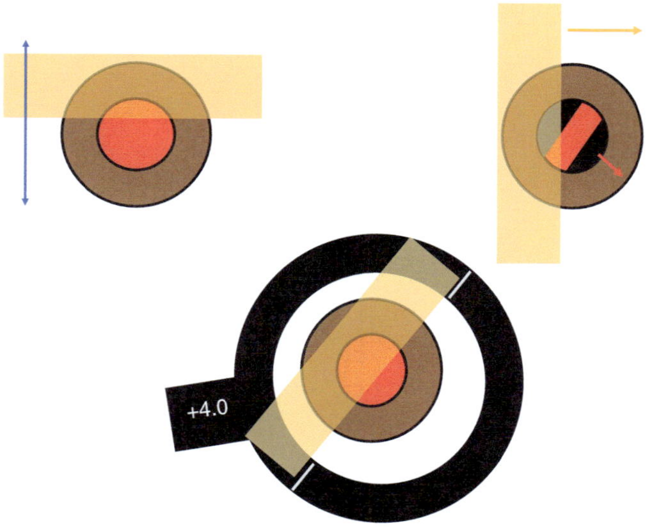

Fig. 14 The reflex is neutralized moving the intercept up and down along the 180-degree axis (top left panel). However, when the streak is placed in the 90-degree meridian, there is with motion with a tilted red reflex indicating oblique astigmatism (top right panel). With additional plus cylinder placed in the 70-degree meridian (acting at the 160-degree axis), neutralization is observed (bottom panel). After adjusting for WD, the final dispensed refraction will be −1.50 + 4.00 × 70

and we used it on a different lens material. If we measure a lens with index of refraction >1.53, the GLC will read the lens power LOWER than actual; if we measure a lens with index of refraction <1.53, the GL will read the lens power HIGHER than actual.

The GLC is used to measure the **back surface** of a given lens (Fig. 16). Three probes make contact with the surface of the lens. The outer two probes are fixed, while the center one moves (straight blue arrow), retracting as the instrument is pressed down on the lens's surface. As the probe retracts, the hand on the face of the dial turns (curved blue arrow) by an amount proportional to the distance of the central probe movement.

In our previous discussions with Geometric Optics (Chap. 1), we described minus lenses as simple meniscus concave shaped objects (Fig. 17, left panel). The shape of a minus lens in a spectacle frame may surprise some readers (Fig. 17, right panel).

What's the surprise? Notice that the **spectacle minus lens** is actually a thick lens that has a weak plus lens power on the front surface and a stronger minus lens power on the back. The net result is still a minus power lens. There are many

Fig. 15 Four atypical cases: (**a**) Keratoconus scissoring. (**b**) Bull's eye with motion in the middle, against motion in the periphery. (**c**) Posterior capsular opacity. (**d**) Nuclear sclerosis or very high refractive error

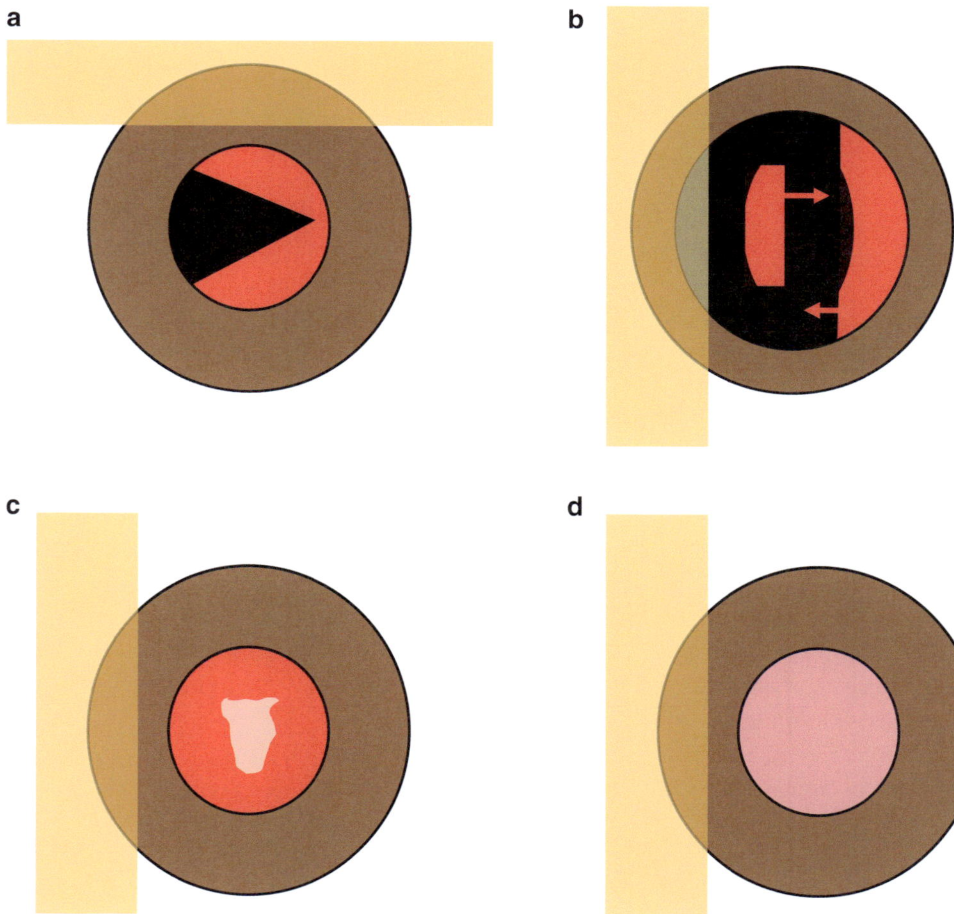

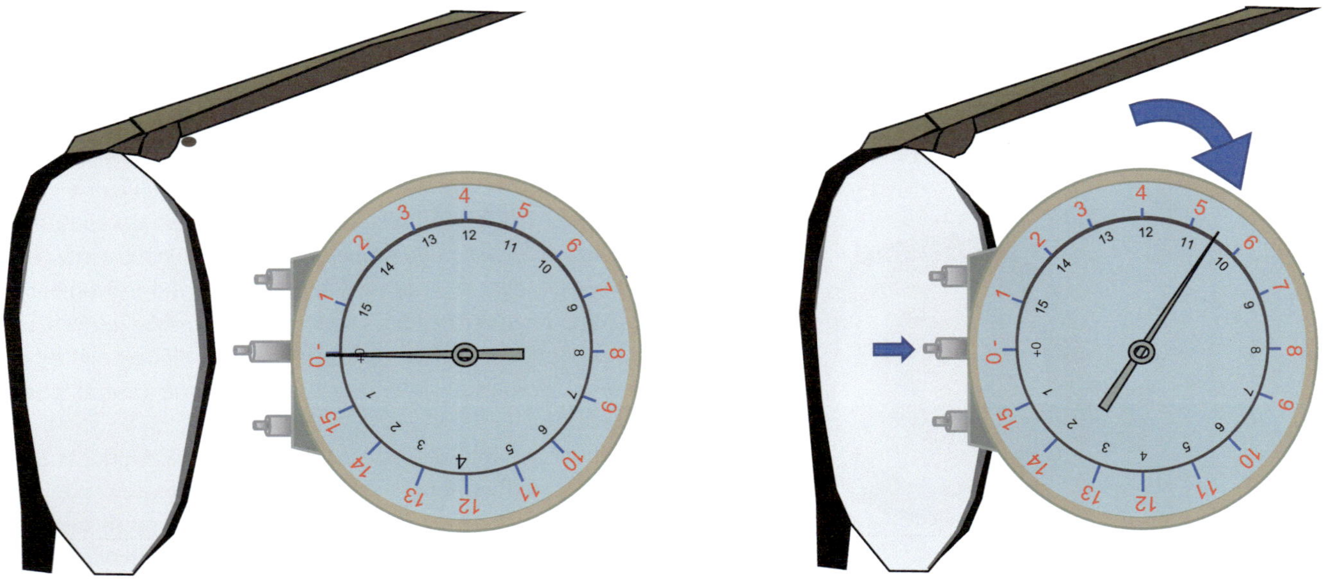

Fig. 16 Geneva lens clock (GLC). The central prong is on a spring and will be pressed differently depending on the curve of the crystal. When the GLC is placed on the optical center perpendicular to the posterior surface, it reads: −5.5D refractive power (on the red scale) along 180-degree axis of these glasses. The black scale is used for the front surface

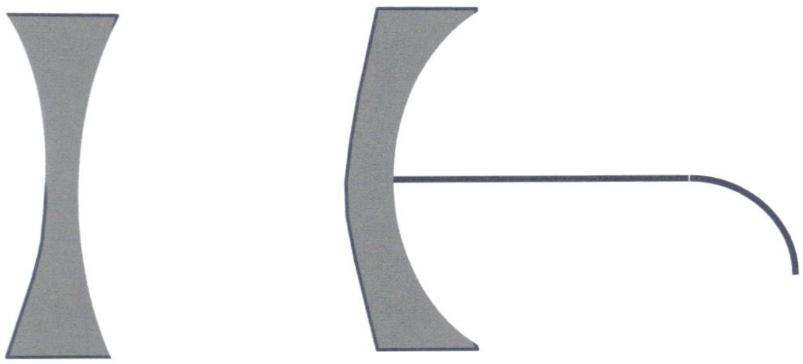

Fig. 17 A theoretical minus lens (used in geometric optics; left panel) and a minus lens used in eyeglasses (right panel)

reasons for this complex construction, such as considerations for manufacturing, historical practices, and the architecture of the eyeglasses.[4] The approximate power of the lens can be calculated by adding the front surface to the back surface. For example, a lens with a + 8D curve on the front surface and a −10D curve on the back surface will have a net power of +8 + (−10) = −2D.

We can also see how varying combinations of front surface and back surface base curves can be used to construct eyeglasses with similar or different powers. For example, the same power of eyeglasses (−1.00D) can be constructed using two different combinations of front surface and back surface base curves (Fig. 18).

[4]For example, having a protruding front surface would make for a cosmetically undesirable lens, in addition to requiring thicker frames.

Different manufacturers may use different front surface and back surface base curves in their lenses. Modern laboratories will typically choose between a limited range of base curves for a given power range in order to minimize peripheral aberrations.[5]

By convention, modern eyeglasses are constructed such that the cylinder is ground onto the back surface.[6] The front surface is therefore usually spherical.

The GLC can help identify different problems with glasses:

A. Suppose a patient is unhappy with a new pair of glasses that he received at his last visit 1 month ago. When the old glasses and new glasses are measured using a lensmeter (see next section), they both read −3.0D total refractive power. At this point, we may be tempted to simply reassure the patient that the glasses were made correctly and send them out of the office. However, if we use a GLC, we may then find that there was previously a − 5.5D posterior curve on the old glasses, but the new glasses have −7.0D D posterior base curve. In this case, the glasses were made "correctly," but the patient

[5]"Lens Form: Sphere, Cylinder, and Axis". https://www.laramyk.com/resources/education/lens-form-and-theory/lens-form-sphere-cylinder-and-axis/. Accessed June 7, 2020.

[6]Historically, this was not always the case. Older texts may reference the idea of "checking to see if the cylinder power was ground into the front surface" when troubleshooting glasses. This is a moot point in modern times since, by convention, modern optical laboratories construct lenses with the cylinder ground into the back.

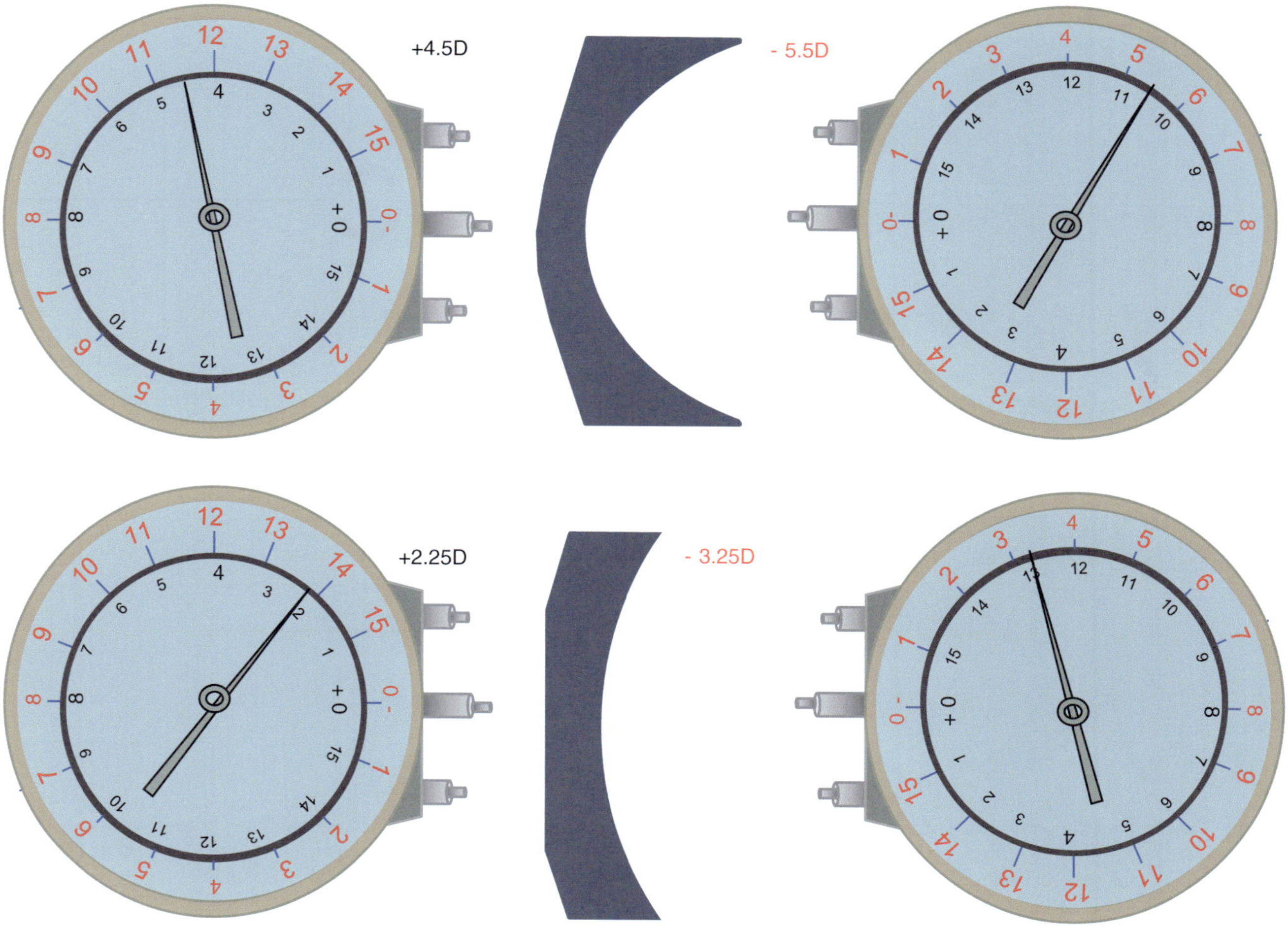

Fig. 18 Graphical example of two potential (and different) ways to construct −1.00D spectacles. In the top panel, a + 4.5D curve on the front and a − 5.5D base curve on the back is used. In the bottom panel, +2.25D curve on the front and a − 3.25D curve on the back is used

describes a fishbowl effect with the new glasses and is unhappy. The solution here would be to rewrite the prescription with instructions given to the optical lab to maintain the old back surface base curve.

B. If assessing an old pair of glasses, the plus cylinder power may have been ground on the front surface or the lenses were placed backwards. This would also have the similar strength on the lensmeter, but the distortion would be noticeable to the patient.

Specially constructed GLCs can also be used to determine the thickness of a gas permeable contact lens.

Finally, when trying to measure the power of a spherocylindrical lens, remember that the posterior surface will contain the cylinder, so we must adjust accordingly when using the GLC (Fig. 19). Suppose when measuring the back surface of the lens, the GLC reads −6.00D along the 90-degree axis (top left panel) and −8.00D along the 180-degree axis (bottom left panel). Assume that the front surface is +7.00D. We can calculate the power of the lens by constructing a power cross to determine that the power of this spherocylindrical lens is −1.00 + 2.00 × 180.[7]

Lensmeter

Introduction to the Lensmeter and the Optometer Principle

Fun fact: "Lensmeter" is the name given for the device used to measure the power of a spectacle lens; the "Lensometer®" is a trade name for a particular brand of lensmeter. You can win friends and be the highlight of social parties by knowing this type of information.

All lensmeters work on the **optometer** principle: if we have a single converging lens with a known power (and known focal length), we can take advantage of this property

[7] See Chap. 10 "Spherocylindrical Lenses", to review this concept.

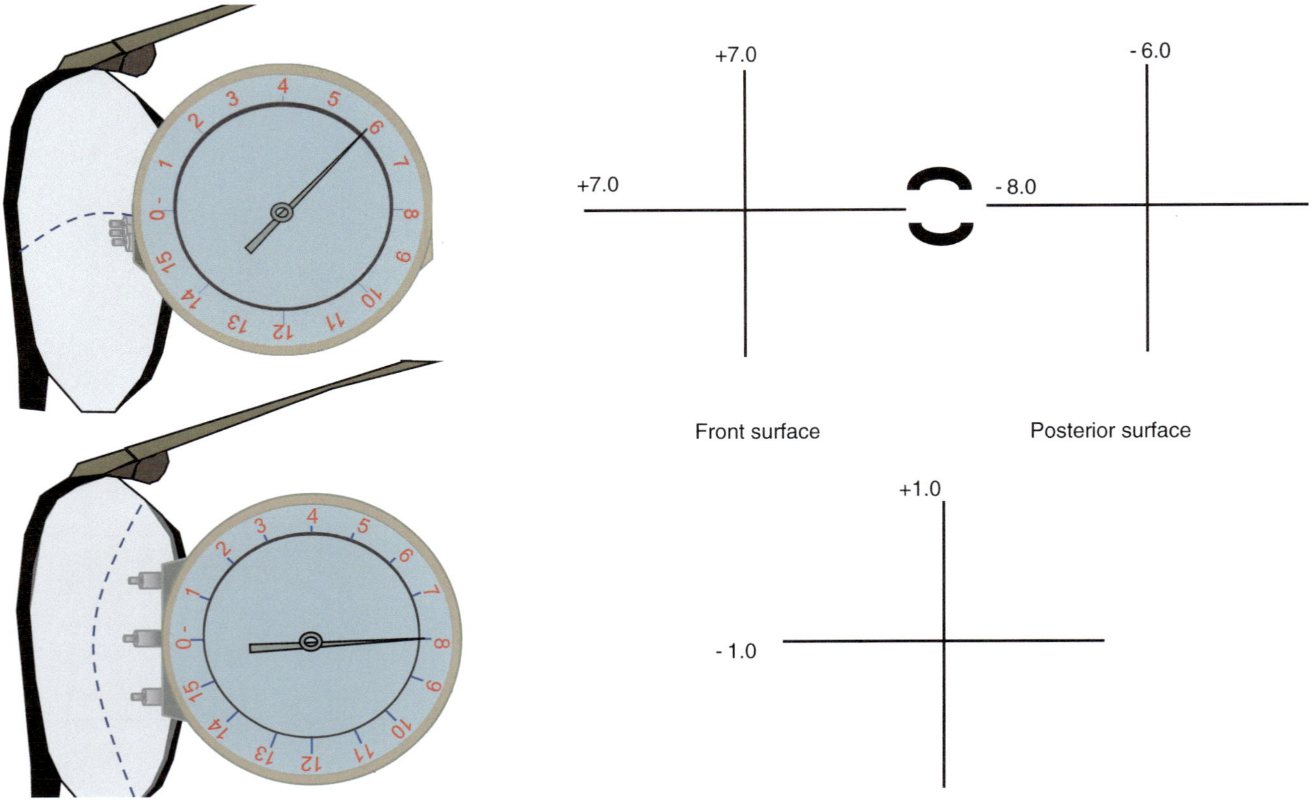

Fig. 19 Determining the power of a spherocylindrical lens. In the top left panel, the GLC reads −6.00D along 90 degrees. In the bottom left panel, the GLC reads −8.00D along 180 degrees. Assume that the front surface is +7.00 D sphere. A power cross may then be used to combine the power of the front surface and back surface to determine the power of the spherocylindrical lens: −1.00 + 2.00 × 180

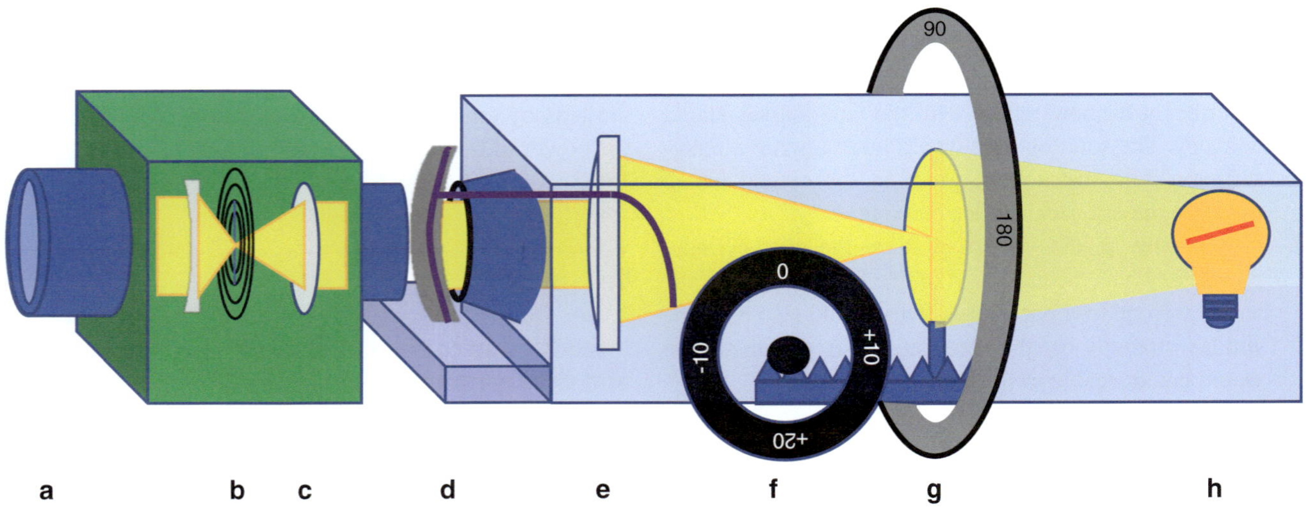

Fig. 20 Lensmeter. (**a**) Adjustable eyepiece. (**b**) Reticle (with prism scale and axis scale). (**c**) Keplerian telescope (green box). (**d**) Spectacle lens. (**e**) Standard lens. (**f**) Power drum. (**g**) Target mire and Axis Dial. (**h**) Lamp collimator (blue box)

by placing an unknown lens and adjusting it until the unknown lens' focal length matches up with the known lens' focal length. We can then back-calculate the power of the unknown lens once the focal lengths of the known lens and the unknown lens match up.

In a typical lensmeter (Fig. 20), the known lens (a.k.a. standard lens) is inside the machine, and a light source illuminates a target behind it. The unknown lens (eyeglasses; we will discuss positioning in a minute) is placed in front of the known lens – that is, closer to the examiner's eye. The examiner can dial in power into the lensmeter until the unknown lens "matches up" (has the same focal length) as the known lens.

A typical lensmeter will also have an astronomical (Keplerian) telescope that allows for precise detection of parallel rays at neutralization. This prevents the examiner's refractive error from causing significant measurement error.

How to Use the Lensmeter: Single Vision Lenses

There are several key steps to follow when using the lensmeter. We can break them down as follows. Let's suppose we are measuring a simple pair of **single-vision lens (SVL) glasses** with distance correction only for starters:

1. Focus the eyepiece: before placing the eyeglasses, turn the power drum until the mires are out of focus to eventually bring them into focus (this avoids error potentially caused by your accommodation). Then, turn the eyepiece in a counterclockwise (CCW) (to add plus power) direction to fog the target. Then slowly move the eyepiece in a clockwise (CW) (to add minus) power until the target is clear. This helps to prevent your refractive error from "skewing" the results. Then, adjust the power drum to focus the mires at a drum reading of zero (plano).
2. Position the eyeglasses: for SVL glasses, position them with the **temples facing away from you**. Remember that since the majority of the eyeglass power is ground on the back surface, it is closer to the lensmeter aperture. Align the SVL lens so that the mires cross in the center of the target.
3. Measure the sphere:
   (a). Focus the **single lines** by rotating the drum CCW while simultaneously rotating the cylinder axis wheel so that the single lines are perpendicular to the triple lines (widely spaced triple mires).
   (b). If the single lines and triple lines come into focus at the same time, then the SVL glasses only have spherical correction. Pat yourself on the back and move on.
   (c). However, if only the single lines focus, record this as the sphere power, and we must now measure the cylinder.
4. Measure the cylinder:
   (a). Move the power drum further CCW (adding more minus) to bring the **triple lines** into focus.
   (b). Calculate the difference: the power at which the triple lines focus – the power at which the single lines focus – this is the plus cylinder power for the SVL glasses.
5. Read the axis from the axis wheel.

If you want to further summarize this: (1) Rotate the axis so that the thin guys are parallel (thin lines are parallel). (2) Rotate the drum so that the thin guys are in focus (sphere power). (3) Rotate the drum so that the fat guys (thick triple lines) are in focus. (4) The difference between the fat guys and thin guys is the plus cylinder power.

Bifocal Lenses: Measuring Add Power

Suppose we want to measure a pair of **bifocal lenses**: the biggest thing to remember is that for the distance portion of the lens, we must still position the glasses so that the temples are facing away from you. However, if you want to measure the **bifocal add power** very precisely, especially in high power lenses, you have to turn the glasses around so that the **temples are facing toward you.** Why is this? Recall that the *bifocal power is ground on the front surface* of the glasses, so we want this portion to be closer to the lensmeter aperture. Then, we can follow these steps:

1. Center the bifocal add and refocus the thin triple lines
2. The difference in the triple lines power measured for the bifocal add and the power measured when measuring the distance portion is the add power.
3. If we are dealing with a trifocal lens, we can repeat this same procedure with the intermediate portion: refocus the triple lines for the intermediate segment; the difference between the distance portion power and the intermediate segment power is the actual "intermediate add" power.
4. Progressives are a bit more of a challenge to measure and add in. That is why many manufacturers will etch a small (~1 mm) two-digit number in the margin of the lens (Fig. 21). Spectacles with +1.75 add will have a "1.7"; spectacles with +3.0 add will have a "3.0."

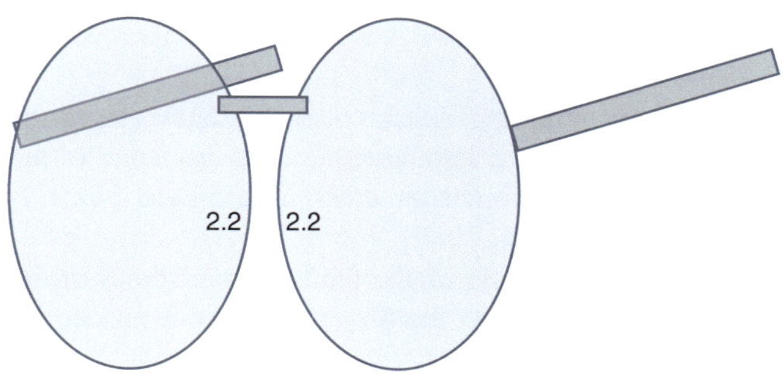

Fig. 21 Progressives lenses will have a small two-digit number (in this example, "22") etched. This is an example of spectacles with 2.25 add

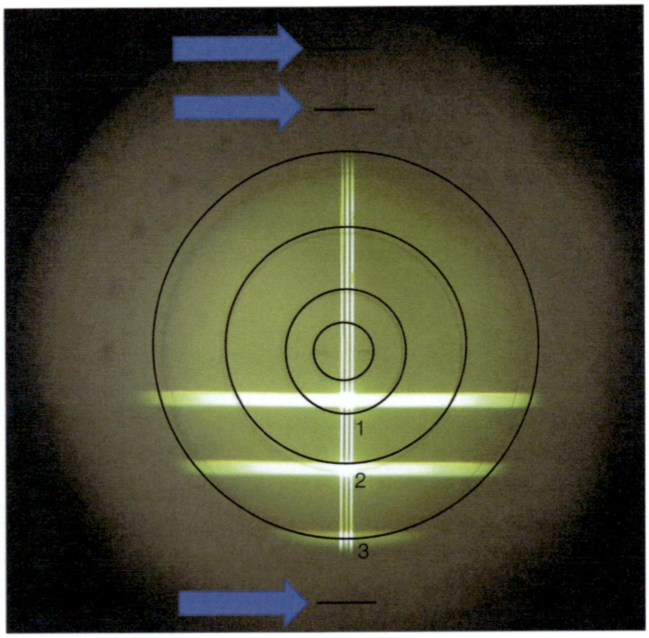

Fig. 22 View through a lensmeter demonstrating a spectacle lens with BD prism. In a patient with 2 BD prism, regardless of whether this is a right lens or left lens, no matter how the spectacle lens is moved, the intersect of yellow lines remains at the 2nd dark ring. There are two additional dark lines (blue arrows), not circles at 12 and 6 o'clock representing 4 and 5 PD, respectively

Measuring Ground-In Prism

What happens if you have a fancy pants patient with prism in his/her glasses? Send them to your local neuro-ophthalmologist colleague?[8] Sure, but you can also follow these steps to measure the prism power and orientation:

1. Mark the pupillary center (position on the glasses through which the patient is viewing while looking straight ahead) using an erasable marker. Center this mark on the lensmeter target. This assumes that the glasses were made correctly with the optical center of the glasses at the center of the pupillary axis. Most manufacturers have markings on the eyeglass lenses that can be used in conjunction with stencils to find the true optical center of the eyeglass lenses.[9]
2. Count the number of black concentric circles from the central cross of the lensmeter target to the center of the vertical and/or horizontal cross mires. Each circle is equivalent to 1 PD.
3. Record the direction of the thick portion (base) of the prism by determining the **direction** of the displacement of the mires. For example, if the mires are displaced **upward**, then this is a **base-up** prism, etc. In Fig. 22, notice the central thick mire (among the three thick mires) is used to count the downward displacement circles. Since this intersection point is "two-circles down," this indicates there is 2 PD base-down in this lens. In Fig. 23, notice the intersection of the mires has been shifted to the right (relative to the examiner) when measuring the right lens of a pair of glasses. Since the *shift is relative to the examiner*, we can determine that there is 2 PD base-in (not base-out). If the mires had been shifted to the left (relative to the examiner, not pictured), then we can determine that there is 2 PD base-out in the right lens.

Other fun facts about the lensmeter: there is a knob at the top of some lensmeters that you can spin and rotate in any direction to measure up to 15 PD of prisms (Fig. 24). If no knob is present, a trial prism can be placed between the spectacle and the telescope to compensate for the deviated image.

The dark rings can also help determine if the pupillary center does not match the optical center in patients without ground in prisms. In this situation, if the lens spectacle is placed on the lensmeter so that the pupillary center mark is centered, the yellow lines would be off center. The view would be similar to Fig. 23, but moving the spectacle would actually move the yellow lines to the center.

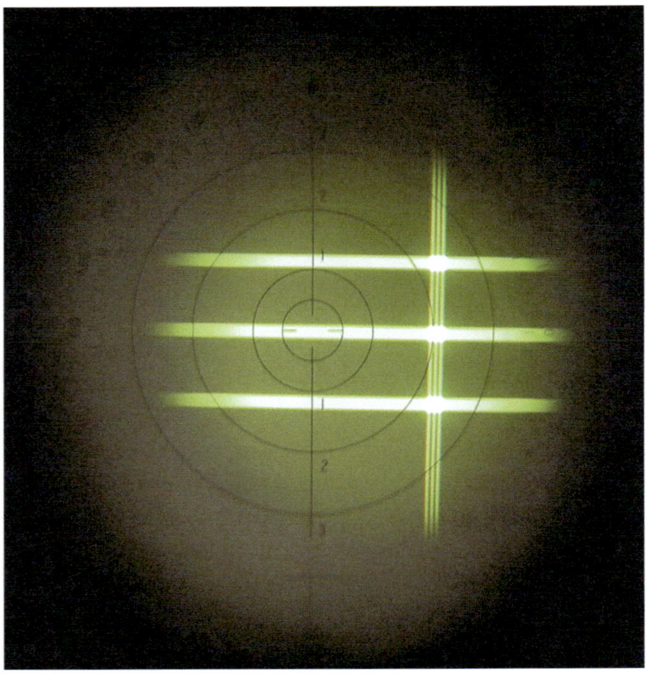

Fig. 23 View through a lensmeter with a right lens spectacle with 2 PD base-in ground in prisms. Note that the orientation of the prism (base-in vs. base-out) is determined by the shift relative to the examiner. No matter how the spectacle is moved, the intersect of yellow lines remains at the 2nd dark ring

[8]This is a surefire way to lose your favorite neuro-ophthalmologist accepting your other referrals.

[9]See Chap. 16 Construction of Glasses: Ophthalmologists as Opticians, for further details

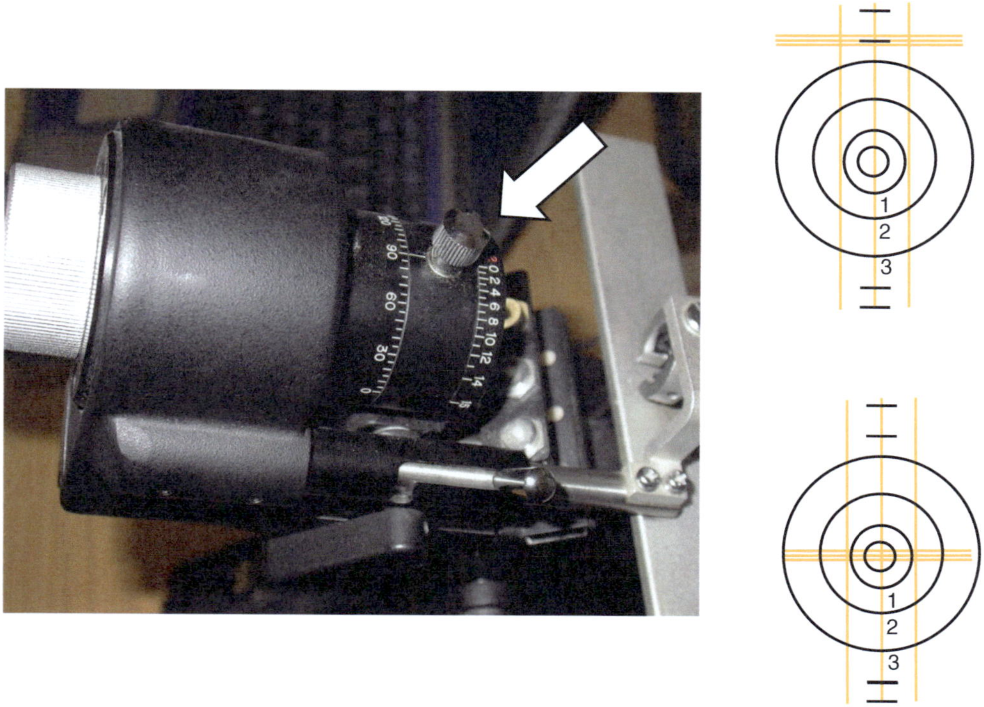

Fig. 24 Prism knob on a lensmeter (white arrow) can be spun and rotated to bring the displaced image (top right panel) to the middle of the target mires (bottom right panel)

Phoropter

Fun fact: the phoropter also relies on the optometer principle. In fact, "phoropter" is actually a contraction of "phoro-optometer." The history of how this device came into origin and its evolution over the years is a fascinating rabbit hole that you can read about online on your own time.

The phoropter allows the clinician to quickly assess the refractive error of a patient but may also be used to detect heterophoria, horizontal/vertical vergences, and accommodative amplitudes. The main usefulness of the phoropter is that instead of an examiner having to slowly take out one lens at a time, as if you are trying to pick the right wand for a young wizard, multiple lenses can quickly be dialed in and out during the course of a clinical refraction.

Let's review some phoropter anatomy:

We have previously discussed how to use the phoropter during the course of a routine subjective manifest refraction in Chap. 15 "Glasses in Clinical Practice."

The phoropter may be considered as an optical Swiss army knife because it has so many functions and capabilities. Of course, we rarely use them, but there are several features we can point out about the phoropter that may be useful in certain select situations:

- The vertex distance can be measured through the vertex distance mirror, and it can be adjusted by moving the patient's forehead rest (see Fig. 25, I). The distometer (see Sect. VII, Distometer) can also be used.

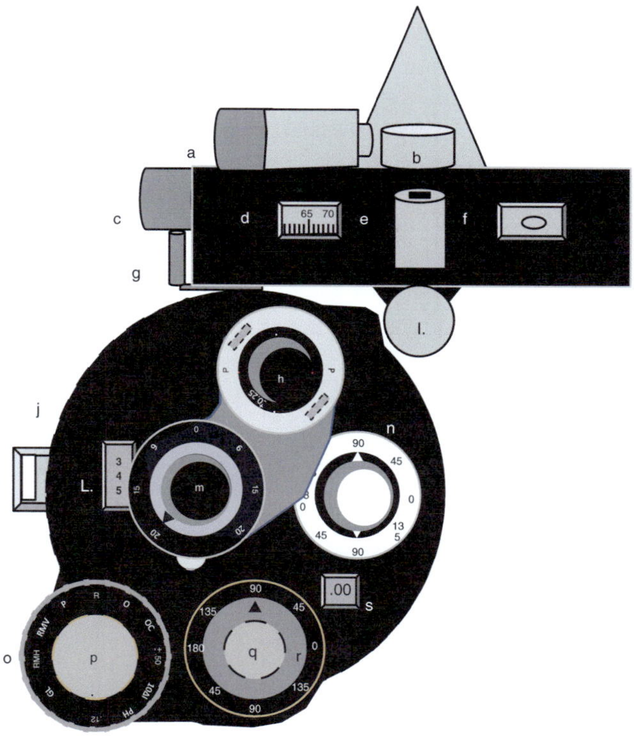

Fig. 25 Phoropter. (**a**) Leveling knob. (**b**) Rotation adjustment knob. (**c**) Pupillary distance knob. (**d**) Pupillary distance scale. (**e**) Near rod holder. (**f**) Level bubble. (**g**) Convergence setting. (**h**) Jackson cross cylinder. (**i**) Vertex distance forehead rest knob. (**j**) Sphere power dial. (**k**) Vertex distance mirror. (**l**) Sphere power scale. (**m**) Risley prism. (**n**) Cylinder axis scale. (**o**) 3D sphere power change. (**p**) Auxiliary lens knob. (**q**) Cylinder power knob. (**r**) Cylinder axis knob. (**s**) Cylinder power scale

- Setting the auxiliary lens knob on "*R*" places a + 1.5D lens in the patient's view. This would allow retinoscopy to be done without having to subtract a working distance. It will also fog the patient.
- The sphere power can be adjusted +/– 0.25D at a time using the sphere power dial (see Fig. 25, J.) or the large dial (Fig. 25, O.) around the auxiliary lens knob to change 3D at a time.
- We can look at the **auxiliary dial** (for the left eye) in closer detail (Fig. 26):

Note: The right auxiliary dial is similar to the left auxiliary dial with the following notable differences. First, instead of a 10ΔI there is a 6ΔBU option. Second, instead of a GL (green lens), a RL (red lens) option can be used to simulate glasses used in Worth 4 Dot (W4D) testing. Finally, instead of WMH/WMV options, a RMH/RMV (red Maddox rod horizontal/red Maddox rod vertical) option is present.

The following features are present in the auxiliary dial:

- The fused cross cylinder (±0.50) setting can be used to measure the required add power. See Chap. 15, Glasses in Clinical Practice, for more information on how to use the fused cross cylinder setting to determine the required reading-add power.
- The **10ΔI** on the right dial and a **6ΔBU** on the left **dial can** be used to dissociate the patient's vision. This is useful in binocular balance and in patients who might be malingering. A full discussion regarding binocular balance is beyond the scope of this text. For a brief discussion on malingering, see Chap. 21 Clinical Problems with Optics and Refractive Manifestations.
- **0.12** setting may be used only on picky "type A" patients, who would like to see if additional −0.25D is better than −0.12D after their 4th LASIK surgery. It is not used very often because most patients may not be able to tell a 0.12D difference. For practical purposes, most optical laboratories are unable lenses in powers smaller than 0.25D steps.
- **RL** (red lens) is on the patient's right, and **GL** (green lens) is on the patient's left. This can be used in W4D testing to look for suppression scotomas or diplopia. It is important that the color of the W4D matches the colors of the lens filters; otherwise, this may lead to false "fusion" readings.
- The Maddox rods **RMH, RMV** (on the patient's right) and **WMH, WMV** (on the patient's left) can help test the patient for torsional diplopia, but they do not rotate so they cannot be used to quantify the amount of torsion. For example, a patient with a right superior oblique palsy with right hypertropia and right excyclotorsion looking through RMH and WMH would describe a tilted red line going from her right shoulder down to her left hip; the red line will be below the white line.[10]
- If you can't find those plastic polarized glasses that came with the stereoacuity book, the polarized filters **P** in the phoropter are useful when checking binocularity.

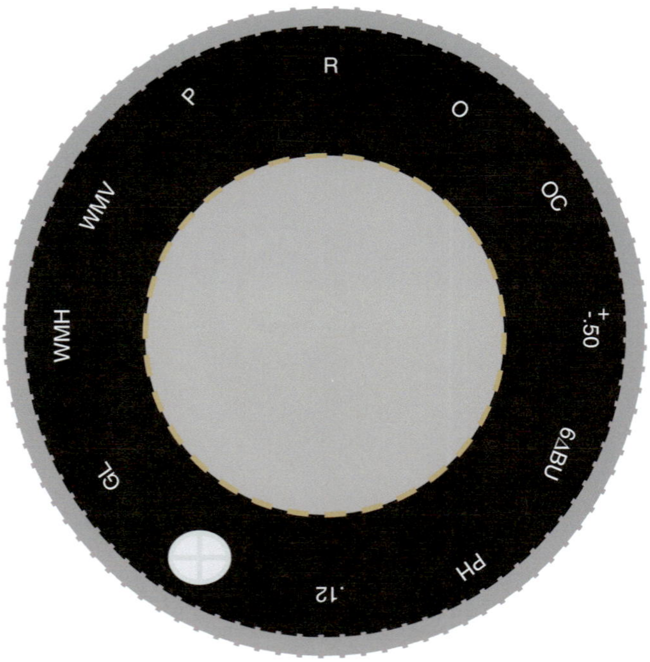

Fig. 26 Auxiliary lenses for the left eye: **R**, Retinoscopy. **O**, Open. **OC**, Occluded. **+ − 0.50**, Jackson cross. **6ΔBU**, 6 Diopter base-up prism. **PH** Pinhole, 0**.12** 0,12 D lens, **GL** Green lens, **WMH** White Maddox rod horizontal, **WMV** White Maddox rod vertical, **P** Polarized lens

The final tool is the Risley prism with a range from 0 to 20 PD that can be found on both sides (Figs. 25, H, and Fig. 27). Each consists of two wedge prisms inside the cylinder that can be rotated to be used as horizontal or vertical prisms. With the "0" in the horizontal position, up to 20 PD BU and BD prism can be dialed in (indicated by a black arrowhead); with the "0" in the vertical position, up to 20 PD BI and BO can be dialed in. This is a very useful tool to measure phorias, tropias, and vergence amplitudes in patients with diplopia and strabismus. Patients can even adjust the small dials (green double-ended arrow) to find the prism power they like best.

Trial Frames

Trial frames allow the patient to try their refraction prior to purchasing lenses. They should be considered in certain clinical situations, such as:

[10]This is somewhat counterintuitive, but we assure you that we have checked this in the clinical setting and is not a typo.

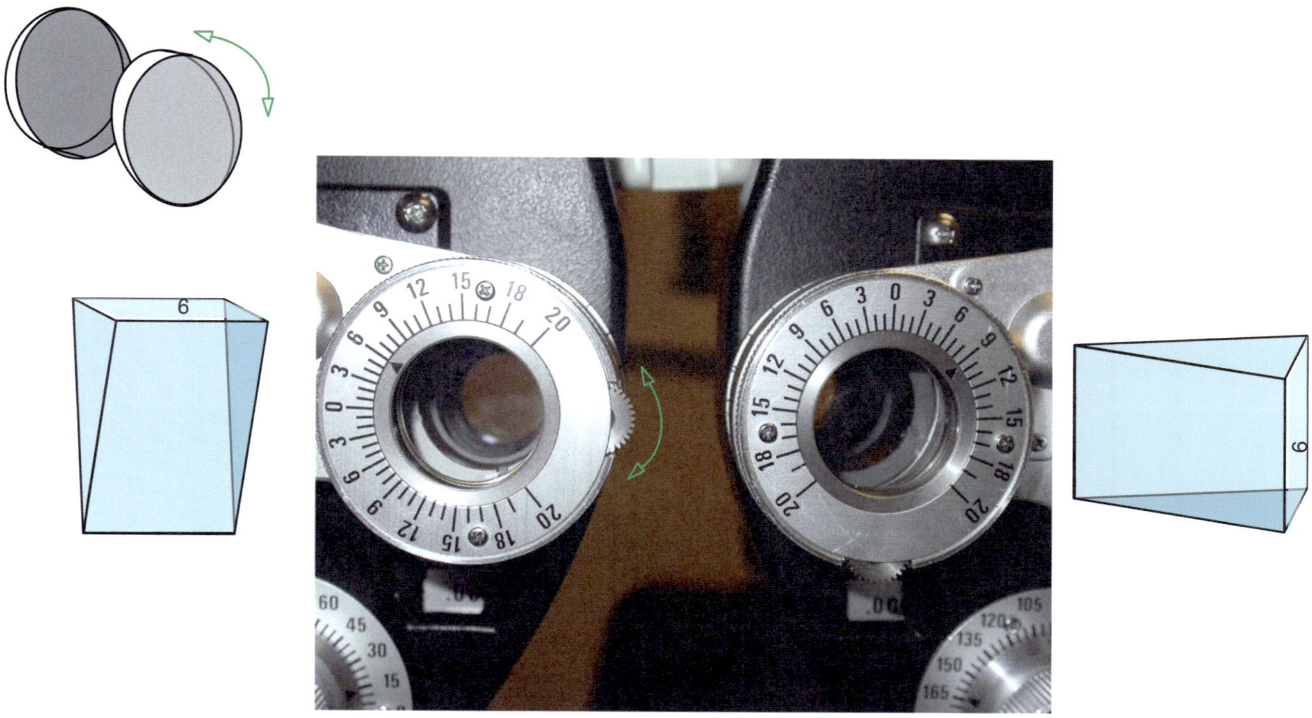

Fig. 27 A Risley prism combination consists of two wedge prisms inside the cylinder (top left panel). In this example, the phoropter Risley prism on the left side of the figure shows a 6 PD base-up setting, and the Risley prism on the right side of the figure has 9 PD base-out setting. The small dark triangles on the silver ring show the base of the prisms is "up" on the left and "out" on the right side

- To help decide on whether or not it is worth changing their glasses
- If the new manifest refraction reveals a significant change in the axis of astigmatism
- If the new manifest refraction is a borderline anisometropic prescription (approaching ~3D between the two eyes)
- To appease very picky, highly demanding patients
- To trial prism lenses for correction of diplopia prior to dispensing
- To be used for double Maddox rod testing

If a patient is taking an excessive amount of time in deciding between lens options during a manifest refraction, the trial frames allow for patient flow as well. We may give the new prescription in a trial frame and tell the patient to walk around for a bit as we continue to see other patients.

Trial frames have several disadvantages, including but not limited to not fully simulating dispensed spectacles, having difference in base curves, and limited field of vision.

When using trial frames, we can take note of three "slots" (cells) (Fig. 28). In general, the highest sphere power obtained during manifest refraction should go in the rear cell. The cylinder power should go in the middle cell, and the axis can be adjusted accordingly. Finally, low power sphere lenses (e.g., −0.50D and +0.50D) or prisms can be placed in the front cell. This allows for easy swapping in and out of low sphere power to titrate the final refraction while minimizing effects of longer vertex distance.

Distometer

The vertex distance is the distance from the cornea to the back surface of the spectacle lens. For most low-moderate refractive errors, a standard distance of 12.5 mm vertex distance is used. For higher powers (both high minus and high plus), changing the vertex distance will affect the power of the lens (See Chap. 6 Lens Effectivity).

When dispensing glasses, and especially for higher power prescriptions, we must ensure that the vertex distance is the same as the old prescription. This can be measured using the phoropter or a device known as the **Distometer** (Fig. 29). Notice that the distometer is used with the patient's eyelid closed – this is a nice way to prevent iatrogenic corneal abrasions! In terms of accuracy, the device is calibrated to assume an upper eyelid thickness of 2 mm so that the measured vertex distance does not need to be further adjusted by the examiner.

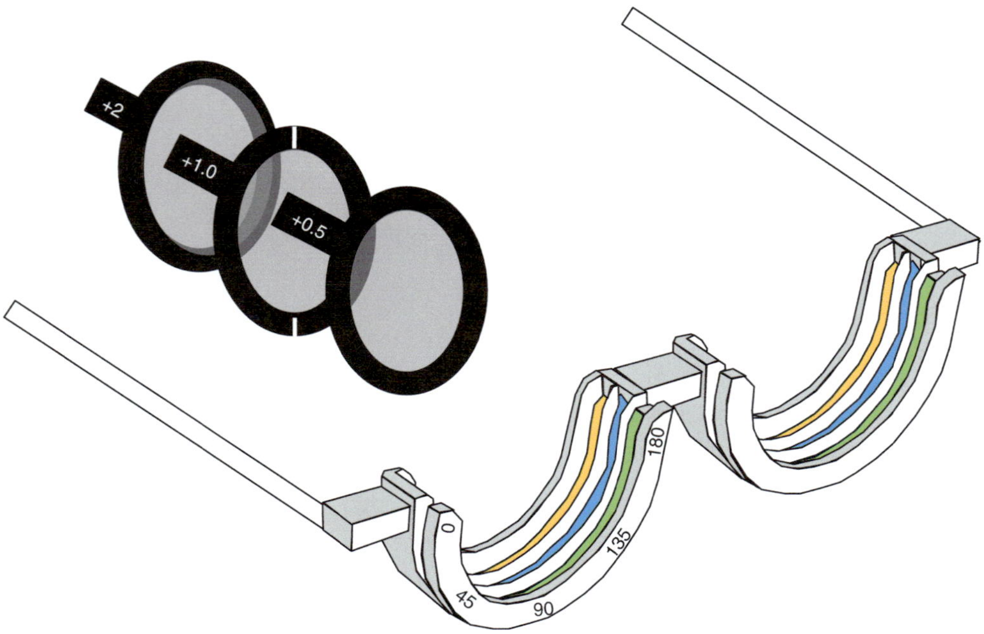

Fig. 28 Trial frames will have three cells. High power trial lenses should go in the most posterior cell (yellow). Cylinder power is placed in the middle slot (blue), and low spherical power (e.g., −0.50D and +0.50D) is placed in the front slot (green) to allow for easy exchange

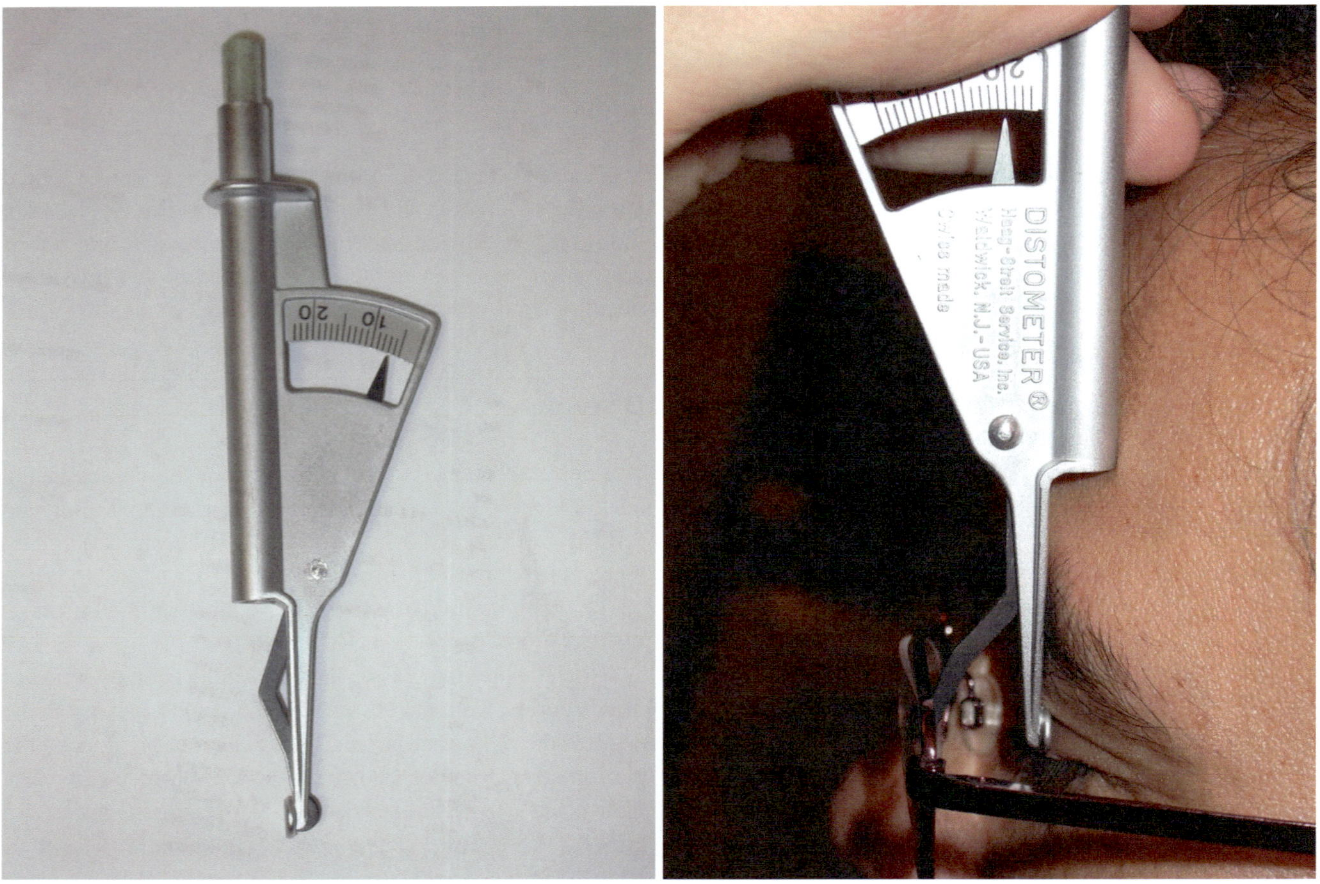

Fig. 29 This distometer is used to measure the vertex distance. Notice that the patient's eyelid is closed. The device is calibrated to assume approximately 2 mm thickness of the upper eyelid. The measured reading therefore does not need to be further adjusted to calculate the correct vertex distance

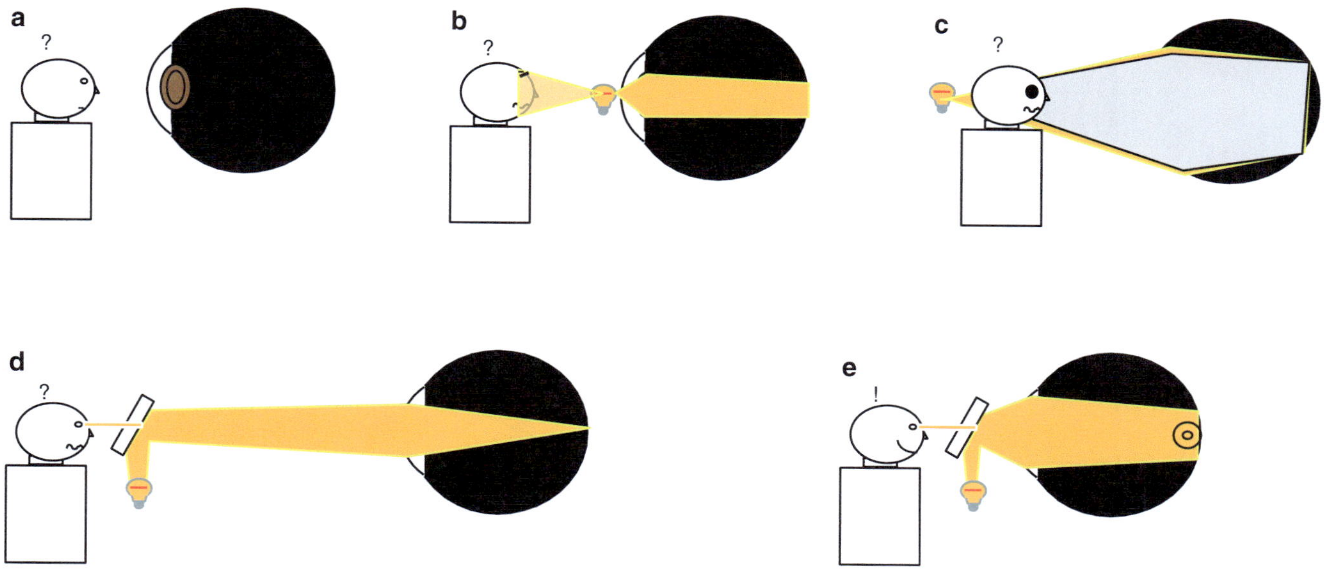

Fig. 30 In ambient light conditions (**a**), the examiner is unable to visualize the patient's retina. If a light source is placed between the examiner and the patient (**b**), the light will illuminate the patient's retina but would cause glare to the examiner and preclude his/her view. If the examiner sits in front of the light (**c**), then the light is effectively useless and creates a situation similar to (**a**). A 45-degree mirror and prism combination can be used to project light onto the patient's retina while allowing for the examiner to simultaneously observe the illuminated posterior segment. If the examiner is too far away from the patient (**d**), he/she will not be able to examine the patient properly. When the examiner is viewing the patient's eye from close range (**e**), he/she will be able to examine the patient's retina

Direct Ophthalmoscope

The direct ophthalmoscope: a neuro-ophthalmologist's second favorite instrument for viewing the optic nerve. (The −55D Hruby lens attached to some slit lamps is the preferred.) This instrument uses the built-in optics of the patient's own eye. Remember that an emmetropic human eye acts as a + 60D lens (see Chap. 7 "Schematic Eye"). We can also take advantage of **angular magnification** to visualize the posterior segment (see angular magnification section below).

The humble ophthalmoscope has quite the history in ophthalmology. It was first developed in the 1800s by Cambridge mathematics professor Charles Babbage (1791–1871) and then by German physicist Hermann von Helmholtz (1821–1894) in 1915. Later, William Noah Allyn (yes, the same of the company fame) developed the world's first handheld direct illuminating ophthalmoscope.[11]

Let's think of this as a superhero origin story! The device overcame a simple problem of how to look through a dark pupil as no one had been able to do this before. Since the posterior segment is relatively dark, an observer would need a light source that was bright enough to illuminate the retina while simultaneously allowing enough reflected rays to exit the eye and create a conjugate retinal image outside the eye, preferably on the observer's retina (Fig. 30). If the observer sits behind the light, the light blocks the observer's view and produces a lot of glare. If the observer sits in front of the light, then the observer blocks the light.

The ophthalmoscope overcomes this problem by having an internal light source perpendicular to the examiner that is then redirected to the patient. Originally, a 45-degree mirror with a small opening in the center was used, and later a prism was added to modify the original design. This construction allows the examiner to project light into the patient's eye paraxial to the examiner's line of sight without blocking the view or causing glare.

Modern ophthalmoscopes will have a light source that is coaxial to the observer's line of sight (without blocking it) and small diameter compensating lenses to focus a virtual **upright image** of the patient's retina onto the observer's retina. In contrast, an *indirect ophthalmoscope* (see next section) will form an *aerial inverted image* in front of the observer.

This simple model works as long as the patient and the examiner are emmetropes (Fig. 31). However, if either one has a significant refractive error (hyperopia or myopia), then the compensating lens power must be dialed into the ophthalmoscope accordingly. Multiple compensating (plus and minus) lenses can be placed into a dial (similar to the phoropter) (Fig. 32). The aperture size can be varied, and the source of light can be made to seem as if it originates at the 45-degree two-way mirror.

[11] Ophthalmoscopy. https://en.wikipedia.org/wiki/Ophthalmoscopy. Accessed June 7, 2020

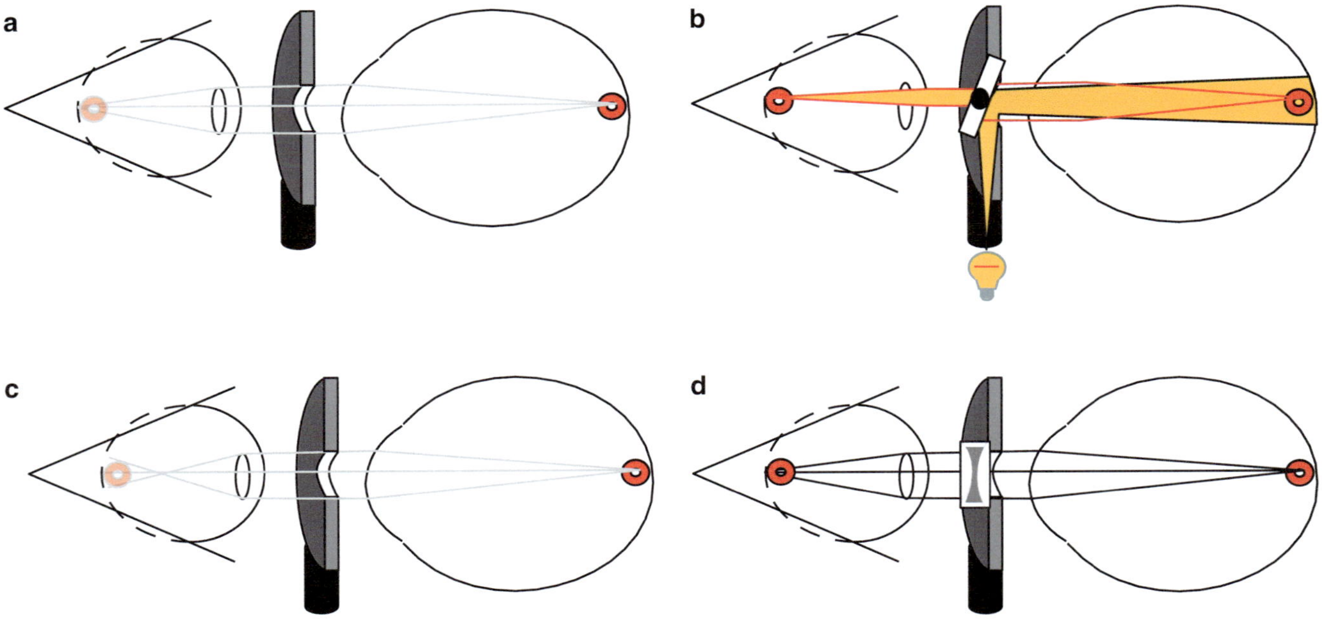

Fig. 31 Direct ophthalmoscope compensating lens. (**a**) If the patient and the observer are emmetropes, then a conjugate image of the patient's retina will form on the observer's retina, but a stronger light is needed to see it. (**b**) A bright light source and a two-way mirror illuminate the retina and create a bright image on the observer's retina. (**c**) If the patient is ametropic, the conjugate image will be out of focus. (**d**) If a small compensating lens is dialed in, then a focused image can be formed on the observer's retina

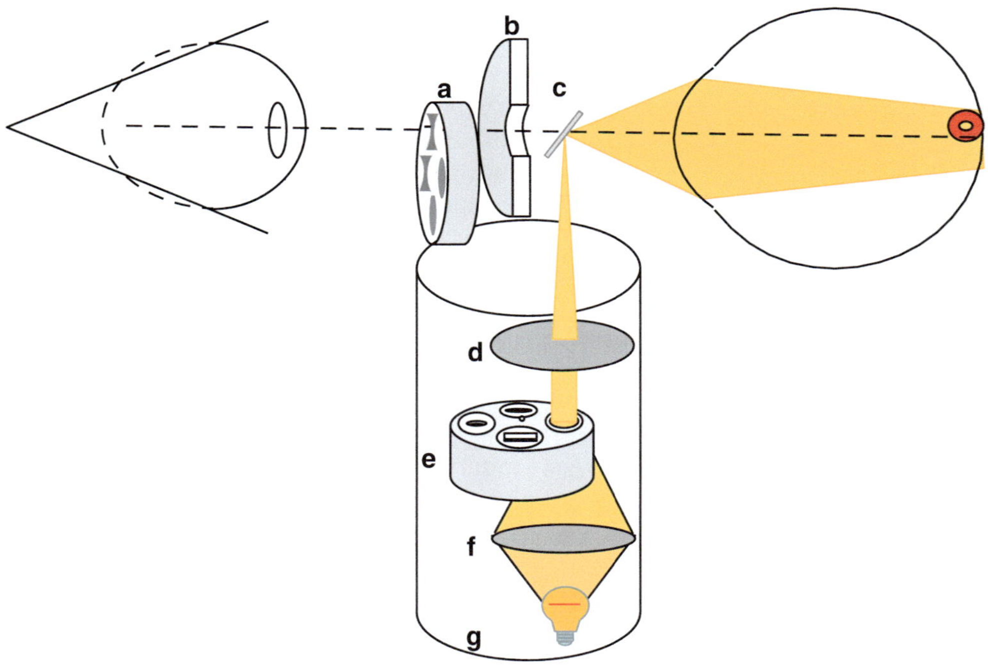

Fig. 32 Direct ophthalmoscope components: (**a**) Lens wheel with compensating lenses. (**b**) Peephole. (**c**) 45-degree two-way mirror. (**d**) 2nd condensing lens. (**e**) Aperture wheel. (**f**) 1st condensing lens. (**g**) Light source

The second converging lens (Fig. 32, D) will focus the light source on the mirror. If this light source were far away, then the light rays entering the eye would be parallel and focused on a single point on the retina. Since a wider area of illumination is desired, a diverging ray is preferred. A pharmacologically dilated pupil will also allow more light into the patient's eye and increase the illuminated area to 3 mm. The power of the compensating lens will depend on the patient's refractive error and the distance to the patient. The examiner may use the ophthalmoscope and continue to wear his/her glasses as a result.

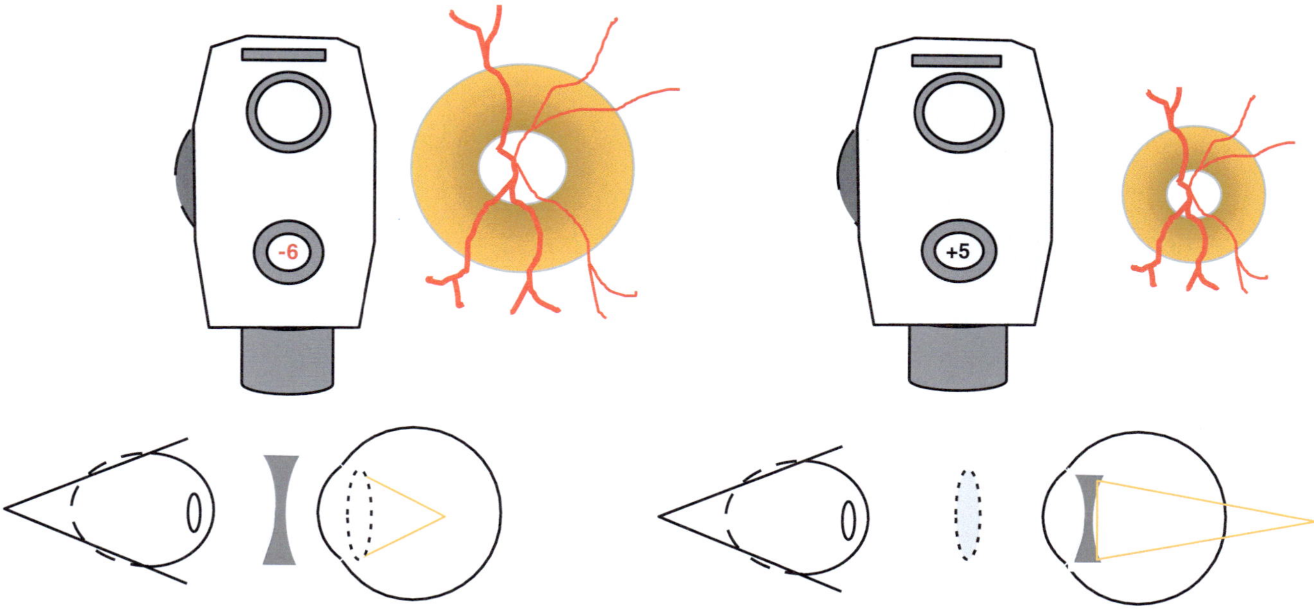

Fig. 33 Left panel shows a plus-power internal refractive error in a myopic patient and a minus-power lens dialed into the ophthalmoscope which creates a magnified image through a Galilean telescope (minus-power eyepiece and plus-power objective lens). Right panel shows a minus-power internal refractive error in a hyperopic patient and a plus-power lens dialed into the ophthalmoscope which creates a minified image through a *reverse* Galilean telescope (plus-power eyepiece and minus-power objective lens)

The direct ophthalmoscope will use the optical properties of the patient's eye to magnify the image as well.[12] While ray tracing would show no magnification, angular magnification causes a 15-fold magnification (60D/4) in an emmetropic patient. When examining myopic patients, the examiner will notice extra magnification due to the Galilean telescope formed by the minus-power compensatory lens dialed into the ophthalmoscope and the plus-power internal refractive error of a myope. Similarly, when examining a hyperopic patient, a reverse Galilean telescope is formed, and the patient's retina may be less magnified (though this may give a secondary advantage of increased field of view). As always, you cannot escape geometric optics! (Fig. 33)

Several miscellaneous notes to finish this section:

- To avoid touching noses with the patient, the examiner should use his/her right eye to examine the patient's right eye and vice versa.
- To better see the optic nerve, the examiner should position himself/herself approximately 15 degrees to the temporal side of the patient.
- The ophthalmoscope may also be used to compare the red reflex of both eyes simultaneously from a distance.
- The ophthalmoscope may also be used to test for eccentric fixation as well as use the slit feature to perform a Watzke-Allen test to assess for macular pathology – proving that if one has excellent clinical exam skills, one doesn't always to have order an OCT of the macula!

PanOptic Ophthalmoscope

The PanOptic™ is a modified ophthalmoscope (Welch-Allyn, Skaneateles Falls, NY, USA) that provides good visualization of the posterior segment and may be preferred by both examiners and patients.[13] Using a longer working distance, it provides a larger, 25-degree field (similar to a binocular indirect but maintains an upright image of the posterior pole) through an undilated pupil (Fig. 34). The examiner can also stand further away from the patient, which is handy in the era of social distancing! The simplified internal optics includes 3 plus-power lenses and a light source that is focused on the cornea.[14] This allows illumination through a small pupil and avoids reflections from other anterior structures. A light aperture that is conjugate with the pupil blocks extra reflections as well.

[12]For a review of angular magnification, see Chap. 8 "Magnification and Telescopes"

[13]Petrushkin H, Barsam A, Mavrakakis M et al., Optic disc assessment in the emergency department: a comparative study between the PanOptic and direct ophthalmoscopes. *Emerg Med J*. 2012;29(12):1007–1008. https://doi.org/10.1136/emermed-2011-200038

[14]If you pay close attention to the diagram, you can see this is a modified astronomical telescope with an additional plus power lens to "re-invert" the inverted image.

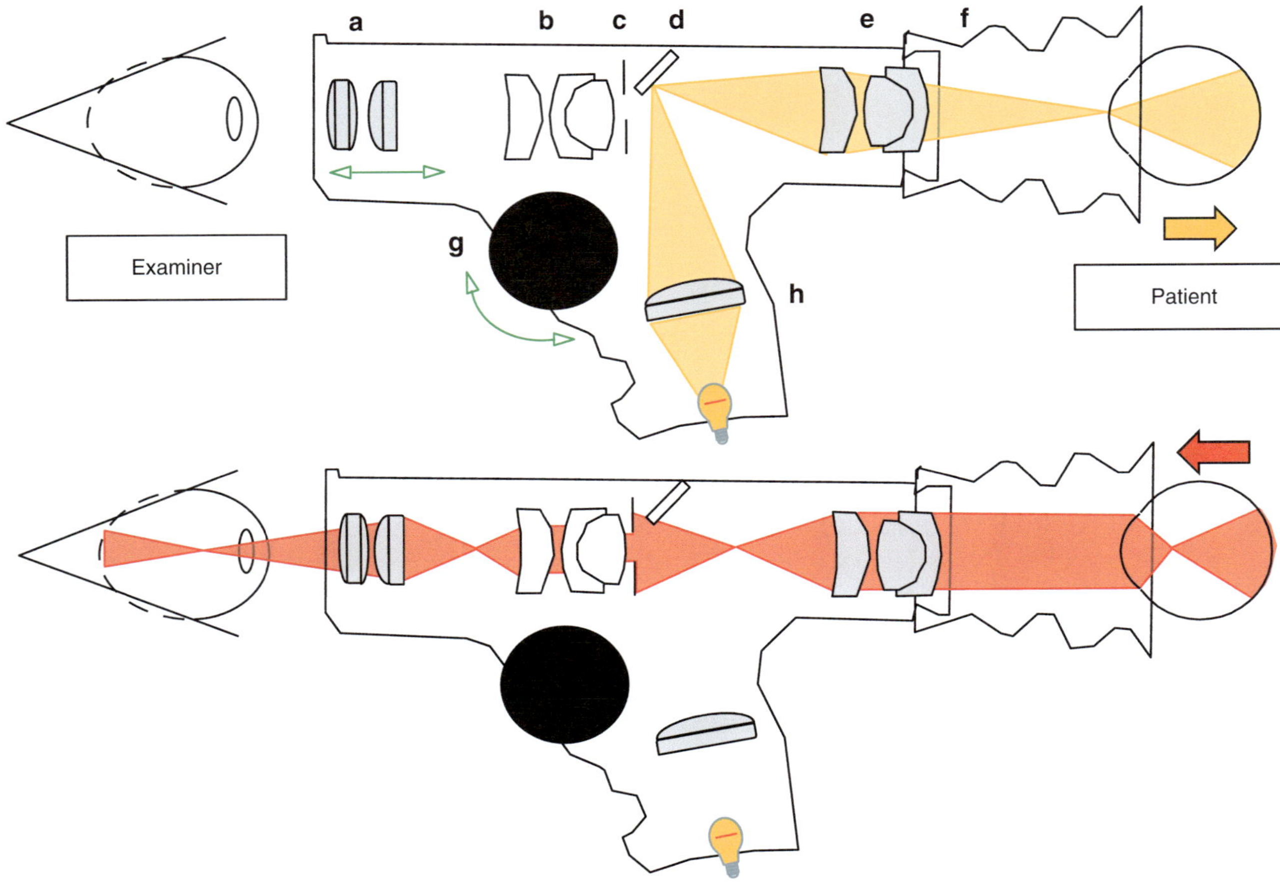

Fig. 34 PanOptic™ ophthalmoscope. The top panel shows the Illumination system, the bottom panel shows the viewing system. (**a**) Eyepiece. (**b**) Imaging lens ~ + 40D. (**c**) Incoming light aperture. (**d**) Mirror to reflect light source. (**e**) Objective lens ~ + 40D. (f) Soft extensor to block other light sources. (**g**) Focus dial to move eyepiece. (H) Condenser lens focuses light onto the mirror

Binocular Indirect Ophthalmoscope (BIO)

While the direct ophthalmoscope has its many advantages, the examiner is limited by a small, two-dimensional view of the patient's fundus. Wouldn't it be even better to have an instrument that allowed us examine a patient's eye, confers a three-dimensional view, and also frees up our hands? By now you can tell that we enjoy giving a historical context to the instruments we use.

In the 1930s, a young Belgian medical student was trained as an ophthalmologist at Moorfields Hospital in England. He saw his life upended by the German invasion of Belgium during War World II. First, he joined the Belgian air force and then joined the resistance. After his second capture, he fled to France with his wife and two children and joined the resistance there. Posing as a lumber mill operator, he helped smuggle over 100 refugees across the Pyrenees while under the nom de guerre Jacques Pérot. After being discovered by the Gestapo, he fled to England where he began work on the binocular indirect ophthalmoscope (BIO). In 1947, he emigrated to the USA and started the first retina service at the Massachusetts Eye and Ear Infirmary. His name: Professor Charles L. Schepens, MD.[15]

Compared to the direct ophthalmoscope, the BIO has certain notable features:

- Larger field of view (25 degrees vs. 7 degrees).
- Allows examination of the peripheral retina.
- Decreased magnification from 15× to 3× (when using a 20D lens) (60/20 = 3×).
- Better view of the fundus in patients with media opacities.
- The line of sight of both of the observer's pupils enters the patient's pupil in a paraxial fashion but through a slightly different path than the illumination. This reduces reflections and back scatter.[16] The narrower new pupillary

[15] "Charles L. Schepens, MD". https://eye.hms.harvard.edu/charlesschepens. Accessed June 7, 2020

[16] This reflex-free system was designed by Gullstrand. Yes, the same optics genius who won a Nobel Prize for the reduced schematic eye (See Chap. 7, "Schematic Eye").

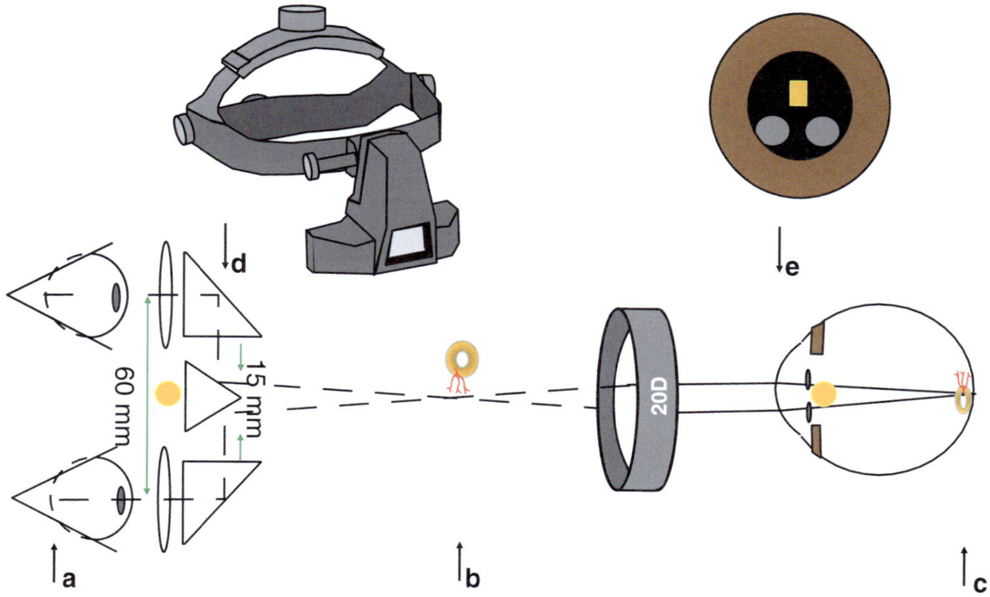

Fig. 35 Binocular indirect ophthalmoscope (BIO). The binocular eyepiece reduces PD to about 15 mm. Using a 20D condensing lens, an aerial, inverted, real image will form 5 cm anterior to the lens. (**a**), (**b**), and (**c**) planes are conjugate. (**d**) The faceplate and (**e**) the patient's cornea are conjugate; an image of the patient's pupil will form on the faceplate, and an image of the faceplate will form on the patient's pupil. (**e**) shows the image of the observer's pupils (gray circles) and the light source (yellow square) that are formed on the patient's cornea, within the pupil. Light rays and image rays between the 20D lens and the cornea will be parallel

distance will reduce stereoacuity, but this is compensated for by axial magnification (Fig. 35).

- The BIO is more useful in a wiggly pediatric patient than the direct ophthalmoscope. Clinical pearl: animal crackers have been used by our authors for years to improve cooperation of young patients.

We can examine the construction of the BIO in greater detail (Fig. 35). The BIO's binocular eyepiece reduces the examiner's pupillary distance (PD) to approximately 15 mm. When examining an emmetropic eye, an inverted, real image will form 5 cm anterior to the 20D lens. Notice that examiner's eyes, 20D lens, and patient's eye will form a conjugate plane. An image of the examiner's eyes and light source will form on the patient's cornea (Fig. 35, E).

The power of the condensing lens will determine three things:

- Viewing distance
- Field of view
- Magnification

Thanks to the laws of similar triangles,[17] an easy rule of thumb when it comes to magnification of the handheld lens is to divide the refractive power of the eye (60D) by the power of the lens. Let's use a 20D lens as our examining lens. We can use the laws of similar triangles to determine the magnification of the image (Fig. 36). The focal length of the lens is 1/20 = 50 mm; the focal length of the eye (using the RSE) is 17 mm.[18] We can convert the focal length into power to make the math easier:

Transverse magnification = power of the eye/power of the lens = 60D/20D = 3×

Therefore, a 20D lens would magnify the retina 60/20 = 3×; a 30D lens would have a larger field but less magnification 60/30 = 2×. The 20D lens is the most commonly used lens for BIO in adults. For examination of pediatric patients, especially patients with retinopathy of prematurity (ROP), a 28D lens is preferred as zones 2 and 3 will be easier to see.

Earlier, we stated that the BIO reduces the pupillary distance from +60 mm to 15 mm. One would expect normal stereopsis to be reduced as well by 4×. However, as mentioned above, axial magnification compensates for this. Using a 20D lens, we can calculate the axial magnification = (transverse magnification)^2 = $(3\times)^2$ = 9×. Now applying the reduction of PD (4×), we can calculate the final magnification obtained when using the BIO as:

Final magnification with BIO = 9/4 = 2.25×.

[17] See Chaps. 7 and 8 "Schematic Eye" and "Magnification and Telescopes".

[18] We could also divide the focal length of the lens by the focal length of the eye: 50 mm / 17 mm = 3.

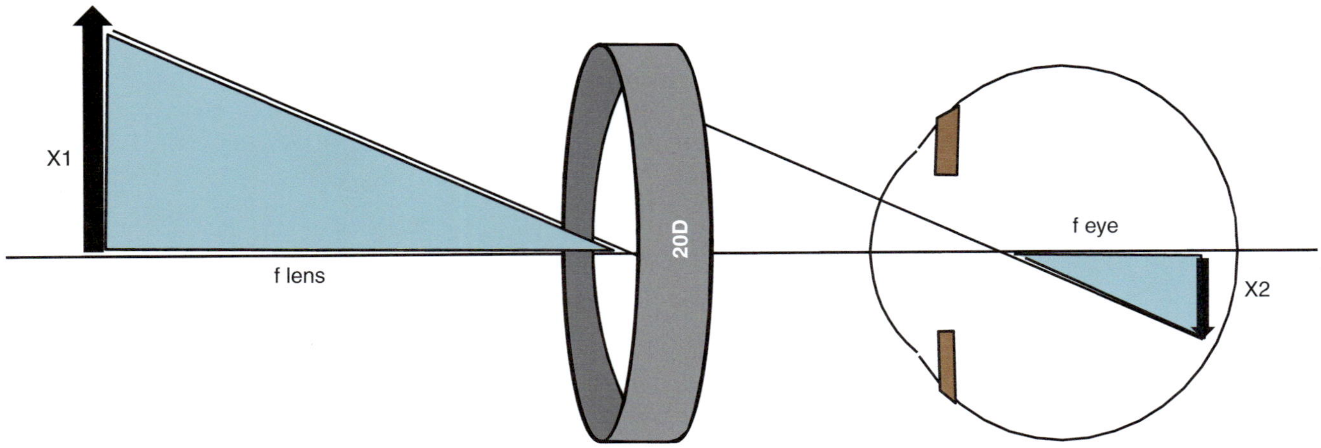

Fig. 36 The laws of similar triangles help us determine the magnification of the image

Operating Microscope

Here's another instrument we couldn't live without. If we approach this tool from a problem-based perspective, we would need an operating microscope with the following features:

- Provides adequate and adjustable magnification
- A light source that provides sufficient illumination without causing thermal and photic injury to the patient's eye
- Makes all rays parallel and paraxial to avoid shadows, glare, and other optical aberrations
- Maintains binocularity and stereoacuity while magnifying a very small area
- Hands-free control of magnification, focus, light, and X-Y-Z axes
- An observer scope to help first-year ophthalmology residents lubricate the cornea with *just* the right amount of BSS
- Cup holder (optional) and music player (advanced models only)

While there are many brands of operating microscopes currently available, all of them are built upon the following optical principles that address surgeons' needs (Fig. 37)[19]:

- A light source is located in the floor stand far away enough to not heat up the surgeon's forehead. A fiber optic cable can be used to bring the light onto the field.[20] As with other microscopes, the light is coaxial – parallel to the line of sight, but not in the same spot. Once again, Gullstrand's reflex-free system is used to our benefit. A nearly collimated light beam or a focused light beam may be used.[21] (For those of you who are too embarrassed to ask, collimating means to make rays parallel, close to zero vergence.)
- Binoculars to allow stereoscopic vision.
- Magnification changer and a collimating lens.
- Beam splitter allows a second person or camera to have a view as well.
- Foot pedal to control X/Y/Z axes, magnification, focus, and lighting.

From an ophthalmic optics standpoint, we should appreciate that many of the previously discussed concepts are used in the modern operating microscope, such as lenses, mirrors, total internal reflection, Galilean telescope, and magnifiers. Further subtopics regarding the operating microscope, such as optimizing visualization, avoiding photic damage, etc., are beyond the scope of this text. You may wish to consult the operating manual of a given microscope and/or consult other available resources for more information.

Slit Lamp Microscope

Built upon similar principles as the ophthalmoscopes, the slit lamp has three main components: an illumination system, a stand, and an observation system. We can use the schematic used in the commonly encountered Haag-Streit slit lamp (Haag-Streit, Switzerland) as an example (Fig. 38).

[19]Cordero I. Understanding and caring for an operating microscope. *Community Eye Health*. 2014;27(85):17

[20]Fiber-optic cables use total internal reflection (TIR) to transmit light. See Chap. 1 "Geometric Optics", for more on TIR.

[21]Cionni RJ, Pei R, Dimalanta R, Lubeck D. Evaluating Red Reflex and Surgeon Preference Between Nearly-Collimated and Focused Beam Microscope Illumination Systems. *Transl Vis Sci Technol*. 2015;4(4):7

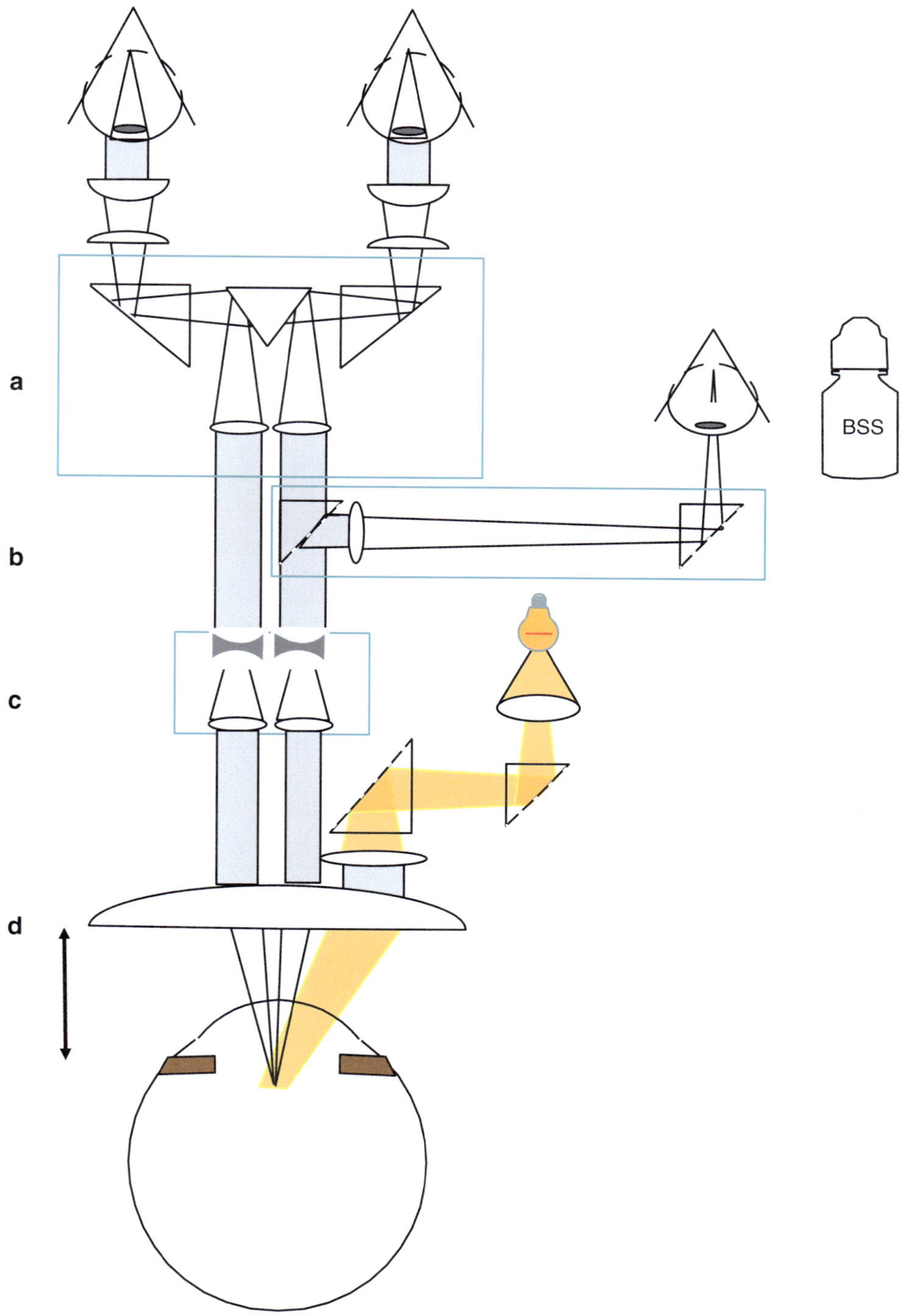

Fig. 37 Operating binocular microscope. (**a**) Binoculars include eyepieces, objective lenses, and mirrors to narrow the pupillary distance. (**b**) Beam splitter uses a 45-degree two-way mirror. (**c**) Magnification changer using a Galilean microscope. (**d**) Main objective lens with a fixed working distance 15–20 mm (dark arrow). Gray areas show parallel rays. Assistant's bottle of BSS not included

Again, notice the many familiar components we have previously discussed, including mirrors, Galilean telescope, and prisms.

Illumination System

A beam of light in the shape of a thin slit coming in at an angle will allow the observer to see small details and depth better than a wide beam of light aimed straight on. Imagine a quiet, dark cabin with a curtain slightly open and a ray of sunshine illuminating the dust particles floating in the air as the observer ponders the secrets of optics.[22] To form an evenly illuminated slit beam, an occluder with a thin linear opening is placed between a condenser lens and an objective lens (Fig. 39). This is known as the Kohler illumination principle, wherein the occluder is analogous to the diaphragm aperture in a camera.

[22]Who said that optics can't be poetic?

Fig. 38 Haag-Streit slit lamp microscope schematic. (**a**) Illumination source. (**b**) Patient's eye. (**c**) Tilted mirror. (**d**)+10D objective lens. (**e**) 16× Galilean telescope. (**f**) Porro-Abbe prism. (**g**) Adjustable eyepiece. (**h**) Observer

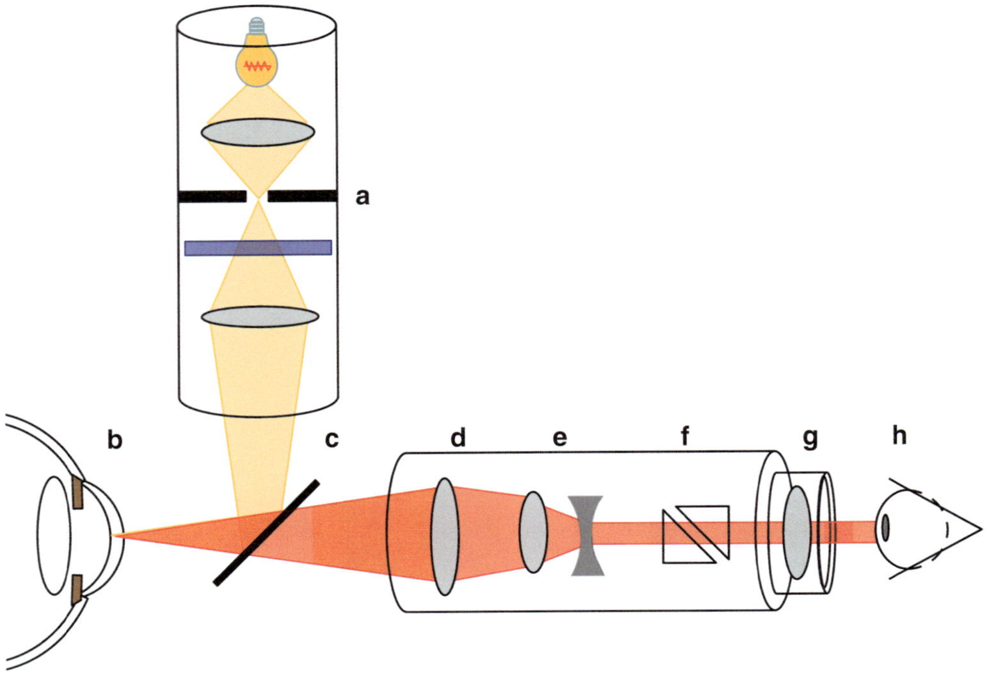

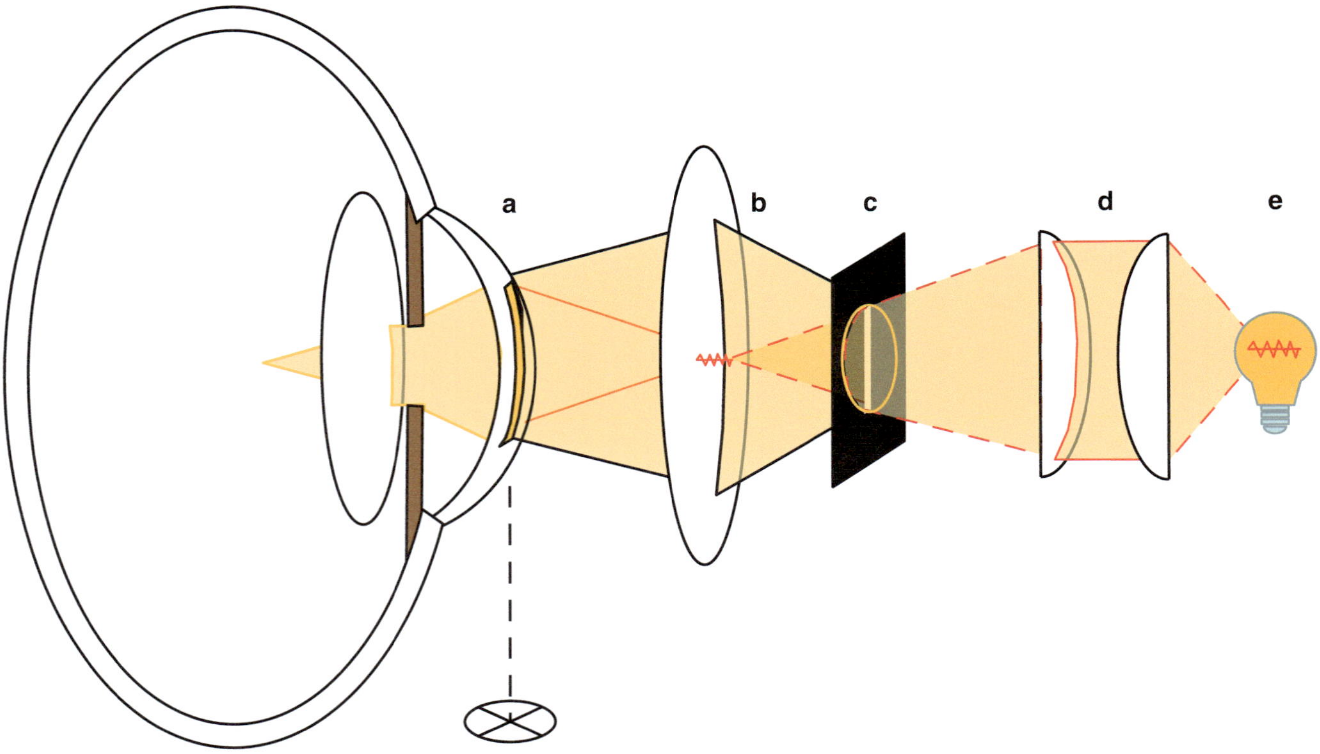

Fig. 39 Kohler illumination principle within a slit lamp. (**a**) Image of slit/optical section over the common pivot point of the viewing and illuminating arms. (**b**) Objective lens with an image of the filament. (**c**) Occluder with slit opening. (**d**) Condenser lenses. (**e**) Light source. Notice **a** and **c** are conjugate planes (dark lines) as are **b** and **e** (red dashed lines)

Due to the refractive power of the cornea and the lens, light does not reach the fundus without a diverging lens such as a handheld lens (+90D, +60D) or the attached Hruby lens. The Hruby lens is a −55D lens that is found as an attachment on some slit lamps that can be slid into view in order to examine the fundus. Note that it will provide an upright image of the patient's retina (mnemonic: Hr**u**by = **u**pright)

The incoming light may be located below the examiner (as in the Zeiss slit lamps) or above the examiner (as in the Haag Streit slit lamps). The light and viewing systems may be arranged in a parfocal setting with both systems focused

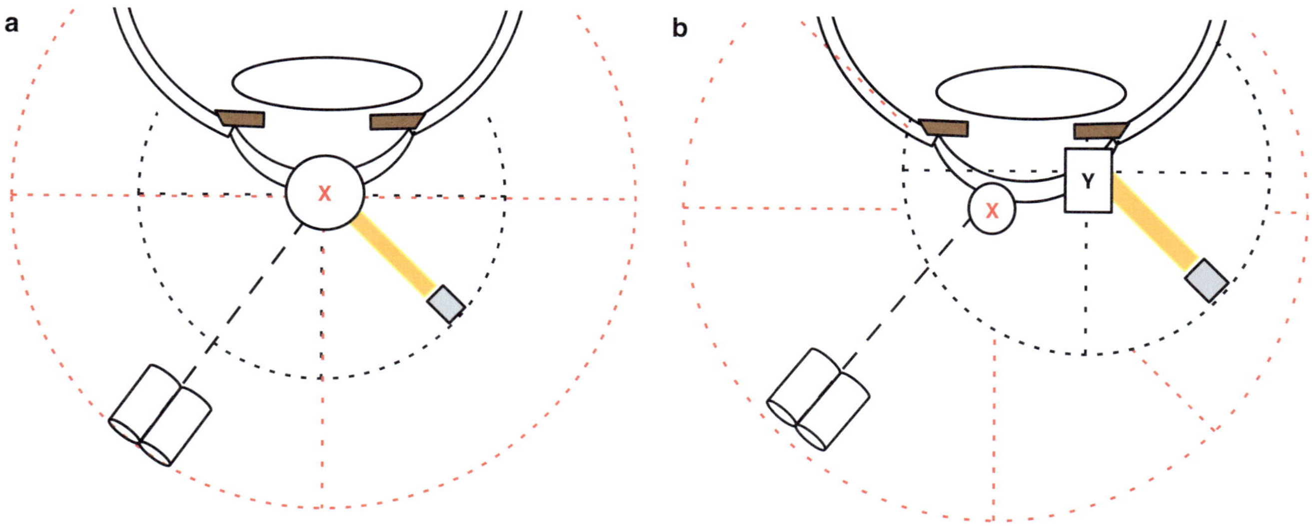

Fig. 40 Parfocal vs. non-parfocal settings. Panel A shows an example of the viewing system and the illumination system in a parfocal setting, both focused at the same location of interest. Panel B demonstrates a non-parfocal setting wherein the viewing system is rotating around point "*X*" and the illumination system is rotating about point "*Y*." This may be helpful in certain clinical situations, especially if the examiner wishes to evaluate peripheral corneal or anterior chamber angle pathology

on the same plane on the eye or non-parfocal setting (Fig. 40). A non-parfocal setting may be useful to examine pathology located in the far periphery of the anterior segment (cornea, angle anatomy).

Using different techniques (with varying angles and illuminations), clinicians can examine the anterior segment with various illumination methods, including direct focal illumination, diffuse illumination, specular reflection, transillumination, indirect lateral illumination (retroillumination), and sclerotic scatter. A full discussion regarding the appropriate application and advantages of each technique are beyond the scope of this text. However, there are several optical principles we can appreciate:

- Specular reflection relies on a non-parfocal setting in order to examine the peripheral endothelium.
- Sclerotic scatter involves aiming intense light at the limbus from an incoming angle that is greater than the critical angle. The cornea will reflect this light according to the principle of total internal reflection. This also requires a non-parfocal setting.
- Several light filters are selectable with each viewing method. For example, the red-free (green) filter can be used to visualize the nerve fiber layer and intra-retinal hemorrhages by filtering out undesirable wavelengths of light. The cobalt blue filter (450–500 nm) will function similar to the excitatory blue filter used in fluorescein angiography to improve visualization of topical fluorescein.[23]

[23]Refer to the discussion in Chap. 14 "Physical Optics and Advanced Optical Principles".

Stand

The stand may include:

- Comfortable and stable rest surface for patient and observer
- Joystick to control *X, Y, Z* axis
- Control of illumination and magnification
- Power source
- Applanation tonometer
- Fixation lights (select models)
- Protective shield (very important in a post-COVID world!)
- Cell phone charger (deluxe models only)

As we mentioned previously, the observer should be careful with their posture to avoid chronic cervical problems from repeated use.

Observation System

The observation system of a slit lamp is very similar to an operating microscope (see Fig. 37); it will have several familiar optics devices:

- Stereoscopic eyepieces
- Magnifying Galilean telescope
- Objective lens
- A Porro-Abbe prism is used to reinvert the image. This unique glass prism is constructed such that four right-angled prisms are joined face-to-face fashion.

Incoming light undergoes total internal reflection four times (ensuring no loss of right-left orientation) within the prism before exiting in the same orientation as the incoming light.[24] The image is rotated 180 degrees as a result – in some ways, this functions as an astronomical telescope to "re-invert" the returning image to the examiner.

The aforementioned Galilean telescope component therefore maintains the "re-inversion" caused by the Porro-Abbe prism, yielding an overall upright image with maintained left-right orientation.

Keratometer

Purkinje Images

Before discussing the construction and application of the keratometer, it is important to first discuss the concept of Purkinje images. There are four main Purkinje images – each image is a reflection of incoming light from an internal structure within the eye:

- P1 (aka corneal reflection or glint): Reflection of light from the anterior corneal surface. This is the brightest of the four images and used in keratometry and topography.
- P2: Reflection of light from the posterior corneal surface. This is the dimmest of the four images.
- P3: Reflection of light from the anterior crystalline lens surface. This is the largest of the Purkinje images.
- P4: Reflection of light from the posterior crystalline lens surface. This is the only "inverted" image and has a brighter intensity than P3. For cataract surgeons, this is of significant importance because the position of P4 (compared to P1) can be used for intraoperative assessment of IOL position and pseudophacodonesis (Fig. 41).

For all intents and purposes, we can combine P1 and P2 into a single image since they are almost completely superimposed. P1 and P4 are usually used to determine eye position, though some devices may use the third image as well.

As an aside, in modern surgical microscopes that use three lights, P1, P3, and P4 may appear as a triangular cluster of lights (P1 and P3 would appear like an upright pyramid whereas P4 would appear as an inverted pyramid). Interestingly enough, under certain lighting conditions, you may be able to visualize P3 and P4 as this

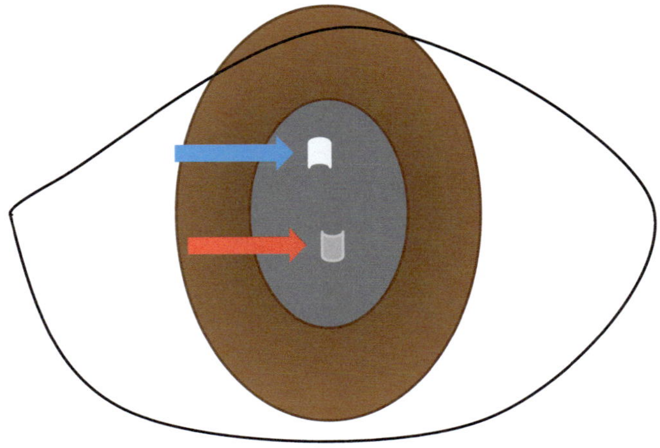

Fig. 41 Purkinje images seen on slit lamp examination. The first and second Purkinje images (P1 and P2, blue arrow) usually appear as a superimposed figure in the superior pupillary space. The fourth Purkinje image (P4, red arrow) is usually seen in the inferior pupillary space. P4 is inverted relative to the other images. P3 is not shown in this figure.

reflected light may be "reflected back into the eye" from the posterior corneal surface creating an entoptic phenomenon. Finally, P3 and P4 in a pseudophakic eye come from the anterior and posterior optic of the IOL; these can vary widely from case to case based on the IOL size, material, toricity, and other factors. A more detailed discussion of Purkinje images and their intraoperative role in cataract surgery can be found in Chap. 28, Intraoperative Optics for Cataract Surgery.

Manual Keratometer

Also known as an "ophthalmometer," the manual keratometer measures the curvature of the cornea and its refractive power. This is useful in various clinical settings, including but not limited to contact lens evaluations, quantifying keratometric astigmatism, evaluating the health of the tear film, determining the source of a patient's astigmatism, and detecting irregular astigmatism.

Some limitations of the manual keratometer include:

- Limited to two-point measurements at 3–4 mm central corneal zone.
- Does not provide any information about the peripheral cornea.
- Does not account for spherical aberration.
- Susceptible to misalignment and focusing errors.
- Though distortion of mires indicates irregular astigmatism, the presence of distorted mires precludes a quantified, accurate measure of keratometric astigmatism.

[24]Porro-Abbe prism. https://en.wikipedia.org/wiki/Porro%E2%80%93Abbe_prism. Accessed June 7, 2020

- User skill and experience: as automated devices, including corneal topographers, have become popular; performing manual keratometry is quickly becoming a lost art!

The most commonly used manual keratometer uses two formulas to derive the dioptric power of the cornea.

The first formula is our good friend from Chap. 5, Power of Lenses in Different Media, the equation used for determining the refractive power of a spherical surface:

$$D = (n' - n) / r$$

where n' is the index of the cornea, n is the index of refraction of air (1.0), and r is the radius of curvature. Though the keratometer measures the anterior corneal surface, it uses an assumed index of refraction of 1.3375 rather than the actual 1.376.

The second formula is used to find the radius of curvature. If we consider the anterior surface of the cornea as a convex mirror, we can apply the following formula:

$$r = 2^* d(I/O)$$

where "*d*" is the distance from the object to the 1st virtual Purkinje image formed within the eye. Note that this Purkinje image is different from the previously discussed Purkinje images of the cornea and crystalline lens. In this scenario, a ring is placed in front of the keratometer light source that ends up creating a virtual image of this ring posterior to the corneal surface (inside the eye). Because the distance from the mirror (cornea) to the image (*v*) is so small (4 mm), "*d*" can be approximated to just (*u*), which is the fixed distance between the keratometer and the cornea. "*I*" is the image size, and "*O*" is the object size (the size of the illuminated ring(s)) (Fig. 42).

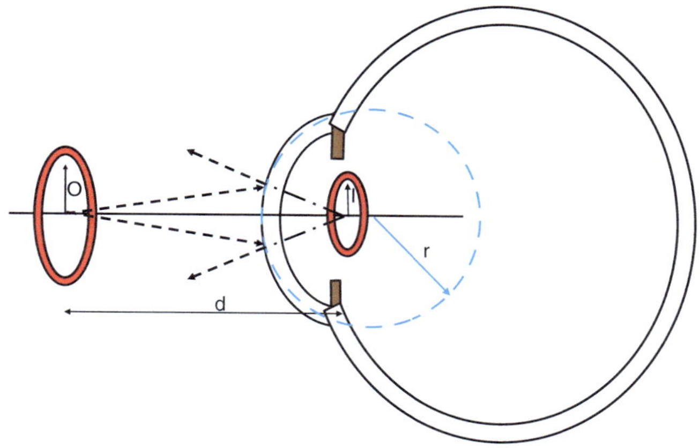

Fig. 42 Keratometry formula. $r = 2 * d\ (I/O)$, **r** radius of curvature of the central cornea (blue arrow and blue circle). **d** Distance between the object and the image, **O** Radius of the object, **I** Radius of the image. Note that the Purkinje image of the ring forms posterior to the patient's cornea (inside the eye)

How to Use the Manual Keratometer

When performing keratometry, the goal is to focus the mires and center the reticle in the bottom right circle (known as the focusing circle) (Fig. 43):

1. Measure the horizontal meridian. Turn the horizontal drum (left drum) to superimpose the plus signs (Fig. 43, Panel B).
2. Measure the vertical meridian. Turn the vertical drum (right drum) to superimpose the minus signs (Fig. 43, Panel C).
3. Record the values of the horizontal drum (meridian closest to 180 degrees) and the vertical drum (meridian closest to 90 degrees). The difference between the two readings is the amount of keratometric astigmatism (in plus cylinder) present in the patient's cornea (Fig. 43).

Practice Questions

1. Which of the following is the most likely cycloplegic refraction if, during streak retinoscopy (at the standard working distance), you observe neutralization while moving the intercept left to right across the 90-degree axis and with motion when moving up and down across 180-degree axis? (Fig. 44)
   A. Plano +1.00 × 180
   B. −1.50 + 2.00 × 180
   C. Plano +1.00 × 90
   D. −1.50 + 2.00 × 90

2. If the Geneva lens clock measures the following:
   What will be the most likely strength of this spectacle lens? (Fig. 45)
   A. −1.00 + 2.00 × 090
   B. −6.00 + 2.00 × 180
   C. +1.00 + 6.00 × 090
   D. +1.00 + 2.00 × 180

3. Where would you place the spectacle lens in this lensmeter? (Fig. 46)
   A. Location A
   B. Location B
   C. Location C
   D. Location D

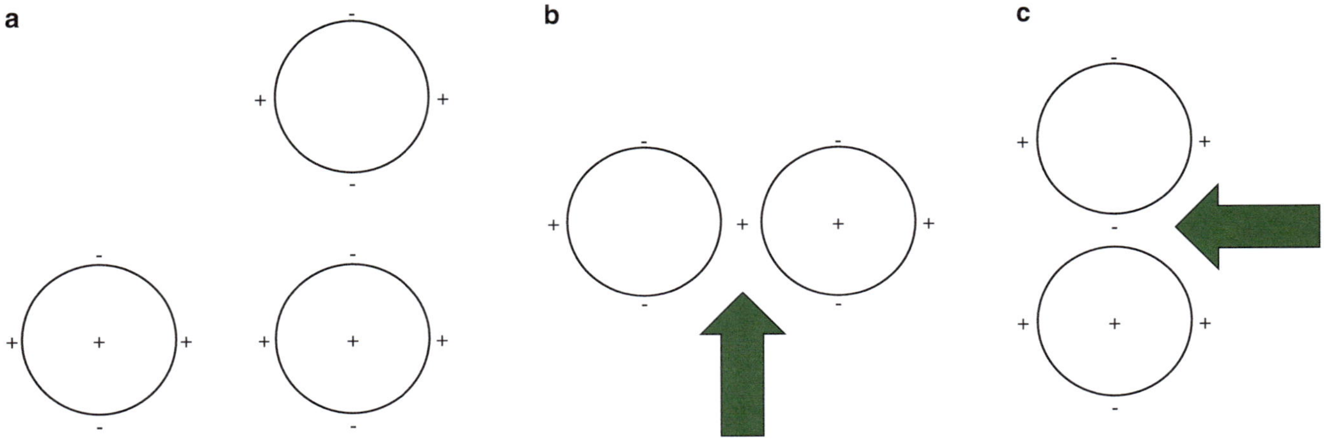

Fig. 43 Sequences for performing manual keratometry. (**a**) The focusing circle (bottom right circle) is used to quantify the amount of keratometric astigmatism. (**b**) The horizontal meridian can be assessed by superimposing the plus signs by rotating the left drum. (**c**) The vertical meridian can be assessed by superimposing the minus signs by rotating the right drum. The difference in the recorded values is the amount of keratometric astigmatism present (in plus cylinder)

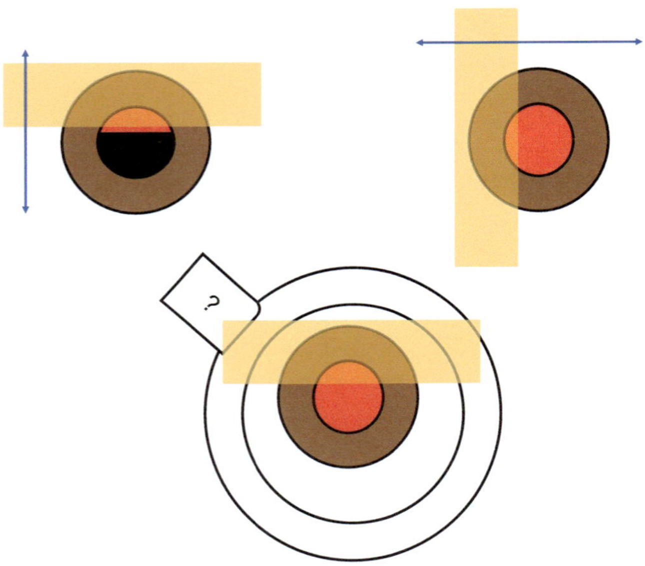

Fig. 44 This patient has a light streak that moves with motion across the 180-degree axis and neutralizes across the 90-degree axis

4. What kind of ground in prism is present in this lens (Fig. 47)?
   A. 3 PD base-down
   B. 4 PD base-down
   C. 4 PD base-up
   D. 5 PD base-down.

5. Using a direct ophthalmoscope, the examiner must dial additional −6.00D compensating lens power to see the patient's uncorrected eye fundus clearly. Will the optic nerve appear more or less magnified than a zero setting in an emmetrope?
   A. More minification
   B. More magnification

Answers

1. Answer: B (−1.50 + 2.00 × 180). If neutralization is achieved across 90 degrees with zero sphere and with motion is observed along 180, then we know that this patient requires a corrective cylinder placed in the 180-degree meridian (in order to act at the 90-degree axis). Though we are not given the amount of cylinder power used, we can see from the answer choices that we can safely eliminate C and D as the correcting cylinder in these choices is placed in the 90-degree meridian (which would act at the 180-degree axis, which is 90 degrees away from where we need the corrective cylinder). Looking at answer choices A and B, we know that we must add an additional −1.50 sphere once the working distance is subtracted. The trial lens used is likely a + 2.00 × 180 cylindrical lens.

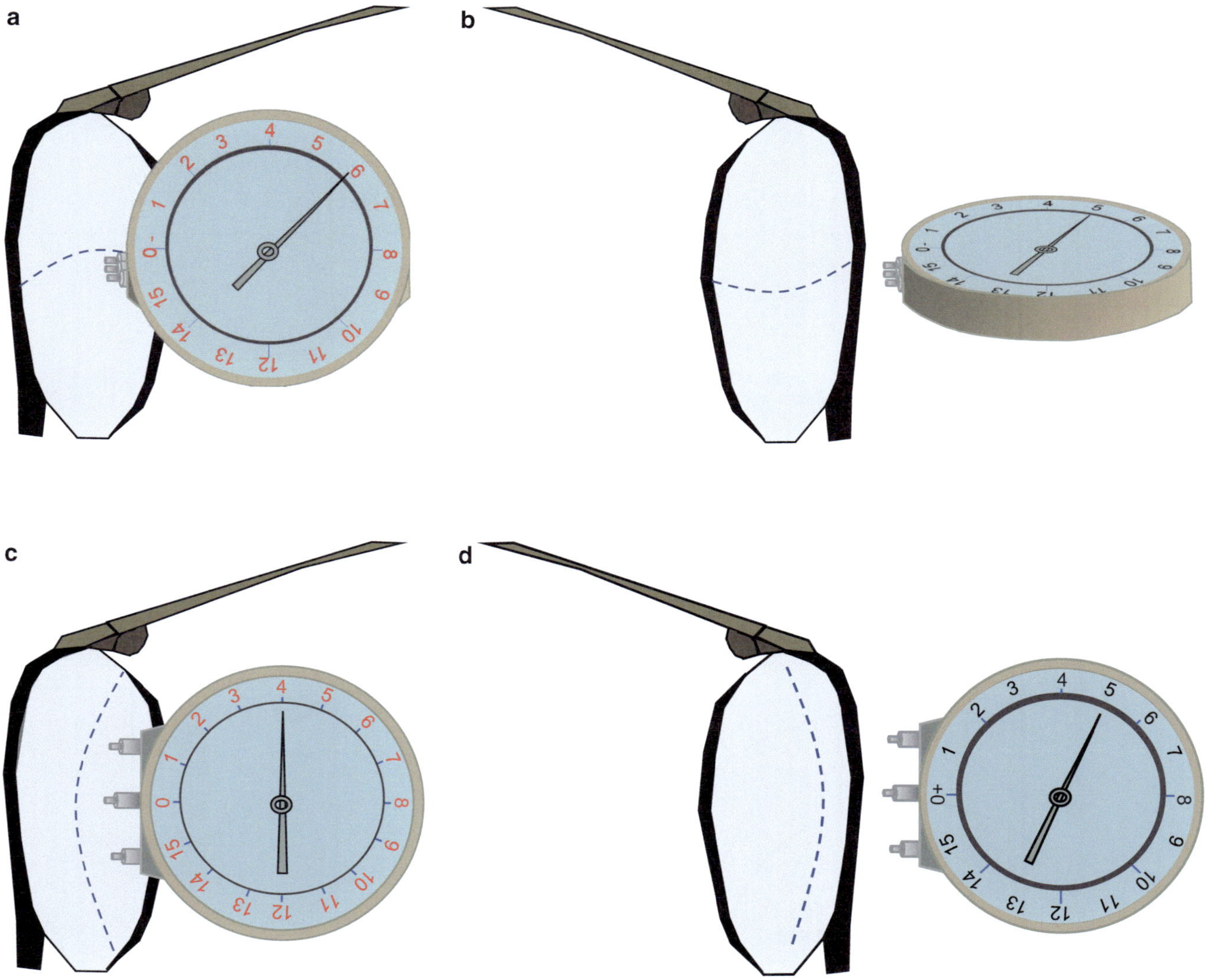

Fig. 45 GLC measurements. (**a**) On the back surface the GLC reads −6.00D along 90 degrees and −4.00D along 180 degrees. The front surface is +5.00D along both meridians

2. Answer: A (−1.00 + 2.00 × 90). We know that the power of the front surface is +5.00D. For the back surface, we basically have −6.00D @ 90 and −4.00D @ 180. We can write this as a power cross as seen in Fig. 48 (top right panel). We can then combine the front surface and back surface power crosses to generate the combined power cross (bottom panel). Then using the double arches method, we can determine that the power of the spherocylindrical lens is −1.00 + 2.00 × 90 (Fig. 48).
3. Answer: Location B. The spectacle lens should be placed where the rays are parallel.
4. Answer: C. Notice that the yellow lines intersect the 1st bar above the 3rd circle representing the amount of prism (4 PD) and location of prism (base-up) relative to the centering circle.
5. Answer: B. Dialing a minus lens within the ophthalmoscope will create a Galilean telescope when we take into account the (+) refractive error within the patient's eye. This will create a magnified image.

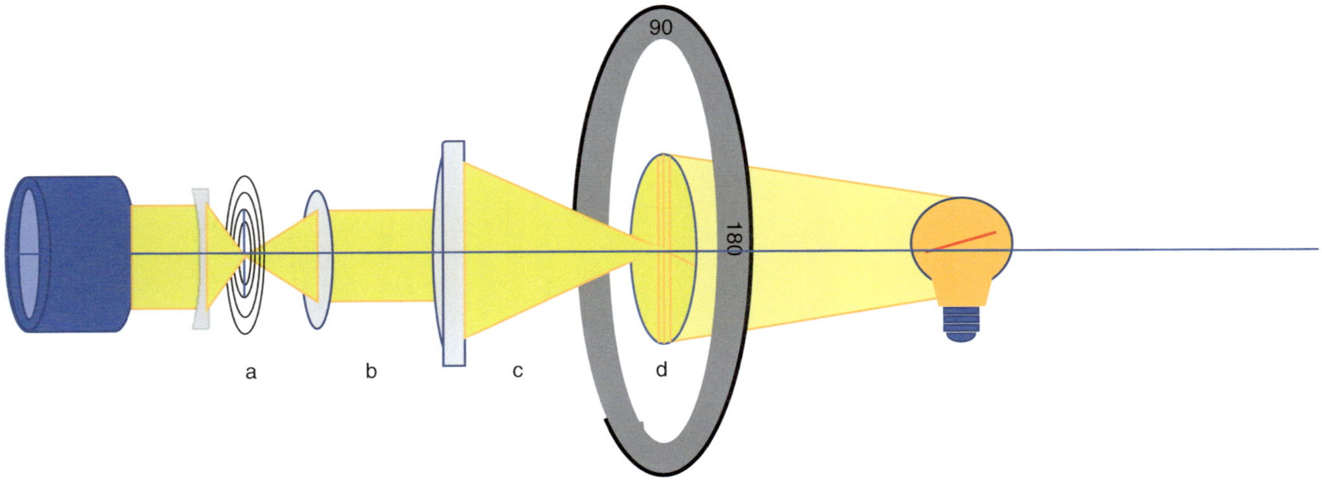

Fig. 46 Cross-section of a lensmeter

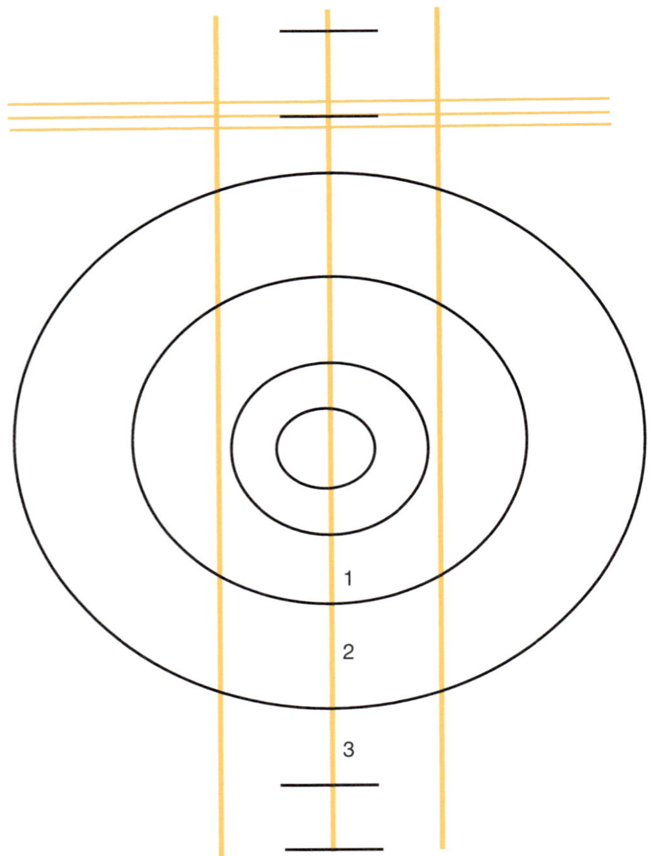

Fig. 47 Observed lensmeter results of measuring an eyeglass lens with unknown prism power

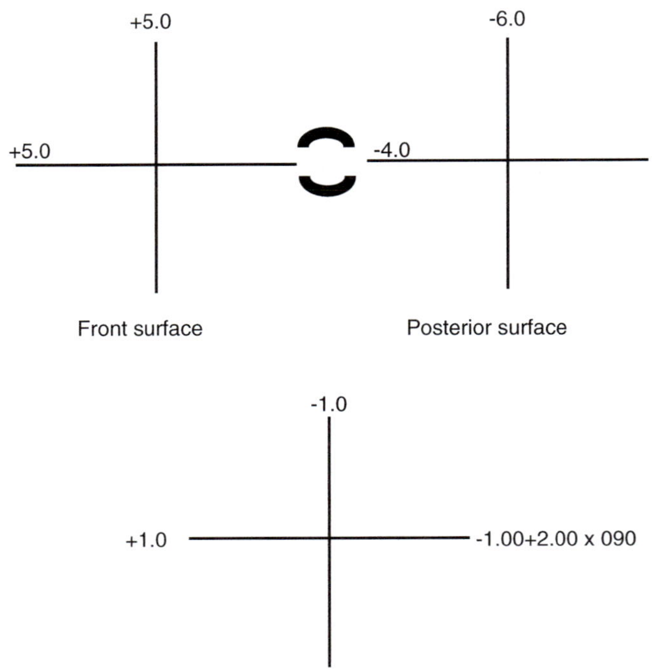

Fig. 48 The front surface is a spherical lens of +5.00D represented by the first power cross. The posterior surface is represented by the 2nd power cross. Adding the two-power crosses produces the power cross on the bottom. This can be used to determine the power of the measured spectacle lens

Visual Acuity Testing and Assessment

Kamran M. Riaz

Objectives

- To define and understand the various methods of visual acuity testing.
- To know the differences between various terms used in visual acuity threshold measurements.
- To understand important principles regarding the Snellen visual acuity and ETDRS visual acuity charts.
- To be able to discuss alternative methods of visual acuity testing in common clinical scenarios.
- To understand the role of color vision testing and binocular testing.
- To describe how contrast sensitivity and defocus curves play a role in visual function and clinical practice.
- To memorize the definition of legal blindness in the United States.

Introduction

Visual acuity testing is like going to the DMV: no one particularly enjoys doing it, but it seems like it is something we all have to do regularly. Even you retina folks may accidentally check visual acuity (which is okay, don't feel guilty; you may have even enjoyed it).[1] Just like at the DMV, we will see many "lines," be given forms to fill out and encounter confusion at nearly every step of the way. Also, similar to visiting the DMV, you may be forced to set aside a Saturday morning when nothing else is going on to read this chapter. Make sure you are well-caffeinated because you may be here for a few hours. However, unlike going to the DMV, we hope that what you learn from this chapter will be helpful your daily practice.

As ophthalmologists, we rely on visual acuity as our main "vital sign" when examining a patient; interestingly enough, the actual testing of visual acuity is a relatively neglected topic. We hope this chapter will clear up some of the key concepts about visual acuity testing, make it less painful to understand, and maybe even teach you something along the way. Let's get in line.

Tests for Visual Acuity

The Four "Targets" of Testing Visual Acuity

Before we even get to our familiar Snellen visual acuity chart, there are some definitions of visual acuity tests that we have to (unfortunately) introduce at this time. We fully understand that some of these terms are abstract and nebulous. Hence, we have listed each term and then given a question (in parenthesis) that you can use to help understand what exactly a given test is trying to accomplish:

- Target Detection: *Do you notice this test object at all?*
  - Examples of this type of testing include the "Tumbling Es" and "Landolt Cs" test. In this type of testing, we rely on the patient's ability to visually detect the location of a gap or break in the test object (either the E or the C). This type of test can be used on a nonliterate English or illiterate adult patient. The patient can be easily instructed to tell the examiner the orientation of the letter, which in turn is an indirect test used to determine whether or not the patient is noticing the gap or break in the letter.
- Target Recognition: *Can you tell me what this test object is?*

[1] On a side note, the authors are working on patenting a light switch and marketing it as "The Retinal Surgeon's Phoropter." Phase III clinical trials are pending… just kidding; we love our retina colleagues!

K. M. Riaz (✉)
Dean McGee Eye Institute, University of Oklahoma, Oklahoma City, OK, USA

K. M. Riaz et al. (eds.), *Optics for the New Millennium*, https://doi.org/10.1007/978-3-030-95251-8_18

   - You are probably most familiar with this type of testing, such as the Snellen and ETDRS Visual Acuity charts. In this test, the patient has to not only "see" the letter, but he/she must recognize the letter as well. The choice of letters, design of the chart, and spacing between the letters are crucial factors to ensure that the letter recognition difficulty is equal for different letter sizes and chart working distances. The ETDRS chart standardizes and fills in the gaps of the Snellen chart – more on this in the sections below. This type of visual acuity testing is the most common method used in clinical and research settings.
- Target Resolution Threshold: *Do you notice the separation between these objects?*
   - This type of testing requires patients to discriminate the separation between elements of a stimulus pattern. We are testing the visual angle (see next section), so it does not require the patient to "recognize" a letter but rather the separation or space between a patterned element. It differs from Target Detection because the stimulus pattern fills up most of the testing screen. Examples of this type of testing include acuity grating testing (such as Teller acuity testing) and checkerboard pattern testing.
- Target Localization: *Do you notice any difference between these test objects?*
   - This type of testing requires patients to tell the difference in spatial positions of a segment of a test object. The most common example is Vernier acuity testing (see next section). A patient is shown lines and asked to point out where exactly he/she notices a misalignment or discontinuity in the line.

Degrees, Minutes, and Seconds of Arc

Before we continue further, we have to define some key terms and principles used in visual acuity testing:

- 1 degree is 1/360 th part of a circle.
- 1 minute is 1/60 th of a degree: this is the most important one to know.
- 1 second is 1/60 th of a minute.

Why is this important? Because all visual acuity testing methods rely on a test object/letter casting a certain angle (referred to as "subtending an angle") onto the patient's retina. The test object/letter is constructed so that each individual component can be related to some fraction of our above circle, usually in minutes of arc (also known as *arcmin*).

Let's use a more familiar example: suppose we ask a patient to look at the letter "E" on the 20/20 line on the Snellen visual acuity chart. If the patient can read the line without any glasses correction, we can pat ourselves on the back for a job well done with cataract surgery. However, what exactly is this 20/20 letter "E" doing? The letter "E" subtending an angle (casting an image with a specific size) onto the patient's retina. We are, in turn, testing the patient's ability to recognize and read it.

If we break this down further, the letter "E" on the 20/20 line is constructed so that the whole letter subtends an angle of 5 *arcmins* when viewed by an observer standing 20 feet (6 m) away; however, the letter "E" is constructed with 5 unique "strokes". Each "stroke" on the letter "E" subtends 1 arcmin as well (Fig. 1).

For an observer viewing the Snellen chart at 20 feet, larger letters will accordingly subtend larger *arcmins* proportional to their size compared to the 20/20 letter "E." For example, since the 20/200 line is 10 times the size of the 20/20 line, we can determine that the 20/200 letter "E" will subtend 10 times the *arcmins* as well: 10 x 5 *arcmins* = 50 *arcmins* subtended by the 20/200 letter "E" when viewed by an observer at 20 feet (Fig. 2). Similarly, the 20/60 letter "E" will subtend 3 x 5 *arcmins* for a total of 15 *arcmins* when viewed by an observer at 20 feet.

We will discuss the Snellen visual acuity chart in the next section, but what we need to understand at this point is that each letter on the visual acuity chart will subtend a certain angle (measured in *arcmin*) onto a patient's retina. When we test a patient's visual acuity, we are basically testing whether or not the patient recognizes these subtended angles.

With this background, we have four more definitions to review. Notice that there is some overlap between these and the ones we previously introduced – remember, this entire chapter is like being at the DMV: it seemingly defies all logic and usefulness, but you just have to get through it.

Four other terms are used in the measurement of visual function. We will group the first three together, and the fourth

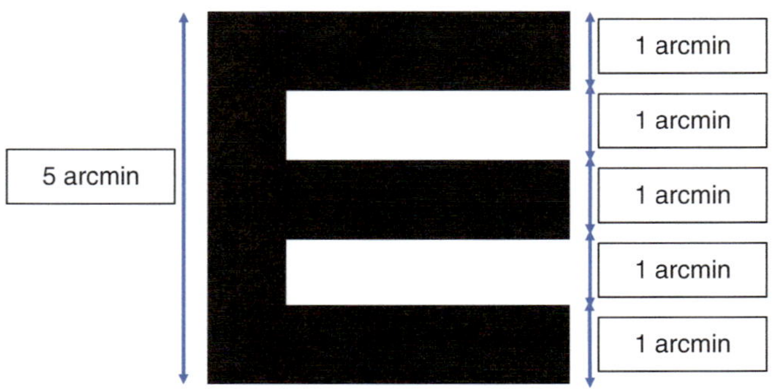

Fig. 1 Each "stroke" on the 20/20 letter "E" subtends 1 *arcmin*, whereas the entire letter will subtend 5 *arcmins* (when viewed from 20 feet away)

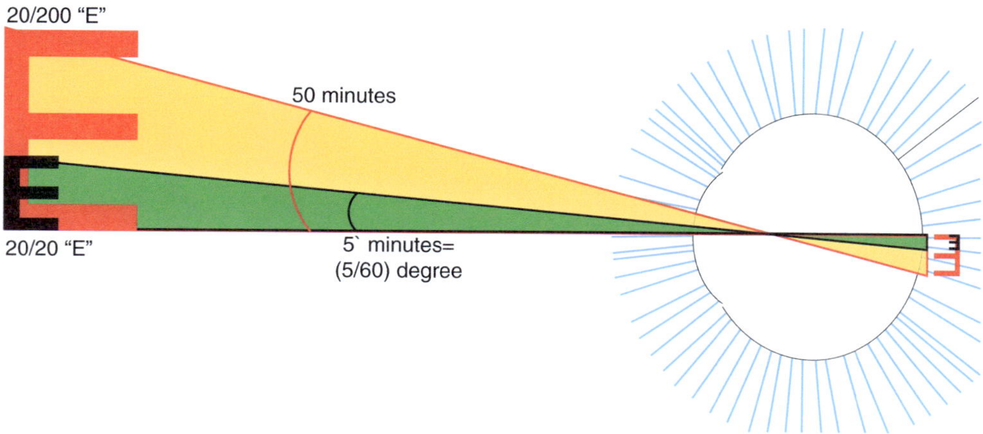

Fig. 2 The 20/20 letter "E" will subtend 5 *arcmins* to an observer viewing the Snellen eye chart at 20 feet. Using this as a reference, we can determine the *arcmins* subtended by larger letters as proportional to the 20/20 letter (5 *arcmins*). For example, the 20/200 letter "E" will subtend 10 times the *arcmins* for a total of 50 *arcmins* when viewed by an observer at 20 feet

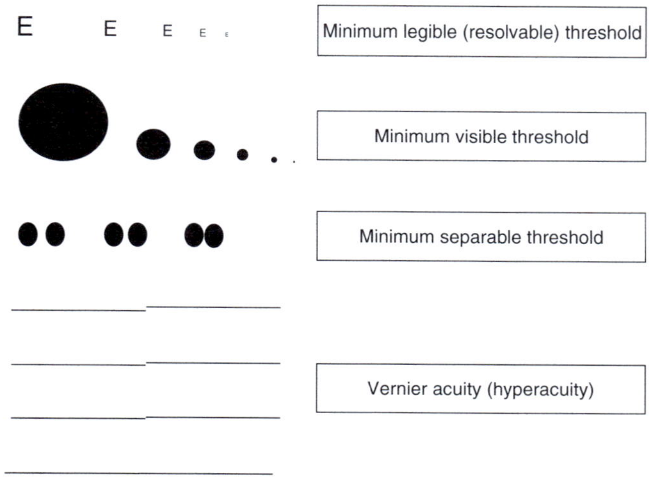

Fig. 3 Depiction of minimum legible (resolvable) threshold, minimum visible threshold, minimum separable threshold, and Vernier acuity. Minimum legible (resolvable) threshold involves testing at the *arcmin* level. Minimum visible threshold involves testing at approximately 10 *arcsecs*. Minimum separable threshold (MST) similarly involves testing at the *arcsec* level (<10 *arcsecs*). Vernier acuity, a subset of MST, is the most sensitive form of visual acuity testing and involves testing at approximately 2–3 *arcsecs*

(Vernier acuity) can be thought of as a subset of the third category (minimum separable threshold) (Fig. 3).

Minimum Legible (Resolvable) Threshold

Minimum legible threshold (a.k.a. minimal resolvable threshold) (MLT/MRT)[2]: This refers to the point at which a patient cannot further distinguish between progressively smaller **subtended angles (using letters or forms)** from one another. In this type of testing, we usually test patients on the *arcmin* level. The Snellen visual acuity chart is the most commonly used tool to determine the minimum legible threshold. For example, if a patient can only read up to the 20/40 line (and can't read any letters on the 20/30 line), we will record the visual acuity as "20/40". This notation is simply a numerical way of saying, "this 20/40 line is the patient's minimum legible threshold."

Minimum Visible Threshold

Minimum visible threshold (MVT)[3]: In some ways, this is a weird definition because we aren't really testing the patient's ability to see letters. Instead, we are testing his/her ability to **distinguish a target from a background**. Typically, a target (or letter) of varying brightness levels against a background is presented to the patient; the patient is asked to indicate which target s/he can no longer see. In this test, we ascertain the viewing angle within which the patient's eye can detect the presence (or absence) of a stimulus. Testing at this level is at seconds of arc (arcsec) and only stimulates a few photoreceptors. Lea Symbols (discussed later in this chapter) are an example of MVT testing.

Minimum Separable Threshold

Minimum separable threshold (MST)[4]: In this kind of testing, two objects are presented to the patient with progressively smaller space in between them; the patient is asked to indicate at which point he/she cannot **distinguish between the two objects (such as dots or bars) separately** because they will seem like the same object. Testing at this level is also at the level of *arcsecs*. Teller Acuity Cards (discussed later in this chapter) are a form of MST testing.

Vernier Acuity

Vernier acuity (a.k.a. hyperacuity): As discussed above, Vernier acuity may be thought of as a subset of MST. However, Vernier acuity is *much more specific than MST* as this type of testing involves asking the patient to **notice "breaks" within**

[2] Some texts may refer to this kind of testing as *recognition acuity*.

[3] Some texts may refer to this kind of testing as *detection acuity*.

[4] Some texts may refer to this kind of testing as *resolution acuity*.

a line or misalignment of line segments. Vernier acuity is the most sensitive type of testing because we are testing at the level of 2–3 *arcsecs* as the break in the line will cast an angle smaller than a photoreceptor. For example, Fig. 4 shows eight different lines constructed with segments that are "closer together" and "farther apart" than their neighbor. If you zoom (not the teleconference application) in closer, you can start to see each segment; but when you step back far enough, all the lines will seem to be straight lines, and the segments will disappear. When you are physically closer to the lines, the segments are casting angles "large" enough to be noticed by your photoreceptors; when you step back, the angles are too small to be noticed by your photoreceptors, so the lines appear to be completely straight lines.

Vernier acuity is used throughout ophthalmology: the keratometer, lensmeter, applanation tonometry, and even the Amsler grid all make use of Vernier acuity! For example, we ask patients to use an Amsler grid because very early retinal neovascularization or an epiretinal membrane that affects a few photoreceptors may not cause enough changes for a patient to incorrectly read letters (because the other photoreceptors may detect the visual stimuli and hide the flawed information from the damaged photoreceptors). However, when we present the familiar checkerboard/grid lines, we can test at the photoreceptor level to detect early pathology. Vernier acuity can therefore detect visual acuity changes before it affects the MLT/MRT, MVT, and/or MST.

For example, suppose you are looking at the image of two lines separated by a space of 3 mm (*x*) from 40 meters away (*y*) (Fig. 5). We can use similar triangles if we want to determine how large this space will be on the retina. Recall our discussions from Chap. 7 "Schematic Eye", we can use the "17 mm" rule as the distance from the eye's nodal point to the retina (*y'*). For exact numbers, we can add the 5.5 mm (distance from the nodal point to the cornea) to *y*, so that 40 meters can be rewritten as 40,005.5 mm. We can then solve for *x'* as follows:

$$x/y = x'/y'$$

$$x' = (x/y)*y' = (3\text{ mm} / 40005.5\text{ mm}) * (17\text{ mm}) = 0.0013\text{ mm}.$$

The width of a retinal cone is approximately 0.004–0.005 mm, so the image can easily be captured by a retinal cone. In other words, Vernier acuity allows this image to be perceived by a single retinal cone when viewed from 40 meters away!

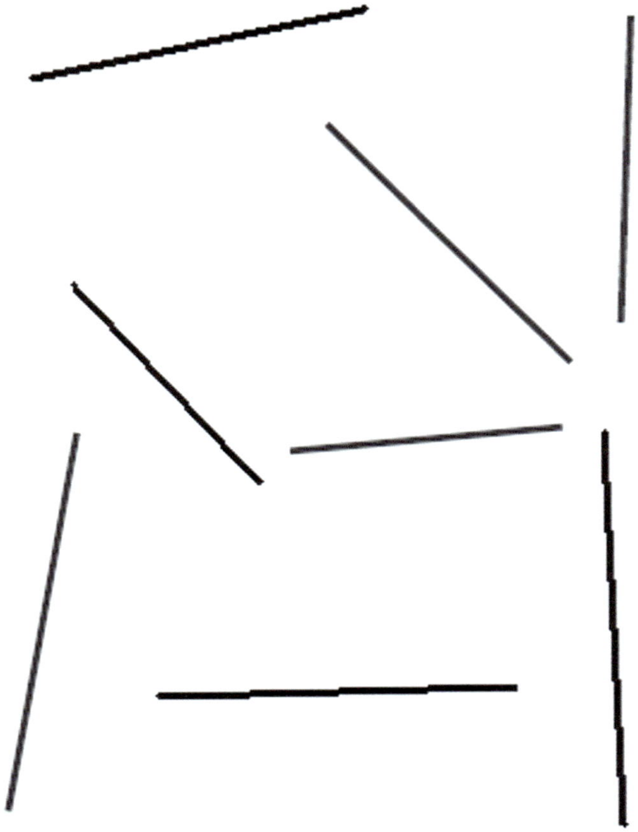

Fig. 4 Vernier acuity tests a patient's ability to discriminate between segments within a line or breaks within a line. When you look at the lines close-up, the lines will appear to be jagged or irregular because the angles cast by each segment are large enough to be noticed by your photoreceptors. As you begin to step back, each line will look like a clear, straight line until all the lines appear to be straight lines

Snellen Visual Acuity Chart

The Snellen visual acuity chart is like your driver's license: you use it every day and don't really think much about it unless you have to use it for a photo ID to get through a security line at the airport or appease the exam center proctor to let you into the testing center to take your board exam. Similarly, we use the Snellen chart all the time in clinical practice and may not give much thought to its development, usefulness, and, most importantly, why it is used to assess a patient's visual function.

Herman Snellen (1834–1908) was a Dutch ophthalmologist who introduced a visual acuity chart that could easily

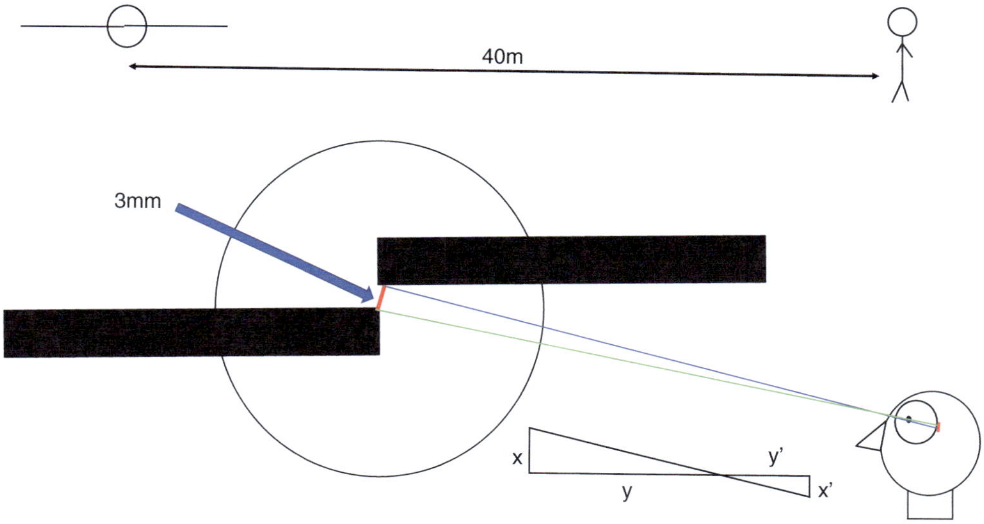

Fig. 5 Vernier acuity allows the observer to spot a small break in the line from 40 m away. The break is magnified in the bottom panel, where similar triangles show the space between the dark lines as a red line projected onto the retina. The retinal image size of a 3 mm break in a line 40 m away is smaller than a single retinal cone

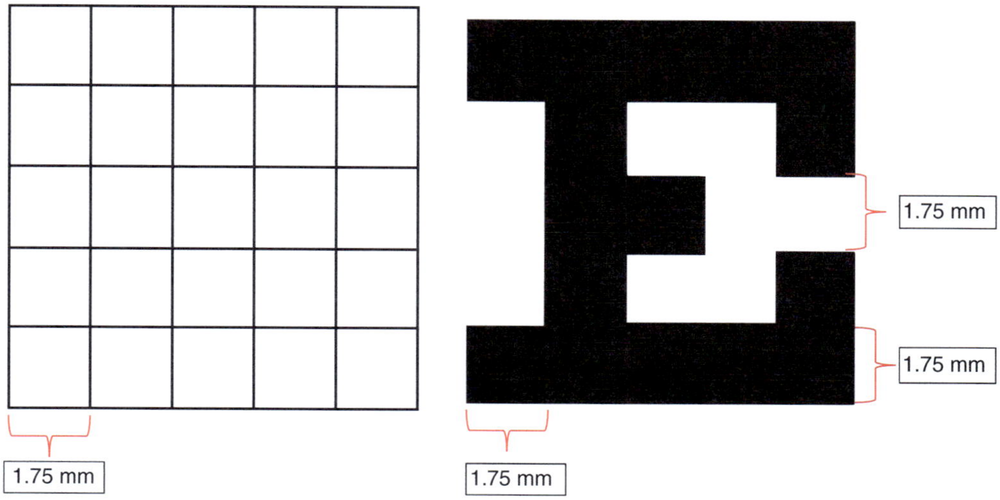

Fig. 6 Snellen letters are actually optotypes: using a 5x5 grid pattern of alternating black and white squares (each measuring 1.75 mm), letters can be generated with standardized heights and lengths, corresponding to a fixed number of *arcmins*

and quickly assess subtended angles (*arcmins*).[5] While other charts had been previously introduced, the Snellen chart was revolutionary. It was the first to use optotypes: using a 5x5 grid pattern, alternating black and white squares could generate letters within this grid (Fig. 6).

Fun fact: Snellen's first chart actually had symbols instead of letters; another early version had the letter "A" (rather than the familiar "E") and numbers as well. The letters are arranged so that the critical detail within each letter (stroke of the letter and gap width) will subtend approximately one-fifth of its total height; the height and width of the optotype is approximately 5 times the thickness of a stroke. Therefore, the Snellen chart tests a patient's ability to recognize an optotype when it subtends 5 *arcmins*, which can only be appreciated if the patient can recognize a letter with a spatial pattern separated by a visual angle of 1 *arcmin*. Snellen's chart included a 7-step sequence (minimum angle of resolution: 10, 5.0, 3.5, 2.5, 2.0, 1.5, and 1.0 arcmins).

We can now measure visual acuity in terms of the visual angle perceived by a patient using optotypes. Notice that it would be extremely cumbersome and awkward to use the previously mentioned *arcmins* to relay information about a patient's visual function: "Mr. Jones is able to see the optotype that subtends 5 *arcmins* at 20 feet."[6] As stated previously, the

[5]Parker P. Heritage of ophthalmology. Herman Snellen, 1834–1908. J Ophthalmic Nurs Technol. 1988 Jan-Feb;7(1):38

[6]The next time you want to tease a junior resident, you can use this nomenclature to indicate that a patient has 20/20 vision.

20/20 optotype is constructed so that each stroke of the letter subtends 1 *arcmin* and the entire letter subtends 5 *arcmins* when viewed at 20 feet (or 6 meters). Snellen letters serve as a proxy that allows us to measure the patient's perception of the visual angle based on his/her ability to read the optotype that accordingly subtends that particular visual angle.

Similarly, each letter on the Snellen chart is designed so that any letter on a given line will subtend 5 *arcmins* when viewed from that distance. For example, the 20/60 letter will subtend 5 *arcmins* when viewed from 60 feet; similarly, the 20/100 letter will subtend 5 *arcmins* when viewed from 100 feet. To determine the number of *arcmins* for every letter larger than the 20/20 line when viewed at 20 feet, the inverse of that line can be multiplied by 5 as follows:

- 20/40 line: inverse = 40/20 = 2 x 5 = 10 *arcmins*
- 20/80 line: inverse = 80/20 = 4 x 5 = 20 *arcmins*
- 20/200 line: inverse = 200/20 = 10 x 5 = 50 *arcmins.*

You may want to grab another cup of coffee and re-read the previous three paragraphs a few times to let all that amazing information soak in.

When we say that a patient has "20/40" visual acuity, for example, we are actually saying that at the standard testing distance (20 feet), the patient can only perceive the optotypes on the 20/40 line that subtend 10 *arcmins*. The denominator can also be considered the distance at which that size letter subtends 5 *arcmins*. If a patient only has 20/40 vision (i.e., able to perceive only 10 *arcmins* from 20 feet away), then when we compare this vision to a patient with 20/20 vision (i.e., able to perceive 5 *arcmins* from 20 feet away), we can compare these two patients' perception of visual angles: the 20/20 patient has double the perception as the 20/40 patient. Finally, another way to think of this (and a way to explain this to patients) is that a patient with 20/40 vision needs to be 20 feet away to see the 20/40 line, whereas a patient with 20/20 vision can see the 20/40 line from 40 feet away.

Enough about visual angles, let's talk a bit about the letter size on a Snellen chart. If we look at the letter "E" on the 20/20 line, the total length of each stroke is approximately 1.75 mm; therefore, the total height of the letter is approximately 9 mm (Fig. 6).[7] Recall that a "stroke" refers to both the shaded portion and the space within a letter. Table 1 shows the height for each letter on a given line on the Snellen chart – please note that this has been given for illustrative purposes only and should not be committed to memory.[8]

[7]The BCSC Clinical Optics (*Clinical Optics: Basic and Clinical Science Course*. American Academy of Ophthalmology, 2020) gives the height of the 20/20 letter "E" as 8 mm. Other sources vary, including 8.73 mm.

[8]International Society for the Enhancement of Eyesight, January 28, 2005. http://www.i-see.org/eyecharts.html. Accessed February 23, 2022.

Table 1 Approximate heights for letters (optotypes) found on the Snellen visual acuity chart

Line on Snellen chart	20/15	20/20	20/30	20/40	20/50	20/60	20/70
Height of letter (mm)	7	9	13	18	22	27	31

Notice that letters on each consecutive line increase in size by approximately 4–5 mm, though from the 20/20 to 20/15 line, the size goes from 9 mm to 7 mm. Thus, there isn't a fixed ratio or pattern of how the height of each line compares to the line before or after it. On most Snellen charts, this progression is irregular and can vary significantly, especially when considering larger letters. For example, there is a 100 percent size increase when comparing the 20/100, 20/200, and 20/400 letters. This non-uniformity (lack of geometric progression) of letter sizes is one major limitation of the Snellen chart – this would lead to the development of more uniform charts, such as the ETDRS chart, which we will discuss in the next section.

Other disadvantages of the Snellen chart include:

- The use of black and white squares to create optotypes also creates nearly 100% contrast of each letter, further amplified when testing in a dark room and using a white computer monitor or background. Thus, we are (potentially) artificially enhancing a patient's actual visual function by adding 100% contrast into the equation. In most everyday visual situations, 100% contrast is nearly nonexistent. This may explain why some patients test several lines better on a Snellen chart but may have worse "functional vision" with their everyday visual tasks in typical lighting situations. See the discussion on Contrast Sensitivity toward the end of this chapter for more information.
- Different rows have different numbers of letters, ranging from 1 to 8 letters per row.
- Not every line is of equal legibility or difficulty as they may not contain an equal number of "easy letters" and "hard letters." Easy letters are considered those letters that don't have many other letters with similar shapes in the English alphabet – for example, the letters A, J, and Z are considered easy letters. Hard letters may have one or more letters with similar shapes – for example, the letters C, D, G, O, Q, U, V, and W share many similar features and are more likely to be confused.
- Memorization bias may play a role when using noncomputerized Snellen charts. This bias is more of an issue when using printed or projected Snellen charts wherein the examiner cannot present multiple varieties of the same line to assess whether the patient can genuinely see the line or has "memorized" the line because he/she has done the test

Table 2 Snellen visual acuity can be readily converted into other nomenclature systems used to report visual acuity, including visual angle (*arcmin*) notation, decimal (Visus) notation, and logMAR notation

Snellen (feet)	Snellen (meters)	Visual Angle (arcmins)	Decimal notation (Visus)	logMAR
20/15	6/4.5	0.75	1.33	−0.12
20/20	6/6	1.00	1.00	0.00
20/25	6/7.75	1.25	0.80	0.10
20/30	6/9	1.5	0.67	0.18
20/40	6/12	2.00	0.50	0.30
20/50	6/15	2.50	0.40	0.40
20/60	6/18	3.00	0.33	0.48
20/80	6/24	4.00	0.25	0.60
20/100	6/30	5.00	0.20	0.70
20/200	6/60	10.00	0.10	1.00
20/400	6/120	20.00	0.05	1.30

so many times.[9] Ironically, as Snellen's original chart (with the E, FP, TOZ, etc. at the top) became a staple in medical offices worldwide, it became so recognizable that some authorities felt it needed to be redone into something less recognizable to avoid unwanted memorization bias. Computerized charts have eliminated this bias since we can show the patient many varieties of the same line.

Nevertheless, the Snellen visual acuity chart remains the most commonly employed method of visual acuity testing in clinical practice outside of the research setting. Snellen acuities can be converted to other commonly used methods of reporting visual acuity, including Snellen in metric notation, visual angle (Arcmins) notation, decimal (Visus) notation, and logMAR. LogMAR notation is particularly useful for comparing the mean Snellen visual acuity in a series of patients and comparing across populations (Table 2). LogMAR notation is commonly used to report visual acuities and refractive outcomes in clinical research publications.

The ETDRS Visual Acuity Chart

The Early Treatment Diabetic Retinopathy Study (ETDRS) is one of those landmark studies in ophthalmology that you should definitely know about. While the study sought to assess the efficacy of scatter and focal photocoagulation to halt the progression of retinopathy, the study also gifted us with the standardization and popularity of the ETDRS visual acuity chart – thanks retina people!

As discussed in the previous section, the Snellen chart has considerable limitations and drawbacks. For example, letters with serifs, or extra strokes at the edges (e.g., underline strokes under the two legs of the letter "A", additional strokes in the letter "E", etc.), may create additional difficulty for a patient to recognize correctly. Thus, vision scientists realized that sans-serif, simplified letters (e.g., DEFHNPRUVZ - Gesundheit!) could be easily recognized with "similar" difficulty. Charts that sought to improve on the limitations of the Snellen chart had been developed prior to the ETDRS study. Louise Sloan (1898–1982) had developed optotype fonts (Sloan letters) to give letters of consistent difficulty that established standards for future clinical studies.[10] Ian Bailey and Jan Lovie-Kitchin at the National Vision Research Institute (Australia) had also previously designed a "logMAR visual acuity chart" built upon the geometric progression of optotypes to standardize visual acuity testing in 1976.[11] Basically, the ETDRS took the Bailey-Lovie chart and made some additional modifications, such as using a 4 m testing distance (instead of 6 m) and Sloan letters (instead of British Standard letters). As the ETDRS had significant implications for the clinical management of diabetic patients, the associated chart also became popular among clinicians and vision research scientists. Today, LogMAR charts, such as the Bailey-Lovie and ETDRS charts, are considered the gold standard for clinical research studies in ophthalmology.

Why on earth did they use this chart? Think of the ETDRS as improving on the flaws of the Snellen chart; in other words, it's like one of those new "REAL-ID" driver's licenses that have advanced features compared to the older driver's licenses. Key features and advantages of the ETDRS include:

- Sans-serif optotypes of letters are used in each line of the chart; this is thought to make each letter equally legible (and equally challenging) when compared to other letters on each line.
- The ETDRS has the same 10 letters introduced by Sloan: CDHKNORSVZ (almost seems like the world's worst vanity license plate!).
- Each line also has the same number of test letters (5) per line.
- The size of every letter on a given line is the same as its fellow letters; each letter is further separated by a white space equal to the size of the letter itself. This arrangement helps to minimize any unwarranted consequences of crowding.
- Each letter has a value of 0.02 log units, so the total value of each line is 0.1 log units. Hence, each line decreases in 0.1 log unit increments, so each line varies from the line

[9]Admit it, many of you nerds have (subconsciously) memorized that the 20/30 line is OFLCT and the 20/25 line is APEOTF.

[10]Finkelstein D, Masoff R. Louse Littig Sloan, pioneer in clinical vision research 1898–1982. *Arch Ophthalmol* 1982; 100: 1347

[11]Bailey IL, Lovie JE. New design principles for visual acuity letter charts. *Am J Optom Physiol* 1976; 53: 740–745

above and the line below in a logarithmic (geometric, fixed pattern) fashion.

- Therefore a **three-line change** (gain or loss of vision) will correspond to **doubling or halving, respectively, of the visual angle**. This relationship makes comparisons of visual acuity across studies more straightforward and more comparable.
- LogMAR notation is actually a measurement of vision loss (Table 2). In other words, like golf, the lower the score, the better. Notice that 20/20 vision corresponds to a logMAR score of zero. *Loss of vision* will correspond to *positive logMAR scores*.
- Visual acuity measurements using a logMAR chart are twice as repeatable as those from a Snellen chart[12] and over three times more sensitive to interocular differences in visual acuity.[13]

ETDRS charts are available for various test distances ranging from 20 feet (6 meters) to 2 meters (6.5 feet). Potential limitations of this chart include its size (physical footprint in an exam lane), cost, and increased testing time (compared to the Snellen chart). On this last point, we can see that the ETDRS chart has 55 letters, whereas the Snellen chart has 36 letters; this explains why it takes longer for a patient to complete the ETDRS.[14]

Assessing Visual Acuity in Nonliterate or Illiterate Adult Patients

For clinical practice and exam purposes, you may need to be familiar with some methods of testing visual acuity in patients who are nonliterate in English or altogether illiterate (in any language). Several potential testing methods include:

- Arabic numerals (0–9) are the most popular number system used worldwide, regardless of a patient's native language. Most visual acuity charts have a "numbers" option to generate optotype numbers as a proxy for letters.
- Picture Methods: Allen pictures, Lea Symbols, Handy Eye Chart, etc. In each of these methods, picture optotypes are used so the patient can easily recognize them. These are especially popular among pediatric patients. You are already probably familiar with the **Allen pictures** commonly used in pediatric ophthalmology clinics – though it is possible that they may need to remove the rotary telephone symbol because kids may no longer recognize it! The **Lea Symbols** test involves giving the patient a sheet with four reference "images" (house, square, circle, and apple) that are then shown as optotypes on a screen; the patient is asked to match what he/she sees on the screen with the symbols on the reference sheet. The **Handy Eye Chart** involves a picture of nearly universal hand gestures and positions as a proxy for optotypes that the patient can then demonstrate using his/her own hand – and before you ask or ponder, no, "flipping the bird" is not considered a universal hand gesture and therefore is not part of the chart.
- Letter Position Methods: Tumbling Es, Landolt Cs, etc. In this test, the patient is shown a letter in different positions and then has to report the letter's position as a proxy for "seeing" the letter. In the **Tumbling Es** test, the "E" can be placed in one of four positions (facing up, down, left, or right), and the patient can similarly use his/her hand to display three fingers up, down, left, or right. The **Landolt Cs** test involves showing the letter "C" in one of 8 possible positions; as a result, there is less chance that the patient "guesses right," as can happen with only four choices on the Tumbling Es test.[15]
- Internet Visual Acuity Charts: Thanks to the magical power of the Internet, several readily available visual acuity charts (especially for near vision) are available in most languages that can be printed out and placed at the recommended testing distance.

Assessing Visual Acuity in Pediatric Patients

We should also be familiar with various testing methods that can be used in pediatric patients. Remember that the bulk of vision development occurs **after** birth. A more detailed discussion of vision development from birth to adulthood is presented in Chap. 23 "Pediatric Optics". Starting from birth (chronologically), the following test(s) may be used at the discretion of the examiner and based on the clinical setting:

- Blinks to light reflex and pupillary light reflex: These two reflexes should be present (almost) immediately after birth.
- Pattern stimulus: By one week of age, infants can distinguish between a gray-shaded stimulus and a black-shaded stimulus at 1 foot away. The examiner can ascertain this acuity by observing if the infant will look (even for a few moments) longer at the patterned stimulus.

[12]Lovie-Kitchin JE. Is it time to confine Snellen charts to the annals of history? *Ophthalmic Physiol Opt* 2015; 35: 631–36

[13]McGraw PV, Winn B, Gray LS, et al. Improving the reliability of visual acuity measures in young children. *Ophthalmic Physiol Opt* 2000; 20: 173–84

[14]Shamir RR, Friedman Y, Joskowicz L, et al. Comparison of Snellen and Early Treatment Diabetic Retinopathy Study charts using a computer simulation. *Int J Ophthalmol* 2016; 9: 119–23

[15]Or as can happen on a multiple-choice exam with four answer choices and you are completely clueless. There's a 25% chance that you may just guess right!

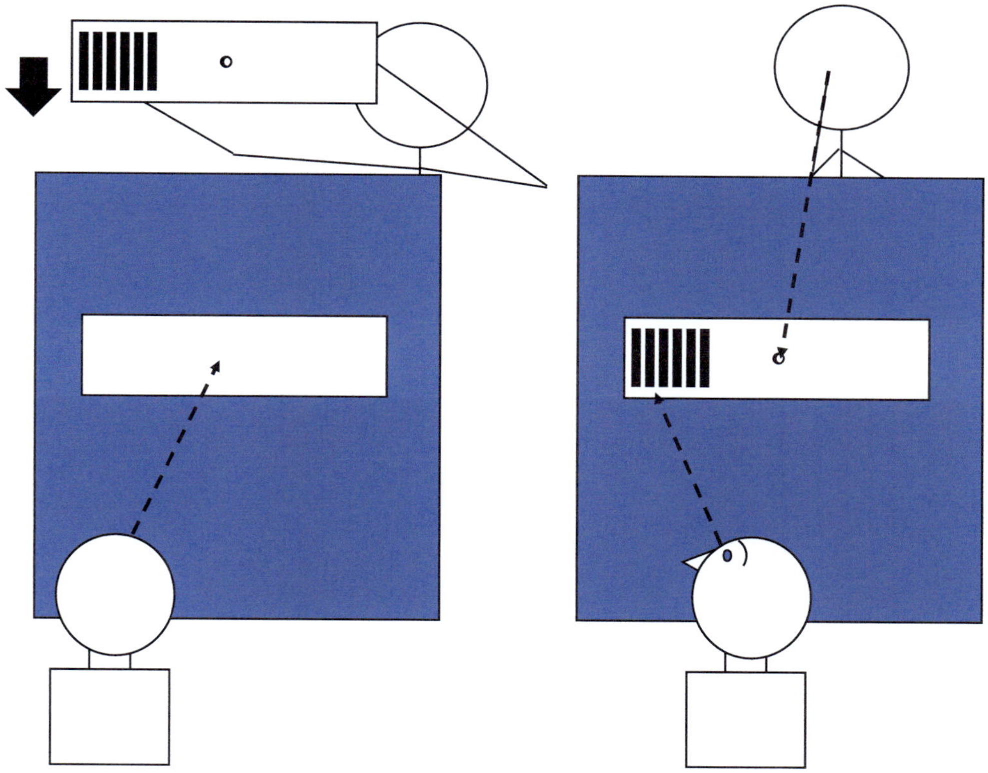

Fig. 7 Teller Acuity Cards. The examiner stands behind a screen and presents cards with varying contrast patterns to the child, observing through a central viewing hole if the child preferentially looks toward the area of the card with the pattern. This indicates that he/she can see the pattern on the card. This response is then translated into an approximate visual acuity

- OKN drum: A nystagmus will be induced if the baby can see stripes and follow the OKN drum. This response indicates the vision is at least 20/200. This ability can be seen at 6 weeks or earlier.
- Equal behavior with either eye covered. If a child cries and fights occlusion when the right eye is covered but does not react when the left eye is covered, they will likely have poor vision in their left eye. This is the child's way of saying, "Stop doing that, I can't see when you cover my only good eye!"
- Fix, follow, and maintain and central, steady, and maintain (FFM and CSM): The "fix and follow" are monocular tests wherein the examiner tests if the child can maintain fixation and follow an object of interest. The smiling face of a quiet examiner will get their attention (no fancy toys are necessary). Similarly, the "central and steady" portions are monocular tests to see if the child can use his/her central vision to fixate on an object of interest and keep the eye steady (i.e., no nystagmus or strabismus eye movements). If an eye is **un**centered due to constant strabismus or eccentric fixation, it would be labeled "**UC**." If the eye is **un**stable due to nystagmus, it would be labeled "**US.**" By covering the dominant fixating eye, the examiner forces the child to fixate with the other eye; then, the dominant eye is uncovered, and the child is allowed to see with both eyes open. If he/she can maintain central and steady fixation on the object with both eyes, then we can say that the child has the "**m**aintained" portion as well. If the eye drifts off and alignment is **unm**aintained due to intermittent strabismus, it would be labeled "**UM**." More specifically, the child's vision can be described as "holds fixation for 2 seconds" or "holds fixation until blink", before reverting to fixation with the dominant eye.
- A 10–15 PD base-down prism or 20PD base-out prism can be used to induce a deviation. If no movement is observed, then the vision in that eye is likely poor.
- Teller Acuity Cards (preferential looking): We will discuss this in more detail later in the chapter ("Contrast Sensitivity"). In brief, this test involves presenting cards with high contrast gratings on one side and no grating (and equal luminance) on the other side. The examiner views the child through the central viewing hole to determine which side of the card is "preferred" by the child. If the child has good visual function, he/she should preferentially look toward the side of the card with more contrast (more pattern) to indicate that he/she can "see it" (Fig. 7).
- Picture optotypes (Allen cards, etc.)
- Letter optotypes with matching (Lea Symbols, "HOTV" testing). Most 2.5-year-old kids can play a matching game with HOTV letters. Even if they are shy or don't know the letters yet, they can understand the concept of matching letters. A single letter is shown at 10 or 20 feet while the child sits on his/her parent's lap and holds a small sheet with the HOTV letters. For the sake of the examiner, animal crackers are an indispensable part of this exam. Families can also practice the matching game at home prior to the appointment.

Age	Pupillary light reflex	Blink to light	OKN drum	Following movements	Fixation	Visual Acuity
At birth	✓	✓	↓			20-1000
2-4 weeks			↓	↓	↓	
6 weeks			↓	↓	↓	
3 months				↓	↓	
6 months						20/400

Fig. 8 Chronological summary of visual acuity from birth to six months. It is clinically relevant to remember this figure when an anxious new parent comes in because their 1-week-old is not fixating on faces yet

- Tumbling E, Landolt C.
- Electroretinography (ERG) test: This test can determine retinal functionality. It gives no information about the anterior eye or the post-retinal visual pathway. Younger kids would have to be sedated to perform this test.
- Visual evoked potential (VEP) test: This test can be used in patients from infants to young kids. Recall that the VEP tests the function of the visual pathway from the retina to the occipital cortex (i.e., "behind" the eye). It does not necessarily give information about the eye per se but more about the functionality of circuitry behind the eye. It can help quantify optic nerve pathology and amblyopia.

A chronological summary of visual acuity from birth to six months is shown in Fig. 8.

Several other principles and pearls may be discussed here regarding checking visual acuity in pediatric patients.

1. As clinicians, we must appreciate that while all patients are concerned about their children's health, if a parent has amblyopia, he/she may be even overly concerned. One of the authors (GVV) had a patient who could do HOTV matching at 15 months of age with a recorded vision of 20/30 on each eye. It turns out that the child's mother had dense amblyopia, and was told that amblyopia could run in families and that it was best caught early. Feeling guilty, she went online and found HOTV and taught her daughter each of the figures in sign language(!). The author thanked the mom, reassured her that her daughter was fine and also explained that we could have detected amblyopia at this age even without sign language. The learning point here is that we should be cognizant of parents' concerns and, therefore, be familiar with various types of visual acuity testing for pediatric patients.
2. It is likely that young patients will at times want to get the correct answer desperately and will cheat around an occluder whenever possible. The examiner has to be alert and ensure the eye is adequately occluded.
3. While this may seem to be a direct contradiction to the previous point, in recent times ("post-hipster era"), it is not uncommon to have a pediatric (grade-school or junior-high) patient who is eager to receive glasses such that he/she <u>intentionally</u> misses the line. This type of malingering may be easily missed if the clinician is unaware of these psychosocial factors. These patients can usually be diagnosed by "bottom-up visual acuity testing," i.e., starting at the 20/10 line and then increasing to the 20/15, 20/20, etc., lines as needed. Similarly, confrontational visual fields may also help detect this subset of patients. Please see Chap. 21, "Clinical Problems with Optics and Refractive Manifestations", for a complete discussion of malingering and its relationship with optics.
4. Young (and adult) patients with amblyopia may experience a crowding phenomenon during visual acuity testing (a.k.a. contour interaction). This phenomenon is due to abnormally large receptive fields of neurons in the visual system of the amblyopic eye. The affected eye may score 20/30 on a Snellen chart with one letter at a time and 20/50 when a line of letters is presented. When recording this patient's vision, should we record it as 20/30 or 20/50? Well, both are correct – it depends on how the visual acuity is recorded. For this reason, it is vital to record the visual acuity with single letters <u>and</u> a line of letters during a visit in order to be able to compare sequential vision measurements. Some visual acuity devices have crowding bars which enable the examiner to present one letter at a time with these crowding bars to minimize the crowding phenomenon.

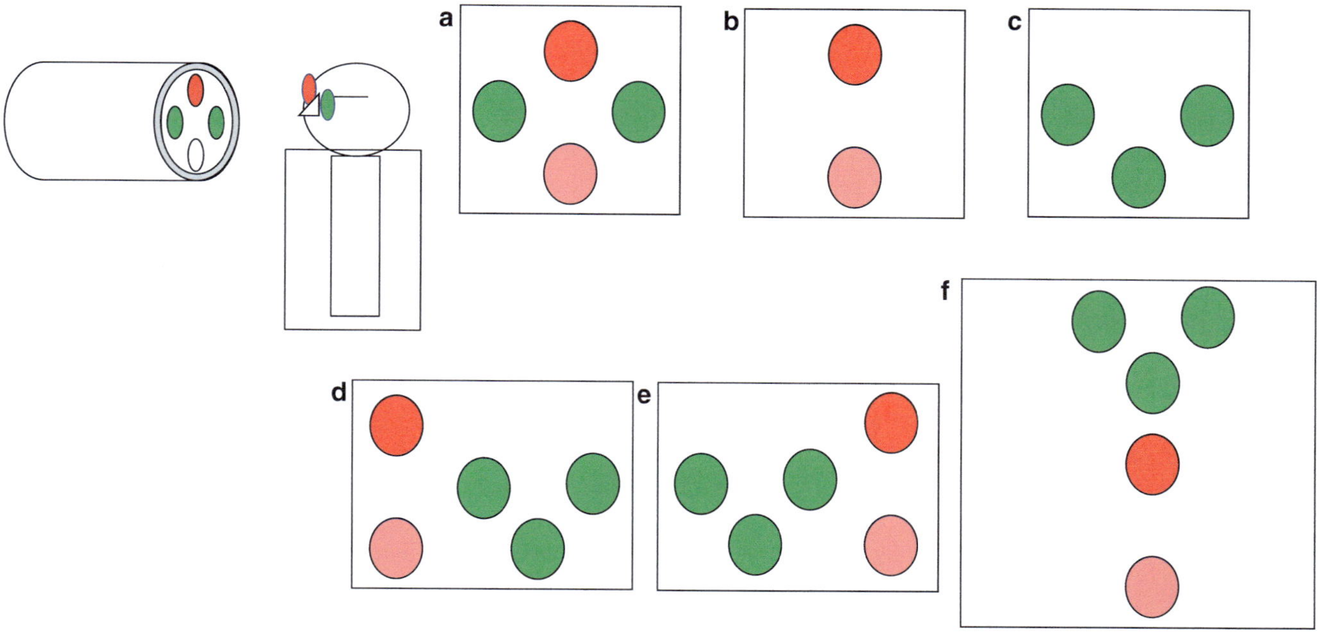

Fig. 9 Worth Four Dot: Patient perceptions. (**a**) Normal binocularity. (**b**) Suppression of the left eye. (**c**) Suppression of the right eye. (**d**) Diplopia due to exotropia. (**e**) Diplopia due to esotropia. (**f**) Diplopia due to right hypertropia

Assessing Visual Acuity in Patients with Nystagmus

Suppose we have a patient with 20/30 vision when tested binocularly and 20/80 vision when tested left eye only. In most patients, we would expect the right eye to test 20/30 because we often assume that the patient's vision is as good as his/her best eye under binocular conditions. However, what if a patient has 20/40 vision with both eyes open and 20/70 with one eye at a time? This seemingly paradoxical finding is a common situation in patients with Congenital Idiopathic Nystagmus (CIN). If vision is tested monocularly, the latent nystagmus will worsen the monocular recorded vision in these patients. To avoid this pitfall and measure a more accurate monocular vision, the examiner has three choices:

- Fog one eye with a lens that is +5.00 D sphere greater than their refractive error *instead of occluding* it.
- Have the patient hold the occluder at arm's length. This distance may allow enough peripheral vision to prevent the latent nystagmus from emerging while still only testing one eye at a time.
- Use a combination of Duochrome letters with red-green filters or polarized lenses. Unlike the standard Duochrome test (which is a monocular test).

Clinically, this has significant implications as it could affect whether a patient can pass a vision screening exam, obtain a driver's license, etc.

Binocular Vision Testing

Worth Four Dot

This simple test requires a Worth Four Dot (W4D) flashlight and red/green glasses (red lens goes over the right eye). The W4D is constructed with a red light at the top, two green lights in the middle, and a white light at the bottom (Fig. 9). The test is performed at 33 cm (near) and at 6 m (distance). Remember that the red lens will only allow in red light; the green lens will only allow in green light. Patients with normal binocularity should see two green lights, one red light, and one pink light at near and distance (Fig. 9, Panel a).

If the patient is suppressing one eye, he/she will only see one set of color dots. For example, if the left eye is suppressed, the patient will report seeing only 2 red dots (top light and bottom light) (Fig. 9, Panel b); if the right eye is suppressed, the patient will see only 3 green dots (the two middle lights and the bottom light) (Fig. 9, Panel c).

If the patient has diplopia, he/she will report seeing 5 dots (Fig. 9, Panel d and e). The alignment of the dots may not be intuitive but much like the Maddox rods, crossed diplopia will cause uncrossed images – what the right eye sees will appears on the right and what the left eye sees appears on the left. However, and this may seem counterintuitive, a right hypertropia will make the images the right eye sees appear lower than they really are (Fig. 9, Panel f).

Patients with monofixation syndrome will have a small tropia (<8 PD), peripheral fusion, and a small central scotoma. They will be able to see all four dots at near when a large image falls on the peripheral macula; however, when they stand further away from the lights, a small image is formed on the fovea, and their small suppression scotoma may impede the patient seeing one of the colors.

Testing of Stereo Acuity

Stereo acuity testing relies on polarization to help to quantify a patient's binocular depth perception. See the "Polarization" section in Chap. 14 "Physical Optics and Advanced Optical Principles", for a full discussion on polarization.

Stereo acuity is measured routinely by pediatric and strabismus specialists as it can help monitor eye suppression and intermittent strabismus. Typically, two slightly disparate images are presented to the retina and integrated in the occipital cortex. Finer stereoacuity is necessary to discern between images as they are presented closer and closer to each other. Stereoacuity can be measured at near and distance. Some tests may have false positives from monocular cues patients can see. One of the most commonly used tests is the stereo fly test. The figure is shown horizontally and slowly rotated to an upright position. As the image of the wings "pop up," a child with intact stereo acuity should be able to reach out and try to grab them.

Other tests of similarly constructed objects (animals, raised dots among a series of dots, etc.) may be used for finer discrimination of stereo acuity.

Color Vision Testing

Before proceeding, you may wish to review the section on "Spectral Sensitivity and Visual Pigments" in Chap. 14 "Physical Optics and Advanced Optical Principles".

Color vision defects can be classified into two categories: congenital and acquired. Acquired defects are usually blue-yellow defects, whereas congenital defects are usually red-green, though they can also include blue-yellow. Historically, there were several iterations of color vision testing beyond the scope of this text. Several commonly-used tests can be used to screen, assess, and quantify color vision defects.

Let's get a definition out of the way: *pseudoisochromatic*. You have probably used this and not given much thought to the word because it sounds intelligent; we suspect that most people in ophthalmology don't know what this word means but use it anyway because everyone else uses it, not knowing that most everyone else may also not know it… confused yet? Pseudoisochromatic refers to colored plates that appear to be the same colored (isochromatic) to patients with color-vision abnormalities and multi-colored to patients with normal color vision. The **Ishihara** and **HRR color plates** are two commonly used methods of pseudoisochromatic color plate testing.

Four commonly used methods for color vision testing are the following:

1. Ishihara color plates: Developed in 1917 by Dr. Shinobu Ishihara, these color plates are perhaps the most popularly used plates for color vision testing. The plates involve using confusion lines among spots with common points (copunctal points) to build patterns of differently colored spots (usually in the form of a number or a line). There are four different types of plates used:
   (a) Vanishing design plates: patients with color vision defects will not see anything at all, whereas color-normal patients will see a sign on this plate.
   (b) Transformation design plates: patients with color vision defects will see a different sign as compared to color-normal patients.
   (c) Hidden digit design plates: patients with color vision defects will see a sign on this plate, whereas color-normal vision patients will not see anything.
   (d) Classification design plates: a vanishing design is used on either side of the plate – one for green vision defects, the other for red vision defects. It can further differentiate between red and green color vision defects.

   Ishihara plates are available in books of 14 plates (most commonly used), 24 plates, and 38 plates. Basically, you should know that individuals with defective color vision may see nothing at all, something different, or something "present" that differs from color-normal patients, depending on the plate being used. As a result, this is a test with good sensitivity for screening color-deficient patients, but it does not specify the deficiency. Finally, a fun fact: the first plate is considered to be the control plate, so both color-normal and color-deficient patients should be able to see it. If a patient says that they can't see the first plate, you may have a malingerer on your hands!
2. Hardy, Rand, and Rittler (HRR) test: This book has 24 color plates; the first four are "instruction plates"; the following six plates are "screening plates" that present the most challenging targets for finding one of the three primary color vision defects (deuteranopia, protanopia, and tritanopia) – if a patient clears these six plates, then he/she is unlikely to be color deficient. The next 14 plates are used to diagnose the exact type of color deficiency and the extent (mild, moderate, or severe). One of the main advantages of the HRR test is its speed: a patient has to

only clear six plates (rather than 14 or more) in order to have "normal" color vision.

3. Farnsworth D-15 test: This type of test involves active participation from the patient to arrange 15-colored discs or patterns in the correct order. If you are feeling incredibly bored at the DMV, you can also try the Farnsworth-Munsell 100 hue test, which involves 100 different plates to be arranged in groups of 20 plates – this test is very time-consuming and fatiguing! The color difference between adjacent plates is approximately 1–4 nm, which is considered as the near- minimum level for an observer to distinguish. Thus, this test is much more *specific* in classifying *which color deficiency* a patient is likely to have. The D-15 is also useful to determine if a patient has a **congenital or acquired color deficiency**. An individual who fails the Ishihara test but passes the D-15 test will probably not have significant color discrimination problems for most visual tasks and vocations.
4. Anomaloscope: This instrument is the most accurate for testing color-deficiency severity and distinguishing between dichromats and anomalous trichromats.[16] As you may have gathered, it's mainly used for research purposes. Basically, the patient is asked to match red and green light sources with a yellow light source. This allows for good detection of all types of red-green color vision deficiency. Some anomaloscopes may also have blue-green matching capabilities. Patients with protanopia will use more red light to match the colors compared to patients with deuteranopia, who will use more green light to match the colors. This instrument can also indicate the severity of the color deficiency based on how a patient performs.

Miscellaneous Topics

Concept of Optical Infinity

We previously stated that the standard testing distance for visual acuity is 20 feet (6 meters). However, even at this distance, there is technically some accommodation present. We can calculate this accommodation: 100/600 cm = 1/6 D. This is unlikely to be significant to most people, but we may still theoretically over-minus a patient, due to rounding the 1/6D to 1/4D, by approximately −0.25D.

Optical infinity is the distance at which accommodation is so negligible that it can't affect the measured refraction. At this point, you might be worried that you will have to find a super-long exam lane to test a patient's visual acuity at "optical infinity". Thankfully, we can find a workaround to limit the accommodation to have a negligible effect on the final refraction. In this case, we will want the accommodation to be <1/8 D to avoid a rounding error and incur the additional −0.25D. Therefore, we should apply the reciprocal of 1/8 = **8 meters** (which is equivalent to **26.25 feet**).

Again, most patients would probably not notice this, but suppose your patient is a smart-aleck optics nerd who comes in for a refraction and scoffs at your 20-foot exam lane as inadequate to test at "optical infinity." You would then have to test this smart-aleck at 26.25 feet if possible – otherwise, send him to your enemy across town and move on with your day. Or ask them to take another step back from the chart, another step back, until they are standing in your least favorite partner's room.

Contrast Sensitivity and Contrast Sensitivity Function (CSF)

Contrast sensitivity is a visual function that is separate from visual acuity, even though it plays a role in a patient's "tested" visual acuity. Simply stated, contrast sensitivity is a patient's ability to differentiate between bright ("white") and dim ("black") components of a target object. When we test a patient's visual acuity using black letters against a white background, we are artificially supplying the patient with near 100% contrast sensitivity. For example, suppose we had a patient with 20/20 vision but presented her with two visual acuity charts at the same distance, one with high contrast and the other with low contrast. She would likely perform better on the high contrast visual acuity chart than on the low contrast visual acuity chart.

In real-world scenarios, a patient with poor contrast sensitivity may have poor visual function due to difficulty seeing the edges of objects, reading black print on colored paper, driving on a "cloudy" day, etc. Similarly, in target objects with low lighting (low luminance), we are more likely to distinguish between shades of gray (as compared to bright luminance conditions) because the subtle differences in shade may be easier to appreciate. In bright luminance conditions, the extra light "washes out" the shades of gray, so we cannot distinguish as easily until the contrast increases (i.e., the target object is closer to having distinct black and white patterns). The **contrast threshold** is the minimum amount of contrast needed for the patient to distinguish between the "light" and "dark" components of an object; *the lower the threshold, the better a given patient's contrast sensitivity*.

We can now build upon this by briefly discussing **spatial frequency**.[17] Imagine we have a grating pattern (basically, think of this as an object with alternating black and white bars), as shown in Fig. 10. Spatial frequency is simply a

[16] As the name suggests though, it is so anomalous that it's never used… see what we did there.

[17] Tutorial on Spatial Frequency Analysis. http://www.psy.vanderbilt.edu/courses/hon185/SpatialFrequency/SpatialFrequency.html. Accessed April 19, 2020

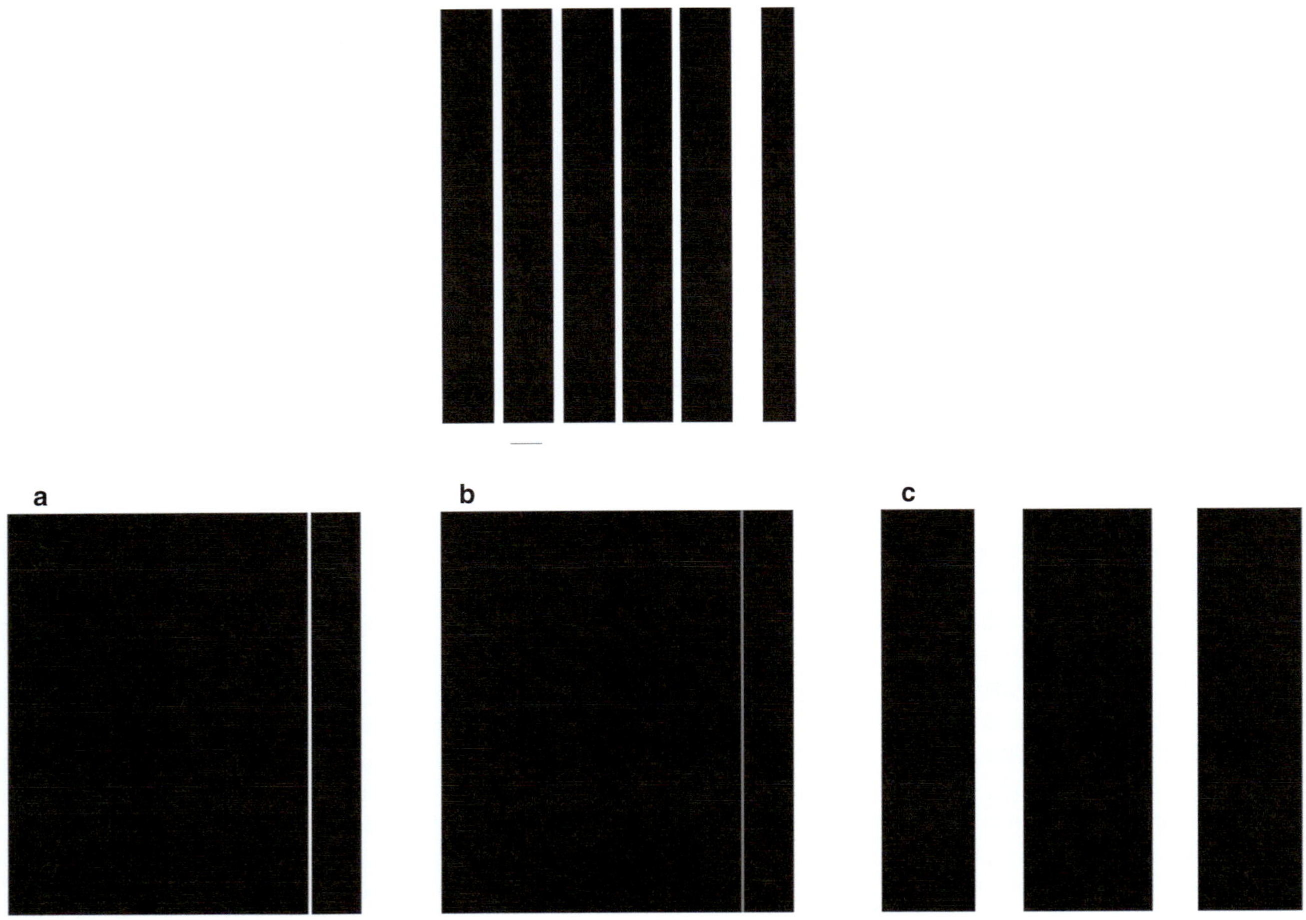

Fig. 10 A sine-wave grating is a pattern of alternating black and white bars that can be used to understand contrast sensitivity and spatial frequency better. In Panel A, the object has been imaged with high spatial frequency and high contrast, thereby giving a good estimation of the original object. Panel B shows how decreasing the contrast while maintaining a high spatial frequency can affect the image quality. Panel C shows an image of low spatial frequency and high contrast

fancy way of saying: *when we look at this object, how many pairs of bars will be imaged within one degree of the visual angle on the retina* (approximately 0.3 mm). For example, viewing your index fingernail at arm's length will cast an image that occupies one degree of the visual angle on the retina. If you move your arm closer or further away, a larger or small visual angle will be cast, respectively. A grating pattern with high spatial frequency will cast many narrow bars onto the retina (Fig. 10, Panel A); a grating pattern with low spatial frequency will cast fewer bars ("fatter bars") onto the retina (Fig. 10, Panel C).

Several possibilities may occur when we view this object: ideally, we would want to visualize the object with high spatial frequency and high contrast (Panel A). However, there is *always a tradeoff between spatial frequency and contrast.* If we image the same object using high spatial frequency and lower contrast (Panel B), the image quality suffers. Similarly, if we image the object using low spatial frequency and higher contrast, the image suffers (Panel C). This relationship between frequency and contrast isn't totally inverse. Instead, the relationship better approximates a curve: up to a certain (high) level of spatial frequency, we can maintain relatively high contrast sensitivity, but after a certain level of spatial frequency, the contrast sensitivity decreases significantly (Fig. 11).

Wake up, you probably dozed off. Any image that we perceive of an object, whether taken by a camera or the human eye, will only capture a certain amount of detail of the object. We discussed this previously with the point spread function (PSF) in Chap. 14 "Physical Optics and Advanced Optical Principles". We can take this one step further by including contrast in this idea: there will always be a ratio of the image contrast compared to the actual object contrast. This ratio is called the **transfer factor**, a proxy for contrast sensitivity – in other words, how much of the actual contrast we are actually "seeing," which we will discuss in more detail in the next section.

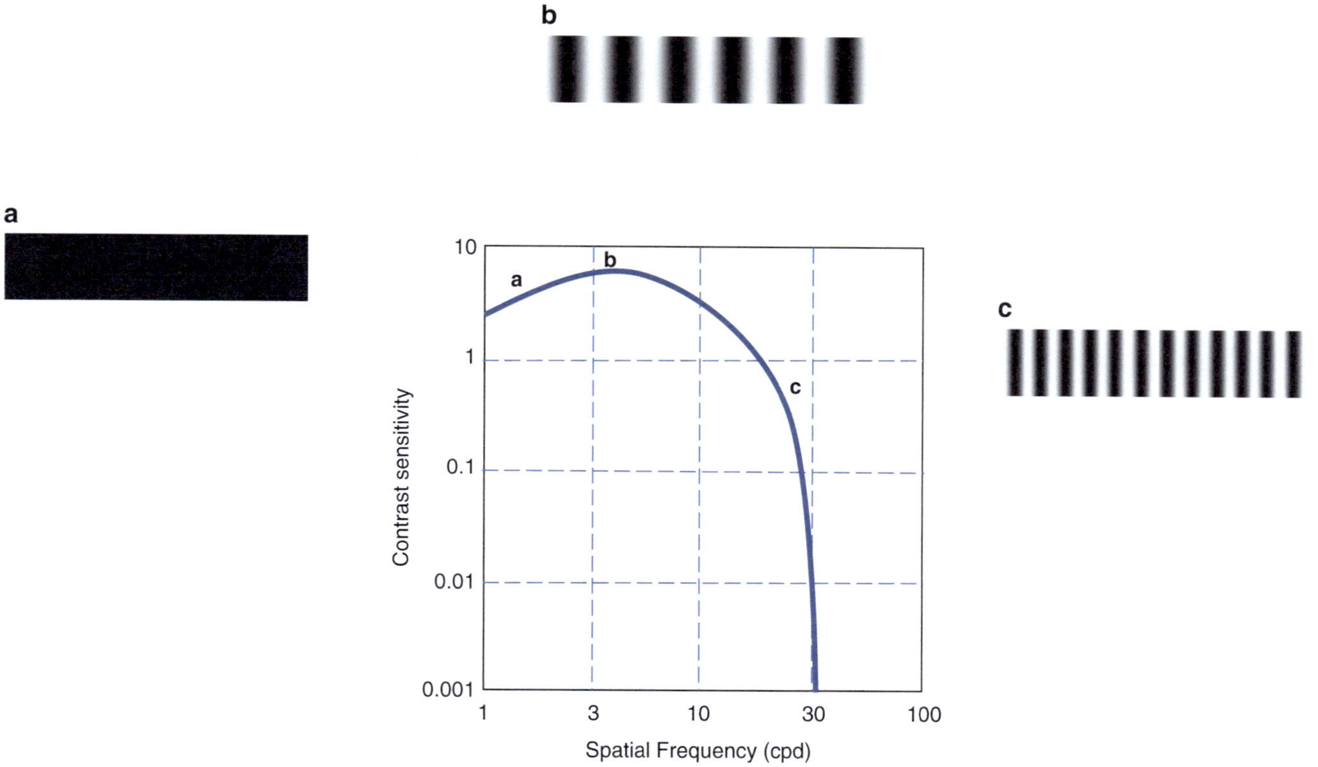

Fig. 11 The highest level of contrast sensitivity (vertical axis) is seen for low (Panel A) to medium (Panel B) levels of spatial frequency. Contrast sensitivity decreases significantly once spatial frequency reaches higher levels (Panel C)

When we view an object, contrast can either enhance or diminish the perception of that object for a given spatial frequency number. In other words, an object may have low spatial frequency, but with good enough contrast, we may be able to see it better (e.g., white text on a black page as compared to black text on a white page). Suppose that by the time we are finished at the DMV, it's nighttime as we are driving home: in low light conditions (with only street lights on), we may not be able to make out high spatial frequencies (such as individual leaves on a tree). However, we can still make out low spatial frequencies (the tree itself) just as well as we can during daytime. But if we turned off our headlights and drove on a road without any lights, it would be difficult to see anything, even trees, because both the spatial frequency and the contrast have become relatively low. Please note that this author does not endorse driving without your headlights turned on at nighttime.

We can formally test contrast sensitivity using charts such as the Pelli-Robson chart that presents various optotypes over a range of contrasts. The patient is shown parallel bars (known as sine-wave gratings) of varying widths (spatial frequency) and contrasts. Medium-level angular frequency (approximately 5–7 cycles/degree) is the sweet spot for optimal detection by most patients; lower and higher frequencies are much more difficult to detect.[18] Specific eye pathologies, such as retinal and optic nerve disease, may asymmetrically affect contrast sensitivity more than visual acuity.

We take advantage of contrast sensitivity and spatial frequencies when performing Teller Acuity testing. We can alter both the spatial frequency (number of bars) and the contrast to see if the child will prefer the grating pattern as a proxy measurement for the patient's visual function. A typical CSF is shown for an infant vs. an adult in Fig. 12. We can see that infants cannot see high spatial frequencies and require more contrast, even for low-intermediate spatial frequencies.

Thus, an infant's visual system is best suited for seeing objects very close with good lighting and high contrast (which makes sense because his/her entire world is located up close). As he/she gets older, the CSF will continue to improve. This CSF improvement, along with the development of the optical system (cornea, lens, retina, etc.), allows for healthy vision development.

Finally, as we age, the CSF at high spatial frequency decreases for various reasons, such as those mentioned above. However, even in the absence of retinal pathology, factors such

[18]Leguire LE, Algaze A, Kashou NH, et al. Relationship among fMRI, contrast sensitivity and visual acuity. *Brain Res* 2011; 1367: 162–69

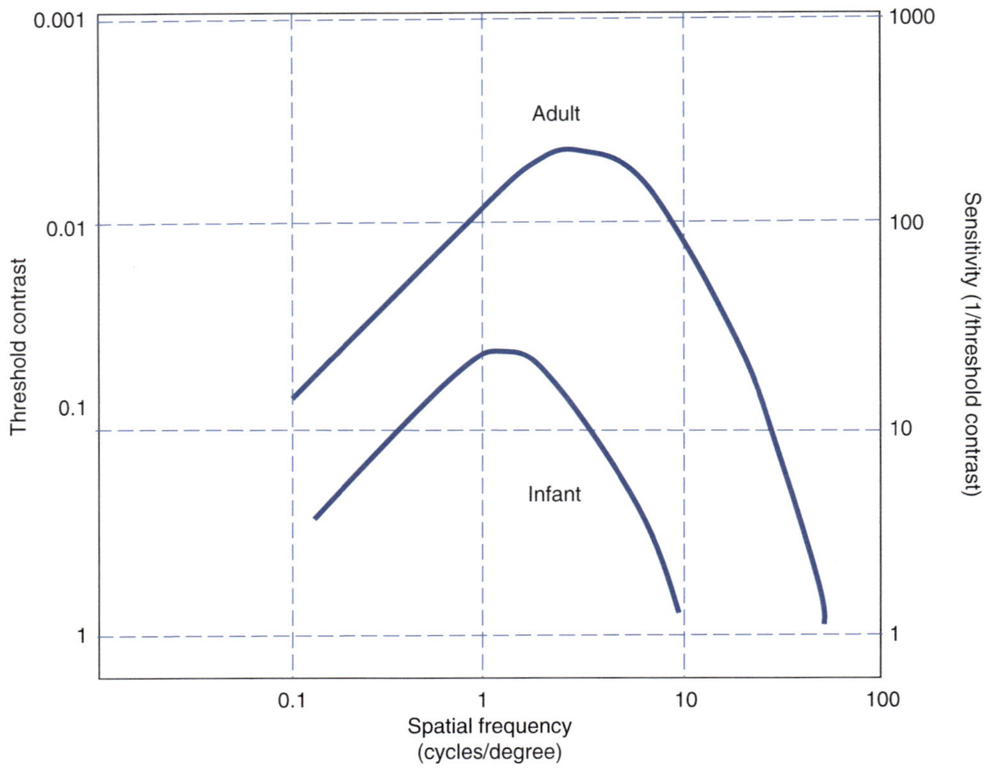

Fig. 12 Contrast sensitivity function (CSF) curves for an infant vs. an adult. Notice that the infant cannot see high spatial frequencies very well and requires much more contrast, even for low-intermediate spatial frequencies

as decreased pupil size also decrease the CSF. Therefore, older patients may need higher contrast for visual objects with high spatial frequencies (such as small print).

Modulation Transfer Function (MTF)

Recall that the transfer factor will decrease as the spatial frequency increases: there is only so much contrast that the eye can faithfully transfer at higher spatial frequencies. Therefore, the **modulation transfer function (MTF)** is a graph that shows how we perceive contrast based on the spatial frequency. It can be used for any optical system, such as a camera or (especially) an IOL.[19] By convention, we refer to this as the **contrast sensitivity function (CSF)** when referring to the human eye: a person with high CSF requires very little contrast to see an object and vice versa. Basically, *you want to have a high CSF because it will give you "better" vision.*

Let's simplify the MTF definition: the MTF is simply a way to describe the CSF for a lens system, whether it is the eye, glasses, or an IOL. A perfect lens would have an MTF of 1 (or 100%); this means that the lens is so amazingly perfect that every single object is faithfully represented in the image. If we have an object with low details (low spatial frequency, such as a sheet of white paper with two black bars), the MTF for any lens should be quite high. This high MTF value makes sense because there is not much detail in the object that needs to be captured by the lens. Therefore, for boring, uninteresting objects with low spatial frequency, the MTF of most lenses should be quite high. If we lived in a stick figure world (such as the two-dimensional world from Edwin Abbott's novel, *Flatland* (1884), then, the MTF would be quite high.

However, we live in a world with complex objects having significant details. When we test visual acuity in the clinic using a Snellen acuity chart, we use high-contrast black and white figures that lack significant complexity. In other words, our assessment of a patient's visual acuity can instead be thought of as: *how well does this patient see a simple image with high contrast?*[20]

[19]The MTF is extremely important when considering favorable optical properties of an IOL, especially presbyopia correcting IOLs such as multifocal IOLs and extended depth of focus IOLs. See Chap. 27 What's on the Menu: An Overview of Currently-Available IOLs and Relevant Optics.

[20]Some boring nerdy stuff: think of optical images (perceptions of a given object) analogous to our perception of sounds: what we hear is a fractional amount (with varying quantity and quality) of the "true sound" of a bird or a Mozart symphony, for example. Similarly, optical images are fractions of the true image: we can represent this mathematically using a sine-wave grating (SWG). The SWG contrast is indicated by the brightness difference between the brightest and darkest parts of an image. SWGs usually show a gradual change of dark/light ratios. A variant of SWGs involves arranging black and white bars with an abrupt change instead. These are known as Ronchi rulings, which are based on a **square wave pattern** rather than a sine-wave. Snellen visual acuity letters are basically Ronchi rulings: high-contrast black and white letters are used to assess a patient's vision without any real assessment of patients' ability to perceive contrast; in other words, these black-and-white visual acuity charts are poor ways to assess a patient's functional visual acuity. See "Modulation Transfer Function (MTF)" by Warren Hill, MD, for more information: https://bit.ly/2MSkNYF

Since objects in the real world have both details (frequency) and modulation (contrast), a faithful image of that object should ideally have as many details and contrast as possible. This is where the MTF helps: for a given frequency, we want to know how much modulation (contrast) is present in the image of the object. Mathematically, the MTF is described by the following equation:

$$MTF\left(u\right) = Mi / Mo$$

where MTF(u) is the MTF at a given frequency, Mi is the modulation of the image, and Mo is the modulation of the object.

If you are ever nerdy enough to look at IOL insert sheets (or FDA approval materials online), you may notice that many IOLs will include these MTF graphs. The MTF of a perfect IOL would be 1 (Mi/Mo = 1), but again, no such IOL exists. Also, at some (low or high) frequencies, no image of the object can be captured, whether by the eye or an IOL.

Remember our discussions on spherical aberration – we warned you that you could never escape this concept in Ophthalmic Optics![21] The net spherical aberration of the eye is slightly positive, which increases as we age. When we do cataract surgery, we remove whatever negative spherical aberration the (cataractous) lens provided, so we further increase the spherical aberration of the patient's eye. This is one reason why aspheric IOLs (with negative spherical aberration) are popular as they seek to "replace" the (cataractous) lens' negative spherical aberration.

Suppose we instead placed a spherical IOL (which has positive spherical aberration) during cataract surgery. The increased net positive spherical aberration will worsen the MTF and subjective visual quality. Higher power IOLs will disproportionately worsen the MTF compared to routinely used power IOLs; for example, a + 36.0D IOL will cause 4 times worse spherical aberration than a + 18.0D IOL. Monofocal aspheric IOLs will either improve or not worsen the net positive spherical aberration; therefore, the MTF values of aspherical IOLs are much higher than the MTF values of spherical IOLs.

MTF is a popularly used and validated metric to quantify the optical performance of an IOL.[22] By using optical bench equipment and an aberration-free model cornea, MTF values for given spatial frequencies (e.g., 50 and 100 lp/mm, equivalent to 20/40, and 20/20 Snellen letters) can be used with fixed pupil sizes (e.g., 3.0 mm and 4.5 mm to simulate photopic and mesopic conditions). The IOL's optical quality can be quantified by dividing the area below the measured MTF curve by the area below the diffraction-limited MTF curve; **a more desirable IOL** will have *higher MTF values* indicating its performance for a given distance. Overall, monofocal IOLs will have high MTF values at distance and low MTF values at near. Presbyopia-correcting IOLs, especially those that rely on diffractive optics (e.g., multifocal, diffractive extended depth of focus, and trifocal IOLs) will usually have lower MTF values at distance but better MTF values at intermediate and near. Wavefront-modifying presbyopia-correcting IOLs, while offering a different philosophical approach to improve intermediate- and near-vision, have very low MTF values.

Thus, the concept of MTF has even greater significance for advanced technology IOLs. Again, if you are nerdy enough to look at the inserts for these presbyopia-correcting IOLs (which you should be if you truly want to be a "refractive cataract surgeon"), you may notice the inclusion of MTF curves tucked away in the device specifications sheet. Depending on the technology of the presbyopia-correcting IOL, the MTF values for distance, intermediate, and near will vary. For example, multifocal IOLs with higher add powers will have better MTF values at near (compared to monofocal and trifocal IOLs). In contrast, trifocal IOLs will have better MTF values at intermediate (compared to monofocal and multifocal IOLs).[23] Ideally, a desirable presbyopia-correcting IOL will have high "average" MTF values for all distances and pupil distances. However, finding this "Goldilocks" IOL remains elusive as all presbyopia-correcting IOLs will have better and worse performances for certain distances and pupil sizes.[24] Finally, MTF values can also be affected by IOL design, material, architecture, and technology platforms. Nonetheless, despite its imperfection, it is one "standardized" metric that can be used to assess the playing field of presbyopia-correcting IOLs. Future versions of presbyopia-correcting IOLs will likely seek to improve MTF values, especially at distance, to improve patients' subjective visual acuity.

Defocus Curves

Defocus curves are of particular interest in the current climate of cataract surgery, especially with presbyopia-correcting IOLs. To simplify, a defocus curve is an objective measurement of how well a multifocal or extended depth of

[21] See Chap. 14 "Physical Optics and Advanced Optical Principles", for more information regarding spherical aberration.

[22] Pieh S, Fiala W, Malz A, Stork W. In vitro strehl ratios with spherical, aberration-free, average, and customized spherical aberration-correcting intraocular lenses. Invest Ophthalmol Vis Sci. 2009 Mar;50(3):1264–70

[23] Son HS, Tandogan T, Liebing S, Merz P, Choi CY, Khoramnia R, Auffarth GU. In vitro optical quality measurements of three intraocular lens models having identical platform. BMC Ophthalmol. 2017 Jun 29;17(1):108. https://doi.org/10.1186/s12886-017-0460-0. PMID: 28662629; PMCID: PMC5492950

[24] Santhiago MR, Netto MV, Barreto J, Gomes BA, Schaefer A, Kara-Junior N. Wavefront analysis and modulation transfer function of three multifocal intraocular lenses. Indian J Ophthalmol. 2010 Mar-Apr;58(2):109–13

focus IOL (MFIOL/EDOF-IOL) is correcting presbyopia by measuring *visual acuity at a range of distances*. Thus, both defocus curves and MTF curves are complementary, like peanut butter and jelly, in assessing IOL performance.

A defocus curve is set up by first correcting the patient's refractive error and giving him/her whatever refractive correction is needed to give the best possible distance visual acuity. This helps to eliminate any positive or negative effects induced by residual refractive errors. For example, residual myopia may artificially make a given IOL test better for near-vision in a pseudophakic patient. After the patient is best corrected for distance, a consecutive sequence of increasing minus-power lenses (starting from +1.0 to −4.0, in 0.5D) is presented to the patient, and he/she is asked to read the smallest line possible.

When the examiner presents these lenses, we can simulate the patient's vision at that particular distance. This concept is easier understood with the minus lenses: for example, the −1.0D lens will simulate vision at 100/1 = 100 cm, the −2.5D lens will simulate vision at 100/2.5 = 40 cm, and the −4.0D lens will simulate vision at 100/4 = 25 cm.

In general, we see that MFIOLs with higher add powers (e.g., +4.0 add) will often give excellent vision at 33 cm and closer; however, patients may lose 1–2 lines of vision (ranging from 20/30 to 20/40) when testing between 50 to 40 cm. Conversely, lower add MFIOLs (e.g., +2.5 or + 3.0 add) will often give better vision in the 33–50 cm range, while causing 1–2 lines of loss of visual acuity at 33 cm and closer.

Given that MFIOLs/EDOF-IOLs with different add powers have different defocus curves, some surgeons take advantage of this disparity by employing a "mix-and-match" approach with presbyopia correcting IOLs. This approach involves placing a lower add MFIOL or EDOF-IOL in the dominant eye (therefore giving the patient better intermediate vision, theoretically) and a higher add MFIOL or EDOF-IOL in the non-dominant eye (therefore giving the patient better near vision, theoretically). This combination allows the "strengths" of one MFIOL/EDOF-IOL to cover up the "weaknesses" of the other.

Legal Blindness

There are some definitions that you simply have to memorize. The definition of legal blindness in the United States (at the time of this writing, April 2021) is that the best-corrected vision in the BETTER eye is ≤20/200 OR the field of vision in the better eye is ≤20°. These requirements do not vary by state. Driver's license requirements do vary depending on the state, so do not waste time memorizing every state's requirement for exams. However, you should know your state's particular requirements for daytime only and unrestricted driving for clinical practice.

It is important to commit this to memory because patients may sometimes ask you to write a letter regarding the legal status of their vision. You want to make sure that in your noble efforts to help a deserving patient use local and federal government assistance programs for low-vision patients, you don't inadvertently help an "undeserving" patient. Another takeaway from this definition is that a monocular patient is not necessarily "legally blind" if he/she still has good BCVA in the better eye. However, a patient with end-stage glaucoma with central visual acuity of 20/50 with a peripheral visual field ≤20° in both eyes is considered legally blind.

Tests for near Vision

The Jaeger chart is the most commonly used eye chart to assess near visual acuity. Other charts include the Nieden and Parinaud near charts. Depending on the model/type of card, the testing distance may vary. Letter heights are not standardized, and there is no logarithmic progression of letters.

For this purpose, a variety of standardized near-reading charts are available to serve as a better proxy for modern optotypes distance acuity measurements, such as the Bailey-Lovie Word Reading Chart and the Colenbrander English Continuous Text Near Vision Cards, and the RADNER Reading Charts. These charts also have logarithmic progression of letters with validated chart design, optotype size, and specified test distance. Moreover, these charts have continuous text with typeset material used such that the distance height of lower-case letters subtends 5 *arcmins*.

Congratulations, you have just completed the visual acuity chapter. It's time to leave the DMV and never return.

Practice Questions

1. Which of the following measurements of visual acuity is the *most sensitive* assessment method?
   A. Vernier Acuity.
   B. Minimum Separable Threshold.
   C. Minimum Visible Threshold.
   D. Minimum Legible Threshold.
2. Which of the following statements is CORRECT?
   A. There are 60 *arcdegrees* in a visual circle.
   B. 360 *arcdegrees* make up one *arcmin*
   C. 5 *arcmins* is equivalent to 1/12th of one *arcdegree*
   D. 60 *arcsecs* is equivalent 10 *arcmins*
3. For an observer standing at 20 feet, how many *arcmins* are subtended by an optotype found on the 20/60, 20/100 and 20/200 line? How many arcmins are subtended by the 20/15 and 20/10 optotypes?

4. If patient 1 (who has 20/15 vision) is looking at an object in full focus from 100 feet away, where does patient 2 (who has 20/20 vision) have to stand to see the same object in full focus?
5. Patient 1 (who has 20/30 vision) can view an object when standing 20 feet away from the object. From how far away can patient 2 (who has 20/20 vision) view the same object?
6. Suppose that a patient's BCVA is 20/80 when tested on the Snellen eye chart in a standard exam lane. How far must the patient move toward the chart to see the 20/20 line?
   A. 5 feet
   B. 10 feet
   C. 15 feet
   D. 17.5 feet
7. Which of the following statements is TRUE about the ETDRS visual acuity chart?
   A. The space between each letter on a given line is approximately half the size of the letter, thereby reducing the unwarranted effects of crowding.
   B. The ETDRS uses 15 letters that have been chosen to be equally difficult in viewing ability to ensure that no one line is easier than the other.
   C. Testing a patient's visual acuity with the ETDRS chart takes less time (when compared to the Snellen visual acuity chart), making it the gold standard for clinical research studies.
   D. Each line on the ETDRS differs from its neighboring line by 0.1 log units.

Answers

1. Answer: Vernier acuity is the most sensitive form of visual acuity assessment; by asking a patient to notice breaks in a line segment, we can test down to the level of 2–3 *arcsecs* (**Answer Choice A**). Minimum Separable Threshold is at a level of >3–5 *arcsecs*; in this method, two objects are presented to the patient with progressively smaller space until he/she can't distinguish any separation between the two objects. Minimum Visible Threshold is similarly at multiple *arcsecs* level; in this method, a target with varying brightness levels is presented to the patient until the patient cannot detect the stimulus any further. Finally, the Minimum Legible Threshold is tested at the level of *arcmins*; in this method, a patient is asked to distinguish between smaller subtended visual angles (such as using letters to test visual acuity).
2. Answer: A visual circle is made up of 360 degrees of arc (*arcdegrees*); each *arcdegree* can be further broken down into 60 *arcmins*; each *arcmin* can itself be further broken down into 60 *arcsecs*. 1 *arcmin* is equivalent to 1/60th of an *arcdegree*, so 5 *arcmins* is equivalent to 1/12th of one *arcdegree* (**Answer Choice C**).
3. Answer: Remember that for an observer at 20 feet, each optotype on the 20/20 line will subtend 5 *arcmins*. To determine the number of *arcmins* for every letter further up the chart, we can take the inverse of that line and multiply it by 5 (which is the number of *arcmins* subtended by the 20/20 line). In this case:
   - 20/60 line = 60/20 = 3 x 5 = 15 *arcmin*
   - 20/100 line = 100/20 = 5 x 5 = 25 *arcmin*
   - 20/200 line = 200/20 = 10 x 5 = 50 *arcmin*
   - 20/15 line = 15/20 = 0.75 x 5 = 3.75 *arcmin*
   - 20/10 line = 10/20 = 0.5 x 5 = 2.5 *arcmin.*
4. Answer: We can take the reciprocal of Patient 1's vision and multiply it by the desired distance. In this case, Patient 1 has 20/15 vision, so: 15/20 x 100 feet = 75 feet away.
5. Answer: Similarly, we have to take the reciprocal of Patient 1's vision and multiply it by the desired distance. In this case, Patient 1 has 20/30 vision, so: 30/20 x 20 feet = 30 feet away.
6. Answer: These types of problems may seem confusing, as there are several ways to solve them. We recommend thinking of these problems as complicated ways of asking you to solve ratio problems.

   Since we know that the patient's BCVA is 20/80 (when tested at the standard testing distance of 20 feet), we need to calculate how many *arcmins* this patient can perceive: 80/20 = 4 x 5 = 20 *arcmins*. We have to determine how close the patient has to be in order to basically see 5 *arcmins*. "X" feet is the distance the patient actually needs to be at:

   - 20 feet/x feet = 20 *arcmin* / 5 *arcmin*
   - 20x = 100, x = 5 feet

   At this point, we may see that we calculated 5 feet, glance up at the answer choices, rejoice that we see "5 feet (answer choice A)," and think we have solved our problem. But this is where these types of problems are devious. Notice that the question said how far the patient must **move toward the chart**. In other words, we know that the patient needs to be 5 feet away from the chart; since he is currently 20 feet away, he must actually move **15 feet closer** (**Answer Choice C**) to be 5 feet away.
7. Answer: As mentioned in the text, there are several features of the ETDRS chart worth committing to memory. The space between each letter on a given line is equal to the size of the letter, thereby reducing the unwarranted effects of crowding. The ETDRS chart uses 10 letters (CDHKNORSVZ). As there are 55 letters on the ETDRS (compared to 36 letters on the Snellen chart), visual acuity testing will take longer on the ETDRS chart compared to the Snellen chart. The biggest advantage of the ETDRS chart is that each line differs from a neighboring line by a fixed logarithmic value of 0.1 log units (**Answer Choice D**). A 3-line change is equivalent to doubling (or halving) the visual angle, making it easier to compare visual acuity across research studies.

Low Vision and Vision Rehabilitation

G. Vike Vicente

Objectives

- To understand how low vision can affect patients' lives
- To have a familiarity with currently available options, including devices and training, on how to improve functional vision in both adult and young patients with low vision
- To know how clinical skills, considerations, and nuances best measure vision and refract low vision patients
- To familiarize the reader with optical and non-optical aides for near and distance tasks

Introduction

Despite our numerous successes with clinical and surgical rehabilitation of patients, we will inevitably be faced with patients whose eye condition(s) cannot be improved. While we ourselves may not be able to help them further, we should be familiar with what our low vision specialist colleagues are able to do for these patients. The skillset required for and routinely employed by these saints is truly remarkable and inspiring – it really takes a special set of skills to patiently work with this patient population.

As ophthalmologists, we may not be personally involved in the low vision rehabilitation of patients. However, we will inevitably be the ones to diagnose and determine when patients may not benefit from any further clinical and/or surgical treatment. Thus, we may be the "gatekeepers" that can appropriately refer these patients to our low vision specialist colleagues. While important for exams, this knowledge is also extremely valuable for clinical practice. We should have a good understanding of various devices, tools, training, and other strategies that can be offered to patients to improve their functional vision for activities of daily living (ADLs).

The authors recommend that ophthalmology trainees should spend at least some time (even for a few days at some point in training) to first-hand observe and appreciate what your local vision rehabilitation specialists do.

Finally, we would like to give a special thanks to Drs. Belinda Weinberg, OD, and Suleiman Alibhai, OD, of Washington, DC, for teaching us how to help our low vision patients (LVPs). We could not have written this chapter without their help.

Definitions

There are several definitions that must be committed to memory as they are often used extensively (and sometimes interchangeably) in the magical world of low vision rehabilitation:

- Vision disorder: This implies progressive, irreversible vision loss due to ophthalmic pathology, such as nystagmus, aniridia, and macular degeneration. Vision disorders can cause *vision impairment*, *vision disability*, and *vision handicap*.
- Vision impairment: This term refers to permanently reduced acuity, loss of visual field, presence of central scotoma, and/or best corrected visual acuity (BCVA) <20/40 in the better seeing eye.
- Vision disability: This term refers to a less severe form for vision impairment. Patients with visual disabilities may have difficulty with vision-intensive tasks, such as seeing the board, reading a book, bubbling a Scantron sheet, and finding a bus.
- Vision handicap: This term refers to vision impairment or vision disability that require low vision assistance, such as preferred seating in classrooms and books on tape.
- Legal blindness: This term is perhaps the most important to know. It is a standard definition for the entire United

G. V. Vicente (✉)
Clinical Pediatrics and Ophthalmology Georgetown University Hospital, Washington, DC, USA

Eye Doctors of Washington, Chevy Chase, MD, USA
e-mail: vvicente@edow.com

K. M. Riaz et al. (eds.), *Optics for the New Millennium*, https://doi.org/10.1007/978-3-030-95251-8_19

States and does not vary state by state.[1] *A patient is considered to be legally blind if the best corrected vision is <20/200 or less in the better seeing eye or if the widest diameter of the visual field around a point of fixation is ≤20°.* For example, if a monocular patient has 20/25 vision in his functional eye, he is not considered legally blind. As another example, a patient with end-stage glaucoma with visual acuity 20/40 in both eyes but a central visual field of 15° in both eyes is considered legally blind.

The Low Vision Patient (LVP)

Sometimes, the eye disease wins. As much as we ophthalmologists pride ourselves in treating cataract, glaucoma, macular degeneration, and a myriad of other eye diseases, we are painfully aware that we cannot win all eye battles.

This doesn't mean that we throw in the towel when we can't improve a patient's objective visual acuity. A patient with a vision disorder (as described in the previous section) not amenable to further clinical or surgical therapy is a low vision patient (LVP). Note: This does not mean this is a *no vision* patient! We can still help a LVP with correct diagnosis, empathy, discussion of further treatment options, and appropriate referrals to low vision rehabilitation resources.

A LVP isn't simply someone with <20/400 visual acuity. There are several additional factors that should be considered as well:

- Visual field loss (central and/or peripheral scotomas)
- Loss of contrast sensitivity
- Loss of color discrimination
- Glare and photophobia

While some of these can be assessed with objective tests (such as visual acuity testing, visual field testing, etc.), a subjective assessment is also required. Specifically, five key (and subjective) areas should be further assessed in LVPs:

- Difficulty with reading tasks (newspaper, email, financial documents, mobile phone, etc.)
- Activities of daily living (see next section)
- Safety issues (reading prescription bottles, house safety assessment, etc.)
- Barriers to social participation (driving, transportation, etc.)
- Psychosocial status (including depression, anxiety, hallucinations (e.g., Charles Bonnet syndrome, etc.), and other psychiatric conditions)

On this last point, we should appreciate that vision loss can be profoundly depressing for many patients (or exacerbate already-existing depression). Some patients with vision loss may experience hallucinations, both with insight (Charles Bonnet syndrome) and without recognition (e.g., dementia, Parkinson's disease). Appropriate referral to a mental health specialist, psychiatrist, and/or neurologist may be life-changing or even life-saving.

Activities of Daily Living (ADLs)

While we use visual acuity to assess visual function in routine ophthalmic clinical practice, a more accurate and comprehensive assessment of visual function of LVPs includes their ability to perform everyday activities.

Thus, activities of daily living (ADLs) is a broad term used to describe *functional vision* required to perform everyday tasks of living such as cooking, grooming, reading mail, and using a telephone. It is difficult to correlate a visual acuity in the office to the effect it has on a given patient's ADLs as other factors, such as comorbid non-ophthalmic conditions, must also be considered. In order to best help a given LVP, we must understand what specific ADLs are impaired due to their decreased vision. In assessing an LVP, a detailed history regarding specific ADLs will help us know what devices and treatments may be offered. For example, an assessment of ADLs requiring distance vision and near vision may be a good starting point:

Near Vision ADLs:

- Reading vision for mail, books, and newspapers
- Near vision for household tasks such as sewing, fixing appliances, and cooking
- Near vision for personal grooming, shaving, and applying make-up
- Near vision for recreational tasks such as using a fishing hook or playing cards
- Near vision for social tasks such as reading a menu at a restaurant
- Near vision technological tasks such as using a computer, cellphone, or handheld device

Distance Vision ADLs:

- Vision required for mobility, such as using public transportation, walking in urban areas, reading street signs, train times, and (most importantly for many patients) driving
- Vision for watching television and movies

[1]Driver's license requirements for both unrestricted and daytime-only driving vary state by state. These should not be committed to memory for the sake of exams, but you should know your state's requirements for clinical practice.

- Vision for other recreational tasks, such as golfing, bird-watching, etc.

Other classifications include assessing daytime/nighttime ADLs, color discrimination, contrast sensitivity, and glare assessment. These last two items are noteworthy because they have an inverse relationship: if a patient has decreased contrast sensitivity, we may be tempted to increase the lighting – but this may worsen the glare! Similarly, if a patient complains of glare and we intervene with decreased lighting or tinting, this may worsen contrast sensitivity. Finding the Goldilocks zone between these two conditions may be an additional challenge for the low vision specialist.

Measuring Visual Function in LVPs

Before discussing low vision aids, we must first discuss several principles for measuring visual acuity and visual field in LVPs.

Visual Acuity

Given that many LVPs may have BCVA <20/400, simply writing "<20/400" is not very helpful. While terms such as count fingers (CF) (at a given distance), hand motions (HM), and light perception (LP) provide everyday functionality, they too lack specificity. Remember that linear or reading visual acuity is more useful than single letter acuity.

For this reason, LVPs may require a different eye chart; many such charts are available.[2] The standard Snellen or ETDRS chart can also be moved closer to the LVP in order to measure a given letter at a lesser distance. For example, CF can be converted into Snellen visual acuity using the following table (Table 1):[3]

Low vision specialists prefer the ETDRS visual acuity chart over the Snellen as the former allows assessment of visual acuity using logMAR notation as well as provides backlighting.[4] Distance visual acuity may also be tested both with and without single and/or multiple pinholes, especially in patients with good central retinal/optic nerve function (e.g., end-stage glaucoma). A Feinbloom number chart is commonly used as it comes in a portable spiral book and is calibrated for 10 feet. This can lead to more precise visual acuity measurement.

Table 1 Comparing Snellen visual acuity and the corresponding "count fingers" distance

Snellen equivalent	Count fingers (CF) distance
20/8000	CF @ 1'
20/4000	CF @ 2'
20/2666	CF @ 3'
20/2000	CF @ 4'
20/1600	CF @ 5'
20/1333	CF @ 6'
20/1143	CF @ 7'
20/1000	CF @ 8'
20/800	CF @ 10'

Computer-driven tests, such as the Grating Acuity Test and Grating Contrast Sensitivity test, may better evaluate an LVP's ability to see both the direction of a grated pattern and its contrast, allowing objective visual acuity measurements as low as 20/4000, compared to 20/1600 with current low vision eye charts.[5]

A few other methods and definitions are useful to better evaluate visual acuity and function in LVPs:

- *Contrast sensitivity (CS)* is a qualitative measurement that may be a better predictor of visual performance than traditional BCVA. Examiners must watch for CS issues when the symptoms are worse than expected given the visual acuity. For example, LVPs may report needing stronger lighting than previous, difficulty with street curbs, finding dark objects on dark backgrounds, etc.
- *Threshold print size* is the absolute smallest size the patient can read.
- *Target acuity* is the patient's goal visual acuity ("I want to be able to read this newspaper," etc.) that may or may not be the same as the objective BCVA
- *Critical print size* is the size the patient can read fluently for brief periods.
- *Enlargement ratio* (ER) = critical print size/target acuity. This is how much bigger the print needs to be for the patient to be able to read it.
- *Acuity reserve (AR)* is the low vision specialist's goal. A patient's critical print size may be 20/80, but we should provide enough assistance so the patient can be an over-achiever and be able to read 2–3 lines smaller. This way they will be able to read the critical print size for prolonged periods of time (e.g., reading a novel, etc.)
- *Metric print size (M)* is a common unit among low vision specialists. 1.0 M = 20/50; Snellen = newspaper print; 2.0 M = 20/100 Snellen.

[2] For example, the Berkley Rudimentary Vision Assessment is popularly used as it allows the examiner to test the LVP's vision at 25 cm for an objective visual acuity measurement as low as 20/16,000.

[3] Modified from "How Visual Acuity is Measured," https://lowvision.preventblindness.org/2003/10/06/how-visual-acuity-is-measured/. Accessed July 19, 2020

[4] See Chap. 18 "Visual Acuity Testing and Assessment", for a discussion on the Snellen and ETDRS charts.

[5] Bittner AK, Jeter P, Dagnelie G. Grating acuity and contrast tests for clinical trials of severe vision loss. *Optom Vis Sci*. 2011; 88(10):1153–1163

- *Continuous text cards* may be used to measure near visual acuity rather than the traditional near vision card. Remember that linear or reading acuity is more useful than single letter acuity.

How can we put all these definitions into practice?

Let's say a patient's measured acuity or critical print size, where they are able to read fluently, is 2 M (metric print size units) at 40 cm with a +2.50D add, but their goal (target acuity) is 0.8 M. Thus, the actual AR would be 0.5 M, 2–3 lines smaller than the target. The enlargement ratio (ER) would be:

ER = measured acuity/acuity reserve = 2 M/0.5 M = 4X. The add power that should be offered is +2.50D × 4 = +10.00D.

Visual Field

We should be quite familiar with objective peripheral visual field testing, such as Humphrey and Goldmann visual fields. For LVPs, central visual field testing devices as macular microperimetry may be useful to objectively locate central scotomas and the patient's retinal point of fixation (preferred retinal locus, or PRL). Recall that these patients may either spontaneously or interventionally develop new (or even multiple) PRLs. In other words, while these patients may have poor exactly-in-the-center central vision, they may have new PRLs slightly adjacent to the central scotoma that can be used advantageously for low vision rehabilitation.

Simple Interventions for LVPs

While most LVPs will benefit from a formal consultation with a low vision specialist, there are some simple interventions that we can offer as ophthalmologists to immediately help patients as they await their low vision referral. Alternatively, some patients may not be able to access a low vision specialist due to distance or financial barriers. Therefore, there are some simple things that we can offer to provide some functional benefits:

Illumination

For most LVPs, simply increasing their ambient lighting (home or office environment) is a simple and effective way to improve functional vision. A simple low vision assessment should include a lighting assessment and demonstration. Don't panic at this physics discussion, but recall that light intensity is the inverse square of distance ($1/r^2$); simply stated, patients may benefit from lighting sources with incoming light that is closer and more directed toward their visual area of interest, especially books. For example, gooseneck lamps are better than regular lamps as they create a focused "spotlight" effect (Fig. 1). Ideally, the lampshade will be lower than eye level and tilted at 45° to reduce glare. High intensity light bulbs such as LEDs may be more useful than traditional bulbs; however, in some patients, it may have a paradoxical effect of "too much brightness."

For a small subset of LVPs (mainly those with glare problems such as patients with oculocutaneous albinism (OCA)), dimmer light bulbs with less intensity may be indicated. Remember that there is often a trade-off between glare and contrast sensitivity.

Tints

For some LVPs, as mentioned above, glare can be more problematic as scattered light will decrease contrast and visual acuity and cause discomfort from photophobia. In addition to modulating the intensity of ambient lighting,

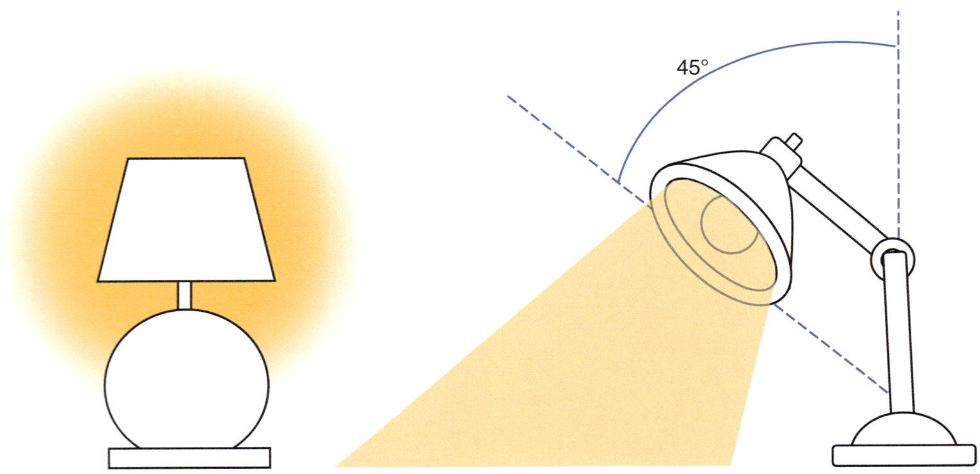

Fig. 1 Preferred lighting. The lamp on the right would provide better illumination for a low vision patient

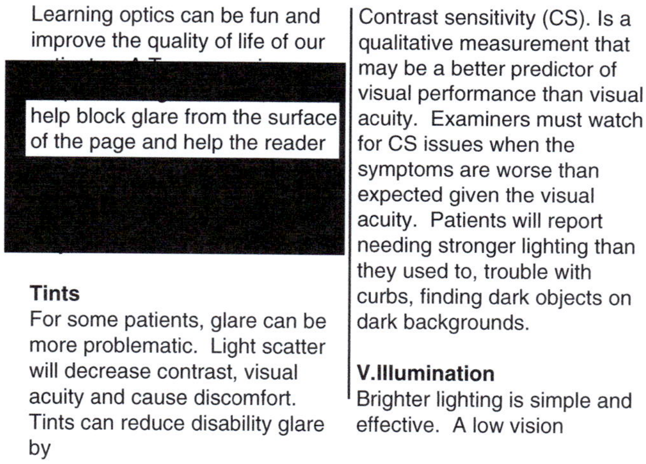

Fig. 2 A typoscope may be helpful for patients who enjoy reading. It functions as a masking device to block glare from the white paper on a page. In addition, it helps patients to focus on the text area of interest by minimizing potentially negative effects of crowding

additional tints can reduce disability glare, for example, by selectively blocking blue light.[6] Yellow, orange, and amber tints may be more useful than simple dark glasses in certain patient populations.

Typoscope

Another useful tool for patients with glare is known as a typoscope. This simple reading shield can help block glare from the surface of the page and help the reader stay focused on the correct line by minimizing potential effects of crowding (Fig. 2).

Refraction in LVPs

Many LVPs may have difficulty in answering questions ("1 or 2") during a subjective manifest refraction as they may not be able to appreciate the differences between the presented options. For example, a patient with 20/200 due to AMD may not appreciate 0.25D of additional cylinder presented – one would be wasting his/her time trying to fine tune a manifest refraction in such a scenario.

As a result, several considerations must be considered in this unique patient population. For example, a Jackson cross

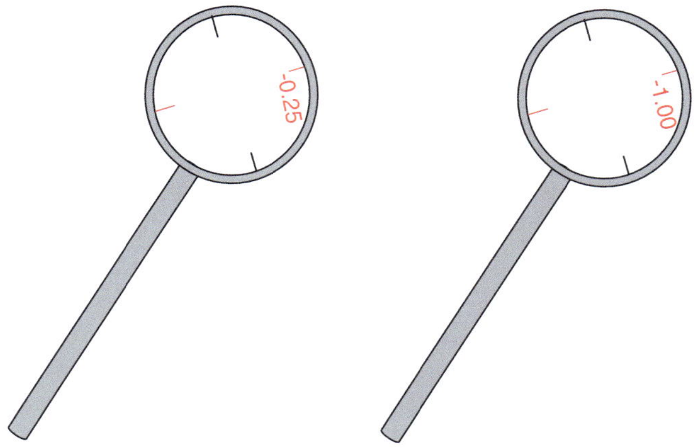

Fig. 3 0.25 D vs. 1D Jackson cross cylinder

cylinder (JCC) with +/− 1D options (instead of the usual +/− 0.25D options) would be potentially more useful, whether used in a phoropter or a trial frame (Fig. 3).

When trying to refine the sphere, rather than agonizing over +/− 0.25D sphere increments, adding −1/+1D sphere at a time may be more effective. One clinically useful pearl to determine how much sphere to add at a time may be to convert the patient's BCVA at 20 feet to 10-feet visual acuity and then divide the denominator by 100. For example, if a patient's BCVA is 20/400:

20/400 → 10/200 (10-feet visual acuity) → 200/100 = 2D. This patient should be offered +/− 2D sphere during manifest refraction.

Remember that reassurance, patience, and compassion are needed in abundance. When scheduling these patients, additional time for refraction should be planned for during their clinic visits.

We can now divide our remaining low vision tools/strategies as "optical" (requiring glasses, lenses, etc.) or "non-optical."

Optical Tools and Strategies

Near Vision and Reading Aids

For many LVPs, optimizing functional near visual acuity is even more important than distance visual acuity. As many LVPs may spend more time indoors/at home, improving functional reading vision may be considered as the most important goal of the low vision specialist. Several options to consider include the following:

[6] See Chap. 16 "Construction of Glasses (Ophthalmologists as Opticians)", for a detailed discussion regarding the usage of tints in glasses.

High Power Plus Single Vision Lenses and Kestenbaum's Rule

High power plus single vision lenses (think "Coke-bottle" glasses) are an excellent option as they are hands-free and provide a wide field of view for near vision tasks. These are available in a range of approximately +4 to +20D lenses; higher powers may need to be custom-ordered. These lenses may be placed as a full-frame or half-frame (similar to a bifocal) in one or both eyes.

Remember that any plus lens will exert base-out prismatic effects when patients look nasal to the optical center.[7] When using high power plus lenses, a significant base-out effect may require the use of *base-in* prism to decrease convergence demands at near.

A rule of thumb for dispensing base-in prisms: *add 2 PD more than the reading portion* (whether a single vision high power lens of a bifocal (see next section)) of the glasses. For example, if an LVP is requiring a +6.00D add, we would need to give approximately 6 + 2 = 8 PD base-in for each eye. A patient with a +10.0D add would require 12 BI prisms over each eye.

A downside of this option is that these glasses have a very short working distance and are extremely heavy. Furthermore, recall that when dealing with higher power prescriptions (both myopic and hyperopic), the effects of vertex distance may be more impactful; a careful measurement and maintenance of vertex distance is necessary, especially when changing frames or updating an LVP's refraction. Finally, these types of glasses are quite expensive.

When discussing high power plus lenses, we can introduce a favorite topic of exams (and senior attendings): *Kestenbaum's rule*. In 1953, the good Dr. Kestenbaum, in a very appropriately named paper ("Reading Glasses for Patients with Very Poor Vision"),[8] described how the clinician can estimate the strength of a high power plus lens needed to read newspaper without accommodation.[9] This elegantly simple rule requires the clinician to measure the *distance* Snellen acuity for the *better seeing eye*, take the reciprocal, and use that as the required add power for both eyes.

For example, if the BCVA in the right eye is 20/200 and left eye is 20/300, then we would apply Kestenbaum's rule to the right eye: 20/200 → 200/20 = 10. We would give both eyes a +10D lens, NOT a +10D, for the right eye and a +15D for the left eye. Of course, we would need to give some base-in prism (12 PD BI to both eyes) to decrease convergence demands with high power plus lenses.

If one wants to further understand how/why Kestenbaum's rule works, read the rest of this paragraph; otherwise, skip to the next section. Basically, in order to read newsprint (8 point), a patient needs to have at least 20/50 linear BCVA to read at 40 cm. Note that this is linear, not single letter, BCVA (remember the previous discussion about the importance of linear visual acuity measurements in LVPs). At 40 cm, a patient lacking any accommodative ability will require a +2.50D lens (100/40 = 2.5). A patient with 20/100 linear BCVA at 40 cm will be able to read 20/50 letters at 20 cm. At this distance, the non-accommodating patient will need a +5D lens for assistance, (100/20 = 5), which would be the same power as the one determined by Kestenbaum's rule.

High Add Bifocal Segments

As the term suggests, some LVPs may require additional add power in a bifocal segment beyond what we could customarily dispense. In general, because these patients often have plus-power distance vision glasses as well, round top or executive style bifocal segments work best. Flat-top segments may not be the best choice for patients with hyperopic glasses due to the debilitating effects of image displacement and image jump.[10] If an LVP requires a myopic prescription, a flat top bifocal segment (available up to +5.00D) would be a reasonable choice. Progressive add lenses may not be well tolerated due to the "transition zone" and oblique astigmatism that would be increased with higher powers; these may be considered for add powers up to +3.5D.

The following table is a starting point reference for how much add power should be given to a LVP with the following "starting" BCVA at 40 cm.

Required Add Chart

VA @ 40 cm with +2.50	Add needed for 20/40	Working distance
20/50	+3.00	33 cm
20/60	+3.75	27 cm
20/70	+4.25	22 cm
20/80	+5.00	20 cm
20/100	+6.25	16 cm

Remember that higher add powers will create a shorter working distance and increase binocular strain due to the

[7] See Chap. 2 "Prisms in Ophthalmic Optics", for a review of this topic.

[8] Clearly, it was much easier to publish academic papers without fancy and creative titles in the 1950s.

[9] Kestenbaum A. Reading glasses for patients with very poor vision. *Am J Ophthalmol*. 1953;36(8):1143–1144

[10] See Chap. 12 "Glasses for Written Exams", for a discussion on bifocal types, image jump, and image displacement. Recall what we have said regarding flat-top bifocals: traditionally, it was taught that flat-top bifocals should not be placed in hyperopic glasses. However, in modern optical practice, flat-top bifocals are cheaper to make, and thanks to advancements in laser-etching technology (edge-to-edge power), flat-top bifocals are nonetheless commonly dispensed in plus-lens glasses.

increased convergence required. Base-in prisms, as discussed previously, should be given in these cases.

"Computer" low vision glasses can also be constructed with an intermediate add as the top portion of the bifocal and the near add as the bottom portion of the bifocal.

High Power Handheld Lenses (Handheld Magnifiers)

Think of these as monocles for the modern age as patients can hold them up to their eye(s) when needed (variable eye to lens distance). They can also hold them near to the page or object of interest – visualize Sherlock Holmes using a magnifying glass. These lenses are available with or without illumination. They allow for different working distances based on the power of the lens but require a steady hand. Their narrow field of view can be increased by holding the lens closer to the spectacle plane. These are available in ranges from +5 to +20D.

One optics-nerd point: We have previously discussed how angular magnification and using a lens as a simple magnifier (held at 25 cm from the object of interest) can be used to provide magnification.[11] For most modern magnifying glasses, because it is difficult to hold the magnifier at 25 cm, it is much easier to hold it closer to the object of interest. Therefore, magnifiers are given a "trade magnification" power that modifies the previous "simple magnification formula (D/4)" as follows:

$$\text{Trade magnification} = \left(\text{power of the lens} / 4\right) + 1$$

For example, trade magnification of a +8D lens is (8/4) + 1 = 3× magnification.

Stand Magnifiers

A stand magnifier can be placed over a text or newspaper and may work better than handheld lenses, especially for patients with tremors. Advantages of these devices include availability of extra illumination and various sizes. Disadvantages include a fixed working distance. These are available in power up to +50D.

Loupes for Near Vision

Close focus telescopes may be worn by patients for reading activities. Like surgical loupes, they have a longer working distance than reading spectacles but allow the patient to use his/her hands for holding the reading material. Disadvantages include a small field of view, limited depth of focus, and precise head positioning. If one recalls how long it took to learn how to effectively work with surgical loupes during residency, now try applying that to an 85-year-old patient with end-stage AMD learning to use loupes. It can be done, but it will take practice – so don't be surprised if your AMD patient learns how to use loupes more effectively than you do!

Video Magnification and Electronic Displays (Tablets, CCTVs)

Though these devices may have traditionally been quite expensive, they have become more affordable in recent times due to cheaper technology and government assistance for eligible patients. These devices can be very effective and helpful in this patient population. Older versions of this technology involved the device scanning, digitizing, and reformatting written text. Due to recent advancements, this process is made much faster and faithfully reproduces written text. These devices can also be connected to the Internet, desktop, or phone to allow patients to read electronic texts/newspapers, etc. Patients can customize their magnification and/or desired contrast levels.

They are especially advantageous in patients with scotomas or eccentric fixation who need high magnification during reading tasks as these patients often have difficulties with beginning and ending of words (Fig. 4). Remember that patients with eccentric fixation would have worse linear visual acuity than single letter acuity due to crowding effect (this is similar to patients with amblyopia) (Fig. 5).

Electronic devices can also incorporate speech-to-text software both as "input" (from the patient) and "output" (from the device) to allow patients to use their voice to accomplish computer-related ADLs. For example, thanks to the magic of speech-to-text software, both you and your 86-year-old AMD geographic atrophy patient can tell Alexa® to download a song, order pizza, or set an appointment on your calendar.

Commonly used electronic devices, such as computers and tablets, now have additional built-in features for

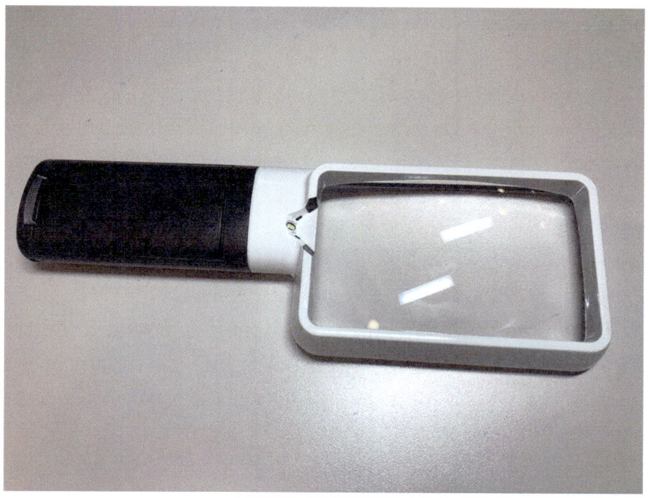

Fig. 4 Handheld magnifier

[11] See Chap. 8 "Magnification and Telescopes".

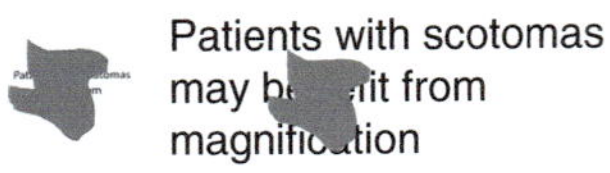

Fig. 5 Patients with central scotomas benefit from magnification of the object. Notice both gray scotomas are the same size

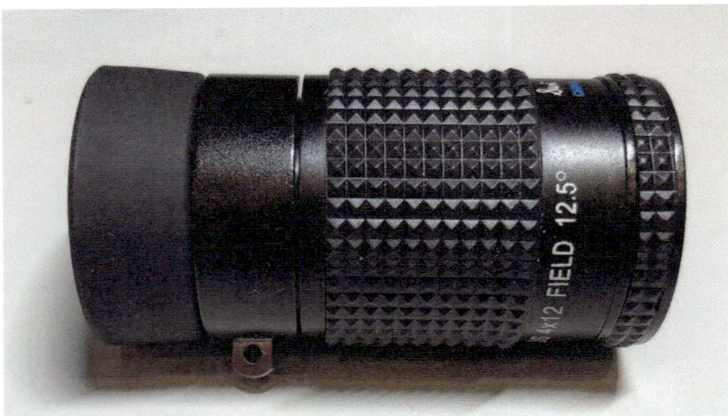

Fig. 6 Low vision telescope

enhanced magnification, speech-to-text, and contrast adjustment.

Distance Vision Aids

Distance activities of daily living to consider for LVPs include seeing street signs, crossing signals, wall-mounted menus, television, theater, and public transportation (bus numbers, train times). In rare circumstances, driving may be considered depending on local state requirements for a driver's license. Each state has its own minimum requirements of BCVA and peripheral visual fields for restricted and unrestricted licenses.

Some simple devices include binoculars and handheld monocular distance vision lenses. A few other devices include:

Telescopes

Telescopes can be very effective for distance vision, me mateys.[12] They can be handheld or placed in the glasses and may be placed in one or both lenses. They can be especially effective for indoor distance activities, such as viewing a TV screen or reading the chalkboard (e.g., a school-age patient with hereditary retinal disease) (Fig. 6).

Galilean telescopes are generally preferred for LVPs: they provide an upright, magnified (2–10×) image with a shorter focal length. The field of view is wide and the weight of the telescope is quite light. Additionally, they are cheaper to make as compared to astronomical telescopes.

Keplerian (astronomical) telescopes may be considered as they can gather more light rays; by using inverting prisms, images can be made upright as well. The magnification is somewhat smaller (2–4×) and the focal length is longer. Furthermore, they are heavier and more expensive than Galilean telescopes, especially the inverting-prism portion. However, the image quality is usually much better than Galilean telescopes.

Some telescopes may have a fine-tuning dial for adjustable focus, similar to the operating microscope. One disadvantage is that the magnification provided is inversely proportional to the field of view: higher amounts of magnification will decrease the field of view, making them suboptimal for tasks that require good peripheral vision such as driving. Another disadvantage is the decreased contrast sensitivity by both kinds of telescopes.

Reverse Telescope

If an LVP has good central vision but significantly reduced peripheral vision, then an off-center reverse Galilean telescope can be mounted on the peripheral part of the eyeglasses to increase/widen the peripheral field of view. Though the use of a reverse Galilean telescope will minimize objects, it may confer the advantage of increased peripheral vision to allow an LVP, for example, to go through doors more easily. A high power (10–30 PD) *base-out prism* can be placed on the temporal portion of each lens to shift the outer field inward (relative to the patient).[13]

Bioptic Telescopes with Driving Glasses

LVPs can use small, bioptic telescopes mounted on eyeglasses (usually the superior portion) to help them drive safely. Similar to the previous option, the small telescope portion is placed away from the optical center and used intermittently when driving to improve perception of the peripheral visual field, similar to how a rearview window is used by all drivers intermittently. Though this device requires considerable training and practice, a magnification of 2–6× is possible. For example, a patient may only see 20/200 BCVA with glasses, but if they can achieve 20/70 through the bioptic portion, this may qualify him/her for a restricted (daytime only) driving in some states. This option may be especially useful in patients with nystagmus as most states allow for restricted drivers licenses with the use of bioptics (Fig. 7).

[12] Recall Chap. 8 "Magnification and Telescopes", for a discussion on telescopes and all things related to pirates.

[13] "Vision Aids for Impaired Peripheral Vision or Tunnel Vision," https://www.schepens.harvard.edu/images/stories/nire/peripheral_vision.pdf. Accessed July 21, 2020

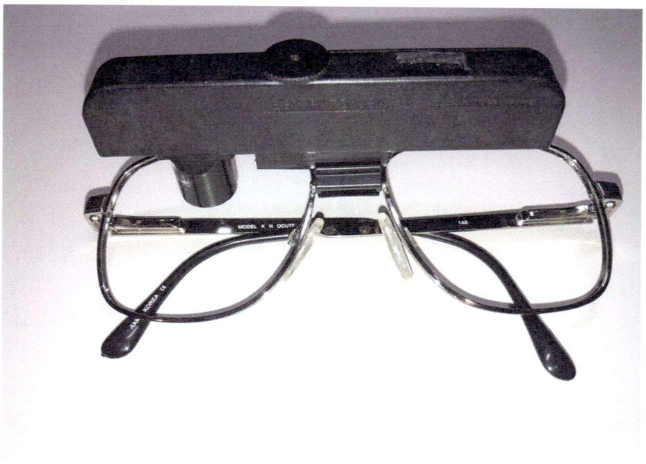

Fig. 7 Bioptic telescope

Surgical Options

Implantable Miniature Telescope (IMT)

The IMT was FDA approved in 2014 as a surgically implanted device to potentially improve vision in LVPs with end-stage AMD. The IMT was designed to enlarge objects in the central visual field and "project" them onto the mid/peripheral (and presumably healthy) retina in order to improve these patients' functional vision. While the device offers a potentially surgical option and may be improved upon in the future, there are numerous hurdles that prevent its widespread use:

- On-label use of the device requires implantation at the time of cataract surgery. Most patients with end-stage AMD are usually pseudophakic for many years (many with open posterior capsule due to YAG capsulotomy). As a result, many potential patients don't qualify due to their prior history of cataract surgery. While one may consider using an IMT in a phakic patient with pattern dystrophy or other central macular disease (North Carolina macular dystrophy, etc.), this would be an off-label use of the device.
- A skilled low vision specialist trained in the rehabilitation exercises necessary after implantation is crucial to a successful visual outcome. Given the scarcity of these sorcerers/sorceresses of vision rehabilitation, it may be difficult to find a skilled and experienced practitioner. Patients must undergo preoperative training with an external telescope to determine whether they qualify or whether adequate vision can even be obtained.
- The fellow eye must have good peripheral vision. Most patients with end-stage AMD usually have significant disease in the fellow eye as well.
- The device itself is quite large (4.4 mm long and 3.6 mm in diameter) and requires a 9 mm sclerocorneal incision (similar to an extracapsular cataract extraction wound).

At this time, there is no significant evidence to assess the effectiveness of the IMT in improving visual acuity in patients with late or advanced AMD.[14]

Another option is to create a "poor man's" version of the surgical IMT by creating a Galilean telescope at the time of cataract surgery. For example, one can plan for a postoperative IOL target of +10D in order to create roughly a −10D eyepiece inside the eye (focal length 10 cm).[15] The patient can then use +5D lenses (focal length 20 cm) held 10 cm away from the eye for 2× magnification.

Future technologies may include retinal implants and cortical visual prosthetic devices; none of these devices are available for widespread use at the time of this writing.

Non-optical Tools and Strategies

There are dozens of non-optical (think: "not glasses") methods that can be used to help LVPs. The following is a non-comprehensive list of tools and strategies that can be considered in addition to the previously mentioned optical tools:

- Devices to help with everyday tasks, such as bold ink pens, large print books, large print playing cards, large print phone dials, etc.
- Services from local institutions, such as requesting utility companies to send large-print bills; requesting banks to issue large print statements and checks with raised lines.
- Referral to state agencies, assisted-living services, occupational therapy, social work, and support groups to help improve quality of life and independence in LVPs.
- Signature guides for legal documents.
- Guide dogs.
- Learning braille.
- Prisms (with eccentric fixation): while theoretically this may make sense (shift the image out of the scotoma into an area of "usable" retina), use of prisms is considered controversial and not frequently used (due to conflicting evidence).

[14] Gupta A, Lam J, Custis P, Munz S, Fong D, Koster M. Implantable miniature telescope (IMT) for vision loss due to end-stage age-related macular degeneration. *Cochrane Database Syst Rev.* 2018;5(5):CD011140

[15] We realize that an IOL target of +10D breaks every rule of cataract surgery.

- Scanning training: training patients to "find" moving objects or objects of interest in the peripheral visual field and indirectly focus on them. Some studies have shown scanning training to be quite effective, especially for patients with stroke-related hemianopia visual field loss.[16]
- Eccentric fixation training: this strategy can be especially useful for young patients with central vision loss and preserved peripheral retina, such as patients with Best's disease.

Just like a certain superhero who cannot see but relies on his heightened sense of hearing to fight evil,[17] sometimes we can take advantage of the preserved sense of hearing to compensate for the loss of vision.[18]

Auditory strategies include National Library Service for the Blind and Physically Handicapped (NLS). Some cities have services wherein volunteers read the local papers and LVPs can call into a toll-free local number to listen to the news being "read aloud."

Other devices and apps that have optical character recognition (OCR) and can read aloud to LVPs include:

- Stand-alone devices that can perform text to speech (e.g., ClearReader+).
- Closed circuit TV (CCTV) e.g., Clearview+ Speech.
- Apps (e.g., Seeing AI) that will describe in audio what is seen on the phone screen that includes currency, bar codes, faces, and emotions.
- Wearable – Orcam. This is a small standalone device with a camera and a speaker that is attached to frames and can recognize text and faces. The user would point to a word on a menu and the device will read the text.

Low Vision Rehabilitation of the Pediatric Patient

While vision loss in any patient is difficult for both the clinician and the patient, it can be even more devastating in pediatric patients. Fortunately, vision loss in the pediatric patient may be especially amenable to low vision therapy. When we work with pediatric patients, we need to keep in mind the child's understanding, apprehension, determination, and acceptance, not to mention the parents' attitude which may range from helpful-motivated, denial, anger, to not-helpful. It may be more difficult to assess the visual potential and visual field of a young child with low vision than an adult.

A low vision evaluation may provide useful information for teachers. Simple questions may include:

- What size print can the child see on the board from the front row (2-inch-tall letters?).
- What is the child's reading speed at 10- or 14-point letter size?
- Does the young patient have a visual diagnosis that would cause them to need more time for certain visual tasks, tests, etc.?
- Can reading be sustained into college years or will audio substitution or braille become necessary?

The clinician should be familiar with what services the county or state can offer young patients. For example, are there pediatric low vision specialists ("vision teachers") available in the local area that can work with the child? Is there an infant and toddler's program that may help?

All of the previously mentioned options may be considered for pediatric LVPs. A few particularly effective strategies and useful considerations in children include:

- Glasses: the full cycloplegic refraction should always be given.
- Telescopes for distance with a goal of 20/40 should be considered. These may be especially useful for classroom situations. Patients with albinism and other congenital retinal diseases may benefit significantly from telescopes.
- Glare control: additional modifications, such as polarized lenses, specialized color tints, and mirror coatings may be effective.[19] Photochromic lenses may also be considered for select patients.
- School activity modifications: for example, using yellow paper to reduce glare or having a specialized computer monitor.
- Just like fitting glasses with kids, frequent follow-ups, adjustments. and alternate devices may need to be used as the child grows older.

Practice Questions

1. Which of the following trial frame choices ("number 1 or number 2") should be offered during a refraction to a patient with 20/100 best corrected vision?
   A. −1.00 D sph vs. −1.25 D sph

[16] Rowe FJ, Conroy EJ, Bedson E, et al. A pilot randomized controlled trial comparing effectiveness of prism glasses, visual search training and standard care in hemianopia. *Acta Neurol Scand.* 2017; 136(4): 310–321

[17] Again, we cannot name this superhero lest we incur copyright infringement.

[18] Apologies to patients with Usher's syndrome

[19] See Chap. 16 "Construction of Glasses (Ophthalmologists as Opticians)", for additional information on glasses modifications, such as polarized lenses, tints, and coatings.

B. −1.00 D sph vs. −1.50 D sph
C. −1.00 D sph vs. −2.00 D sph
D. −1.00 D sph vs. −2.50 D sph.

2. Let's say a patient's measured acuity (critical print size) at which he/she is able to read fluently is 3 M (metric print size units) at 40 cm with a +2.5D add. However, the goal (target acuity) is 1.0 M. Thus, the acuity reserve (AR) would be 0.6 M, which is approximately 2–3 lines smaller than the target. What add would this patient require to be able to read in a sustained, fluid manner?
   A. +2.5D add
   B. +5.0D add
   C. +10.D add
   D. +12.5D add
3. How much base-in prism would you include if the patient requires a +5.0D add?
   A. 4 PD base-in on each lens
   B. 4 PD base-out on each lens
   C. 7 PD base-in on each lens
   D. 5 PD base-in on each lens
4. Which of the following statements regarding optical tools and strategies for low vision patients is TRUE?
   A. The implantable miniature telescope is an effective option as an IOL exchange surgery in pseudophakic patients with end-stage AMD.
   B. A handheld telescope magnifier is an effective option for a patient with Parkinson's disease.
   C. Glasses with telescope magnifiers are an effective option for school-age low vision patients.
   D. When giving high plus power lenses (either as a single vision lens or a bifocal segment), giving a patient additional base-out prism is helpful to decrease the increased convergence demands for near vision.
5. If a patient has a best corrected vision of 20/100, what reading glasses should be offered according to Kestenbaum's rule?
   A. +2.0
   B. +5.0
   C. +8.0
   D. +10.0
6. Which of the following statements is TRUE?
   A. The definition of legal blindness is defined as the vision in the better-seeing eye <20/250 or visual field <25°.
   B. Macular microperimetry is helpful in assessing preferred retinal locus in a patients with Best's disease.
   C. Use of prisms to rehabilitate patients with scotomas and/or hemianopias has been shown to be as effective as scanning training.
   D. Treatments to improve contrast sensitivity will also help with glare symptoms.

Answers

1. Answer: B. Convert BCVA to 10 feet by dividing the BCVA by 2: 20/100 = 10/50. Now divide 50 by 100 = 0.5. This represents the amount of "sphere" difference choices that should be offered to the patient. A 0.25D change may not be appreciated as much by the patient. A full 1D change in choices may end up causing an inaccurate refraction. In general, the worse the patient's best corrected vision, the wider the choices that should be offered.
2. Answer: D. +12.5 D add. The enlargement ratio (ER) would be ER = measured acuity/acuity reserve = 3 M/0.6 M = 5×. The add power that should be offered is +2.50D × 5 = +12.50D. Additional base-in prism (14–15 PD BI) should also be given.
3. Answer: C. 7 PD base-in on each lens. The amount of prism required to ease extra convergence demands due to very short working distance = 2D + add D (+5.0) = 7 PD BI on each lens.
4. Answer: C. The IMT is a potentially effective option for phakic patients with end-stage AMD. At this time, there is no significant evidence to assess the effectiveness of the IMT in improving visual acuity in patients with late or advanced AMD (see Reference 14 cited in the text). A handheld telescope may be difficult to use in patients with significant hand and/or resting tremors, such as in Parkinson's patients. When dispensing high plus power lenses, base-in prisms should be given to decrease convergence demands.
5. Answer: B. According to Kestenbaum's rule, the reciprocal of the vision 100/20 should give you the starting point of what to offer the patient. In this case +5.0D reading glasses. Again, the clinician should strongly consider giving additional base-in prism (in this case, 7 PD BI prisms).
6. Answer: B. Macular microperimetry is helpful to map the location of the central scotoma and assess the location of new PRLs in patients with central retinal disease. The definition of legal blindness in the United States as visual acuity less than or equal to best corrected visual acuity of 20/200 or a visual field ≤20° around central fixation. Use of prisms has not been shown to be more effective than scanning training in patients with hemianopias. In general, treatment strategies to improve contrast sensitivity involve increasing illumination; this usually worsens glare symptoms. Thus, treatment of both entities involves a compromise.

Contact Lenses in Clinical Practice

J. Scott Samples and Kamran M. Riaz

Objectives

- To understand commonly used terms in contact lens design and architecture.
- To understand the advantages, disadvantages, and troubleshooting strategies for soft contact lenses, soft toric contact lenses, and rigid gas permeable contact lenses.
- To have an introductory understanding of advanced contact lens designs available for patients with specific visual needs.

Introduction

We had so much "fun" with contact lenses in Chap. 13 that we felt it was necessary to have a contact lenses chapter in Part II.

In Chap. 13 our discussion on contact lenses primarily focused on calculating the power of three types of commonly used contact lenses: soft contact lenses (SCLs), soft toric contact lenses (STCLs), and rigid gas permeable contact lenses (RGPCLs). You may wish to review this previous chapter (or consult it) as you proceed through this chapter.

Instead, this chapter will focus on the role of contact lenses in clinical practice, with minimal discussion on principles and steps of fitting a given type of contact lens. We will survey the various kinds of available contact lenses, including clinical applicability, strengths, and weaknesses of each lens. Some of you may look at this topic and think to yourself: *but I don't even dispense contact lenses! I refer them to an optometrist or a contact lens specialist!* While that may be true, a basic understanding of contact lenses is essential for board exams and clinical practice. If nothing else, hopefully, this chapter will make you appreciate the skill, experience, and patience required to be an expert contact lens specialist.[1]

Important Definitions

We can group several terms used in contact lens fitting into the following categories based on *architecture*, *materials,* and *surface properties*.

Contact Lens Architecture

- Base curve (BC) (Fig. 1): The curvature of the posterior surface of the contact lens, usually expressed in millimeters. Corneal keratometry measurements (in diopters) can be converted into BC notation to select an appropriately sized lens. Remember this fundamental rule: the *lower the BC value*, the *steeper* the CL, allowing for more vaulting over the corneal surface and avoidance of the central corneal apex.[2]
- Diameter (DIA): The total edge-to-edge length of the contact lens. SCLs will generally have a longer DIA than the corneal diameter as they will encompass the entire cornea (range 13–15 mm). On the other hand, RGPCLs will have a shorter DIA as they will be fit within the cornea (range 9–10 mm).
- Peripheral curve: This curve is the secondary (peripheral) curve of the contact lens that is different from the BC. Given that the cornea is flatter in the periphery than the center, the peripheral curve will also be (generally)

[1] As a cornea specialist, this author (KMR) certainly appreciates the skill of expert contact lens specialists like the co-author (JSS) in dramatically improving visual acuity in complex corneal and anterior segment pathologies.

[2] Recall our discussions of the "SID" rule in Chap. 13 "Contact Lenses for Written Exams".

J. S. Samples (✉) · K. M. Riaz
Dean McGee Eye Institute, University of Oklahoma, Oklahoma City, OK, USA
e-mail: Scott-Samples@DMEI.org

K. M. Riaz et al. (eds.), *Optics for the New Millennium*, https://doi.org/10.1007/978-3-030-95251-8_20

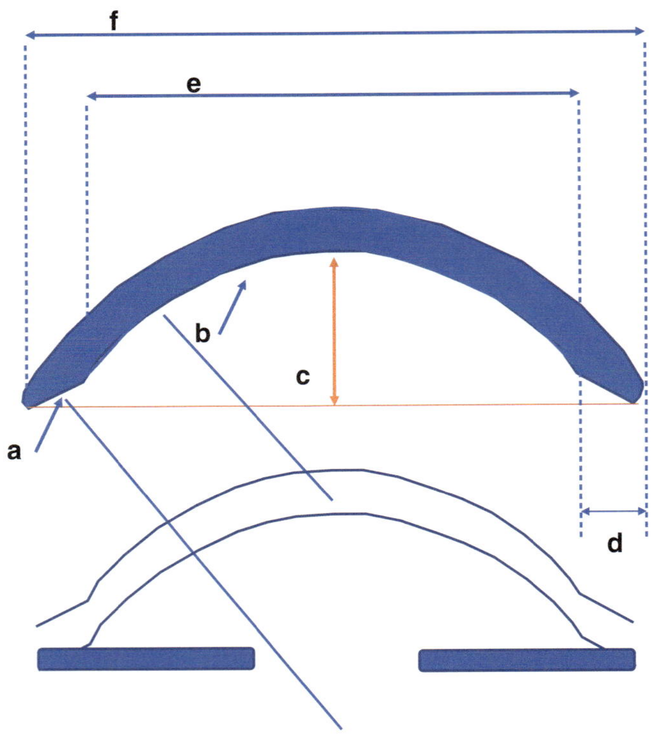

Fig. 1 Contact lens architecture terms: (A) Peripheral curve; (B) base curve; (C) sagittal depth; (D) peripheral curve width; (E) optical zone; (F) diameter

flatter than the BC. The peripheral curve is usually not considered in standard fitting, given that the BC will primarily determine the fit of the given contact lens. The peripheral curve may need to be adjusted to ensure a good fit in advanced cases.

- Optical zone: The central portion of the contact lens – this is where all the refractive action happens as the curvature of the anterior surface primarily determines the refractive power of the contact lens.
- Sagittal depth (a.k.a. vault): Technically, this refers to the distance from the center of the posterior contact lens to a line drawn perpendicular to the edge of the lens. For SCLs, the vault is negligible, but for RGPCLs, the vault must be considered in the context of the resulting tear lens (and its power).

Contact Lens Materials

An ideal contact lens material should incorporate certain favorable qualities:

- Comfortable for patient wear yet durable and resistant to tearing and scratching.
- Surface should allow for optimal lubrication.
- Minimal movement with blinking.
- Resistance to foreign body/deposits forming on the contact lens.
- Transmit oxygen (and nutrients) to the cornea.
- Allow for adequate exchange of tears between the contact lens and the cornea.

Several materials may be used in the construction and design of contact lenses, including:

- Glass: Leonardo da Vinci was the first to describe the idea of using a glass lens with a funnel for pouring water (and therefore altering its power) to be placed on the sclera. Later, Sir John Herschel (1823) described the idea of grinding a glass lens to be fit onto the surface of the cornea using the patient's eye as a model and using a gel to create a protective barrier between the contact lens and the patient's eye. Through the late nineteenth century, this concept began to be refined and used primarily to protect diseased eyes rather than for refractive correction. In modern times, these facts are interesting for historical appreciation only. If you ever encounter a patient with a glass contact lens, he/she may be a time-traveler from the past (or the future?).
- Plastic (polymethylmethacrylate, PMMA): PMMA contact lenses, though highly durable, are relatively impermeable with essentially no oxygen permeability or transmissibility. The tear pump underneath the lens is the only source of oxygen to the cornea with these lenses. These, too, have fallen out of use in modern times.
- Hydrogel polymers (hydroxyethylmethacrylate [HEMA] and silicone hydrogel): These are the most commonly used materials for SCLs, especially silicone hydrogels (introduced in 1998), given several factors:
  - Favorable oxygen permeability (silicone atoms create pores favoring movement of oxygen)
  - Less water content (within the SCL) that allows for better lubrication of the ocular surface[3]
  - Improved patient comfort
  - Resistance to deposits forming on the SCL
  - The ability for extended-wear in select patients
- Cellulose acetate butyrate (CAB): Used primarily in RGPCLs, this material has better oxygen permeability than PMMA but is still much lower than silicone hydrogels. Several modifications can be made:
  - Addition of silicone acrylates: PMMA/silicone can increase oxygen permeability

[3]This may seem counterintuitive but if there is less water within the SCL, then the SCL will be much thinner and much more comfortable. A higher water content SCL will draw out the eye's tears, thus making them more prone to dehydration; they are also much more prone to evaporation from air conditioning and periods of low blinking (computer use, reading this entertaining optics book, etc.)

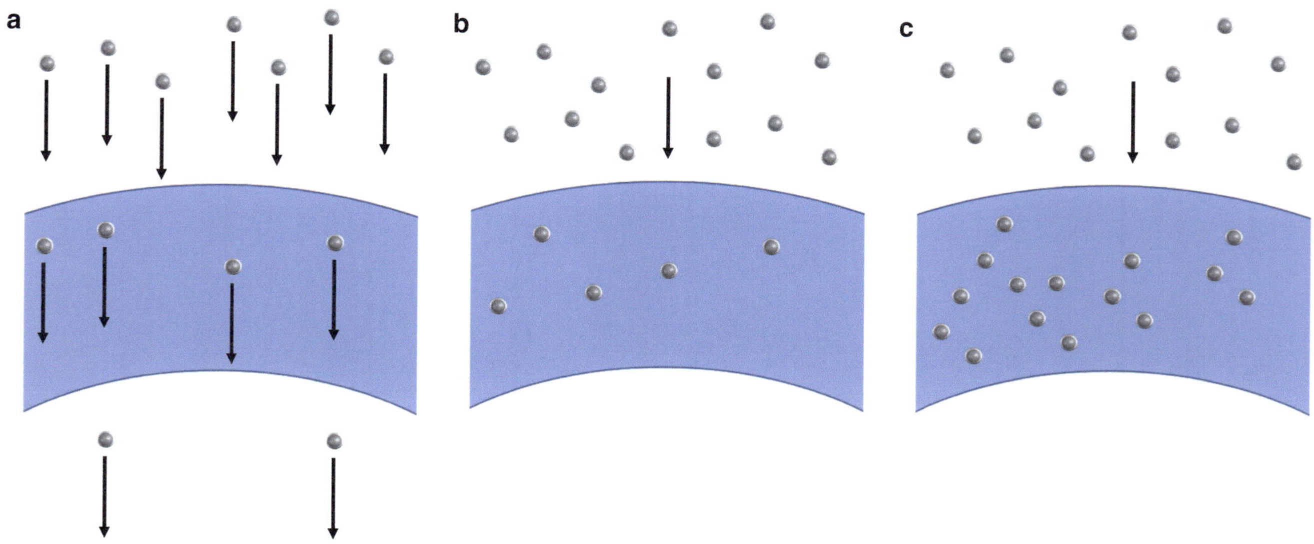

Fig. 2 Visual representations of oxygen diffusion coefficient (D) and solubility coefficient (k). Panel **a** shows the speed of oxygen molecules through a material. The solubility coefficient (k) can be understood as the volume of gas dissolved in a material. Panel **b** shows a material with low solubility coefficient, while Panel **c** shows a material with high solubility coefficient. The Dk value is a measurement of oxygen permeability in a given material. A favorable contact lens material will have a high Dk value

- Fluorosilicone acrylates: Addition of fluorine increases oxygen permeability but renders the RGPCL more fragile. Additionally, fluorine allows mucin to form on the RGPCL, thereby attracting tears and enhancing surface lubrication.

Contact Lens Surface Properties

In the previous section, we discussed several favorable properties of contact lens materials. These materials are especially advantageous because of specific *properties* of the contact lens surface(s):

- Dk: Oxygen *permeability* of a lens material (Fig. 2). *D* is the oxygen diffusion coefficient for a given material, and *k* is the solubility coefficient of oxygen for a given material. In general, these terms are used together as a single entity. A *favorable* contact lens should have a *high* Dk value.
- Dk/t: Oxygen *transmissibility* of a lens material, where *t* is the thickness of the lens material. We can see that lowering the thickness of the lens will therefore increase the Dk/t value (Fig. 3). By convention, Dk/t values are calculated for a −3.00D power contact lens and listed for each lens brand. Myopic contact lenses will generally be thinner in the center compared to hyperopic contact lenses; thus, even if both are made of the same materials, a −4.00D SCL will have a higher Dk/t value as compared to a +4.00D SCL. Thus, a *favorable* contact lens should have a *high* Dk/t value. Modern silicone hydrogels have very high Dk/t values (usually >100) compared to other materials, including other types of hydrogels.
- Wetting angle: This term refers to how water can effectively spread over a lens surface (wettability). Therefore, a *favorable* contact lens should have a *low wetting angle* because it means that water can more easily "flow" across the entire lens surface.

Common Contact Lens Types: Clinical Applications and Troubleshooting

Soft Contact Lenses (SCLs)

In clinical practice, soft contact lenses (SCLs) are the most commonly prescribed contact lenses. Advantages of SCLs include comfort, cost, disposability (especially with daily wear SCLs), availability, and adaptability for patient usage (ranging from refractive to therapeutic). Disadvantages include the inability to correct significant astigmatism, fragility, and potential for misuse.[4]

SCLs are usually the first-line choice for most contact lens wearers. Overall, the Dk (and Dk/t) values of SCLs are quite high (70–140), and thus they offer significant advan-

[4]Though, theoretically, all contact lenses may be abused if in the wrong hands. The popularity and ease of availability of SCLs may falsely skew the "abuse" potential, though any cornea specialist will attest that SCL abuse is the number one cause of clinically encountered corneal infections.

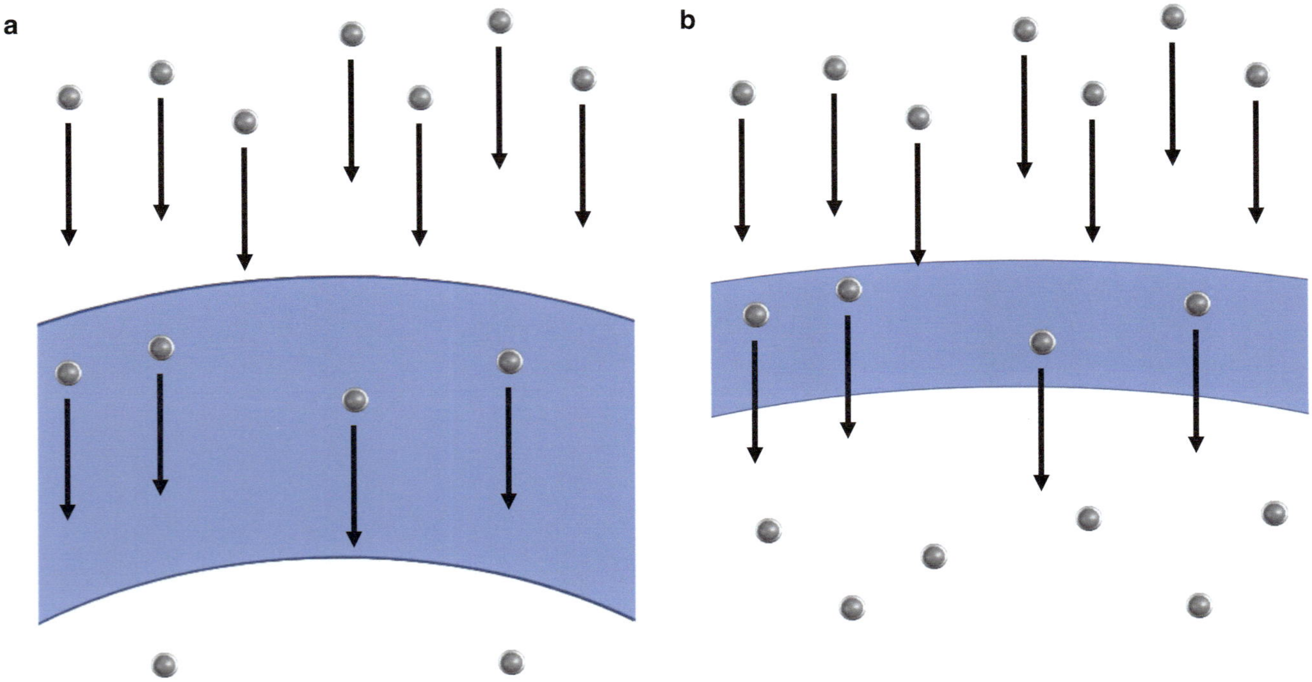

Fig. 3 Dk/t measures the oxygen transmissibility of a lens material. If given two lenses made of the same material, the thinner lens (Panel **b**) will have a higher Dk/t value than the thicker lens (Panel **a**). A favorable contact lens material will have a high Dk/t value

tages in patient comfort and ocular surface lubrication. Different models have varying amounts of the previously discussed features (such as Dk, wettability, etc.). However, what works in one patient may not work well in another patient. Therefore, different models may be tried before the final prescription in a patient. The brand name of the contact lens is a vital part of the prescription! In addition, clinicians may find that certain brands work well for certain patients, while another brand may work well for another type of patient. Contact lens practitioners often have to adopt a "trial-and-error" approach when fitting a patient with SCLs. A complete discussion about every available SCL brand/model is beyond the scope of this text.

SCLs may be worn as daily wear (disposable, removed at night time), 1–2 times weekly, or monthly types, depending on the SCL manufacturer and model. In modern practice, daily disposable SCLs should be recommended to patients to avoid risks associated with improper storage, cleaning, and disinfection associated with extended wear SCLs. The price point of daily disposable SCLs has dramatically dropped in recent years, making them comparable to other SCLs. Monthly wear SCLs are still the most commonly prescribed type of SCL. However, given the high risks associated with extended wear SCLs (and patient abuse of CLs!), daily disposables are rapidly increasing in popularity as a lens of choice for most practitioners in recent years.

Most SCLs are available in select stock BC and DIA sizes. As discussed in Chap. 13 "Contact Lenses for Written Exams", keratometry measurements and slit-lamp examination will help the practitioner choose and adjust an SCL's BC and DIA.

The most commonly available power ranges for SCLs are as follows:

- −6.00D to +6.00D in 0.25D steps
- −6.50D to −12.00D in 0.50D steps
- +6.50D to +8.00D in 0.50D steps

Additional power ranges may be custom ordered from a given SCL manufacturer if needed to correct extreme refractive errors.

Assessing and Troubleshooting SCLs

After performing necessary calculations for the SCL power[5] and selecting an SCL model, further assessment is done as follows:

1. Place the SCL on the patient's cornea *without fluorescein* and assess the fit. An optimum SCL fit will be comfortable for the patient, have good centration on the cornea with approximately 1.0 mm overlapping of the limbus on either side, and 0.25–0.5 mm movement with each blink

[5]This was discussed in Chap. 13, "Contact Lenses for Written Exams". Additionally, a number of online calculators and mobile phone apps are also available to make this calculation of converting the MRx with vertex distance adjustment to SCL power easier in clinical practice (unfortunately, not allowed for exams).

in primary gaze. This is sometimes described as "light 3-point touch" as the SCL *lightly* touches the corneal apex and the limbus at both sides.
   (a) The SCL may be either *too flat (loose)* or *too steep (tight)*.
2. To adjust the fit, we can either change the base curve or the diameter:
   (a) In order to steepen the lens: increase the diameter or decrease the base curve.
   (b) In order to flatten the lens: decrease the diameter or increase the base curve.
   (c) Mnemonic: "Call SID if you have a flat tire": If the lens is flat, we have to steepen it. In order to *s*teepen an SCL, you can *i*ncrease the *d*iameter. If you can remember that silly mnemonic, you can figure out the other three relationships.

Other factors to consider during the evaluation include:

- Assessing vision: If the visual acuity with the SCL is not acceptable, over-refraction may be necessary. If you have done the calculation correctly, the chosen SCL power should be within ±0.75D of the calculated power. If not, further examination or repeat calculation is necessary to account for the discrepancy.
- Comfort: The patient should barely feel the SCL, if at all. For first-time SCL wearers (or switching to a new brand), the patient may benefit from leaving the office and returning in a few hours to "test drive" the SCL before committing.
- Wetness: There should be an even tear film distribution of the SCL surface. Sometimes changing brands may be necessary. If multiple brands are inadequate, we must evaluate for dry eye syndrome/ocular surface disease.

Soft Toric Contact Lenses (STCLs)

STCLs are available in daily, 2-week, and monthly wear options. They are an excellent option to correct 1–2.5D keratometric astigmatism.[6] In addition to choosing an appropriate BC and DIA, the most commonly available power ranges for STCLs are as follows:

- −6.00D to +6.00D in 0.25D sphere steps; cylinder options: −0.75D, −1.25D, −1.75D, −2.25D.
- −6.50D to −9.00D in 0.50D sphere steps; cylinder options: −0.75D, −1.25D, −1.75D, −2.25D.
- STCLs axis values are available in 10° increments.

[6] For astigmatism greater than this, an RGPCL or scleral lens may be required.

Additional power ranges may be custom ordered from a given STCL manufacturer if needed to correct extreme refractive errors.

Recall that STCLs are designed so that the contact lens has minimal movement while on the patient's cornea. If the STCL moved significantly, the cylinder correction would be lost or negatively affected.

Several additional features of an STCL (as compared to an SCL) include:

- Prism ballast and extra weight on the STCL: This allows better alignment and stability of the STCL, especially in the presence of significant corneal astigmatism.
- Thinned out upper and lower edges of the STCL: this allows better contact with the upper and lower eyelids to provide a more secure and comfortable fit.

Assessing and Troubleshooting STCLs

Similar fit/comfort/movement parameters that we discussed for SCLs can be applied to STCLs.

Several other factors to consider include:

- Note that the refractive cylinder is a combination of corneal (keratometric) and lenticular cylinder. If a patient is fit with an STCL but still demonstrates refractive cylinder, there is likely an additional (uncorrected) lenticular cylinder present. For the sake of completeness, it is also possible that the STCL has rotated "off axis." For example, if a patient has MRx: -2.50 + 1.50 x 90 and is fitted with an STCL, but over-refraction shows an additional 1D cylinder, there is likely lenticular cylinder that neutralizes the corneal cylinder to a certain degree. In this case, the patient may be better off with a simple SCL (rather than an STCL or an RGPCL).
- It may take longer for a patient (especially a first-time wearer) to adjust to STCLs compared to SCLs. Additional hand-holding and return visits may be necessary before abandoning a particular STCL model.

Rigid Gas Permeable Contact Lenses (RGPCLs)

Please see Chap. 13, "Contact Lenses for Written Exams", for a full review of the calculations involved in converting a patient's manifest refraction with vertex correction to RGPCL power selection. You may especially want to review the concept of the tear-lens and the "SAM-FAP" rule.

RGPCLs predate the widespread popularity of SCLs. RGPCLs fixed a flaw in previous iterations of hard contact

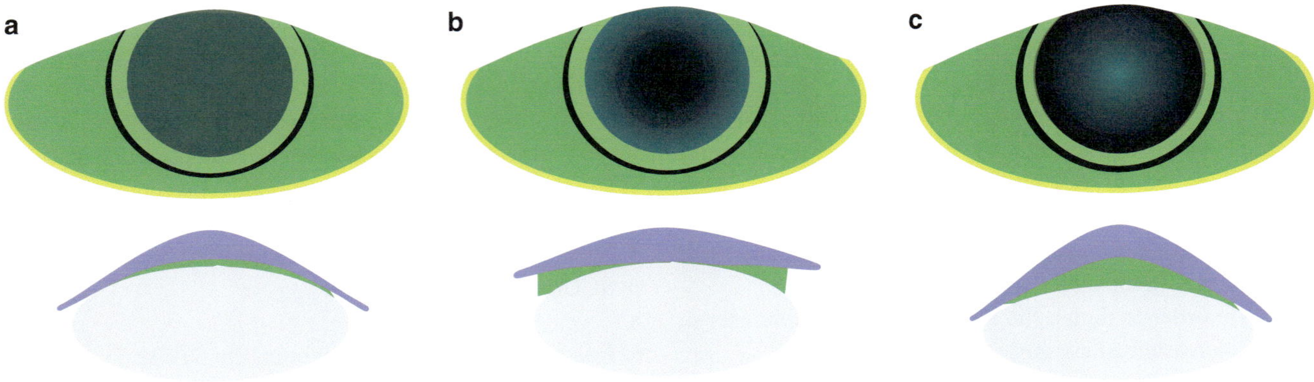

Fig. 4 RGPCL fluorescein staining patterns, Part I (frontal view and cross-section view). Panel **a** shows a good fit with uniform distribution of fluorescein staining underneath the RGPCL. Panel **b** shows a flat fit: notice that the RGPCL is resting on the central cornea with minimal contact with the peripheral cornea allowing for pooling of the fluorescein peripherally (green pooling). Panel **c** shows a steep fit: the contact is extremely tight on the peripheral cornea, preventing peripheral pooling and leading to fluorescein pooling in the middle

lenses. While these lenses (usually made of PMMA) improved patients' vision, the near-complete lack of oxygen permeability led to significant ocular surface issues. The "gas permeable" modification to hard (rigid) lenses allowed them to be worn without unwanted side effects. Thus, the term RGPCL is somewhat of a misnomer because SCLs also allow for oxygen permeability and transmissibility (the previously discussed Dk and Dk/t). In fact, the contact lens community usually refers to "rigid gas permeable" contact lenses as simply "gas permeable (GP)" lenses given the negative perceptions, historically, with the term "rigid." Nonetheless, we will use RGPCLs as a term that encompasses all hard contact lenses.

The beauty of RGPCLs lies in their ability to reshape the tear film, especially in the presence of an astigmatic or irregular cornea, into a spherical shape on the corneal surface. As we have discussed previously (and extensively), the role of the tear film in visual acuity cannot be understated. RGPCLs can normalize the corneal surface and effectively neutralize corneal astigmatism. All else equal, RGPCL wearers often prefer these contact lenses over SCLs, as RGPCLs usually provide sharper and clearer vision.

RGPCLs are generally smaller than SCLs; as a result, they allow for more exchange of tears under the lens with each blink. Modern RGPCLs are made from a firm plastic with minimal water content; as a result, they are much more durable and long-lasting than SCLs. Somewhat paradoxically, a good fitting RGPCL can be much more comfortable than an SCL, especially in patients who have worn them for years.[7]

One critical step in fitting RGPCLs is assessing RGPCL fit *with fluorescein staining* at the slit lamp. Several staining patterns may be observed. Figure 4 shows commonly-encountered RGPCL staining patterns.

- An ideal staining pattern will confirm a good fit with minimal apical clearance (Panel a). As fluorescein will freely diffuse under the RGPCL, a uniform "sea of green" should be observed without any significant intensely green or black areas.
- If the RPGCL fits too flat (Panel B), then this means that the center of the RGPCL and the center of the cornea are making extreme contact such that no fluorescein can enter underneath the lens (central black area). Instead, the fluorescein can freely coat the cornea's peripheral ring where the RGPCL does not fit well. This staining pattern appears like a "green donut," with a peripheral green ring and central black hole.
- If the RGPCL is fit too tight/steep (Panel c), then this means that the center of the RPGCL is so far away from the center of the cornea that all the fluorescein is pooling centrally; since the peripheral cornea and RGPCL are making extreme contact, no fluorescein accumulates peripherally. This staining pattern appears like a "black donut," with a peripheral black ring and central green hole. This pattern is the opposite of the pattern seen in Panel b.

Additionally, several unique staining patterns may be seen in specific patient populations (Fig. 5):

- In patients with significant against the rule (ATR) astigmatism (Panel a) and with the rule (WTR) astigmatism (Panel b), the steep meridian is horizontal and vertical, respectively. Fluorescein will accumulate in the steep areas: thus, it will accumulate horizontally in a "green bowtie" pattern in ATR astigmatism and vertically in a "green hourglass" pattern in WTR astigmatism.
- In patients with oblique astigmatism (Panel c), the RGPCL will primarily "rest" on the flat meridian; therefore, the fluorescein will pool in the areas of the steep

[7]Think back to all those times in the clinic when you have seen an elderly patient who presents for cataract surgery but has worn RGPCLs for 30+ years. These patients are usually quite happy and then unhappy when you tell them that they have to stay out of the RGPCLs for at least 3 weeks prior to biometry measurements (with some practitioners recommending an additional week for every decade of RGPCL use).

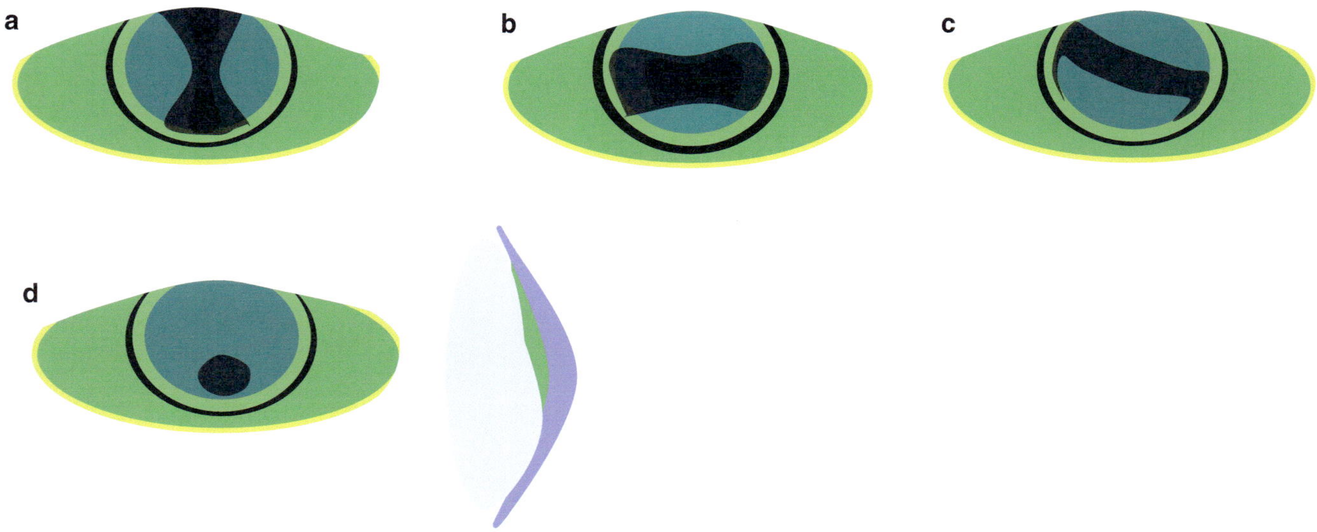

Fig. 5 RGPCL fluorescein staining patterns, Part II. Panel **a** shows a patient with ATR astigmatism: since the steep meridian is along 180 degrees, the RGPCL is making contact with the cornea along the vertical meridian (black) where no fluorescein accumulates. This allows for pooling in the steep horizontal meridian (green). Panel **b** shows WTR astigmatism: an opposite staining pattern is seen (compared to Panel **a**) based on the location of the steep and flat meridians. Panel **c** shows a patient with oblique astigmatism with the steep meridian at 70°: thus, the RGPCL will rest on the flat meridian (160°). Panel **d** shows apical compression in a patient with keratoconus. The RGPCL is touching the bowed-out cornea inferiorly (black area) as the fluorescein pools in the rest of the cornea

meridian. For example, if a patient with oblique astigmatism (steep meridian 70°) was fit with an RGPCL, the staining pattern in Panel c may be seen.

- In patients with corneal ectasia, the area of maximal corneal protrusion will make contact with the RGPCL and prevent staining in this area. Panel D shows a typical staining pattern in keratoconic cornea (inferior steepening) fit with an RGPCL.

In addition to the previously discussed rules on fitting the RGPCL (remember, we usually want to fit slightly steeper than the flattest K), we also have to consider how the RGPCL physically fits with the eyelid(s). An ideal fit is known as an *apical alignment fit* (Fig. 6), wherein the upper edge of the RGPCL fits entirely underneath the upper eyelid.[8] This type of fitting allows the patient to comfortably blink without "touching" the edge of the lens with each blink.

Several modifications can be made for extreme powers of RGPCLs. For example, a high minus-power RGPCL may have a considerable thickness at the edge that may interfere with eyelid movement (e.g., the patient may complain that the RGPCL gets "stuck" to the upper eyelid constantly). In this case, we can ask the optical lab to bevel the lens edge (grind the thick lens edge into a thinner) into a shape known as a "lenticular bevel" (Fig. 7). Similarly, a high plus RGPCL may be too thin at the edge of the lens (compared to its center), and thus, the RGPCL may not make enough contact

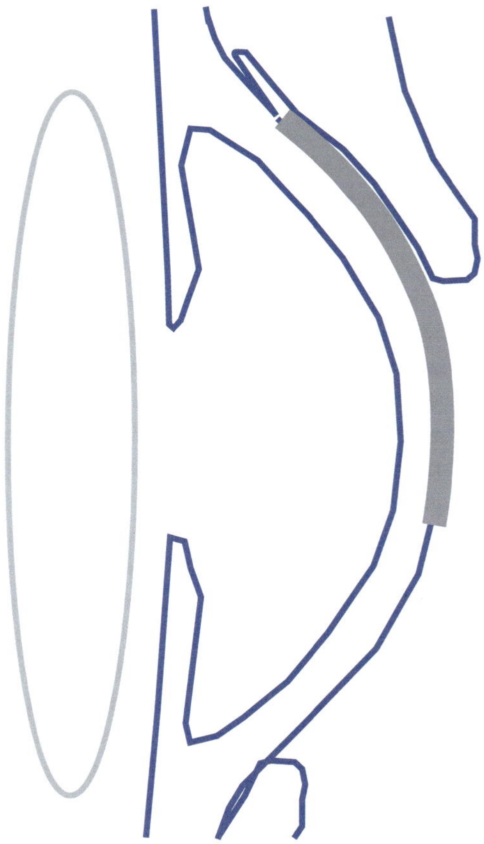

Fig. 6 An ideal fit for an RGPCL is to have an apical alignment fit wherein the upper edge of the RPGCL fits comfortably underneath the upper eyelid

[8]Some practitioners may also refer to this type of fit as "upper lid attachment" fit.

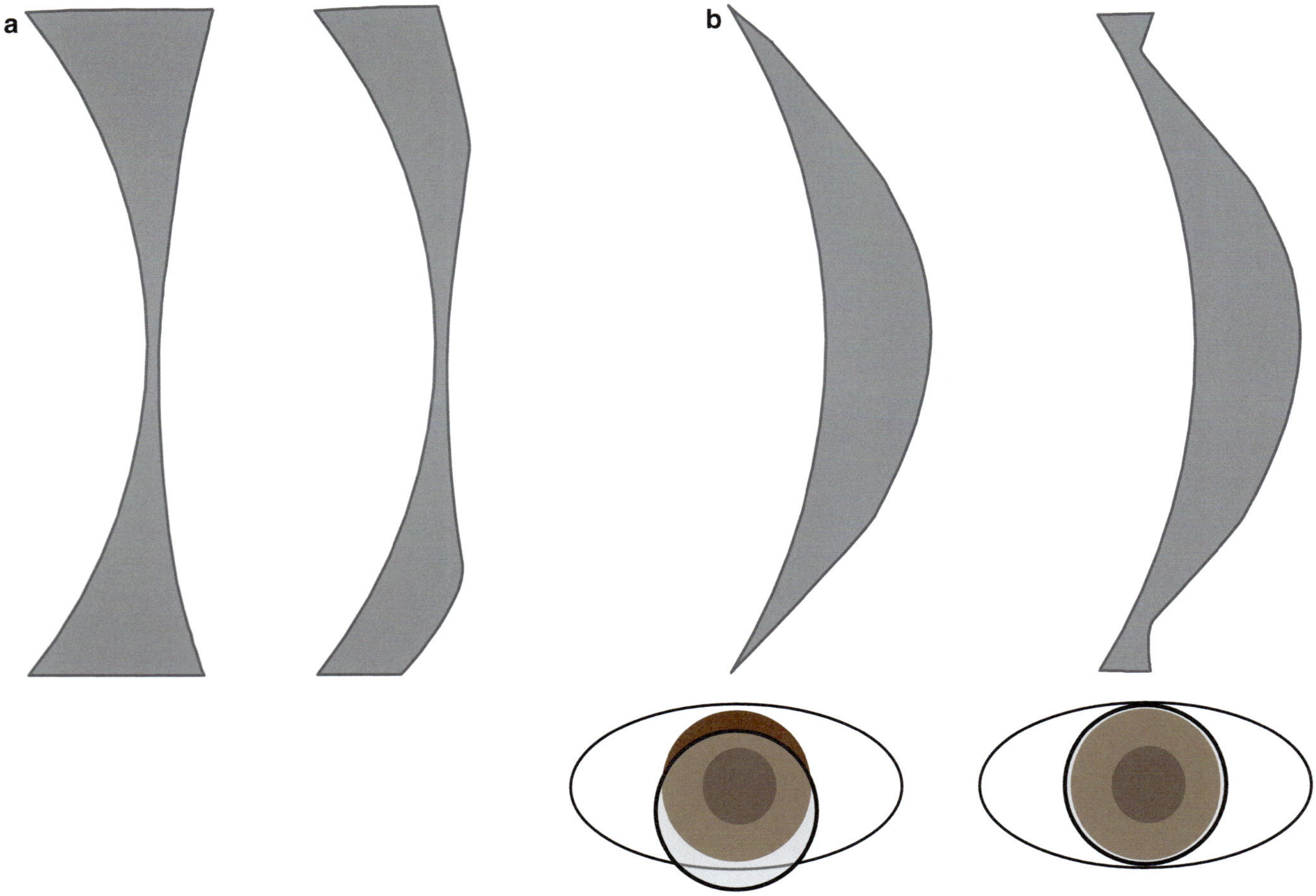

Fig. 7 A high minus RGPCL may be modified with a lenticular bevel to decrease friction with the upper eyelid (Panel **a**). A high plus RGPCL that rides low on the patient's cornea may be modified with a flanged lenticular cut to increase contact with the upper eyelid (Panel **b**)

with the upper eyelid. In this case, we can ask the optical lab to thicken the lens edge into a shape known as a "flanged lenticular cut" (basically make the lens more minus (thicker) at its edges).

Rarely, an interpalpebral (or central) fit may be necessary: in this option, the RGPCL will have an extremely small diameter and rest in between the upper and lower eyelids (without any contact with either eyelid). This fit is slightly more uncomfortable than an apical alignment. It may be considered in special situations, such as extreme hyperopes or unique anatomy (e.g., high upper eyelids [blepharoplasty gone wrong!]).

An RGPCL should be sufficient to correct corneal astigmatism most of the time. However, there may be situations where residual astigmatism is detected on an over-refraction even after placing an RGPCL. This "unruly" residual astigmatism may be due to the posterior corneal surface or lenticular astigmatism. For these situations, special RGPCLs with a "back surface toric" (to match the corneal surface) and a spherical anterior surface may be warranted. Furthermore, "bitoric" RGPCLs (wherein both the anterior and posterior surfaces of the RGPCL have cylinder power) may be needed in advanced cases.

Patient Education

This section may seem unnecessary because most of this is "common" sense information learned during training. However, especially for exams, this section serves as a consolidated, comprehensive laundry list of information that is useful for fitting any type of CLs:

- Educate the patient regarding proper contact lens hygiene: Discussion of simple factors such as washing hands thoroughly before touching contact lenses; disposal of contact lenses cases at periodic intervals; not reusing (or "topping off") contact lens solution; use of hydrogen peroxide solution for extended-wear soft contact lenses; etc.
- This cardinal rule of contact lens hygiene deserves emphasis: Patients should be strongly educated NOT to sleep or swim with contact lenses! Even if the contact lens box (or another eye care provider) tells them it is OK to wear the CL overnight, we should always remind patients that removing the contact lens is always the safest and recommended action. Remember, we are allowed to break this rule to treat corneal disease (such as epithelial defects, etc.), but this requires topical antibiotics for infection prophylaxis.

- Another cardinal rule: Patients should NOT use their own saliva to "re-wet" the contact lens![9] "Homemade" and "organic" contact lens solutions are also a definite no-no. Using tap water is even more of a no-no.
- Educate the patient on proper insertion and removal of contact lenses. A demonstration is usually required for first-time contact lens wearers.
- Remind the patient regarding contact lens replacement schedules. SCLs should be changed per manufacturer recommendations. RGPCLs should be replaced yearly.
- Review signs and symptoms of contact lens-related eye emergencies.
- Arrange for regular follow-up appointments. Well-fitting SCLs can be evaluated on a schedule determined by the provider. RGPCLs, STCLs, and specialty lenses (discussed below) should be evaluated on the eye at least annually.

Miscellaneous Troubleshooting

A few other points may be considered:

- Contact lenses are described by their rear vertex power. Usually, the power of a contact lens may be found on the manufacturer's box. In certain situations, however, the clinician may need to determine the power of a given contact lens. RGPCLs are easily checked by placing the back of the lens in the nose cone of a lensmeter (See Chap. 17 "Optical Instruments and Machines"). This can also be done for SCLs/STCLs but requires an additional liquid chamber with an adjustment for the index of refraction
- An RGPCL may also be used for diagnostic purposes. The tear lens can fill in corneal irregularities for patients with irregular corneas (corneal ectasia, corneal scars, corneal thinning, etc.) as the anterior surface of the RGPCL is evenly coated with tears to create a more stable air-tear film interface. Over-refraction can then be done to determine whether the cause of decreased visual acuity is due to the cornea or other pathology. RGPCL over-refraction is especially useful when multiple ocular pathologies (e.g., aphakia, retinal scarring, etc.) are present, and the clinician is deciding whether anterior segment surgery may benefit the patient. If RGPCL over-refraction significantly improves a patient's vision, then further surgery (e.g., corneal transplant, secondary lens implant, etc.) may be considered as it confirms that the cornea/ocular surface is causing the decreased vision. If RGPCL does not improve the vision, lenticular or retinal pathologies may be more significant than the anterior segment pathologies, and additional surgery may not yield many benefits.

[9] One of the authors may or may not have done this during his high school years and amazingly never developed an eye infection until he learned about contact lens basics during an ophthalmology rotation and realized how lucky he had been his entire life.

Advanced Contact Lens Designs

Presbyopia Correcting Contact Lens Options

Recall from our previous discussions that contact lens-wearing patients may face additional advantages or disadvantages as they approach presbyopic age. For example, myopic contact lens wearers may struggle to read due to increased accommodative demands while wearing SCLs. Conversely, hyperopic contact lens wearers may report an easier time reading in contact lenses (compared to their glasses) due to decreased accommodative demands.

A simple solution to presbyopic contact lens wearers is to simply give them reading glasses, march them out of your office, and tell them to return only when their cataracts have worsened. However, two other options may be considered:

Monovision with contact lenses With monovision, the idea should be to ascertain the dominant eye first and correct it fully with a contact lens. The non-dominant eye can be set for residual -1.50 to -2D myopia, depending on a patient's intermediate/near vision needs. Remember never to assume that the right eye is the dominant eye and the left eye is the non-dominant eye: you must ascertain eye dominance using simple in-office tests. Several monovision contact lens trials may be necessary before finding a combination that works for each patient. Remember that monovision will cause a loss of binocularity and decreased depth perception, so this option may not work for all patients. Patients with intermittent strabismus and stereoacuity should avoid monovision as this can worsen their ability to fuse. Patients who do not have binocularity may be good candidates for monovision.

One trick used by some practitioners to calculate the starting power of the contact lens for the non-dominant eye is as follows: add the spectacle near power to the sphere power and then add additional −0.50D to get the final contact lens power. For example, if a patient wears glasses of −4.00D sphere with +2.00D add, then we can calculate the near eye contact lens power as follows: −4.00 + 2.00 + (−0.50): −2.50 D. We realize this basically leaves the patient with approximately −1.50D myopia, which is what we stated at the beginning, but this rule makes it sound official and sophisticated. Of course, the final power of the CL (for both eyes) can be adjusted as needed depending on the patient's reading distance preferences.

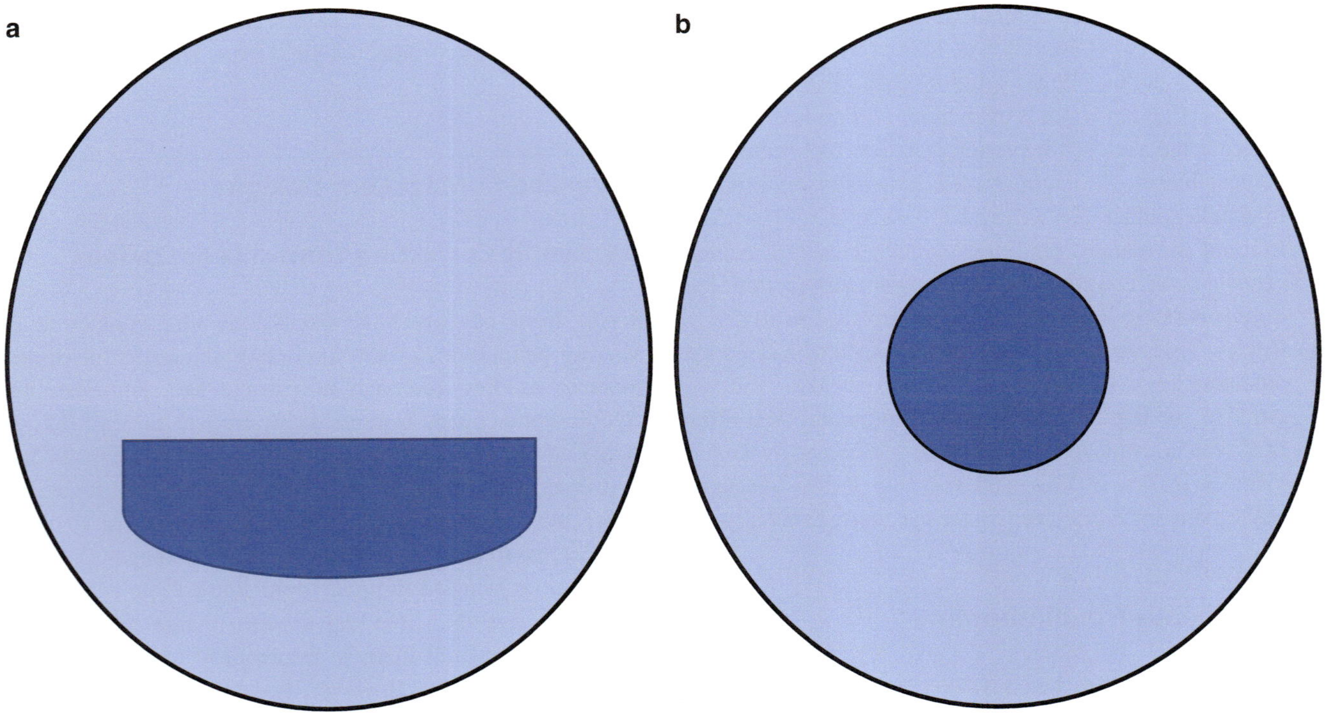

Fig. 8 Multifocal (bifocal) contact lenses, alternating vision style. (**a**) Inferior near add segment. (**b**) Central near add segment

Multifocal contact lenses (MF-CLs) several options may be considered for this patient population:

- Multifocal (bifocal) contact lenses, alternating vision style (Fig. 8): One option involves placing the add power as a "segment" in the inferior portion of the lens (Panel a). When the patient looks down to read (similar to bifocal segments in glasses), he/she will look through the bottom portion of the contact lens. Another option is to place the add power in the central portion of the lens so that when the patient wants to read, the pupil will constrict, and they can focus through the central ("near") portion of the contact lens. The pupil will dilate when the patient wishes to see in the distance, and they can focus through the outer ring ("distance") portion of the contact lens. A variant of this option involves reversing the concentric portions (i.e., the central portion for distance vision, the peripheral portion for near vision).
- Multifocal contact lenses, simultaneous vision style (Fig. 9): These can be used in both SCLs and RGPCLs. Like a multifocal intraocular lens, there is a continuous range of near powers present at various portions of the lens. As a result, the patient will experience some blur due to incoming images from both distance and near. Different add powers may be considered as well, with lower add powers for the dominant eye (to give more distance and intermediate vision) and higher add powers for the non-dominant eye (to give more near vision) in a "mini-monovision" strategy.

MF-CLs may also be found in daily and monthly varieties in a similar range of distance powers as previously discussed SCLs. The add power may be described as "low/medium/high" or may be numerically listed: +1.00D, +1.50D, +2.00D, +2.50D add. Some designs may incorporate additional ring(s) with additional near/distance powers in the center. MF-CLs usually require multiple visits and adjustments. A significant number of patients will not tolerate MF-CLs for various reasons: it is important to warn patients during the "test-drive" phase that this may occur.

Scleral Contact Lenses (ScCLs)

Recently, ScCLs have gained much interest due to their versatility and effectiveness in various clinical situations. This remains an area to monitor closely as future developments with this technology are very likely. ScCLs are made of a rigid gas permeable material; thus, they are technically RGPCLs, just as the corneal RGPCLs we discussed earlier. If we wanted to be very specific, we could call them scleral RGPCLs, but since we refer to them as "scleral contact lenses" in clinical parlance, we will refer to them as ScCLs in our discussion as well.

Think of ScCLs as giant corneal RGPCLs with similar materials and polymers. They are beneficial for the following situations:

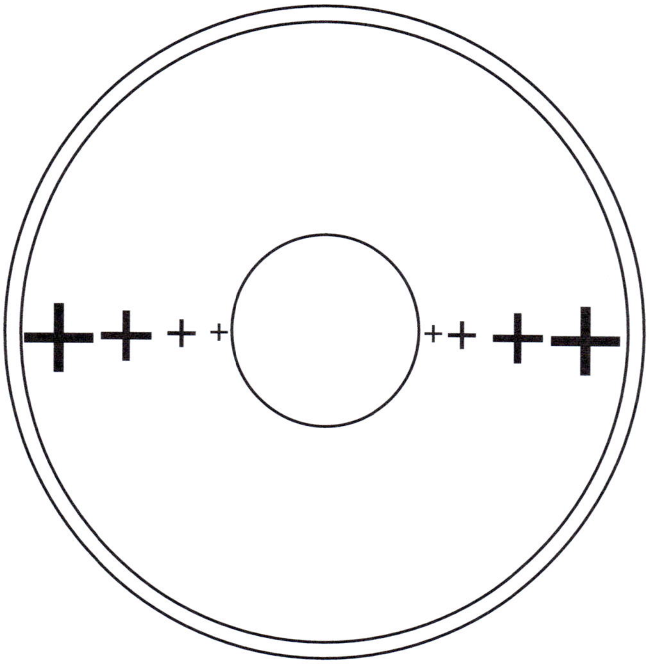

Fig. 9 Multifocal contact lenses, simultaneous vision style. Different add powers are found throughout the contact lens yielding simultaneous near and far vision

- Corrections of high quantities of regular and irregular astigmatism (e.g., corneal ectasia, post-penetrating keratoplasty, etc.)
- Visual rehabilitation in the presence of corneal scars (post RK scars, post-infectious scars, etc.)[10]
- Treatment of ocular surface disease requiring continuous lubrication (advanced dry eye disease, etc.) ScCLs can treat the disease and improve the vision for some patients with advanced dry eye disease.
- Protection of the ocular surface (e.g., non-healing epithelial defects, neurotrophic keratopathy, distichiasis/trichiasis)
- Management of limbal stem cell pathology: as the ScCL vaults over the cornea, it can protect the limbal niche microenvironment, provide lubrication, and improve patients' vision[11]
- Treatment of Type A personalities: patients who are unhappy with both SCLs and RGPCLs

An ScCL consists of three main components (Fig. 10):

- Central optic: The size and shape of the central optic will determine corneal clearance. The base curve is chosen to allow for some vaulting of the ScCL over the cornea to allow for an adequate tear film reservoir
- Peripheral haptic (outer edge design): rests with the scleral surface
- Transitional zone (limbal zone): connects the central optic with the peripheral haptic and vaults over the limbus

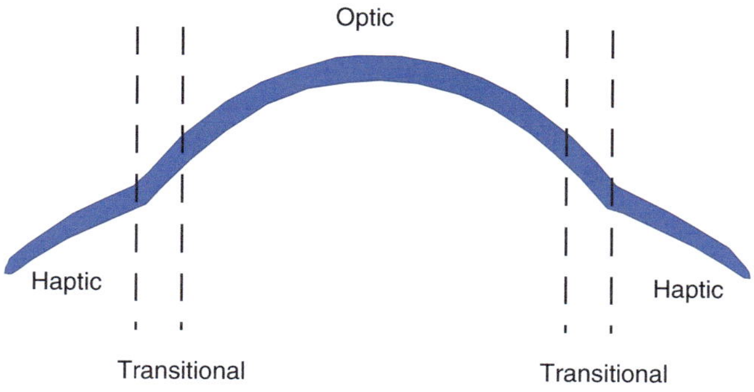

Fig. 10 Components of a scleral contact lens: central optic, peripheral haptic, and transitional zone

ScCLs typically have a large diameter (18–24 mm); smaller variants, known as semi-scleral lenses, are also available. However, fitting is much more difficult because the practitioner has more parameters to consider. A complete discussion of nuances of ScCL fitting is beyond the scope of this text and is best left to an experienced practitioner. However, several considerations should be kept in mind:

- There is no one-technique-fits-all method for fitting ScCLs. Every manufacturer has a guide for their design, and not every ScCL can be adjusted similarly among the various manufacturers.
- A well-fit ScCL does not move much, if at all. Most designs involve a sealed off edge with no tear flow under the ScCL. This requires a "Goldilocks" fit of the ScCL: tight enough to avoid movement but not too tight to cause conjunctival ischemia and blanching. If the ScCL is too flat, the ScCL will have excessive movement with blinking, cause physical irritation, and allow for unwanted tear-fluid exchange.
- The patient will have to "fill" the ScCL with sterile saline or specially approved solutions (e.g., ScleralFil [Bausch and Lomb] and Nutrifill [Contamac Solutions]).
- The ScCL itself has a toric profile: when fitting the ScCL, a specific portion of the ScCL may require additional steepening while flattening the portion 90° away.
- While a well-fit ScCL can help treat limbal pathologies, an ill-fitting ScCL can cause compression on the limbus, leading to unwanted limbal stem cell deficiency and/or corneal neovascularization. Similarly, if the ScCL is too loose at the limbus, it may inadvertently cause conjuncti-

[10]For these two reasons, ScCLs are a cornea specialist's best friend.

[11]Grodsky JD, Doshi R, Riaz KM. Medical management and visual rehabilitation of limbal niche dysfunction. *J Cataract Refract Surg*. 2020;46(2):312–316

val prolapse underneath the lens and onto the corneal surface. This is usually painless for the patient but may affect the vision and drain the fluid reservoir prematurely.

- The central optic should similarly vault the cornea enough to create an adequate fluid reservoir but not too much to prevent comfortable blinking. Different practitioners have different patterns and preferences for the ideal vault; frequently, scleral lens fitters will rely on the manufacturer-recommended ideal vault as a target (usually 200–400 microns) and adjust as needed. One important distinction is that the vault is measured from the highest (steepest) point on the cornea, not necessarily the corneal center. This detail is crucial when assessing the vault in patients with ectatic disease where the steepest part of the cornea is usually shifted away from the center. After the lens is worn for several hours, some of the fluid reservoir may decrease, and the lens may only vault ~100 microns.
- If the ScCL is too thick and the vault is too much, this may artificially affect the "functional" Dk/t of the ScCL, leading to problems such as corneal hypoxia and edema, as shown by mathematical Dk/t models.
- ScCL fitting often requires multiple visits with adjustments. Though time-consuming, it can be gratifying for the patient to experience improved visual acuity and ocular surface comfort with a well-fit ScCL. Often, a well-fit ScCL can obviate the need for surgery, including corneal transplantation. While corneal surgeons enjoy performing transplant surgery, they also enjoy their patients' seeing better, especially without surgery!

Contact Lens Fitting Considerations in Select Situations

Several commonly encountered situations may benefit from contact lens fitting by a skilled and experienced practitioner:

1. Corneal Ectasias (Keratoconus, Pellucid Marginal Degeneration, etc.)

   While many patients with corneal ectasia may require and benefit from RGPCLs or ScCLs, other options may be necessary:

   - Reverse geometry RGPCLs (RG-RGPCLs): This design may be considered for patients with extremely oblate corneas (excessive central flattening with steep periphery). RG-RGPCLs have a *flat central zone* compared to the peripheral curve, allowing for a better fit with oblate corneas.
   - Intralimbic contact lenses: These are specialized RGPCLs with large optical zones (>11 mm).
   - Hybrid contact lens: these custom lenses have a central RGPCL portion and a peripheral SCL skirt. This arrangement combines the optical superiority of an RGPCL with the comfort of an SCL.
   - Piggyback contact lenses: The patient will first wear an SCL for comfort and protection of the ocular surface/cornea. Then, an RGPCL is worn on top to combine the optical benefits of an RGPCL and comfort of an SCL. Some practitioners have even used an SCL to facilitate wearing an ScCL or other advanced geometry contact lenses.

2. Use of Contact Lenses as Bandage Contact Lenses

   Contact lenses, usually SCLs, may help facilitate corneal epithelial healing in the presence of a corneal epithelial defect (e.g., post-PRK, post-superficial keratectomy, treatment of recurrent corneal erosion syndrome, treatment of bullous keratopathy, etc.). Usually, an SCL with high Dk/t approved for extended wear is used and kept in place for 1–4 weeks. The power of the bandage SCL is negligible (usually plano or −0.50D). Topical antibiotics are usually given as prophylaxis.

3. Orthokeratology (Ortho-K)

   Ortho-K is a controversial topic.[12] The basic premise of Ortho-K involves using RGPCLs for overnight wear to cause corneal flattening, thereby secondarily treating myopia temporarily (up to 24 hours). Ortho-K is primarily used to correct myopia in children, and this theoretically allows patients to use Ortho-K during the night to avoid having to use glasses during the day. Previously, it was thought that this strategy is not effective as it does not treat axial myopia: however, newer research has shown that Ortho-K may prevent myopic progression in pediatric patients.[13]

   However, as with any type of overnight contact lens wear, there is a significant increase of potential infectious keratitis, corneal abrasions, corneal hypoxia, etc. This treatment, including determining patient candidacy and appropriate lenses, is best left to experienced practitioners.

[12] See Chap. 24 "Myopia Control", for additional information about this topic.

[13] VanderVeen DK, Kraker RT, Pineles SL, et al. Use of Orthokeratology for the Prevention of Myopic Progression in Children: A Report by the American Academy of Ophthalmology. *Ophthalmology*. 2019;126(4):623–636

Practice Questions

1. Which of the following statements is CORRECT?
   A. The base curve of a contact lens refers to the edge-to-edge length of the contact lens.
   B. The peripheral curve of a contact lens is usually steeper than the base curve as the peripheral cornea is generally steeper than the central cornea.
   C. The sagittal depth refers to the distance between the posterior contact lens and a line drawn perpendicular to the edge of the lens.
   D. The diameter of an RGPCL will usually be longer than the diameter of a SCL.
2. Which of the following materials is most commonly used in the construction of modern-day SCLs?
   A. Hydroxyethylmethacrylate (HEMA)
   B. Silicone hydrogel
   C. PMMA
   D. Acrylic
3. Which of the following combinations of values is the *most ideal* for a SCL?
   A. High Dk value, high wetting angle
   B. High Dk/t value, high wetting angle
   C. High Dk/t value, low wetting angle
   D. High Dk value, low wetting angle
4. If after placing an RGPCL, there is a noted staining pattern of a black peripheral ring and a central green zone, which of the following conclusions can be made?
   A. The patient has WTR astigmatism.
   B. The patient has oblique astigmatism.
   C. The RGPCL is too tight.
   D. The RGPCL is too loose.
5. Which of the following statements regarding contact lens use in presbyopic patients is TRUE?
   A. A monovision contact lens strategy may give good range of vision with some compromise of binocularity and depth perception.
   B. Multifocal contact lenses are generally tolerated and accepted by patients in a short time after first fitting.
   C. Multifocal contact lenses offer crisp vision at all distances: distance, intermediate, and near.
   D. A "mix-and-match" strategy for multifocal contact lenses may involve giving a higher add power to the dominant eye and a lower add power to the non-dominant eye.

Answers

1. C. This is the definition of sagittal depth. The base curve of a contact lens is a measurement of the curvature of the posterior surface of the contact lens (expressed in millimeters). The peripheral curve of a contact lens is usually flatter than the base curve, as the peripheral cornea is usually flatter than the central cornea. An RGPCL is usually smaller than an SCL and, therefore, will usually have a smaller diameter as well.
2. B. HEMA was the most commonly used material in SCLs until the 2000s.
3. C. While both a high Dk and high Dk/t are preferred, a higher Dk/t is preferable to only a high Dk value. A low wetting angle allows for the effective spread of water over the lens surface ("wettability").
4. C. This is the description of a tight-fitting RGPCL. The described staining pattern gives no information about the type of corneal astigmatism present.
5. A. Monovision may be an excellent option for patients who are okay with sacrificing some binocularity in exchange for a range of vision and avoidance of glare/halos. In general, multifocal CLs (MF-CLs) take a significant time for adjustment, and multiple attempts may be necessary to find the ideal add power for a given patient. All MF-CLs have some compromise of visual clarity in exchange for a range of visual acuity. A mix-and-match strategy involves giving a lower add to the dominant eye (for distance and intermediate vision) and a higher add to the non-dominant eye (for distance and near vision).

Acknowledgments The authors are grateful to Rachel M. Caywood, OD, FAAO, for her critical review of this chapter.

Clinical Problems with Optics and Refractive Manifestations

Daniel Wee and G. Vike Vicente

Objectives

- To recognize causes of commonly encountered acquired refractive errors (myopic, hyperopic, and astigmatic) in clinical practice, including vision-threatening and life-threatening etiologies
- To understand the effect of corneal sutures on the development of refractive errors and appropriate clinical management
- To recognize clinical presentations of acquired diplopia, including options for clinical management and alleviation of symptoms
- To define asthenopia, recognize its symptoms, and identify potential causes and treatment strategies
- To become familiar with problems experienced by aphakic patients and clinical options for the treatment of aphakia
- To effectively diagnose and treat malingering, including medicolegal considerations

Introduction

This chapter will cover common and uncommon clinical problems that may present with primary or secondary issues related to optics and refractive errors. While many of these disease entities may have other pathognomonic signs and symptoms, optics and refractive error symptoms may be the primary (or only) presenting symptoms. The topics discussed in this chapter are not only high-yield for clinical practice but are also especially useful to know for certification exams.

As ophthalmologists, we rely on clinical exam skills, imaging, and ancillary tests to make a correct diagnosis and develop an effective treatment plan. While one may think of "optics" as merely limited to updating a patient's glasses, there may be scenarios where the clinician must think critically. As we will see in the next sections, there may be scenarios where new or changing refractive errors may not only blind a patient but may even (gulp) kill a patient.

In each section, you may notice that while we have given a differential diagnosis ("laundry list") of etiologies to know, we have also created clinical scenarios of high-yield etiologies in each category that will hopefully reinforce some of these critical teaching points.

Acquired and Clinical Myopia

While there are many causes of acquired myopia, there are two broad categories to consider in the clinical setting: (1) *increased refractive power* of the eye (refractive myopia) and (2) *increased axial length* (axial myopia). The following classification tree lists common reasons for each category:

- Increased refractive power of the eye:
  - Increased corneal power, such as corneal ectasia (keratoconus, etc.), though this will usually be accompanied by a concurrent increase in astigmatism
  - Lens shape changes
    - Cataract, diabetes, ROP, lenticonus
  - Lens repositioning (forward shift)
    - Drugs (chlorthalidone, sulfonamides, tetracycline, carbonic anhydrase inhibitors)
    - Toxemia of pregnancy
    - Anterior lens dislocation
  - Ciliary muscle tone/excessive accommodation
    - Students, spasm, inadequate fogging by examiner
    - Drugs (antihistamines, miotics, sulfa, tetracycline, topiramate)
- Increased axial length
  - Posterior staphyloma
  - Congenital glaucoma

D. Wee (✉)
Center for Sight, Stockton, CA, USA

G. V. Vicente
Clinical Pediatrics and Ophthalmology Georgetown University Hospital, Washington, DC, USA

Eye Doctors of Washington, Chevy Chase, MD, USA

K. M. Riaz et al. (eds.), *Optics for the New Millennium*, https://doi.org/10.1007/978-3-030-95251-8_21

– Scleral buckle
– Idiopathic progressive myopia

Let's discuss some high-yield clinical scenarios to highlight a few important items from our above "laundry list":

Scenario #1: The Unhappy Middle-Aged Patient with Frequent Glasses Prescription Changes

A 55-year-old man comes in to the clinic and the following scene ensues:

Patient: "Doc, I do not want to see a resident today. I want to talk to the boss doctor."
Resident: "Ok, can I just ask what is going on?"
Patient: "Every time I come here, I get a new doctor, and a new glasses prescription, and after two months the glasses do not work anymore! This is the third time this year!"
Resident: "No problem, I'll get the attending, let me just take a look at your glasses and our notes for a minute."

March:		
Glasses worn:	OD: −1.00 sph (20/25)	OS: −1.50 sph (20/30)
Manifest refraction	OD: −1.25 sph (20/20)	OS: −1.75 sph (20/20)
Glasses issued:	OD: −1.25 sph	OS: −1.75 sph
June:		
Glasses worn:	OD: −1.25 sph (20/30)	OS: −1.75 sph (20/30)
Manifest refraction	OD: −1.75 sph (20/20)	OS: −2.25 sph (20/20)
Glasses issued:	OD: −1.75 sph	OS: −2.25 sph
October (present day)		
Glasses worn:	OD: −1.75 sph (20/40)	OS: −2.25 sph (20/40)
Manifest refraction	OD: −2.50 sph (20/25)	OS: −2.75 sph (20/25)

Exam findings are unremarkable other than trace nuclear sclerosis.

Resident: "Sir, I think I know what is going on. Can I ask you two quick questions?"
Patient: "Fine."
Resident: "Have you been thirstier lately? Do you have to urinate more frequently?"
Patient: "Yes, why do you ask?"
Resident: "In addition to correcting your glasses, I think it is important that we set up an appointment for you to see your primary care doctor soon."
Boss Doctor Attending: "Good job being a real doctor in addition to being an eye doctor, young apprentice. Now go fetch me a coffee."

Remember that a progressive, binocular myopic shift in a middle-aged patient in a few months' time should clue us into a strong suspicion for *type 2 diabetes*. A typical example of this is a 40–50-year-old patient who presents over the course of several months with increasing myopic correction in glasses as described above. The patient may report that the glasses work for a few months before requiring a higher myopic correction. Exam findings may be completely normal, especially in the early stages prior to the development of any diabetic retinopathy. Recall that hyperglycemia may cause swelling of the crystalline lens, which leads to increased refractive power of the lens and progressive myopia (usually with minimal change in astigmatism). Anatomical conditions are unlikely to cause bilateral refractive changes. In this setting, as an ophthalmologist, we can treat the eye (glasses, dilated fundus exam) but should order the initial workup for diabetes, arrange for prompt evaluation with an internist/endocrinologist, and counsel the patient about the need for regular eye exams.[1]

In other cases, acquired myopia is expected, such as post scleral buckle (as the buckle causes axial compression along the equator), leading to increased axial myopia.

Scenario #2: The 1-Year-Old with Constant Tearing

A 12-month-old child is referred by her pediatrician for tearing in both eyes with the working diagnosis of likely nasolacrimal duct obstruction (NLDO). Family history is negative.

- Slit lamp exam: high tear film noted OU
- Cycloplegic refraction: +0.50sph OU
- Dilated fundus exam: normal

The patient undergoes uncomplicated NLD probing and irrigation under anesthesia. Postoperatively, the patient continues to experience epiphora and undergoes another NLD probing procedure. This too fails, and the patient has a third procedure to place an NLD stent. The stent is eventually removed at age 2.5 years, and at this time, the patient's mother states her child has been holding objects rather close lately.

- Repeat exam (patient age 3) including dilation reveals:
- Cycloplegic refraction −7.00D sph OU
- Dilated fundus exam: C:D 0.8 OU

In this case, the patient had an atypical cause of infantile glaucoma which usually causes buphthalmos. However, this child was not light-sensitive nor did the corneas appear large or cloudy. A significant bilateral myopic shift occurred in a

[1]Order a fasting blood glucose, HbA1C, CBC, and BMP so that by the time the patient presents to the internist/endocrinologist, he/she is impressed that you as an ophthalmologist actually remember real doctor stuff.

relatively short period of time. Ideally, the optic nerve pathology would have been appreciated during the first two NLD probing procedures. The learning point here is that *infantile glaucoma* may present with rapidly increasing myopia and accompanying epiphora – diseases don't read textbooks!

Scenario #3: The Young Adult with a Recently Started Medication

A 28-year-old patient presents with complaints of difficulty driving over the past 10 days after she was started on a recent medication. The patient reports she never wore glasses previously.

Exam today:

Visual acuity, sc	OD: 20/50	OS: 20/50
Manifest refraction:	OD: −2.50 sph (20/20)	OS: −2.50 sph (20/20)
SLE: unremarkable OU		

Upon further questioning, she cannot recall the name of her new medication but states she was previously taking gabapentin for control of her seizures. A call to her neurologist reveals that she was recently started on topiramate.

This clinical case scenario is a curveball on the more well-known phenomenon of acute angle closure glaucoma (AACG) secondary to topiramate. In this example, the topiramate induced anatomical changes that stopped just short of inducing AACG (drug-induced myopia). Recall that while the exact mechanism of topiramate's evil effects on the eye is unknown, the prevailing theory is that the drug induces changes in the membrane potential leading to abnormal fluid movements: a combination of uveal effusion and ciliary body edema lead to myopic shift, anterior chamber shallowing, and eventual AACG.

What should we do as ophthalmologists? Should *we* stop the medication? No, remember we are not real doctors! Instead, we must immediately contact the primary care provider and advise immediate cessation of the drug and concurrent alternate medications. If we simply stopped the drug without this discussion with the primary doctor, it is possible that the patient may undergo a severe seizure attack such that by saving the eyeball we ended up sacrificing the patient herself.[2] We should *not* stop the medication without having an alternative treatment plan in place with the primary provider. In terms of the eye, we must educate the patient about AACG symptoms and advise her to come in immediately if such symptoms develop. We should do a daily follow-up with a low threshold for prophylactic laser peripheral iridotomy if the angle doesn't deepen. Usually, with prompt cessation of the drug, AACG can be avoided and the vision recovers in a few weeks' time.

[2]Obviously, not good to save the eyeball at the cost of killing the patient

Acquired and Clinical Hyperopia

As a rule, hyperopic shifts are much more concerning than myopic shifts as they can be vision (and life) threatening – as such, they are a favorite topic for exam purposes.

Similar to the previous discussion on myopia, there are two broad categories to consider in the clinical setting when encountering acquired hyperopia: (1) *decreased* refractive power of the eye (refractive hyperopia) and (2) *decreased* effective axial length (axial hyperopia). The following classification tree lists common reasons for each category:

- Decreased refractive power of the eye
  - Lens changes
    - Aphakia (crystalline lens or IOL dislocation)
    - Pregnancy (both myopic and hyperopic changes are possible)
  - Poor accommodation
    - Tonic pupil and Adie's syndrome
    - Third nerve palsy
    - Trauma
    - Drugs (chloroquine, phenothiazines, antihistamines, anticholinergics, benzodiazepines, marijuana)
    - Pregnancy.[3]
- Decreased effective axial length
  - Tumor (choroidal or orbital)
  - Central serous retinopathy
  - Severe papilledema

Let's discuss some high-yield clinical scenarios, including ones that should definitely not be missed on exams:

Scenario #1: The Happy 50-Year-Old with Miraculously Improved Vision

Patient: "Doctor, I did not come in the last couple of years because my eyes have been doing so well. I stopped wearing the glasses you gave me, and my eyesight has gotten better. I don't even need those lousy bifocals anymore!"

Doctor: "Really?"

Examination today:

Previous manifest refraction OD:	−1.50 sphere 20/20	OS: −0.75 sphere (20/20)
	+2.00 add OU	
Today's manifest refraction OD:	−1.50 sphere 20/20	OS: plano (20/20)

[3]Note that pregnancy can cause myopic changes (as discussed in the previous section) and hyperopic changes. The latter changes can happen both due to crystalline lens changes as well as accommodation changes.

On first glance, we can see that this patient is likely happy because he has basically developed monovision. Should we pat him on the head, thank him for coming in, and send him on his way?

No, while the patient may be happy with his monovision, a closer look at his current refractive error indicates that he has had a hyperopic shift in his left eye that has made him plano. This warrants further clinical examination, including possible imaging.

For this patient, suppose during the dilated fundus exam of the left eye, we observe posterior choroidal folds in a centripetal pattern around the fovea. A CT of the orbits shows an *orbital mass (metastatic tumor)* pushing against the posterior pole.[4] This is a life-threatening diagnosis. The patient will require a multidisciplinary approach with referral to oncology and neurosurgery, among other "real-doctor" specialists. As ophthalmologists, we can continue to assist the team by continuing to perform timely exams and ocular imaging, especially for monitoring the (currently) unaffected eye and treating any ocular involvement in the future.

Scenario #2: The Case of the Unhappy 58-Year-Old Attorney

Patient: "I can't read my legal briefings anymore! I have to close my left eye and simply use my right eye lately. I used to just take my glasses off and read. Sign me up for LASIK now!"

Doctor: "Oh really?"

Examination today:

- Previous manifest refraction (3 months ago): −3.00 sphere OU (20/20)
- Today's manifest refraction: OD: −1.25 sphere (20/40), OS: −3.00 sphere (20/20)

Similar to the last patient, this patient has had a unilateral hyperopic shift in his right eye. Unlike the last patient, this patient is unhappy; presumably, because of his −3.00D myopic error, he was able to take off his glasses to read previously but now is unable to do so. Again, a thorough exam, including dilated fundus exam and potential ophthalmic imaging is necessary. Suppose that the exam of the macula shows an elevated, dome-shaped ring of fluid surrounding the central fovea. OCT of the macula shows a collection of subretinal fluid below the neurosensory retina.[5]

Thankfully, we did not sign up this patient for LASIK! Instead, this is a classic presentation of *central serous chorioretinopathy (CSCR)*. You may wish to review the full pathophysiology, diagnostic tools, and treatment options from other sources, but suffice it to say that this disease can classically present with a unilateral hyperopic shift.

Finally, if a *bilateral hyperopic shift* were to occur, the clinician should have a strong suspicion for *medication-induced retinal edema*.[6] A full list of medications is beyond the scope of this text, but some common and high-yield medications include thiazolidinediones, fingolimod, tamoxifen, niacin, MEK inhibitors, and ketamine. This type of edema usually presents like a CSCR type of macular edema. Treatment options range from simple observation to intravitreal injections, and long-term visual effects range from transient to sight-threatening.

Scenario #3: The 36-Year-Old with Miraculously Improved Vision after Trauma

Patient: I joined a special club two days ago with other like-minded individuals where we beat each other up for fun. I wish I could tell you more about it, but the first rule is that we do not talk about this club. It was my first night, so I had to fight. I'm not sure what happened because the other guy knocked me out pretty badly, but I realize that I don't need glasses for my left eye anymore. I told you this club is amazing!

Doctor: Oh really…?

Examination today:

- Previous manifest refraction: −14.00D sphere OU
- Today's manifest refraction: OD (cc) 20/20 (−14.00D sphere); OS (sc) 20/20 (plano)

Has this patient miraculously improved his vision by getting into this mayhem-filled fight? We should investigate further. Suppose that slit lamp exam is significant for a totally *subluxated crystalline lens* into the vitreous with resulting aphakia in the left eye. While aphakia typically causes a hyperopic shift, in this patient, the aphakia has caused a hyperopic shift of his pre-existing myopia such that he is now basically plano.

Obviously, we cannot simply pat him on his head and send him on his way. In addition to counseling him about not partaking in underground boxing clubs, this is a surgical emergency that needs prompt vitrectomy, lensectomy, and possible secondary IOL placement.

[4]Note that a choroidal melanoma (another favorite exam question) may appear with similar exam findings, though the clinical appearance of a gray-green mass may be seen on fundus exam.

[5]And yes, we could obtain an FA/ICG to confirm the "smokestack" pattern here as well, but none of the authors are retina specialists.

[6]Makri OE, Georgalas I, Georgakopoulos CD. Drug-induced macular edema. *Drugs*. 2013;73(8):789–802

Acquired and Clinical Astigmatism

We previously discussed various types and classifications of astigmatism in Chap. 11 "Astigmatism". When formulating a differential diagnosis for causes of acquired astigmatism, we can divide it into *corneal* or *lenticular* astigmatism. Retinal astigmatism, while theoretically possible, is nearly non-existent.

Differential Diagnosis of Clinical Astigmatism

One way to classify corneal and lenticular astigmatism is to think anatomically: start from the front of the eye and work your way backwards.

A partial differential diagnosis for acquired astigmatism is as follows:

- Corneal
  - Lid/adnexa (compressive etiology)
    - Ptosis
    - Blepharophimosis
    - Chalazion or lid masses
    - Congenital fibrosis of extraocular muscles
  - Conjunctival surface
    - Pterygium, ocular surface tumors
  - Corneal
    - Lesions/masses: pterygium, dermoid, CIN
    - Dystrophies: EBMD, keratoconus, pellucid marginal degeneration, etc.
    - Latrogenic: post-LASIK ectasia
    - Degenerations: Terrien's, Salzmann
    - Scarring secondary to trauma or infections
  - Congenital
    - Fetal alcohol syndrome, albinism, Alport syndrome, infantile nystagmus syndrome, retinopathy of prematurity, Kabuki syndrome, Ehlers-Danlos syndrome (EDS) type 1, Down syndrome, sclerocornea
- Lenticular
  - Compressive: ciliary body tumors (watch for sectoral cataract!)
  - Anterior polar cataracts
  - Cortical cataracts

Let's discuss some high-yield clinical scenarios, including ones that should definitely not be missed on exams:

Scenario #1: The Middle-Aged Female Who Is Unhappy with Her Glasses

A 45-year-old female complains that she can't see well near or far with the glasses you gave her 2 years ago

Current prescription:	OD: −2.00 + 0.50 × 180 (20/50)
	OS: −2.50 + 0.50 × 180 (20/25)

Today's manifest refraction:	OD: −2.00 + 4.00 × 075 (20/25)
	OS: −2.50 + 0.50 × 180 (20/25)

We should note from comparing the two refractions that the patient has experienced a significant shift in refractive cylinder (and axis) in the right eye. This acquired astigmatism must be coming from either the cornea or the lens. Corneal topography or keratometry should be pursued next:

Topography/keratometry: 44.00 × 44.50 @ 180 OU. This confirms that the acquired astigmatism isn't coming from the cornea.

Suppose we now proceeded with the slit lamp exam. Gonioscopy reveals a pale, fleshy lesion in the angle, and a sectoral cataract is present in the right eye. Before dilating the patient, we can get ocular imaging (such as AS-OCT or UBM). Suppose that the UBM confirms a *ciliary body tumor* in the right eye.

Along with the previous case regarding choroidal melanoma, this diagnosis should definitely not be missed as it can lead to blindness or even death. You may wish to review how to diagnose ciliary body tumors (gonioscopy, UBM, AS-OCT, or anterior segment FA) and their treatment (iridocyclectomy, etc.). Remember that a multidisciplinary approach is necessary, including neuroimaging, oncology consultation, and systemic workup/imaging.

Suture Management

In a perfect world, every eye surgeon would be able to place corneal sutures that are robust enough to ensure wound closure but also delicate enough to not cause any astigmatism whatsoever. Obviously, this never happens. Recall that a tight suture placed on or close to the cornea can induce astigmatism (best understood by conceptualizing this as inducing plus-cylinder) by warping the corneal curvature at that location (Fig. 1). Tight sutures located closer to the central cornea will induce more astigmatism than sutures located closer to the limbus.

Topography/keratometry can be very useful to quantify suture-induced astigmatism that may be difficult to detect on clinical exam alone. For example, in this topography-obtained post-penetrating keratoplasty (Fig. 2), there are tight sutures (Panel a, left panel) causing 20.37D of astigmatism at 8°. After removing multiple tight sutures, the astigmatism has decreased to 7.75D (Panel b, right panel). Additional sutures can be removed to further reduce the astigmatism as needed.[7]

[7]While corneal surgeons' preference for the timing of suture removal varies, most surgeons would remove tight sutures starting at 3 months postoperatively after penetrating or deep anterior lamellar keratoplasty. Removing too early may lead to instability of the graft-host junction, including wound rupture and graft dehiscence. Waiting too late (e.g., after 12 months) may reduce the potential benefits of suture removal due to scarring and fibrosis. Most surgeons will continue removing sutures until the astigmatism is <2D and/or the BCVA is acceptable to the patient.

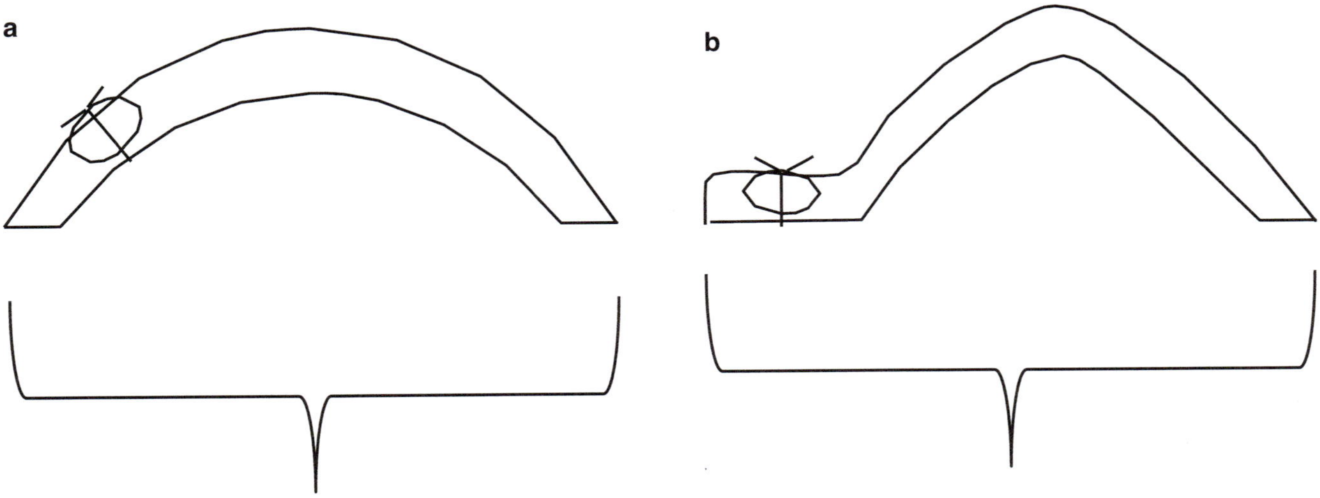

Fig. 1 Tight sutures and astigmatism. A tight suture will induce plus cylinder in the meridian in which it is located. Panel **a** shows an ideal suture that does not distort the corneal curvature. Panel **b** shows a tight suture that flattens the periphery and steepens the central curvature. Notice that the interlimbal distance does not change in either situation

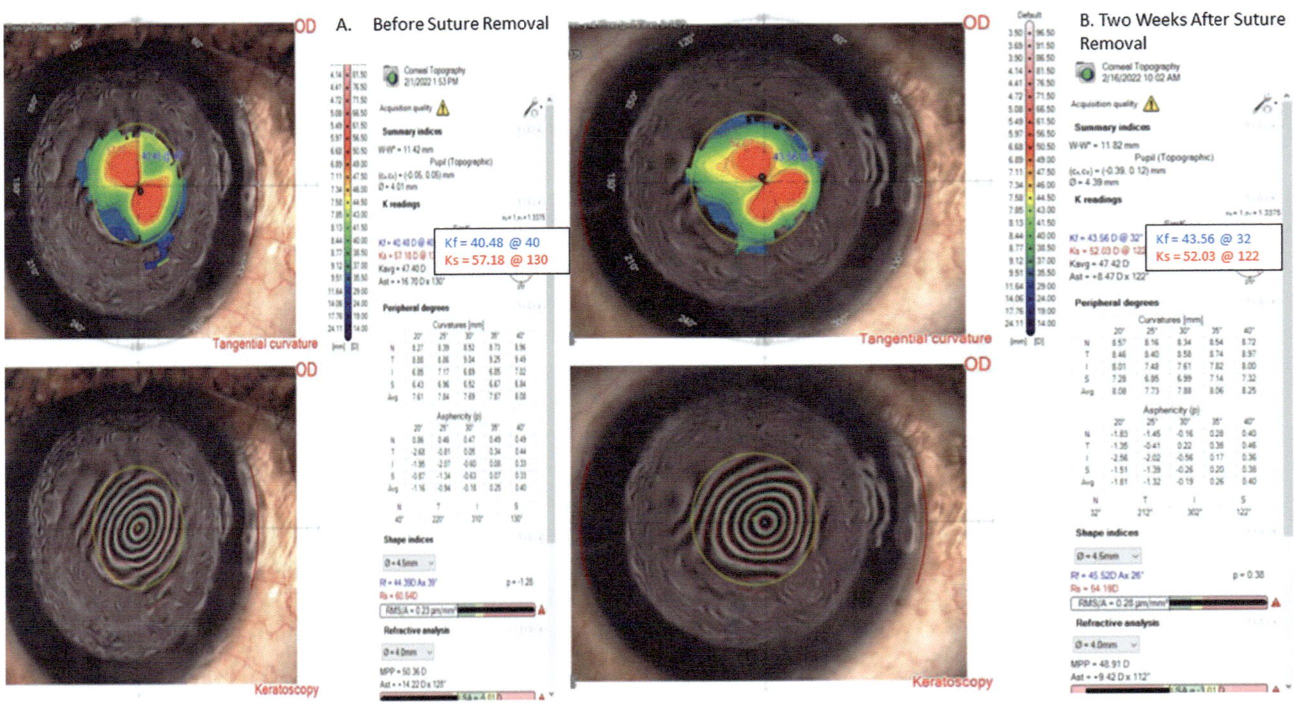

Fig. 2 A tight suture(s) can induce significant amounts of astigmatism. In Panel **a** (left panel), tight sutures are causing 16.7D of astigmatism(!). After suture removal and repeat topography 6 weeks later (Panel **b**, right panel), the astigmatism has reduced to 8.47D. Additional suture removal can be done as needed at this time

Sutures placed at the time of cataract surgery can similarly cause significant amounts of astigmatism. For example, suppose that a 70-year-old patient presents for her one-month postoperative visit after planned extracapsular cataract extraction (ECCE) requiring a wide superior limbal incision. The patient is now pseudophakic in both eyes.

She asks: "I would really like to get my glasses prescription today for my right eye because it's still very blurry. I've been getting by with my left eye for a few weeks now. Will I finally get my glasses prescription today?"

Manifest Refraction today (1 month after ECCE):

$$\text{OD}: -2.00 + 4.00 \times 135 \ (20/40)$$
$$\text{OS}: -1.00 \text{ sphere } (20/20)$$

A (cartoon) clinical exam and topography are shown in Fig. 3. It appears there is a steep suture (marked in red) that

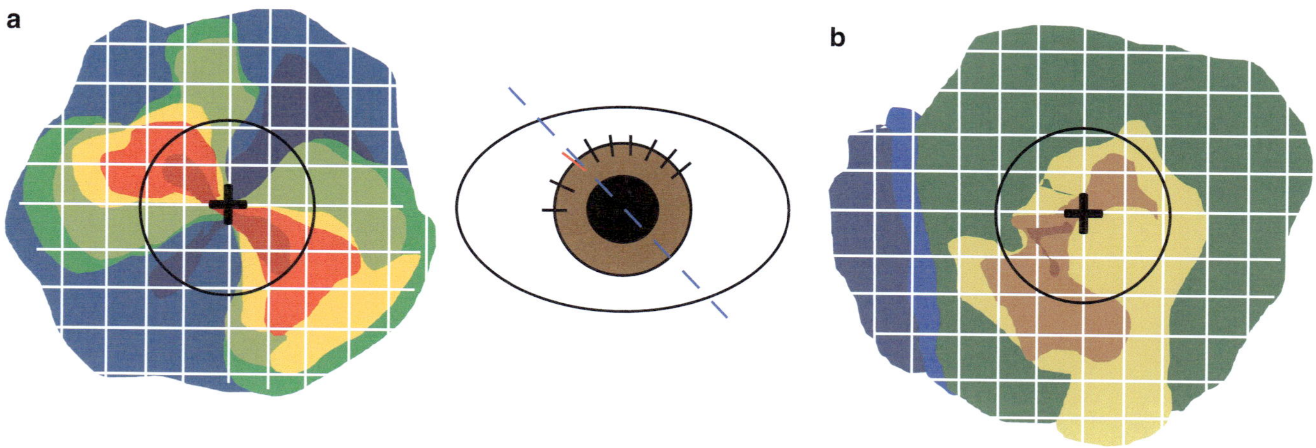

Fig. 3 Topography of the patient's right eye (panel **a**) shows steepening along the 135-degree meridian, which corresponds to the refractive cylinder and location of the tight suture seen on clinical exam. After the suture is cut, repeat topography taken 1 month later shows steepening 90° away of approximately 1 diopter

corresponds to the corneal astigmatism seen on topography at 135°, which also matches the refractive cylinder values. Notice that the spherical equivalent of the manifest refraction of the right eye is plano, which suggests that the patient has excellent vision potential once the astigmatism is reduced.

Suppose we determine that the suture at 130° is tight and we decide to remove it. We reassure the patient that additional time is needed for healing, and we schedule the patient for a return visit in 4–6 weeks.

At the following-up visit 6 weeks later, we can repeat the manifest refraction:

$$\text{OD}: -0.50+1.00\times 45\ (20/20).$$

Repeat topography now corresponds to Panel b in Fig. 3, indicating approximately 1D of astigmatism at the 45-degree meridian. Depending on the needs of the patient, we can either dispense the glasses at this time or consider additional suture removal.

Notice that spherical equivalent is still plano, which is the same as the spherical equivalent noted at the previous visit. Recall that the principle of coupling applies for suture removal as well: flattening in a given meridian will cause steepening of the meridian located 90° away.

In certain situations, the presence of sutures should not preclude other previously discussed causes of acquired astigmatism. Let's see an example of this:

An 80-year-old patient underwent ECCE 1 month ago and was found to have 3D astigmatism at the 135-degree meridian. Suture removal was done and the patient now presents 6 weeks later. Repeat manifest refraction today shows the same amount of refractive cylinder at the 135-degree meridian. What else could be going on (Fig. 4)?

In this situation, the suture removal didn't improve the astigmatism. We have to probe further: dilation reveals that the IOL has dislocated (tilted) causing lenticular (pseudophakic astigmatism).[8] Depending on the situation, treatment options at this time range from simple observation, glasses, contact lenses, IOL repositioning, and/or IOL replacement (with appropriate fixation).

Acquired Causes of Poor Accommodation

Similar to the previously discussed acquired refractive errors, poor accommodation can have a variety of causes. A sample list follows:

- Age, normal presbyopia
- Latent hyperopia
- Medications (parasympatholytics, phenothiazines, tranquilizers, chloroquine, antihistamines)
- Systemic illness (hypothyroid, anemia, myasthenia gravis, diabetes)
- Prior encephalitis or meningitis
- Tumor
- Head trauma – post-concussion syndrome.[9]
- Tonic pupil
- Topical and systemic medications.[10]

[8] See Chap. 11 "Astigmatism", for a discussion on how a tilted/dislocated IOL can induce refractive and astigmatic errors.

[9] Raghuram A, Cotter SA, Gowrisankaran S, et al. Postconcussion: Receded Near Point of Convergence is not Diagnostic of Convergence Insufficiency. *Am J Ophthalmol*. 2019;206:235–244

[10] Smith JL, Buncic JR. Drugs which can affect near vision: a useful list. https://uwpress.wisc.edu/journals/pdfs/AOJ_49_178.pdf. Accessed August 10, 2020

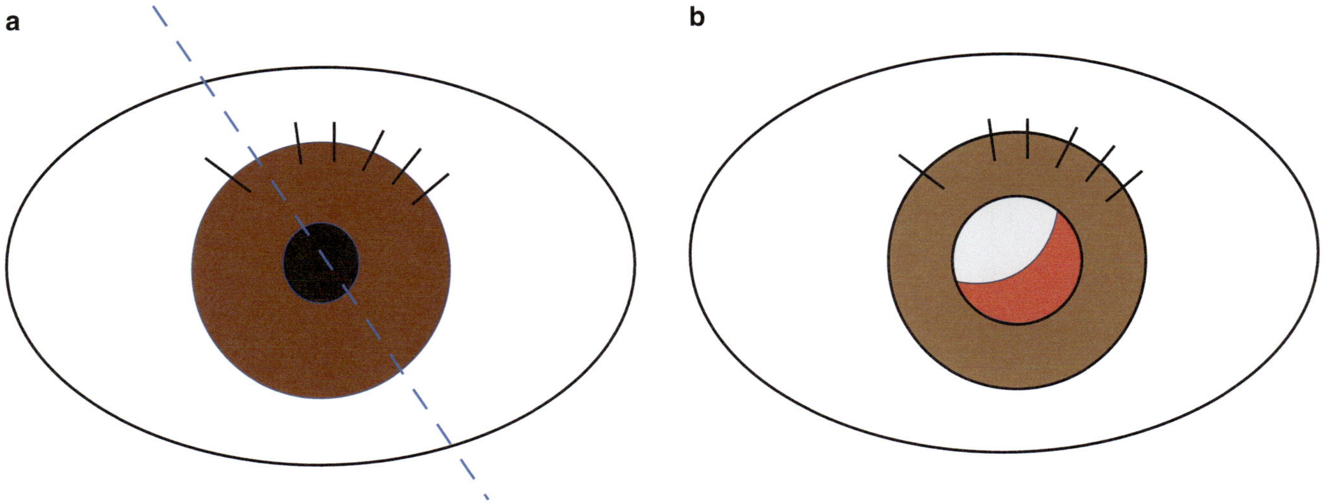

Fig. 4 After suture removal (Panel **a**), there is still refractive cylinder present in the meridian of the removed suture. Dilated exam (Panel **b**) shows a dislocated IOL causing lenticular (pseudophakic) astigmatism

- Ocular trauma
- Down syndrome around 6 years of age.[11]

Let's discuss some high-yield clinical scenarios:

Example #1: The Unhappy Bank Teller

A 39-year-old bank teller complains of poor vision, especially for near tasks, for more than a year. Previously, he reports he never had to wear glasses. For the past year, he has been given several pairs of glasses by various providers, but none of these seem to be working more than a few months.

Exam today:	Uncorrected distance visual acuity: 20/20 OU
	Uncorrected near visual acuity: J7 OU
	Manifest refraction today: +1.75 sphere OU (20/20)

At this point, we may be tempted to dispense the glasses prescription and send the patient on his merry way because he can see 20/20. However, we should remember that his main complaint is with his near vision tasks, especially given his profession. Furthermore, he was already 20/20 at distance without any glasses; a manifest refraction today simply revealed that he had a mild hyperopic correction.

What else could be going on? This is a potentially classic presentation of a patient with *latent hyperopia* who is now having problems with accommodation due to aging. At this time, we need to perform some additional, not-commonly-performed tests, such as measuring the amplitude of accommodation (AOA) and performing a cycloplegic refraction. Suppose the AOA is 6D in each eye, and the cycloplegic refraction is +4.00D sphere OU.

This confirms our suspicions regarding the diagnosis of latent hyperopia. The patient has been hyperopic his entire life, but he was managing when younger because he was able to generate the necessary accommodation. However, now that he is getting older, his AOA is decreasing and he is not able to generate the accommodation that he needs; thus, he is fatiguing quickly, especially given his high demands for near-vision tasks given his profession. Recall that patients can comfortably use one-half their AOA.[12] Therefore, he can comfortably generate 3D of accommodation at this time but it is likely that he will continue to lose his AOA over the next few years. Eventually, he will require the full cycloplegic refraction but will likely not tolerate the full refraction at this time.

One approach is to give these patients one-half the cycloplegic refraction (e.g., +2.00D sphere OU) and slowly increase this over time to allow the patient to "adjust" to the prescription.[13] We could also consider atropinization to force him to use the full cycloplegic refraction, but we should consider the side effects. Another option is to use bifocal glasses or even contact lenses – recall that presbyopic hyperopes

[11] Cregg M, Woodhouse JM, Pakeman VH, et al. Accommodation and refractive error in children with Down syndrome: cross-sectional and longitudinal studies. *Invest Ophthalmol Vis Sci*. 2001;42(1):55–63

[12] See Chap. 9 "Accommodation and Presbyopia", for a review of this topic.

[13] A silly (but hopefully useful) analogy for the latent hyperope is to consider them like a heroin addict: you can't stop them "cold turkey"; you have to transition them off the heroin (accommodation) with a less-harmful substitute, such as methadone (one-half the cycloplegic refraction, in this analogy). Eventually, the goal is to wean these patients off their "love for accommodation" by slowly building up the hyperopic correction over a period of several months or years. We apologize for this analogy as drug addiction is a serious problem in real life, and we don't wish to make light of it as it affects many people. Over the years, we have found that students respond well to this analogy because it is a "memorable" one. We should emphasize that our intent with this analogy is to educate, above all else.

have decreased needs of accommodation when using contact lenses.

Example #2: The Unhappy Social Media Influencer

A 32-year-old female who has built her career on being a "social media influencer" presents with complaints of reading her cellphone over the past week. She reports that if she closes her left eye, she can still read with her right eye only. She is extremely unhappy as her cellphone is her primary means of "letting her followers know what to buy and what is trending."

- Distance visual acuity (uncorrected): 20/20 OU
- Near visual acuity (uncorrected): OD: J1 OS: J10

How should we proceed? In this case, the clinical exam will shed light on the diagnosis. Suppose that in room light conditions, the right pupil is 2 mm whereas the left pupil is 8 mm. When we shine a light into both eyes, the left pupil minimally reacts, but when asked to read the near card, the left pupil constricts to approximately 6.5 mm with a slow re-dilation.

This is a classic presentation of *Adie tonic pupil.* A full review of this entity is beyond the scope of this text, but it should be remembered that decreased near vision in one eye may often be the presenting symptom to the clinician. Hopefully, you can make the correct diagnosis and treat her symptoms so that your social media accounts will also gain thousands of followers.

Asthenopia

Sometimes in ophthalmology, when we want to sound intelligent, we come up with fancy sounding words to describe symptoms and problems that can be easily described in everyday English.[14] *Asthenopia* is no different: it simply means eyestrain, usually due to excessive accommodation, that manifests as subjective, episodic, and often vague symptoms of eye fatigue, discomfort (including intraocular and extraocular), headaches, photophobia, intermittently blurry vision, and difficulty keeping the eyes open. It can be considered a diagnosis of exclusion but also a concurrent diagnosis (with other more readily diagnosed conditions). Asthenopia can results from a combination of etiologies, including excessive accommodation, imbalance of extraocular muscles, organic nervous system disease, and/or improper illumination. It can be a frustrating condition for both the patient and the examiner.

Clinically, we can work up the various symptoms of asthenopia by ruling out/in common causes. We will focus our discussion on asthenopia to etiologies related to refractive errors and glasses. Several useful categories of questions/tests to perform include:

A. Asthenopia due to errors in refraction:
   (a) Was the patient over-minused causing the need for excessive accommodation, especially in a young myope? A duochrome test or cycloplegic refraction may be helpful.
   (b) Is there latent hyperopia present that can only be measured after a cycloplegic refraction, as discussed in the previous section?

B. Asthenopia due to poorly made/functioning glasses:

For example, suppose a 55-year-old engineer comes in for his third refraction in 2 months.[15] He states that "something is wrong with these glasses." You perform another long refraction until your shoulder hurts, but the repeat manifest refraction today is exactly the same as the prescription ground into the patient's current (new) glasses. Before labeling this patient "difficult" and referring them to your least favorite colleague, you may want to review the differential for this problem.[16]

If the repeat manifest refraction matches the current glasses' prescription, then a summary list of what to do next includes:

1. Pupillary distance (PD): Mark the location of the pupillary axis on the lenses, and check the optical center through a lensmeter.[17] Does it line up with the pupils? Is the new glasses' PD the same as the old glasses or the PD used in the phoropter during today's repeat refraction?
2. Base curve: Using a Geneva lens clock, check the old versus new base curves.
3. Is the cylinder ground onto the back surface of the lens, or is the lens backwards?
4. Is the progressive or bifocal segment height okay? Is it affecting chin posture?
5. Is the frame alignment okay? Is the pantoscopic tilt >7°?
6. Does the vertex distance of the glasses match the vertex distance used in the phoropter? This may particularly be a problem with higher power lenses.
7. Has there been a large change in the axis of the astigmatism?

[14] For example, we use the term "ocular straylight" to refer to "glare."

[15] By now, you should have gathered that anytime an engineer comes in for an eye exam in these hypothetical clinical cases, you should buckle up because it's going to be a while.

[16] Similarly, you may wish to review Chap. 15 "Glasses in Clinical Practice" and Chap. 16 "Construction of Glasses (Ophthalmologists as Opticians)" for a full discussion on the topics of prescribing, dispensing, and troubleshooting glasses.

[17] Consult Chap. 17 "Optical Instruments and Machines" for a review on how to use the lensmeter and Geneva lens clock.

8. Has there been a change in lens material? High index lenses are thinner and lighter, but they have more chromatic aberration and a smaller sweet spot.
9. Finally, does the patient not like the frame design but is too embarrassed to say they changed their mind? "Do you think you might see better with a different frame?"

Of note: This question is one of the most common clinical scenarios asked by senior attendings! Other educational instructions to patients include ensuring adequate lighting, limiting screen time (especially with cell phones/tablets), and keeping a diary of symptoms to elicit triggering/alleviating factors. The key feature of all these therapies is to reduce the amount of accommodation done by the patient. The classic trifecta of warm compresses, lid scrubs, and tears may also be used for management of non-vision-threatening symptoms.

As mentioned above, non-glasses-related causes of asthenopia are numerous, including undiagnosed strabismus, dry eye, screen fatigue, and CNS issues. If adjusting the refraction and/or glasses fails to improve the patient's symptoms, additional testing, imaging, and lab workup may be necessary.

Other Commonly Encountered Clinical Problems with Refractive Considerations

There are a few additional scenarios that don't fit nicely into one of the previously mentioned categories but warrant additional discussion.

Night Myopia

Night myopia is the tendency for most people to develop myopia in low illumination settings. Interestingly, soldiers experiencing night myopia during World War II brought additional attention to this topic as observers noticed that additional minus-powered lenses were needed for sighting stars and other objects of interest during nocturnal missions.[18] While a variety of historical theories have been proposed for this phenomenon, we will instead focus our attention to how a patient might present to your office with complaints of night myopia symptoms.

Suppose that a 24-year-old medical student presents to your office complaining of poor night vision. She feels that while she can see well during the day, her vision is particularly worse when she drives home at night time. Her route home involves more than an hour drive through dimly lit roads.

Exam:	Distance vision (uncorrected) 20/20 OD and OS
	Manifest refraction: −0.50D sphere OU (20/20)

What else could be accounting for her symptoms?

This is a classic presentation of *night myopia*. When considering this diagnosis, ophthalmic diseases, such as retinitis pigmentosa, vitamin A deficiency, and congenital stationary night blindness, can be determined by basic exam and clinical testing. If no organic pathology is found, then *five* different reasons may account for these findings.

1. Pupil dilation under scotopic light conditions (Fig. 5): Recall that as the pupil dilates, more light rays will pass through the peripheral cornea and lens in low-light conditions as compared to bright-light conditions. These light rays will be bent more strongly than central light rays (spherical aberration), leading to a myopic shift.[19] Wave front testing or ray-tracing imaging may further quantify the amount of spherical aberration present.
2. Limitations of the refraction lane: The standard lane is 20 feet (6 m) long which is shorter than the distance to test optical infinity.[20] In order to correct for infinity, we have to add an additional −0.25D to the final refraction to avoid under-correction.
3. Purkinje shift: in low light conditions, shorter wavelengths of light will converge more. Simultaneously, as the rods take over at night time, these photoreceptors are more sensitive to blue light. Thus, there is a tendency for the peak luminance sensitivity of the human eye to shift toward the blue end of the color spectrum in scotopic-mesopic light conditions.
4. Loss of accommodation targets: since the patient has a lengthy commute in dimly lit roads, there may be no targets to "anchor" accommodation, such as street lights or road signs. As a result, she may be generating additional accommodative (plus) power and inadvertently "fogging" herself while driving.
5. Spasm of accommodation due to daytime activities: as the patient is a medical student trying to ace her STEP exams to get into ophthalmology, she may be spending most of her day accommodating while reading.

We can help the patient by any of the following methods:

1. Additional myopic correction for "nighttime" glasses to use while driving. For example, instead of simply dis-

[18] Otero JM, Plaza L, Salaverri F. Absolute thresholds and night myopia. J Opt Soc Am. 1949 Feb;39(2):167–72

[19] See Chap. 14 "Physical Optics and Advanced Optical Principles", for a review of spherical aberration.

[20] See Chap. 18 "Visual Acuity Testing and Assessment".

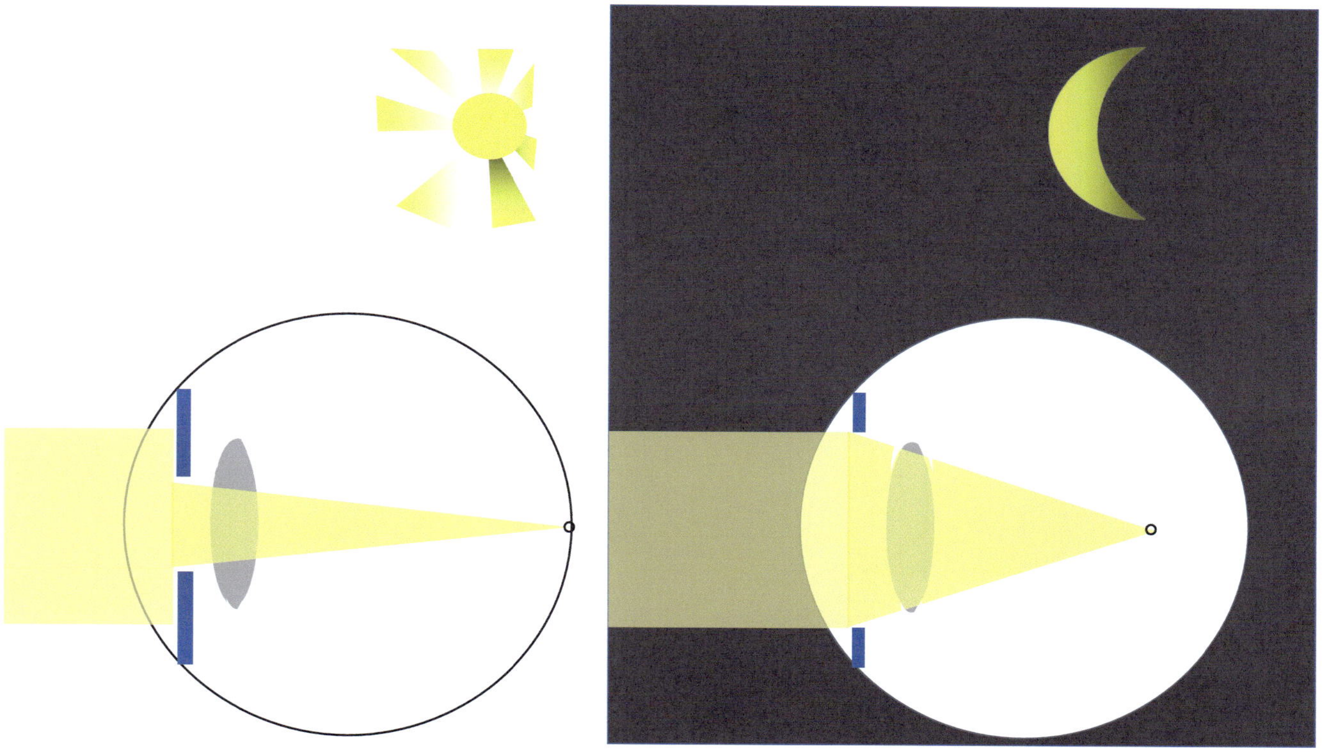

Fig. 5 Spherical aberration contributes to night myopia. Pupillary dilation under mesopic lighting conditions will allow more peripheral rays to pass through the cornea and crystalline lens. These peripheral rays will be refracted much stronger than central rays and will "land" in front of the retina, inducing a myopic shift

pensing −0.50D sphere OU, we can give −1.00D sphere OU that the patient can wear during her commute home.

2. Advise the patient to take study/rest breaks during the day. The "20/20/20" rule can be used to remind patients that every 20 minutes, they should look at a target 20 feet away for at least 20 seconds to break accommodation.
3. A mild pupil constrictor, such as dilute brimonidine/pilocarpine, can be given before her commute home to decrease myopic shift from spherical aberration.

Management of Aphakia

We have previously discussed how hyperopia/aphakia causes problems with magnification leading to anisometropia and aniseikonia.[21] Several options exist for the management of aphakia, ranging from clinical to surgical:

1. Glasses: for one eye or both eyes. If given for both eyes, the patient may do just fine. However, if only one eye is aphakic, certain issues may occur with aphakic spectacles (see below).
2. Contact lenses: contact lenses may be an excellent option for patients with unilateral aphakia. Recall that magnification with contact lenses is less pronounced as compared to the magnification experienced with glasses. This may decrease the negative effects of aniseikonia.
3. IOLs: both ACIOLs and fixated-PCIOLs may be considered, especially if the previous two options are intolerable.

Patients with spectacles for unilateral aphakia will experience similar problems as patients who wear hyperopic glasses:[22]

- Ring scotoma secondary to prismatic effects of the lens periphery
- Jack in the box phenomenon: sudden appearance of objects that jump out of the scotoma
- Magnification (Fig. 6)
- Pincushion distortion (Fig. 7)
- Extra weight of the aphakic lens, which can make the spectacles lopsided and difficult to wear
- Higher cost

[21] See Chap. 8 "Magnification and Telescopes".

[22] See Chap. 16 "Construction of Glasses (Ophthalmologists as Opticians)", for a more detailed review of these topics.

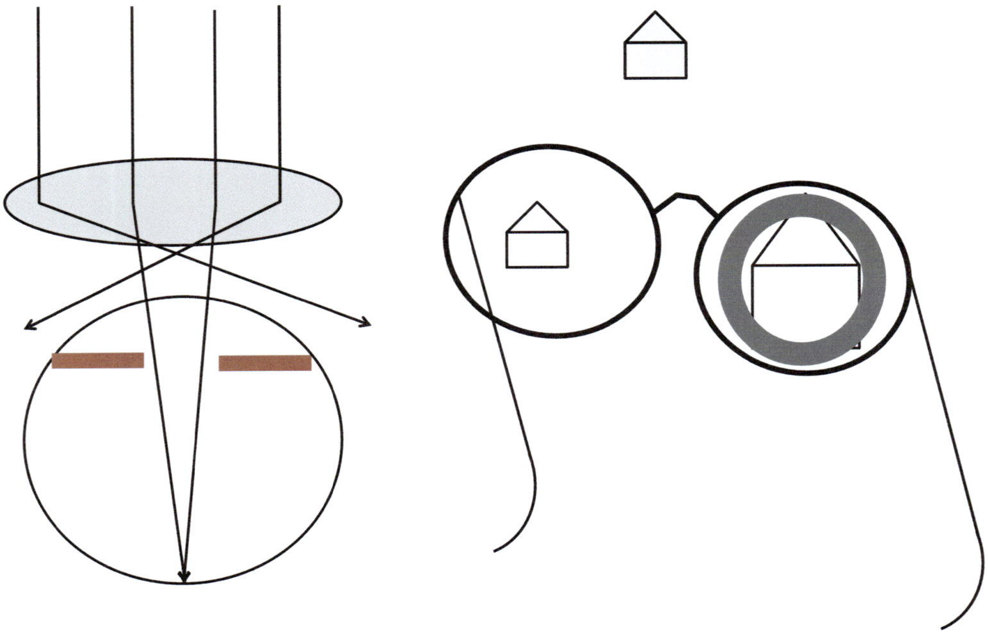

Fig. 6 A high plus-powered lens given to the aphakic eye (right eye) will cause significant magnification and extra weight and induce a ring scotoma. The ring scotoma is caused by light rays that strike the peripheral edge of the lens never reaching the visual axis due to the effects of refraction

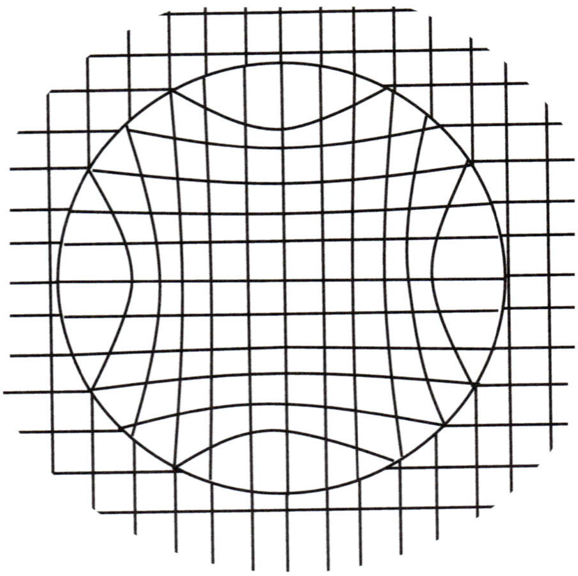

Fig. 7 Pincushion distortion induced by an aphakic lens

Nonorganic Visual Loss (NOVL)[23]

A 7-year-old wakes up on a fine Sunday morning frantically telling her parents that she cannot see: "I think I've gone blind." Her family takes her to a local optometrist who agrees the child is blind but cannot tell why. They refer her to a general ophthalmologist who diagnoses a likely occipital stroke given the child is blind and the eyes appear normal. The child is then referred to a university hospital ED for a stat MRI of the brain.[24] The patient's mother is charged $4000 on her credit card because they cannot obtain an insurance referral. The MRI is normal and the on-call ED attending calls you, asking, "What should we do now?"

This scenario was a real case experienced by one of the authors recently.[25] We will first discuss an increasingly common entity known as nonorganic visual loss (NOVL). NOVL includes both volitional (e.g., malingering) and non-volitional (e.g., factitious disorder, hysteria, etc.) causes. In other words, sometimes the patient is intentionally faking it, but other times, the patient may not be purposely faking it.

NOVL is defined as a decrease in visual acuity or visual field without an identifiable organic cause. It may be present in 0.5–5% of the patient population, and early teens and middle age patients may be the most affected.[26] We have personally observed a 1–2% prevalence in our pediatric practice, with the highest rate among 7-year-olds who would like to wear glasses because it's "the cool thing to wear."

An in-depth review of NOVL is out of the scope of this text, though it is important to distinguish between those conditions in which the patient is *consciously aware (volitional)*

[23]Many thanks to Robert W. Enzenauer, MD, MPH, MSS, MBA, Professor of Ophthalmology and Pediatrics, Chief of Ophthalmology, Children's Hospital of Colorado for his assistance and contributions to this section.

[24]Of course, modern medical practice is that any patient that enters a university ER must get a CT and/or MRI…just kidding.

[25]We will disclose how this case was handled in the end-of-chapter questions.

[26]Lim SA, Siatkowski RM, Farris BK. Functional visual loss in adults and children patient characteristics, management, and outcomes. *Ophthalmology*. 2005;112(10):1821–1828

of his/her deception and those in which the patient *believes their signs and symptoms are caused by a real condition (non-volitional).*

(a) *Volitional: malingering, Munchausen syndrome, etc.*

A patient may pretend to have or exaggerate symptom(s) in order to achieve some tangible or intangible gain. For example, a young child may intentionally fail a vision test because he wants to wear glasses. Another common example is a soldier who intentionally fails a vision test in order to avoid active combat duty.[27]

Munchausen's syndrome is a particular type of volitional (factitious) disorder in which the person wants to assume the role of the sick patient, often for tangible gains such as disability insurance. Munchausen by proxy is a variant of the classical Munchausen's syndrome; in this scenario, someone else (a parent) may make the patient intentionally sick in order to seek attention. These cases may also involve child abuse; a high degree of clinical suspicion and tact is therefore necessary when encountering these patients.

(b) *Non-volitional: conversion disorder, hysteria, etc.*

Patients with a conversion disorder or functional somatic syndrome truly believe their symptoms are real and are caused by a medical problem. These patients are not necessarily "faking" as they may even have had an injury (minor or in the past) that they believe is affecting their eyes. For example, one of the authors had a patient who had minor eye injuries after an oil-rig explosion in the recent past. The patient had no findings on the exam and visual acuity was 20/20 in both eyes. However, the patient was totally convinced that his eyes were damaged from the traumatic injury. He was not seeking any disability insurance or filing a lawsuit. He continued to work at the oil-rig but was convinced that he was going blind. For these patients, validation and reassurance without judgment is extremely crucial (along with lots of preservative-free tears as in the case of the oil-rig patient). Ultimately, a psychiatry consultation or cognitive behavior therapy may be necessary, along with patience and the tincture of time, for resolution of symptoms.

Regardless of volitional/non-volitional causes, all NOVL patients must have thorough workups to rule out organic causes. While it may seem like a waste of time, money, and resources, there are medicolegal considerations as well: we cannot simply pass off someone as a "faker" only to find out that a true organic pathology exists! All variants of NOVL are therefore diagnoses of exclusion. Knowing which tests to order may limit unnecessary testing without missing a subtle degenerative condition such macular dystrophy, inherited optic nerve pathology, or amblyopia.

It is more difficult to diagnose NOVL patients who complain of seeing "blurry" rather than those patients with profound vision loss. Similarly, it is difficult to separate NOVL patients who are exaggerating a symptom with a true underlying organic pathology. In a young patient, it may be easier to diagnose malingering by simply asking "What do you think would help?" They will often tell you: "Glasses!"

The following combination of clinical exams, tools, and imaging may be utilized in the diagnosis and management of NOVL patients. Some of these tests may not only be diagnostic but may be therapeutic as well.

In the following examples, let's assume the patient states his/her RIGHT EYE is blind.

Monocular Blindness Tests

A. Red-Green Glasses and Worth Four-Dot (W4D) Testing

Test setup: The *r*ed lens goes over the *r*ight eye; the green lens goes over the left eye. The W4D light is held 3 feet away.

(a) If the right eye is truly blind, the patient would only see 3 green dots, i.e., the three lights perceived by the left eye.
(b) A patient with normal vision would see 4 dots: one red, two green, and one that is red/green.
(c) Even a patient with amblyopia or monofixation syndrome with a suppression scotoma should be able to see the dots at near, but miss one of the colors at distance.

B. OKN Drum

Test setup: The "blind" right eye is open and the "healthy" left eye is covered. The drum is rotated along its vertical axis in front of the right eye.

(a) If the right eye is truly blind: no nystagmus is observed.
(b) If a horizontal nystagmus is induced, this indicates at least 20/200 vision or better.

C. Base Down 4 Diopter Prism

Test setup: This can be tried under monocular or binocular conditions. A 4 PD base-down prism is moved in front of the affected eye.

(a) If the right eye is truly blind, then no movement will be observed.
(b) A patient with normal vision will move their eye upward to maintain fixation on a target. Again, recall that a virtual image is moved toward the apex so the eye will "move" up to "catch" the virtual image if it has normal vision (this movement is relative to the examiner).

[27] Broderick KM, Ableman TB, Weber ED, Enzenauer RW, Wain HJ, Wroblewski KJ. Nonorganic Vision Loss in the Afghanistan and Iraq Conflicts. *Neuroophthalmology*. 2017;41(4):175–181

D. Mirror Test

Test setup: The "blind" right eye is open, and the "healthy" left eye is covered. A handheld mirror is aimed at the patient so he/she can see his/her own reflection and is then moved around as the examiner says, "I'm going to reflect some light onto your eye":

(a) If the right eye is truly blind, it will not follow the mirror.

(b) A patient with normal vision will follow himself. You can try this at home: it is really hard not to follow the mirror. Since human vanity is second only to human stupidity, a malingering patient will involuntarily look at the mirror to see his/her own reflection.

E. Fogging

Test setup: Both eyes are open in the phoropter, and successive lenses are changed over either eye until the normal eye is fogged with plus lenses and the "bad" eye is not.

(a) If the right eye is truly blind, then the patient will not be able to see through the phoropter.

(b) A patient with normal vision should still be able to see well even if the opposite eye is fogged.

F. Stereoacuity

Test setup: With the patient's near correction refraction in place, both eyes are kept open, and a set of stereoacuity lenses (polarized or red/green) is held over each eye.

(a) If the right eye is truly blind, the patient cannot discern the 3D images.

(b) A patient with normal vision should be able to see the 3D images under binocular conditions.

G. Color Vision Testing: The first plate in the Ishihara plates is considered to be a control so that both color-normal and color-deficient patients should be able to see it. If a patient states he/she can't see the first plate, then you may have a malingerer on your hands.

Binocular Blindness Tests

A. Simple observation of the patient ambulating the room, missing obstacles:

(a) If acute loss of sight is reported, the patient would be expected to be in an anxious state or bumping into objects.

B. Bringing fingertips together from opposite hands across the torso or finger-to-nose testing: Since this relies on proprioception, even patients with actual blindness should be able to do these tasks. If a patient is unable to do these tasks, there may be volitional NOVL present.

C. Using plano trial lenses and rechecking vision ("bottom-up visual acuity"): This is particularly effective in young children around age 7 years who would like to try glasses. This can be combined with showing the patient progressively larger lines on the Snellen chart: for example, starting with the 20/10 line, the examiner can dial in "strong" plano lenses and then show the 20/15 or 20/20 line. The patient will think he/she is getting stronger lenses and will read the larger lines.

D. Confrontation visual field testing: This is also particularly effective in young malingering children; they may lie that they can't see the fingers. If a patient's vision is worse than count fingers, then he/she should also have trouble ambulating and recognizing faces.

E. Averse light reaction: If a patient is truly blind, then suddenly shining a bright light should not cause him/her to suddenly flinch away from the light.

F. Autorefraction/streak refraction: If a patient intentionally performs poorly on subjective manifest refraction, then an autorefraction or streak refraction can be performed to detect the true refractive error of the eye. For example, if the patient pretends that he/she cannot see any better despite any combination of lenses you display on the phoropter, but the autorefraction and streak refraction show a refractive error of −1.00D sphere OU, then you may have a faker on your hands!

G. Corneal topography: Similarly, this may help to show how much corneal astigmatism is present and whether this matches the refraction.

H. OCT macula: This may help rule out any retinal pathology.

Visual Field Loss Tests

I. Visual field testing (Humphrey): A clover-leaf pattern indicates inattentiveness, which may be intentional. Patterns inconsistent with logical scotomas and high false-negatives may also be seen on testing. Remember that central scotomas are extremely rare in NOVL and warrant further evaluation.

J. Tangent screen tests and Goldman visual fields at different distances: Watch for spirally enlarging visual fields ("spiraling isopters"), overlapping isopters, or visual fields that become smaller as the screen is placed further away.

K. Visual evoked potential (VEP) testing: While this may be a fantastic waste of healthcare resources, VEP testing may be needed in certain cases for medicolegal purposes to confirm the diagnosis of NOVL. It is not practical to use VEP testing as a primary diagnostic tool.

Once NOVL is diagnosed, reassurance may be the best initial remedy for many of these patients, as up to 50% of patients may have improvement of symptoms over time. For some patients, especially young children, it may not be helpful to be confrontational (other than the visual fields, see what we did there) with them as there may be underlying psychological or social factors present. A separate discussion with parent(s) may be necessary as well. One option may be to offer over the counter reading glasses and ask the parents to inform them if the vision gets worse despite the placebo glasses. This is relevant, as up to 2% of patients in one study went on to be diagnosed with an organic illness, and up to 40% of adults may have a concurrent psychiatric illness.[28] If a patient is reaching out for medical attention, it may be because they are afraid of complaining about what really bothers them. A multidisciplinary approach may at times be necessary.

Practice Problems

1. If a patient with Marfan syndrome is found to have the right crystalline lens dislocated superotemporally on clinical exam, which of the following refractive errors is most likely present?
   A. −2.00 + 2.00 × 90
   B. −2.00 + 2.00 × 120
   C. −2.00 + 2.00 × 60
   D. −1.0 sphere
2. A 30-year-old professional tennis player complains that she cannot see the ball that well while playing outside at nighttime even when outdoor lights are on. Vision with −2.00 D sphere OU contact lenses is 20/20 OD and OS. A manifest refraction, including Duochrome test, over the contacts is plano. What is the appropriate next step?
   A. Reassure patient nothing is wrong, her best corrected vision in 20/20.
   B. Order an ERG to rule out nyctalopia.
   C. Try −2.50D sphere contacts for nighttime sports activities.
   D. Try −1.50 D sphere contacts for nighttime sports activities.
3. A patient comes in for a 4-week postop appointment after his planned ECCE. Manifest refraction OD shows +4.00D cylinder at 80° (Fig. 8). Which suture can be considered for removal at this time? The suture at:
   A. A
   B. B
   C. C
   D. D
   E. E
4. A 7-year-old wakes up on a Sunday morning blind in both eyes. Her family takes her to a local optometrist who agrees the child is blind but cannot tell why. The patient is then referred to a general ophthalmologist who diagnoses a likely occipital stroke, given the child is blind and

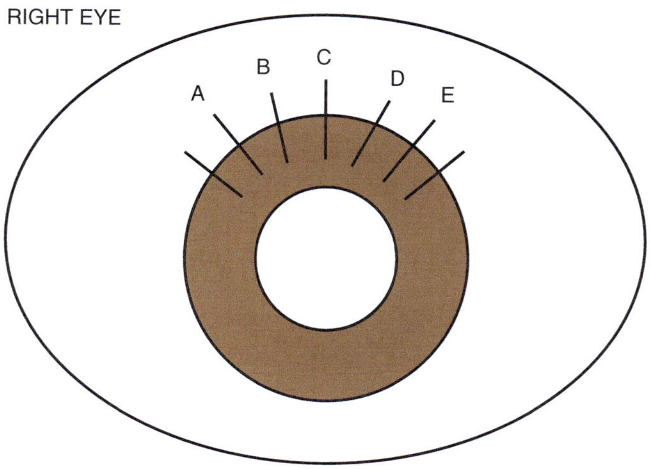

Fig. 8 Which of the following sutures should be cut if the postoperative manifest refraction shows +4.00D cylinder at 80°?

the eyes look normal. The child is then referred to a university hospital ED for a stat MRI of the brain. The patient's mother is charged $4000 on her credit card because she cannot obtain a timely insurance referral because it's a Sunday. The MRI is normal. The child is happily chatting with her mother in the ED room. The ED doc calls you, asking "what should we do next?" (You may recall this is the clinical scenario presented in the chapter text.)
   A. Order an MRA-angiogram.
   B. Observe the child: are they ambulating okay; are they in any stress?
   C. Ask the child what she thinks is wrong or may help.
   D. Order an OCT of the macula.
   E. B and C
5. Which of the following conditions is the LEAST likely cause of acquired unilateral hyperopia:
   A. Adie's tonic pupil
   B. Choroidal melanoma
   C. Diabetes
   D. Central serous retinopathy
   E. Ciliary body tumor

Answers

1. Answer: B. A dislocation (and presumed tilt) of the crystalline lens superotemporally of the right eye will induce plus cylinder (and associated myopic sphere to compensate) in the direction of the tilt. Correcting cylinder (plus cylinder) will be needed in the meridian corresponding to the dislocation/tilt that will act at the axis located 90° away (at 30°).
2. Answer: C. The patient is likely experiencing night myopia and may appreciate a little stronger myopic pre-

[28] Enzenauer R, Morris W, O'Donnell, T, Montrey J. (2014). Functional ophthalmic disorders: Ocular malingering and visual hysteria. https://doi.org/10.1007/978-3-319-08750-4

scription just for her nighttime outdoor sports. As discussed in the text, a clinical examination and thorough history should be sufficient to rule out organic causes of nyctalopia. However, if the patient has a peripheral visual field defect or complains of seeing very poorly for all activities in the dark, then an ERG may be considered.

3. Answer: D. A tight suture at approximately location "D" corresponds to 80°. Cutting the suture at C (approximately 90°) or E (approximately 60°) may also be considered in the future, but at this time, cutting the suture at location D may have the most therapeutic effect.
4. Answer: E. As a follow-up from the clinical scenario presented in the text, the child was sitting happily on her mother's lap in the ED room. When asked by the clinician, "What do you think would help?," her excited response was "Glasses!" It turns out that the child wanted to wear glasses because her friends all wore glasses. A very expensive workup could have been avoided by asking the right questions and keeping the diagnosis of NOVL (whether intentional or unintentional) in the back of one's mind when encountering acute bilateral vision loss.
5. Answer: C. While diabetes can cause acquired bilateral myopia, it is an uncommon cause of acquired hyperopia, especially unilateral hyperopia. Adie's tonic pupil and central serous retinopathy are both (relatively) benign causes of unilateral hyperopia. Choroidal melanoma is a vision-threatening (and potentially life-threatening) cause of unilateral hyperopia. A ciliary body tumor is more likely to cause astigmatism with compensatory myopic sphere.

Optics for Clinical and Surgical Management of Strabismus

G. Vike Vicente

Objectives

- To apply previously discussed optics principles necessary for the proper dispensation of spectacle correction to patients with strabismus
- To troubleshoot glasses in patients with strabismus
- To understand the effect of refractive errors on the measurement of strabismus prior to surgery

Optical Dispensing for Clinical Management of Strabismus

While many patients with clinically significant strabismus may ultimately require surgery, initial treatment consists of various nonsurgical strategies, including glasses, patching, and use of therapeutic prisms. Examples of clinical prisms are addressed in further detail in Chap. 2 "Prisms in Ophthalmic Optics". Patching and other occlusion therapies are beyond the scope of this optics text. Therefore, we will focus our attention on clinical management using glasses and other optics principles previously discussed.

Note that there may be some overlap of material in this chapter and the next chapter, given that many patients with strabismus will inevitably be pediatric patients. These two chapters should be read consecutively so that the material from one chapter complements your understanding of the material from the other chapter.

Accommodative Esotropia (AET)

Accommodative esotropia (AET) usually presents around 2–3 years of age (range 6 months to 7 years). AET can be familial, present acutely or slowly, and demonstrate clinically significant esotropia (20–30Δ). It can occur with any refractive error including myopia or emmetropia, though moderate hyperopia (approximately +4D) is most common.[1]

The differential diagnosis must include infantile esotropia (primary esotropia), cranial nerve six palsies, Duane's syndrome, and neoplastic causes, such as posterior fossa tumors. Patients with AET usually will have full ductions but may have inferior oblique overaction.

There are several clinical examination considerations with optics relevance when evaluating AET patients:

- Prior to dilation, the strabismus should be <u>measured at near and distance</u> and with a + 3.0 D lens.
- Dynamic retinoscopy should be performed while focusing on an accommodative target at near (e.g., a small sticker). The examiner should watch for with motion which may help quantify the amount of hyperopia present.[2]
- It is crucial to fully cycloplege the patient in order to measure the full amount of hyperopia as the eventually dispensed glasses should match the full cycloplegic hyperopic refractive error. For example, if +3.00D sphere OU is measured during the cycloplegic refraction, then +3.00D glasses should be issued. Do <u>not</u> reduce or adjust the power of the glasses for AET patients.
- Dilation of AET patients involves using three sets of cyclopentolate drops given every five minutes and waiting at least 40 minutes for its full effect. Be wary of the overzealous resident who dumps an entire bottle of dilating drops while doing a half-nelson wrestling choke on a screaming 2-year-old!
- Watch for anticholinergic effects of the administered drops (psychosis, tachycardia, gastroparesis, dryness, flushing).

G. V. Vicente (✉)
Clinical Pediatrics and Ophthalmology Georgetown University Hospital, Washington, DC, USA

Eye Doctors of Washington, Chevy Chase, MD, USA
e-mail: vvicente@edow.com

[1] American Academy of Ophthalmology. Basic and Clinical Science Course, Section 6 Pediatrics, 2020–2021. San Francisco, CA: American Academy of Ophthalmology, 2021

[2] Recall the "SPAM" mnemonic from Chap. 15 Glasses in Clinical Practice: "**<u>S</u>**ame (with) motion, add **<u>P</u>**lus; **<u>A</u>**gainst motion, add **<u>M</u>**inus"

K. M. Riaz et al. (eds.), *Optics for the New Millennium*, https://doi.org/10.1007/978-3-030-95251-8_22

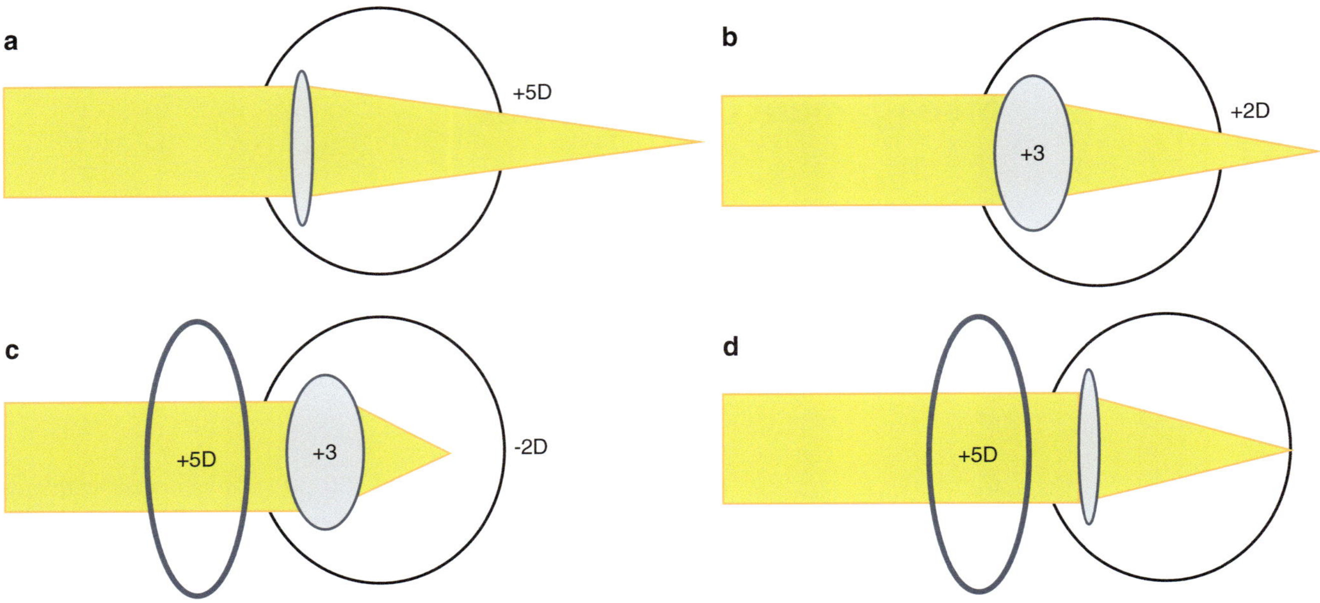

Fig. 1 Panel A represents a + 5D hyperopic eye with relaxed accommodation (i.e., no accommodation generated by the patient). Note the significant uncorrected refractive error. Panel B represents the child generating 3D of accommodation constantly, decreasing the refractive error to approximately +2 D. Blurry vision still remains. In Panel C, suppose that this child is given +5D glasses, she will initially continue to accommodate +3D. Therefore, initially, with the +5.0D glasses and generating +3.00D accommodation, she will see like a − 2.0D myope and complain of blurry distance vision. In panel D, atropine has been given so that the child is no longer in a constant accommodative state and is able to see clearly at distance with the +5.0D glasses

It is important to discuss the following points with the parents of the child:

- It may take some time for the child to adjust to the glasses. The child who has been constantly accommodating will continue to do so, even with the glasses in place, causing an initial period of blurry distance vision. The child may initially (and correctly) observe, "Mommy, everything far away is blurry with these glasses on!" In turn, the mom (or dad) may think to herself/himself, "Well, the glasses do seem rather thick and might be too strong, and the eye doctor seemed very young… Maybe they gave my child the wrong prescription or maybe the optical lab messed up the glasses?" To avoid this scenario, a short course of cycloplegic drops may be helpful: 1 drop of atropine 1% OU once a day for 1–3 days. Some doctors even recommend placing the atropine drops on the same day the child comes back to pick up the frames. Fig. 1 graphically displays the effects of immediate, persistent accommodation of a child with +5D hyperopia after receiving the full correction glasses.
- Remind the parent that wearing the glasses cannot harm the child. However, not wearing the glasses will permanently harm the child by worsening amblyopia and stereo acuity. If AET is not treated, then a non-accommodative surgical esotropia may develop in addition to the existing AET.
- Educate the parent that over the next few months, it is normal to see worsening of eye-crossing when the glasses are not worn.
- If the glasses do not control the AET, then strabismus surgery may be necessary within 6 months. Reassure the parents that it is not their fault that this condition occurred. It wasn't screen time or dim light or anything the parents did.
- Some kids may outgrow this condition over the next ten years, especially if one of the parents is a high myope. Kids who do not tolerate weaning the glasses may wear contacts or undergo excimer laser refractive surgery (ELRS) as adults if they are suitable candidates.
- The doctor may need to try several different strengths of glasses even after the initial dispensed glasses, including potentially prescribing bifocal glasses (especially in the presence of high AC/A ratio, which is discussed in the next section).
- Historically, the teaching was that glasses do not affect the amount of hyperopia; the hyperopia may fluctuate until age 7 and then slowly decreases, regardless of

whether the child wears the glasses or not.[3] However, recent studies have called this teaching into question.[4]

After the initial dispensing, the child will need to be followed up within 4–6 weeks. At this visit, in addition to making sure the frames fit the child well, several other considerations should be kept in mind:

- If the strabismus is fully controlled at near and distance when the glasses are worn, then the patient should continue wearing glasses full time and follow up every 6 months to continue to check for amblyopia, strabismus, and change in hyperopia. A cycloplegic refraction is typically performed every other visit to measure the latter.
- However, if there is still crossing at distance and the child has been diligently wearing the glasses, then a second cycloplegic refraction with atropine (instead of cyclopentolate) should be performed to try to unmask any latent hyperopia not detected during the original visit. If the previous refraction is confirmed, then the patient may have partially accommodative esotropia (see below) and require glasses and strabismus surgery. If additional hyperopic refractive error is found, then the stronger glasses should be issued.
- If the patient is orthophoric at distance but still has esotropia at near when the glasses are on, then the patient has a high AC/A (accommodative convergence/accommodation ratio).

Patients with High Accommodative Convergence/Accommodation Ratio (High AC/A)

This type of patient is a subset/variant of AET. In brief, if the patient is orthophoric at distance but still has intermittent ET at near, then it is likely that a high AC/A ratio exists.[5] These patients often have an average of +2.25D hyperopia[6] but over-converge for a given amount of accommodation, especially when compared to the previously discussed AET patients. Therefore, our goal should be to reduce the patient's exuberant convergence that happens during accommodation by giving additional plus power for near vision tasks. High AC/A patients will benefit from a flat top bifocal prescription (+3.00 add) that intersects the pupil.[7] Unfortunately, a very common error is for the optical shop to make the glasses with the usual "short" bifocal segments given to adults (Fig. 2).

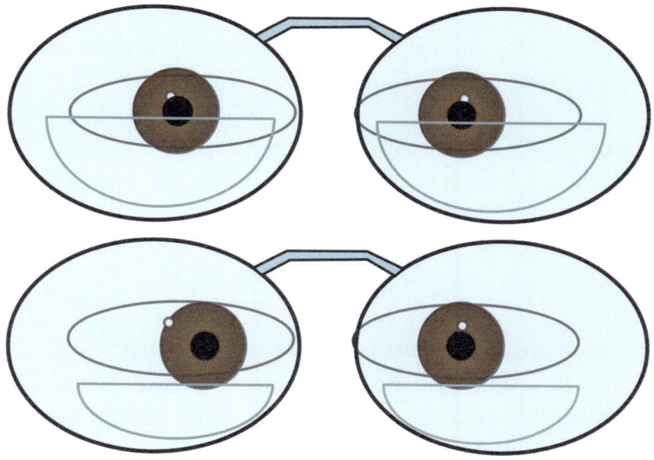

Fig. 2 A bifocal segment that is too low (bottom figure) will not help control the esotropia in patients with high AC/A. The bifocal line must intersect the pupil

Long term, if the child is now a tween and still needs an add at near to control their AET, then a progressive style lens could be used but with great care. The progressive add should be fitted 4 mm higher than an adult lens. Is the child still ortho and with good stereoacuity at near with the new glasses on? Is accommodation and reading okay?

Partially Accommodative Esotropia (Partial AET)

If esotropia at near or distance persists despite glasses with the full "cycloplegic refraction," a second cycloplegic refraction (including potential use of atropine 1%) should be considered. During this repeat refraction, if significant diplopia or crossing (>8PD) persists at near and distance, then partial AET is likely present, and strabismus surgery may be necessary in addition to glasses. Most surgeons base the amount of surgery on the near deviation present with glasses, while others may base their amount of surgery on the distance measurement and use a Faden procedure if the crossing at near is greater than the crossing at distance. A full discussion of the preferred surgical technique is beyond the scope of this text-

[3]Atkinson J, Anker S, Bobier W, Braddick O, Durden K, Nardini M, Watson P. Normal emmetropization in infants with spectacle correction for hyperopia. Invest Ophthalmol Vis Sci. 2000 Nov;41(12):3726–31

[4]Chang JW. Refractive error change and vision improvement in moderate to severe hyperopic amblyopia after spectacle correction: Restarting the emmetropization process? PLoS One. 2017 Apr 19;12(4):e0175780

[5]A mild degree of esophoria is acceptable at near with the glasses on, but there should be no actual esotropia or intermittent esotropia.

[6]This is a key difference between AET patients and AC/A patients. AET patients usually have higher amounts of hyperopia, whereas AC/A patients have low-moderate amounts of hyperopia.

[7]As you read this, you may be wondering if we are violating our rule from Chap. 12 Glasses for Written Exams, wherein we said to avoid giving flat-top bifocals to hyperopes whenever possible. However, there are several important considerations when considering pediatric patients. First, image displacement is better tolerated by kids as compared to adults. Second, prevention of amblyopia supersedes subjective visual complaints. Finally, in real-world optical practice, flat-tops are more commonly prescribed, regardless of refractive error, because they are cheaper to make and the problem of image displacement is thankfully not as visually debilitating as it theoretically seems. Recent advancements in lens construction, such as "digital lenses" (laser-etched lenses), have further minimized previous generation image jump and displacement effects.

book. Instead, you should know that a percentage of patients will likely fail nonsurgical interventions as described above and may eventually need strabismus surgery.

Adults with Accommodative Esotropia

It is not uncommon for AET to recur or worsen in patients in their late 20s. These patients may require a bifocal or readers at a younger age than their peers. Advanced cases of recurrence may ultimately require surgery as well.

Other Considerations for Patients with AET

There are several other considerations for patients with AET, especially as they get older and present for contact lenses, ELRS, and/or cataract surgery.

- Avoid monovision, whether through contact lenses, ELRS, or cataract surgery, in patients with good stereoacuity and intermittent strabismus. The difference in refractive error between the two eyes induced by the intervention may impair fusion and worsen their control on the intermittent strabismus. However, if the patient has a history of suppression, amblyopia, and/or well-controlled strabismus, monovision may be an option. It is crucial for the non-strabismus ophthalmologist to be aware of these conditions prior to any surgical intervention to avoid an unhappy patient (and eventual referral to a neuro-ophthalmologist or strabismus specialist)!
- It is important to avoid prolonged postoperative blurry vision in patients with intermittent strabismus. For example, if an unexpected refractive error occurs after first eye cataract surgery, the patient may need temporary glasses or contact lenses until the appropriate intervention (e.g., IOL exchange, piggyback IOL, staged ELRS, or second eye cataract surgery) can take place. Additionally, prolonged corneal edema may worsen strabismus control – surgeons may wish to use additional topical steroids and/or hypertonic saline to accelerate resolution of corneal edema.
- In myopes with a history of AET, it is important to avoid even slight hyperopic over-corrections with ELRS and/or cataract surgery. Postoperative hyperopia may lead to greater accommodative demand and recurrent ET. Therefore, erring for slight myopia (−0.25 to −0.50D) may be a safer surgical option, even for ELRS surgery.

Adult Esotropia (Adult ET)

While there are many causes of adult esotropia (adult ET), we will focus on those related to optics.

For example, some strabismologists have noticed an increased prevalence of adult ET in early presbyopes. One possible explanation is that some patients have a chronic activation of the near triad due to uncorrected accommodative needs.[8] This may occur either due to poor compliance with reading glasses or because their progressive glasses are not meeting their accommodative needs. As such, the increased accommodative demand can lead to worsening esotropia. These adult ET patients may be told by initial providers that reading glasses should be worn as needed for reading; however, if there is any esotropia present, then they must be encouraged to wear dedicated reading glasses (single vision reading glasses), bifocal or progressive with a high add, and a segment of proper height.

Convergence Insufficiency (CI)

Convergence insufficiency (CI) has a bimodal distribution, affecting both young and old patients. In younger patients, CI may not become symptomatic until 7–10 years of age, when convergence demands for near tasks (such as reading in school) exceed the patient's ability to converge. In older patients, CI may occur as a result of natural aging but also with pathological disease such as brainstem disorders and Parkinsonian neurodegenerative disorders.

CI can be diagnosed in the office with a good history and two simple tests. Important questions to ask during the history include:

- Asking the patient about fatigue or binocular diplopia during reading
- Asking about asthenopia symptoms (see Chap. 21 Clinical Problems with Optics and Refractive Manifestations)
- Asking the patient if he/she tends to close one eye when reading.
- Asking the patient and/or parent how long does it take for the symptoms to occur. For example, if little Suzy is able to play a game she enjoys on her mom's cellphone for two hours but then complains of "reading problems" after 5 minutes, then maybe it's not her eyes.
- Obtaining a good medical history (e.g., asking about hand tremors) and family history (e.g., history of relatives with Parkinson's disease, etc.)

Two in-office tests are especially useful:

1. The easiest is the near point of convergence (NPC) test, which is **not** the same as the optical near point. The NPC can be found by first having the patient wear his/her habitual near correction; the examiner can then move an

[8] Guyton DL. The 10th Bielschowsky Lecture: Changes in strabismus over time: The roles of vergence tonus and muscle length adaptation. Binocular Vision & Strabismus Quart 2006; 21:81-92

accommodative target (e.g., a target with small print) slowly closer to the patient until one eye drifts out or the patient reports seeing double. Most patients can sustain converging their eyes up to 5 cm from their nose; patients with CI may report symptoms (or you may notice eye drift) at a longer distance (range 10–30 cm).

2. The second test is the convergence amplitude (CA) test. The CA test is performed by using a **base-out** horizontal prism bar (in a pinch the rotary prisms in a phoropter may work too). The prism bar's 2 PD segment is held in front of either eye, while the patient is focusing on a near target using their normal reading correction. The bar is then slowly raised up to 35 PD. Most patients should be able to maintain a single object up to this prism. Patients with CI will have one eye drift out and see double when the bar reaches 10 or 15 PD base-out.

Here are two real scenarios in which optics may be helpful for patients with CI:

Scenario #1 A 22-year-old cramming for the LSAT exam reports: "Doctor, I see double when I read more than 30 minutes. I have my exam in 3 weeks, I do not have time for eye exercises to work."

In this scenario, in order to meet the immediate, time-sensitive needs of the patient, we can prescribe a pair of monofocal reading glasses with 5–7 PD base-in prism OU in order to help alleviate his symptoms in the short term. The patient can try these "reading glasses" in a trial frame in the office. We can first have the patient read for ten minutes with their usual correction and then offer the trial frame with additional prism power to see which strength is preferred. Another option may be to give a reading add, though this may be difficult for a non-presbyope to adjust in a short period of time. Finally, habitual modifications, such as advising the patient to hold books further away, may additionally help decrease convergence demands for near.

Scenario #2 A 78-year-old with a hand tremor complains, "Doctor, I'm having a hard time reading the paper. Closing one eye helps but my face gets tired after a while so I gave up reading."

In this scenario, novice practitioners would simply hear "I can't read" and give an additional reading add (e.g., a + 3.00D add instead of the +2.50D they had). But you, dear reader, are no novice! Suppose that the patient returns 1 week later, now complaining: "Doctor, with these new glasses I have to hold the paper closer and the double vision is worse!"

What happened? Closing one eye is a sign of diplopia; it is possible that the +3.00D add essentially shortened the working distance and actually made the convergence symptoms worse!

So what should the "non-novice" practitioner do? Some additional palliative options for this patient can be tried, in the following order:

1. Offer a **lower** + 2.00 add which will create a longer working distance. You can reassure the patient he/she can still read larger font but may have difficulty with extremely fine print: "You may not be able to read the stock pages but you will see less double." This may be especially useful in current times since many older patients are using electronic tablets and reading devices to make the font larger.
2. Try 5–7 PD base-in prisms OU in single vision reading glasses in the office in trial frames; if helpful, the patient can then purchase the glasses.
3. Try 8–12 PD Fresnel base-in prisms that are cut in such a manner so as to only cover the reading segment over the non-dominant eye (for more on prisms please see Chap. 2 "Prisms in Ophthalmic Optics").
4. Taping one bifocal segment with opaque tape. This should be the last resort.

Additional CI treatment options consist of convergence exercises using stereograms that can be performed by the patient at home. It is important to note that pediatric CI patients respond better to exercises as compared to adult CI patients – as the saying goes, "you can't teach an old dog new tricks." These can be provided by an orthoptist, an ophthalmologist, a developmental optometrist, or a pediatric optometrist. For pediatric CI patients, convergence exercises can be done as "outpatient therapy" in the office; as these are quite expensive, they should be reserved primarily for patients with poor home compliance.[9]

This last point is somewhat counterintuitive but bears worth mentioning. Some specialists may actually prescribe **base-out** glasses (as compared to the previously discussed base-in prisms) in order to treat pediatric CI. While the base-out glasses do not help the symptoms (they may initially worsen the symptoms), they may force the patient to converge and develop larger fusional amplitudes. Think of this approach like sending the patient to the gym: you have to break down muscles in order to build them up. Similarly, base-out glasses will force the pediatric patient to develop "stronger" convergence abilities. This approach is not very helpful with adult CI patients.

[9]Convergence Insufficiency Treatment Trial Study Group. Randomized clinical trial of treatments for symptomatic convergence insufficiency in children. Arch Ophthalmol. 2008 Oct;126(10):1336–49

Exotropia and Over-Minus Lenses

As with many things in life, we are initially taught certain rules should never be violated, only to later learn that there are exceptions to this rule. For example, as first-year residents, you may recall being taught that you should never over-minus a patient; this is a sin second only to sleeping with contact lenses overnight.[10]

However, there are two notable exceptions to this rule. The first exception is "extra-minus" correction given to night time athletes or for the treatment of night myopia, as discussed in Chap. 21 Clinical Problems with Optics and Refractive Manifestations. The second exception is for a young patient with intermittent exotropia (XT) who already wears minus glasses.

As residents we are taught to never ever over-minus a patient. However, there are two exceptions to this rule. The first, night time athletes, night time pilots, or truckers are addressed in the Night Myopia section. The 2nd exception is a young patient with intermittent exotropia who already wears glasses.[11]

For example, consider an 8-year-old patient who is a − 1.00D sphere who also has intermittent XT. This patient may be given 2–4D of "extra" minus power in both eyes. This "base-out" effect at distance caused by the over-minused glasses may then stimulate increased convergence to combat the induced worsening of the XT to neutralize the divergent strabismus. It is important to note that this approach will usually work only with younger patients; patients after age 20 may get headaches and may not be able to generate the needed convergence to combat the worsened XT.

As for hyperopic young patients with XT, they should be given partial strength glasses (approximately 2.0D less than the hyperopic cycloplegic refraction if they have >4.0D of hyperopia or 1.5D of hyperopic anisometropia). This is another one of those rare situations where less than the full cycloplegic refraction is given to a hyperopic patient with strabismus.

Use of Prisms for Clinical Management of Strabismus

Please see Chap. 2 "Prisms in Ophthalmic Optics", for additional discussion of using prisms in clinical practice to manage strabismus.

[10]Actually no, sleeping with contact lenses is the only unforgivable sin in ophthalmology. Everything else is negotiable.

[11]Watts P, Tippings E, Al-Madfai H. Intermittent exotropia, overcorrecting minus lenses, and the Newcastle scoring system. J AAPOS. 2005 Oct;9(5):460-4

Considerations for Strabismus Surgery in Patients with High Refractive Errors

For patients with minimal refractive errors, strabismus measurements taken while a patient is wearing his/her glasses may not be significantly different from measurements taken without glasses. However, in the setting of high refractive errors, especially myopia, measurements with glasses may significantly vary from measurements without glasses. Recall that both plus and minus lenses can be thought of as two prisms arranged together; the prismatic effect is especially pronounced when patients look away from the optical center (Fig. 3).

Consider a high myope patient wearing his/her glasses without strabismus. When this patient looks through the optical center of the glasses, there is essentially no prismatic deviation induced. However, now consider the same high myope patient with either an esotropia (ET) or exotropia (XT); given that the patient will look nasal or temporal to the optical center, respectively, this patient will have additional prismatic deviation as mentioned in previous discussions on Prentice's Rule.

Now suppose our myopic patient had a significant XT: this means that our patient will basically be looking through the temporal portion of the minus lens, which will cause additional base-out effect and **worsen** his XT. If we measure this patient's deviation with his glasses on, we will not only have to neutralize the pre-existing XT but also have to neutralize the "additional" XT caused by the glasses. Therefore, if we measured his XT with the glasses on, we will falsely over-measure this patient's XT.

This leads us to a simple but important rule: "*Minus measures more*." In other words, if a patient is wearing his/her myopic correction glasses and we measure the strabismus with the glasses on, we will falsely over-measure the patient's true deviation.

Forgetting this rule may lead to the following scenario:

Dr. Ima Havingabaday gets a call from his 1-day post-op myopic patient who had a bilateral lateral rectus recession for 60 PD of intermittent XT. The patient frantically exclaims over the phone: "Doc, I am seeing a lot of double vision. You said that could happen but I look very crossed-eyed!" Dr. HBD, as she is known around these parts, agrees to have the patient come in urgently. Repeat examination today confirms that the patient now has 12Δ of consecutive esotropia and will likely need to go back to the OR. The patient appears crestfallen and reaches for his phone to start an angry online review…

What may have happened? When Dr. HBD reviewed the chart, the optics mistake became all too clear. The patient's strabismus was measured while the patient was wearing her −10 D glasses. For example, consider that our patient actu-

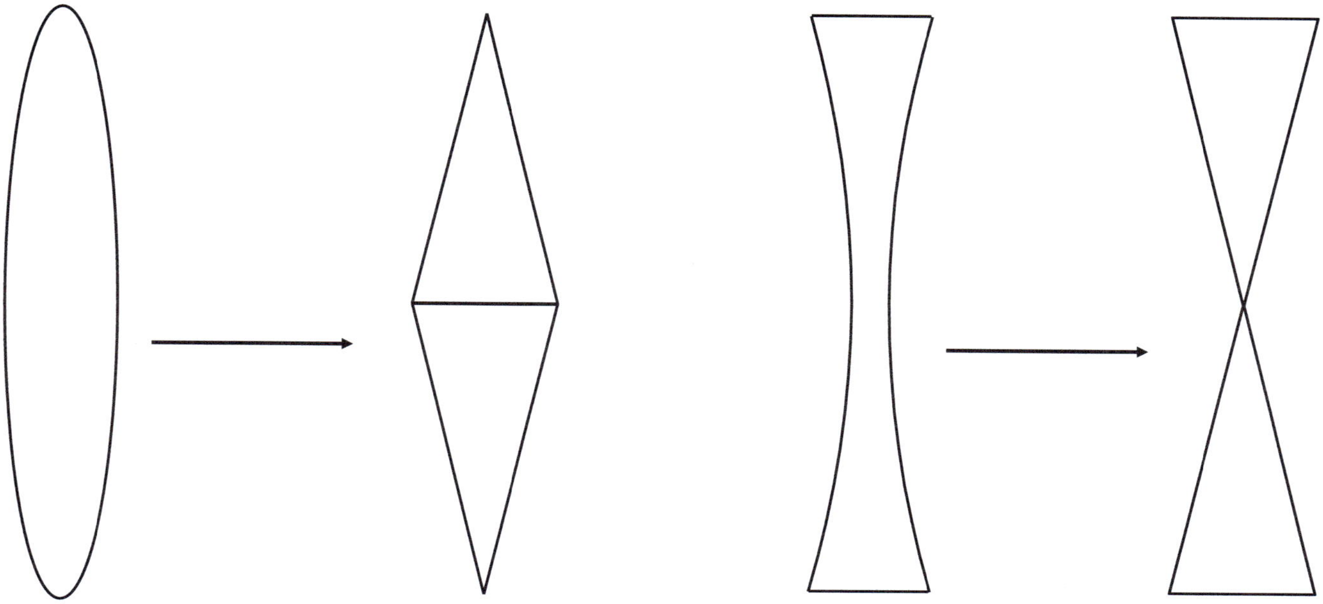

Fig. 3 Prismatic effects of plus and minus lenses. Note that the prismatic deviation increases as the patient looks further away from the optical center of the lens.

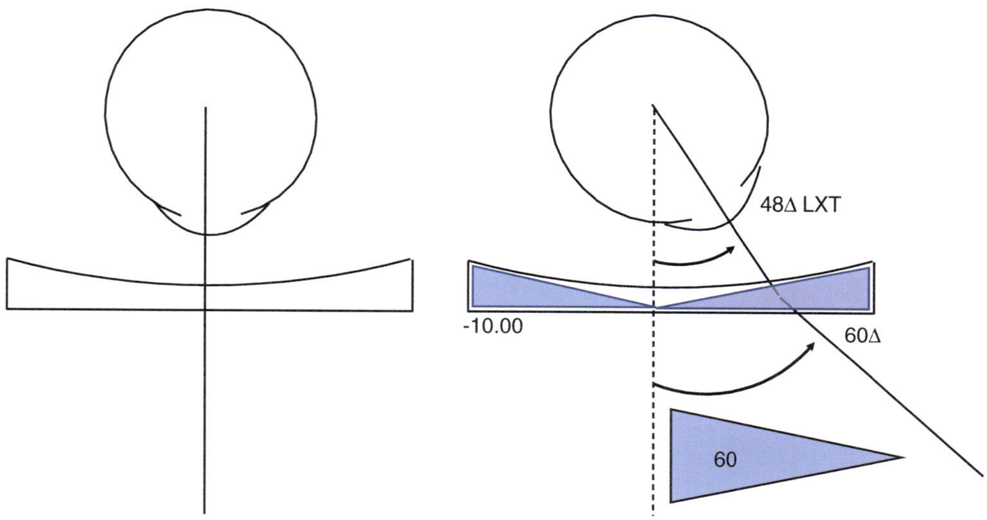

Fig. 4 "Minus Measures More." In this example, the −10 D sphere glasses confer a base-out effect given the pre-existing exotropia that causes the patient to look temporal to the optical center. Therefore, the measured exotropia (approximately 60 PD) is significantly more than the actual exotropia (48 PD)

ally had approximately 48 PD of exotropia without his glasses on. However, when wearing his −10D glasses, the measured exotropia increased due to the base-out effect of the high minus lenses (Fig. 4).

The 60 PD that were measured were therefore "too much" – instead of performing surgery for 48 PD XT, Dr. HBD accidentally did surgery for 60 PD XT, leading to the surgical over-correction, consecutive esotropia, and a poor online review.

So far, we have said that "minus measures more." But how much more? A detailed discussion on this quantification is best left for a strabismus text, but for now, we can use the following approximation:

$$\text{Prismatic effect} = (2.5) * (D)\%$$

where D = spectacle power. We can see that higher refractive errors will cause a higher prismatic effect. For our previous patient, these −10D sphere lenses will have a 25% prismatic effect on the measurement. We can then calculate:

$$0.25^{*}\ 48\Delta = 12\,\text{PD}$$

This minus lens will measure 12 PD additional XT on top of the actual 48 PD XT, leading to the erroneous measurement of 60 PD XT.

Interestingly, minus lenses will have the same effect whether the patient has an XT or ET! For our second example, let's suppose a new myopic patient has a 48 PD LET. Given her LET, our patient will look nasal to the optical center of the left lens (Fig. 5). However, in this example, there is additional **base-in** effect from the minus lens. It will appear to the viewer and the patient that there are 60 PD ET instead of the true 48 PD ET. This would lead to a similar surgical overcorrection of this patient as well.

Plus lenses have the opposite effect of minus lenses. For our third example, suppose we have a hyperopic patient wearing +10D sphere glasses with a 60 PD LXT. Due to the LXT, our patient will look through the temporal portion of the left lens, which would confer a **base-in** effect (Fig. 6). This would actually reduce the measured prism to approximately 48 PD. The examiner must realize that there is a prismatic effect due to the glasses in addition to the actual LXT. If the "glasses-on" measurements were used, there would be a surgical under-correction of the LXT.

In order to avoid this problem, we can either apply the above formula (preferred) or measure the strabismus without glasses. However, this might not be possible in patients with large refractive errors, especially hyperopic refractive errors, because without glasses, the patients may accommodate and

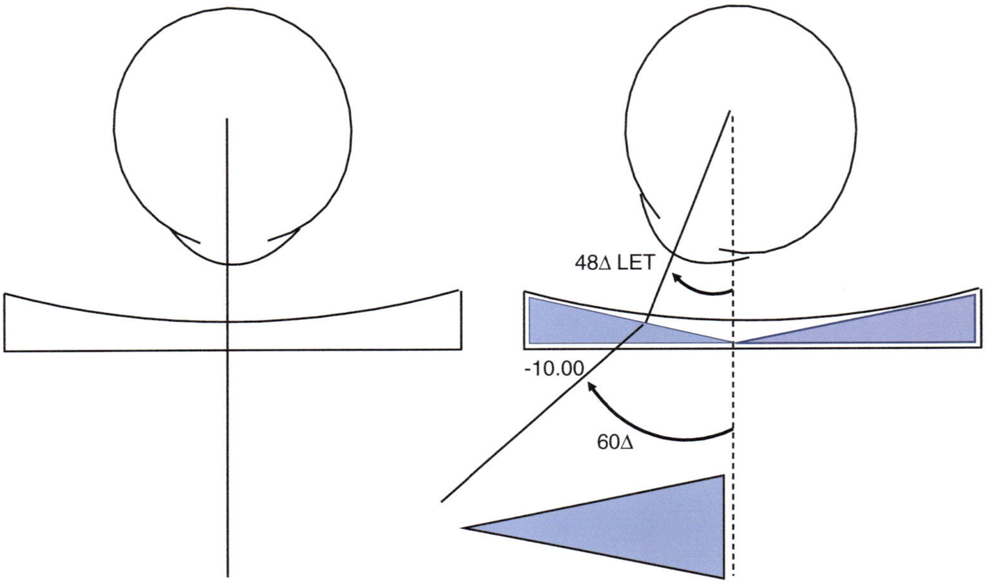

Fig. 5 "Minus Measures More." In this example, even if the same left eye were esotropic, the patient would be looking through the base-in prism portion of this myopic lens. This would similarly lead to a false over measurement of their strabismus

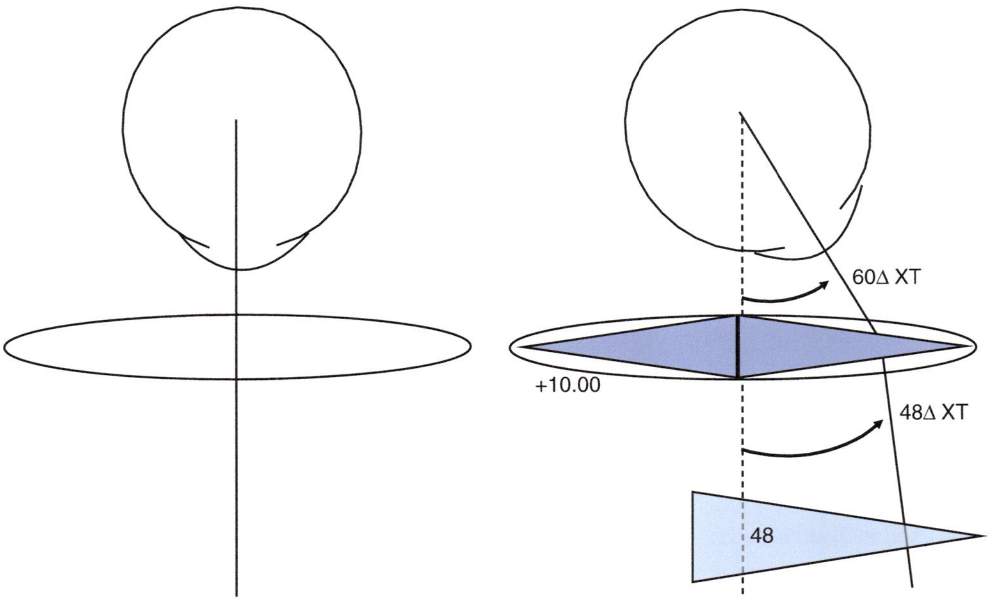

Fig. 6 Effect of plus lenses on measured strabismic deviation. In a hyperopic patient with LXT, the left eye will look through the temporal portion of the lens. The induced base-in prism will cause an underestimation of the true amount of XT

converge, further muddying the measurements. A third strategy may be to measure the strabismus while having patients wear contact lenses as a compromise between maintaining correction of refractive error while avoiding unwanted prismatic effects.

A final note on this subject: even though minus lenses measure more strabismus, it is important to note that the minification effect of high minus lenses will minimize the **appearance** of strabismus. Hyperopic lenses will exaggerate the **appearance** of strabismus due to their magnifying effect, while decreasing the amount of strabismus measured.

Practice Questions

1. If a −16D sphere OU esotropic patient measures 42 PD ET with her glasses on, what angle of deviation would you operate for?
   A. 54 PD ET
   B. 30 PD ET
   C. 32 PD ET
   D. 25 PD ET
2. If a + 10D aphakic OU patient measures 15 PD XT, what amount of deviation would you operate for?
   A. 20 PD XT
   B. 25 PD XT
   C. 10 PD XT
   D. 12 PD XT
3. A 3-year-old comes back for a 6-week follow-up after purchasing his first pair of glasses for accommodative esotropia. His parents state he refuses the glasses. You measure the glasses and they are made correctly: +3.50 D sphere OU and are equal to your last cycloplegic refraction. The frame appears to fit the child well. You measure the child's vision:
   - VA sc 20/25 OD and OS
   - VA cc 20/40 OD and OS
   - He is orthophoric with his glasses on and has 25 PD of Esotropia at near and distance without glasses. Your next step should be:

   A. Re-refract the patient and confirm if the previous cycloplegic refraction was correct.
   B. Tell the parents to insist on the child wearing the glasses.
   C. Consider bilateral medial rectus recession because the glasses are not working.
   D. Give a drop of atropine 1% OU to help relax his accommodation and transition into his hyperopic correction.

Answers

1. Answer: B. Prismatic effect % = (2.5) * (*D*) %, 2.5 X 16D = 40%; thus, a −16D will have a 40% increase in the measurement. Therefore, the true measurement was 30 PD, 40% of 30 = 12PD, Minus Measures More, 30 + 12 = 42 PD.
2. Answer: A. 2.5 X + 10D = 25% prismatic of under-measurement. If the true deviation was 20PD, then 20 X 0.25 = 5PD prismatic effect. (Plus Measures Less) 20−5PD = 15 PD measured XTcc.
3. Answer: D. The child is fogging himself by chronically accommodating; one or two doses of atropine 1% should help. Re-refract if this does not work or if there is still crossing at distance with the glasses on. Strabismus surgery is NOT indicated because the glasses are controlling the esotropia when they are worn.

Pediatric Optics

G. Vike Vicente

Objectives

- To discuss the importance of treating refractive errors, including hyperopia, myopia, and astigmatism to prevent amblyopia in pediatric patients
- To review several special circumstances wherein extra consideration for the construction of glasses may be needed, such as bifocals for aphakia, accommodative insufficiency, and treatment of accommodative esotropia
- To highlight important features of constructing and dispensing glasses in children
- To introduce key principles of contact lens dispensation in pediatric patients
- To briefly discuss advanced topics, such as myopia control, which are of significant interest among practitioners currently

Introduction

One of the most common questions from my comprehensive ophthalmology colleagues is: If a child has "x" cycloplegic refraction, what prescription should I actually give? Is it "x" or do I need to change it to "y"? While the dispensation of glasses and contact lenses has been previously discussed in Chap. 15, "Glasses in Clinical Practice", this chapter will instead focus on a very cute, very unique (and occasionally frustrating!) segment of the human population that is not old enough to drive but makes it all worthwhile if you can successfully improve their vision.

Uncorrected Ametropia and Risks of Amblyopia

Adults with refractive errors (ametropias) may primarily complain of blurry vision; usually, with successful refraction (glasses or contact lenses), the refractive error is neutralized and patients have excellent vision, even if they have gone months or years without glasses. In children, especially from birth to puberty, significant ametropias (especially uncorrected unilateral refractive errors) may lead to permanent visual loss in the form of amblyopia or loss of stereoacuity.

As with the rest of medicine, doctors should intervene if something is bothering or harming the patient. This applies to issuing glasses in children. Most adults wear glasses because the uncorrected refractive error bothers them. With children, we must be aware that uncorrected refractive errors can cause permanent harm to a child's sight in the form of amblyopia or loss of stereoacuity.[1] Thanks to the use of photo-screeners and primary care vision screening, many children with amblyopia risk factors are found early enough to treat successfully.[2] Children with a diagnosis of amblyopia, or with significant risk factors for amblyopia, should be treated without delay in order to prevent any or additional irreversible vision loss.

G. V. Vicente (✉)
Clinical Pediatrics and Ophthalmology Georgetown University Hospital, Washington, DC, USA

Eye Doctors of Washington, Chevy Chase, MD, USA
e-mail: vvicente@edow.com

[1] DeSantis D. Amblyopia. Pediatr Clin North Am. 2014 Jun; 61(3):505–18.

[2] Koo EB, Gilbert AL, VanderVeen DK. Treatment of Amblyopia and Amblyopia Risk Factors Based on Current Evidence. Semin Ophthalmol. 2017;32(1):1–7

K. M. Riaz et al. (eds.), *Optics for the New Millennium*, https://doi.org/10.1007/978-3-030-95251-8_23

Criteria for Unilateral Versus Bilateral Amblyopia

Amblyopia can occur in one eye or both the eyes. Unilateral amblyopia is defined as patients with an amblyogenic factor and:

- Asymmetrical objection to monocular occlusion or
- Failure to initiate or maintain fixation or
- Interocular difference of two or more octaves with Teller fixation preference cards or
- Interocular difference of two or more lines in visual acuity charts.[3]

Bilateral amblyopia is defined as:

- Limited best corrected visual acuity <20/50 in patients 3–4 years old
- Worse than 20/40 in patients 4–5 years old and
- Worse than 20/30 in patients older than 5 years old

Risk Factors for Refractive Amblyopia

The type and quantity of refractive error increases the risk of amblyopia depending on the patient's age. Some types of refractive errors are more dangerous than others! Table 1) below lists cut-off values and guidelines for which clinicians should be concerned about a significant risk of amblyopia. Note that these values are based on consensus as there are not many rigorous published data for guidance. Ultimately, the clinician should use these guidelines and customize monitoring and therapy based on each individual patient. For example, the cut-off values should be lower if a child has anisometropia *with strabismus*.

The key point here is that if refractive amblyopia is caught early (when the vision is better than 20/80), it can often be treated with glasses alone.[4] Therefore, it is important to remind patients that glasses are primarily treating (and preventing) amblyopia, not just the refractive error. If the amblyopia does not improve with glasses alone, then further intervention (such as patching and use of cycloplegics) may be necessary.

Table 1 Guidelines for refractive correction in infants and young children

Refractive error (diopters)				
Condition	< 1 year	1–2 years	2–3 years	3–4 years
Isometropia				
Myopia	−5.0	−4.0	−3.0	−2.5
Hyperopia without esotropia	+6.0	+5.0	+4.5	+3.5
Hyperopia with esotropia	+2.0	+2.0	+1.5	+1.5
Astigmatism	3.0	2.5	2.0	1.5
Anisometropia without strabismus				
Myopia	−4.0	−3.0	−3.0	−2.5
Hyperopia	+2.5	+2.0	+1.5	+1.5
Astigmatism	2.5	2.0	2.0	1.5

Reproduced with permission from the American Academy of Ophthalmology Pediatric Eye Evaluations Preferred Practice Patterns 2017 Guidelines

Dispensing Glasses in Children

Please review the section in Chap. 15, "Glasses in Clinical Practice", that discusses considerations for prescribing glasses in children, such as principles of frame fitting and sizing. In this section, we will discuss several additional key principles.

Visual Acuity Needs in Children

For children without amblyopia or strabismus, there are no set guidelines regarding how much or what kind of refractive error merits glasses correction. Most clinicians will dispense glasses if a child's refractive error is causing symptoms, such as blurred uncorrected near or distance vision <20/40. Wearing glasses is optional as long as the uncorrected refractive error is not harming the child's vision or affecting their learning.[5] This threshold may change with time; for example, an older child may be more discerning than a younger one, as they may have to read smaller print on a classroom board or a page.

In kindergarten (age 5–6 years), most activities are hands on and up close; this keeps the child's attention primarily for near vision tasks. Patients with low myopic refractive errors may not complain of any difficulty with these tasks (especially if given the chance to play with mom or dad's cell

[3]Wallace DK, Morse CL, Melia M, Sprunger DT, Repka MX, Lee KA, Christiansen SP; American Academy of Ophthalmology Preferred Practice Pattern Pediatric Ophthalmology/Strabismus Panel. Pediatric Eye Evaluations Preferred Practice Pattern®: I. Vision Screening in the Primary Care and Community Setting; II. Comprehensive Ophthalmic Examination. Ophthalmology. 2018 Jan; 125(1):P184–P227.

[4]Cotter SA; Pediatric Eye Disease Investigator Group, Edwards AR, Wallace DK, Beck RW, Arnold RW, Astle WF, Barnhardt CN, Birch EE, Donahue SP, Everett DF, Felius J, Holmes JM, Kraker RT, Melia M, Repka MX, Sala NA, Silbert DI, Weise KK. Treatment of anisometropic amblyopia in children with refractive correction. Ophthalmology. 2006 Jun;113(6):895–903

[5]Interestingly, as discussed in Chap. 21, these days there may be a fair number of school-age children who present actually *wanting* glasses because it is the "cool" thing to wear in school...

phone!). However, when the child is presented with distance vision tasks, such as looking at the teacher or blackboard, he/she may complain of blurry vision. Also, objects in the periphery may distract the child.

Langford et al. showed that most distance visual acuity demands in KG through second grade are comparable to 20/200 vision; in grades 3–5, 20/80 visual acuity is needed.[6] For near activities (approx. 16 inches) in this age range, the visual acuity demand ranges from 20/100 to 20/500. This is helpful not only for dispensing glasses, but also vision rehabilitation needs. For example, most low vision specialists will try to achieve at least 20/40 vision for the patients through optical aids, such as loupes or telescopes for patients in this age range. Please refer to Chap. 19, Low Vision and Vision Rehabilitation for more information on this topic.

As children continue to grow older (after age 10), visual acuity needs are approximately the same as adult patients.

A child who appreciates the glasses will confirm the physician's suspicion that the benefit in vision outweighs the nuisance caused by the frames. However, there may be a significant number of pediatric patients that do not accept wearing glasses for other reasons as discussed in Chap. 15, "Glasses in Clinical Practice". To summarize, if the refraction is accurate and the child refuses to wear the glasses, other factors to consider include the following:

- An error in the lenses
- Poor fitting frames
- Cosmetic reasons
- Psychosocial reasons
- Poor parental compliance and/or parental support
- Somewhat simple, but paradoxical: the child may feel that his/her uncorrected blurred vision is not bothering him/her that much

Hyperopic Refractive Errors

Most children are born with low levels of hyperopia: this may be benign and asymptomatic, especially as the eye continues to grow.[7] As discussed above, kids with moderate hyperopia or anisometropic hyperopia should be given glasses to prevent amblyopia. Children older than 4 years may require hyperopic correction if they have symptoms with near vision. Checking near vision and dynamic retinoscopy (See Chap. 17, "Optical Instruments and Machines") prior to dilation is very useful in assessing if a child has

Table 2 Comparison of measured in-office cycloplegic refraction for hyperopic pediatric patients and glasses dispensed

Patient age (Years)	Cycloplegic refraction OU (D)	Glasses to be dispensed
2, no strabismus	+4.0	None
2, with strabismus	+4.0	+4.0
2, no strabismus	+7.0	+5.5

enough accommodation to compensate for his/her hyperopia. As children can accommodate easily, most physicians will "shave off" 1.5–2.0D from the cycloplegic refraction when dispensing glasses. If patients have concurrent hyperopia with accommodative esotropia (AET) then the full cycloplegic hyperopic refraction is issued. See Chap. 22, "Optics for Clinical and Surgical Management of Strabismus", for a more detailed discussion regarding AET.

Table 2 may be helpful to illustrate the in-office cycloplegic refraction (CRx) vs. the dispensed glasses. Note that in patients *without* strabismus, the CRx is adjusted; however, in patients *with strabismus*, the full CRx is given.

Remember that a young patient without strabismus, who is incorrectly issued the full cycloplegic refraction will (unintentionally) continue to accommodate and fog themselves by 1.5–2D, thus seeing blurry at distance with the glasses just like an uncorrected −1.5D myope. See Fig. 1 in Chap. 22, "Optics for Clinical and Surgical Management of Strabismus", for a detailed illustration of this concept.

If a child with strabismus needs to wear his/her full CRx glasses, then a drop of atropine 1% may be placed in both eyes at the time he/she receives the glasses to help relax accommodation and transition into the full-strength hyperopic glasses. Arm splints have fallen out of favor (thankfully!).

Finally, it is important to reassure the parents that it may take a few days for the child to get used to wearing glasses, regardless of whether or not the child has any concurrent strabismus.

Myopic Refractive Errors

While common in teens and adults, myopia in young children (including toddlers and infants) is less common; these patients should undergo a comprehensive workup to rule out any lens, glaucoma, collagen, and/or retinal abnormalities, especially if there is no family history of early myopia. As the world of young children is mainly focused at near, low to moderate myopia is often asymptomatic, well-tolerated and does not merit glasses. If the child is symptomatic, if the refractive error exceeds −1.0D, or the child has <20/40 uncorrected vision in the better eye, glasses may be strongly considered.

[6]Langford A, Hug T. Visual Demands in Elementary School. J Pediatr Ophthalmol Strabismus. 2010;47:152–156.

[7]The commonly heard phrase, "Johnny grew out of his glasses," may apply here.

Table 3 Comparison of measured in-office cycloplegic refraction for myopic pediatric patients and glasses dispensed

Patient age	Cycloplegic refraction OU (D)	Glasses to be dispensed
3	−10.00	−8.00
4	−0.50	None
5 (with intermittent XT)	−2.00	−4.00
6	−1.25	−1.25

As discussed in Chap. 22, "Optics for Clinical and Surgical Management of Strabismus", young patients with intermittent exotropia (XT) may be given extra-minus ("over minused") power glasses to help control the strabismus.[8] Wearing an additional -2D more than the myopic refractive error will stimulate the patient to accommodate and induce convergence. For example, if a child with intermittent XT has −1.5D of myopia, −3.5D lenses may be tried. Studies have shown that wearing this "extra" minus power did not accelerate or worsen myopia in these patients.[9]

For most patients, the full amount of myopia measured with a cycloplegic refraction is issued. However, in patients <4 years old with severe myopia (e.g., > -6D sphere), the final dispensed refraction can be reduced by 1–2D since most of the child's attention is at near, not distance. For example, a 2-year-old child who is a -10D may be issued a -8D glasses instead of the full -10D glasses.

Table 3 may be helpful to illustrate the in-office refraction vs. the recommended dispensed refraction in myopic patients.

Now for some controversy: there is much debate among pediatric ophthalmologists regarding whether or not to *intentionally under correct myopia* with the long-term goal of slowing myopic progression – sort of a short-term pain for long-term gain approach. The idea behind this thinking is that intentional under-correction of myopia will limit accommodative demand and accommodative lag at near. The other school of thought advocates an approach to *intentionally over correct the myopia* with glasses so that they last longer. Some studies have shown an increased myopic shift when young myopic patients are under-corrected.[10]

[8]Rowe FJ, Noonan CP, Freeman G, DeBell J. Intervention for intermittent distance exotropia with overcorrecting minus lenses. Eye (Lond). 2009 Feb;23(2):320–5

[9]Kushner BJ. Does overcorrecting minus lens therapy for intermittent exotropia cause myopia? Arch Ophthalmol. 1999 May;117(5):638–42

[10]Vasudevan B, Esposito C, Peterson C, Coronado C, Ciuffreda KJ. Under-correction of human myopia--is it myopigenic?: a retrospective analysis of clinical refraction data. J Optom. 2014 Jul-Sep;7(3):147–52.

Table 4 Comparison of in-office refraction versus the recommended dispensed refraction based on different refractive errors

Patient age (years)	Cycloplegic refraction OU (D)	Glasses to be dispensed
1	+1.00 + 1.00 × 90	None
1	+1.50 + 3.00 × 90	Plano +3.00 × 90
1	Plano +3.00 × 90	−1.50 + 3.00 × 90
1	−2.00 + 3.00 × 90	−2.00 + 3.00 × 90

Astigmatic Refractive Errors

In general, younger patients tolerate glasses with the full astigmatism correction (regardless of type and/or quantity) better than adults. Recall that with adults, it is acceptable to reduce the astigmatism correction to ensure better tolerance, especially with high amounts of astigmatism and/or oblique astigmatism.

With kids, it is a different story: we want to ensure that amblyopia does not set in, so it is crucial to give the full astigmatism correct, regardless of the cylinder amount or the axis of astigmatism. One rule of thumb recommended in these scenarios: if the spherical equivalent (SE) is plano or hyperopic, then we can reduce the sphere by 1.5D (i.e., additional minus sphere correction).

Table 4 may be helpful to illustrate the in-office refraction vs. the recommended dispensed refraction in an imaginary pediatric patient (age 1 year) with significant astigmatism and various spherical refractive errors.

Prescribing Bifocals in Children

Bifocals are rarely required in young patients. If a bifocal is prescribed, the reading segment should intersect the pupil. See Chap. 22, "Optics for Clinical and Surgical Management of Strabismus", for a detailed discussion regarding when bifocals may be needed.

The following types of pediatric patients may benefit from bifocals:

- Patients who have aphakia or pseudophakia (see the below sections for more information on these special situations).
- Accommodative esotropia (AET) with high AC/A (accommodative convergence over accommodation). In some patients with AET, spectacles with the full cycloplegic refraction will help control the strabismus for distance, but they will not work as well at near and a residual esotropia may be present. In this case, a + 3.00D sphere add OU may be required.
- Accommodation Insufficiency (AI). This can be checked with a near vision card, and/or dynamic retinoscopy

where the undilated child is trying to focus on a near accommodative target next to the retinoscope. If "with motion" retinoscopy is present, then accommodation is insufficient at that distance and a bifocal should be included in the glasses.

- Patients with Down's Syndrome may experience early AI around the time they reach school age.[11]
- Patients who have had a concussion may as well have AI.[12]

Anisometropia and Aniseikonia in Children

See Chap. 8, "Magnification and Telescopes", for additional discussion regarding anisometropia and aniseikonia. We will refrain from making any more pirate jokes in this chapter even though, deep down me hearties, we all enjoy such humor.

Recall that anisometropia is when the quantitative refractive error between each eye is more than 3D. Anisometropia leads to aniseikonia, which is the difference in *size perception* due to anisometropia. Most adult patients can only tolerate a 6–7% size difference between the two eyes.

In pediatric patients, anisometropia and aniseikonia are not as significant as they are in adults; remember that uncorrected refractive errors, especially unilateral ones, may lead to amblyopia. In addition, kids tend to tolerate the subjective difference between the two eyes much better than adults. For example, we can assume that a pediatric patient with anisometropia (e.g., OD: +1D, OS: +4.50D) will fixate with the better seeing eye (OD). Since accommodation is usually simultaneous and bilateral, we can also assume that the non-dominant eye will be accommodating as well.

We can use some examples to highlight this concept:

Anisometropia without Strabismus

Example #1

Suppose we have an 18-month-old child without strabismus with the following CRx:

$$\text{OD}: +1.00\,\text{D sphere}$$

$$\text{OS}: +4.00\,\text{D sphere}$$

This patient will be fixating with his right eye (likely the dominant eye based on the refractive error) and generating +1.00D accommodation in both eyes; this is the bare minimum accommodation needed to see clearly with the right eye without any correction. As such, the "effective" uncorrected refractive error in the left eye is actually +3.00D. This has a high risk of causing refractive amblyopia.

Therefore, we can dispense glasses with the following prescription:

$$\text{OD}: \text{plano}$$

$$\text{OS}: +3.00\text{D sphere}$$

Note that the dispensed glasses prescription for the left eye is not equal to the CRx because of the principles we discussed above.

Example #2

Suppose we have an 18-month-old child without strabismus with the following CRx:

$$\text{OD}: +4.00\text{D sphere}$$

$$\text{OS}: +7.00\text{D sphere}$$

The following glasses prescription should be issued:

$$\text{OD}: +2.50\text{D sphere}$$

$$\text{OS}: +5.50\text{D sphere}$$

Note that this patient has anisometropia. However, since the patient does not have any strabismus, we can reduce the CRx by approximately 1.5D in both eyes with the assumption that the child can easily generate this accommodation on his own. The patient still has anisometropia, which is acceptable to leave as is in this age group.

Example #3

Suppose we have (yet another) 18-month-old child without strabismus with the following CRx:

$$\text{OD}: +1.00 + 1.00 \times 90\ (\text{SE}: +1.5\text{D})$$

$$\text{OS}: +4.00 + 1.00 \times 90\ (\text{SE}: +4.5\text{D})$$

This patient is likely to fixate with her right eye and is used to accommodating +1.5D with both eyes to see clearly at a distance without correction. As such, the effective uncorrected refractive error in the left eye is +2.50 + 1.00 x 90 (SE: +3.00), which will cause refractive amblyopia.

Therefore, we should issue glasses with the following prescription:

$$\text{OD}: -0.50 + 1.00 \times 90$$

$$\text{OS}: +2.50 + 1.00 \times 90$$

[11]de Weger C, Boonstra N, Goossens J. Effects of bifocals on visual acuity in children with Down syndrome: a randomized controlled trial. Acta Ophthalmol. 2019; 97(4):378–393.

[12]Green W, Ciuffreda KJ, Thiagarajan P, Szymanowicz D, Ludlam DP, Kapoor N. Accommodation in mild traumatic brain injury. J Rehabil Res Dev. 2010; 47(3):183–199.

Anisometropia with Strabismus

Example #4

Suppose we have a 24-month-old *with 25 PD LET* with the following CRx:

$$OD: +1.00 + 1.00 \times 90$$

$$OS: +4.00 + 1.00 \times 90$$

For this patient, we have two choices: (1) Dispense the full CRx (because the patient has a significant LET) and (2) adjust the dispensed CRx with the assumption that the patient can comfortably accommodate +1.5D on her own:

Therefore, our two choices are:

$$\text{Choice}\#1: OD: +1.00 + 1.00 \times 90, OS: +4.00 + 1.00 \times 90$$

$$\text{Choice}\#2: OD: -0.50 + 1.00 \times 90, OS: +2.50 + 1.00 \times 90$$

This scenario is a bit more complicated because we did not specify if the LET was an accommodative ET (AET) or sensory ET. If further examination revealed that the patient had an AET, then the *full cycloplegic refraction* should be given. However, if we were certain that this is a sensory (refractive) ET, then it is acceptable to reduce the prescription to allow the patient to accommodate and see if that is enough to control the esotropia.[13]

Considerations for Dispensing Contact Lenses in Children

Contact lenses (CL) may be required for children with aphakia after cataract surgery without IOL placement, as in the case of infantile cataracts or trauma.

In infants and toddlers with unilateral aphakia, while inserting the CL may be initially challenging, the CL may provide better compliance and vision than glasses alone. As we have mentioned several times in the chapter (intentionally), a young child's attention is primarily focused at near. The refractive goal with a CL should therefore aim for intentional low-myopia, approximately −1 to -3D in both eyes.

For example, if the CRx of the left eye of an aphakic 1 year old is +20D, then a + 23D CL can be dispensed to yield approximately -3D "corrected" refractive error. This allows the child to maintain some myopia to focus on objects at near.

In older (school age and beyond) patients, contact lenses may be prescribed on a case-by-case basis. Several important questions to consider:

- Is the child responsible enough to remove and clean the contacts nightly? Remember the cardinal sin of ophthalmology: sleeping with contact lenses. A good question to assess whether the child is ready for this responsibility may be, "Can the child brush his teeth nightly without being nagged?" If a child demonstrates good compliance, motivation, and responsibility, CLs can be cautiously tried in these patients. Ironically enough, corneal ulcers due to irresponsible use tend to occur in *older* patients, not responsible 9-year-olds![14]
- Similarly, it is important to *not force* a child who is not motivated to wear CLs.
- Affordability: CLs are (usually) more expensive than spectacles. Some clinicians encourage older children to raise some of the money required to instill a sense of responsibility towards CLs.
- CLs may also be used for myopia control. This has become a very popular topic in recent years and will be discussed in greater detail in the next chapter.
- Since CLs decrease the negative effects of anisometropia and aniseikonia, stereoacuity may be significantly improved with CLs vs. glasses. School age patients who play sports that require fine motor skills and rapid hand-eye coordination (e.g., baseball and hockey) may benefit from CL use during these activities.

Practice Questions

1. An 18-month-old patient without strabismus has a cycloplegic refraction (CRx) of: +7.00 D sphere OU. What glasses should be dispensed?
   A. +7.00D sphere OU
   B. +5.50D sphere OU
   C. +2.00D sphere OU
   D. No glasses at this time.
2. A 24-month-old patient with 20 PD of esotropia at near *and* distance has a CRx of: +3.50 D sphere OU. What glasses should be dispensed?
   A. +3.50D sphere OU
   B. +2.00D sphere OU

[13] Admittedly, you may need to read this example a few times to fully appreciate and understand the nuances behind it. One suggested way: try to teach this to your significant other or a group of friends – if they can understand it, you probably understand it well! We do not take any responsibility for your popularity level plummeting as a result of this nerd maneuver, however.

[14] Chalmers RL, Wagner H, Mitchell GL, Lam DY, Kinoshita BT, Jansen ME, Richdale K, Sorbara L, McMahon TT. Age and other risk factors for corneal infiltrative and inflammatory events in young soft contact lens wearers from the Contact Lens Assessment in Youth (CLAY) study. Invest Ophthalmol Vis Sci. 2011 Aug 24; 52(9):6690–6.

C. +3.50D sphere OU with +3.00D add bifocal OU
D. The patient will not benefit from any glasses at this time and will instead need to undergo strabismus surgery.

3. A 24-month-old patient is wearing +2.00D sphere glasses OU and has a CRx of +2.00D sphere OU. She is orthophoric at distance but has 20 PD of esotropia at near with her glasses on. What is the appropriate next step?
   A. Continue with the current glasses full time
   B. Plan strabismus surgery
   C. Schedule MRI and further neurological workup to rule out intracranial mass.
   D. Change current glasses to a + 2.0 sph with a + 3.0 bifocal add OU.
4. A 24-month-old patient with 30 PD of esotropia at distance is orthophoric at near. He has a cycloplegic refraction of +2.00D sphere OU. What is the appropriate next step?
   A. Observe for now, continue to watch for amblyopia.
   B. Plan strabismus surgery.
   C. Schedule MRI and further neurological workup to rule out intracranial mass.
   D. Try +2.00D sphere glasses.
5. A 10-month-old patient has a − 3.00D sphere OU CRx. What glasses should be dispensed?
   A. None
   B. −1.00D sphere OU
   C. −3.00D sphere OU
   D. −4.50D sphere OU
6. A 3-year-old patient has a CRx:
   OD: +3.00D sphere (VA 20/25)
   OS: +5.00D sphere (VA 20/70)
   Examination reveals that there is no strabismus present. Which of the following choices represents a reasonable choice for the dispensed prescription glasses?
   A. +3.00D OD, +5.00D OS
   B. +1.50D OD, +3.50D OS
   C. +3.00D OU
   D. +5.00D OU
7. A 5-year-old patient has a CRx:
   +1.00 + 4.00 × 90 OU.
   Examination reveals that there is no strabismus present. What glasses should be dispensed?
   A. +1.00 + 4.00 × 90
   B. −2.00 + 4.00 × 90
   C. −0.50 + 4.00 × 90
   D. +1.00 + 2.00 × 90
8. A 3-year-old patient without strabismus has a CRx:
   OD: Plano, OS: +4.00D sphere
   What glasses should be dispensed?
   A. OD: -1.50D, OS: +2.50D
   B. OD: Plano, OS: +4.00D
   C. OD: +4.00D, OS: +4.00D
   D. OD: Plano, OS +4.00D; with +3.00D bifocal add OU
9. A 5-year-old patient without strabismus has a CRx:
   −2.00 + 4.00 × 180 OU
   What glasses should be dispensed OU?
   A. −3.50 + 4.00 × 180
   B. −1.00 + 2.00 × 180
   C. −2.00 + 2.00 × 180
   D. −2.00 + 4.00 × 180
10. A 6-month-old is aphakic in her right eye. She is wearing a + 20 D contact lens in her right eye. A cycloplegic over-refraction over her contact lens shows +1D sphere OD. What contact lens power should be prescribed?
    A. +19 D
    B. +20 D
    C. +21 D
    D. +24 D

Answers

1. **Answer: B.** If the child has >5D of hyperopia and no esotropia is present, then 1.5D sphere can be reduced ("shaved off") off the measured CRx. Note that this would not apply if the child had any tropia on exam.
2. **Answer: A.** If the child has a hyperopic refractive error and esotropia is present, then the full CRx is prescribed.
3. **Answer: D.** This patient has residual esotropia that is worse at near. This is likely a case of accommodative esotropia (AET) with high AC/A ratio, which means that the distance power is not enough to control the esotropia when focusing at near. Thus, a + 3.00D bifocal add OU would be a reasonable choice at this time.
4. **Answer: C.** This patient has divergence insufficiency, where the esotropia is worse at distance. This patient is at high risk of a cranial six nerve palsy and should have a neurological workup.
5. **Answer A.** The myopia present in this infant is not high enough to cause amblyopia or significant symptoms at this time. However, a patient with this amount of myopia at this age is concerning. A thorough workup is indicated though to rule out causes of high early myopia such as infantile glaucoma. The patient should be monitored at frequent intervals and may need glasses in the future.
6. **Answer: B.** Because this hyperopic patient does not have strabismus, 1.5D should be reduced ("shaved off") from both lenses.
7. **Answer: C.** Because this hyperopic patient does not have strabismus, 1.5D should be reduced ("shaved off") from both lenses. It is important to note that the *full cylinder* is prescribed.

8. **Answer: B.** This patient will be fixating with the right eye without having to generate any accommodation. Therefore, the left eye will have an "effective" uncorrected refractive error of +4.00D sphere that will cause amblyopia. Issuing a prescription that covers the uncorrected amblyogenic error is appropriate. Given the age of the patient, we do not have to worry about any anisometropia or aniseikonia issues; preventing amblyopia supersedes any other considerations.
9. **Answer: D.** The spherical equivalent of this patient's CRx is plano. The full CRx should be offered.
10. **Answer: D.** The +1D over-refraction tells us this infant has +21D of hyperopia but is only corrected for +20D. Since the infant's world is mostly at near, the goal should be to leave this patient with a small amount of myopia with the contact lens in place. The ideal over-refraction would be −3.0D. This can be achieved by a + 24.0 D contact lens.

Acknowledgments Special thanks to Ann Yen, Mara Robinson, and Mike Robinson for their insights on early elementary classroom learning and Dr. Suleiman Alibhai, O.D, F.A.A.O, for his help in understanding the needs of low vision students.

Myopia Control

G. Vike Vicente

Objectives

- To discuss current ideas regarding established and recent etiologies of myopia in children.
- To understand the concept of peripheral defocus and its role in the myopia control.
- To discuss various philosophical approaches towards halting myopia progression, including glasses, contact lenses, pharmacological therapies, and surgical intervention.
- To discuss which methods have been shown to produce positive results, especially in light of recently published literature.

Introduction

Genetics and Environment

In the last 30 years, childhood myopia rates have increased by approximately 66% in the United States; this rate may be even higher in other countries. Myopia is believed to have both a genetic and environmental component.[1] For example, studies in twins have shown high rates of myopia regardless of twin type. Identical twins usually have very similar refractive errors, whereas the magnitude of refractive error may vary among fraternal twins.[2] Additionally, pediatric myopia risk increases if one or both parents are myopic.[3] However, no known single gene or particular mutation directly causes juvenile-onset myopia.

However, even with the strong evidence of genetics, myopia prevalence has dramatically increased in the recent years, suggesting environmental factors may play a stronger role than previously recognized.[4] Furthermore, ethnic and geographic variations may play a supplemental or separate role in the development of myopia among children. For example, ethnic Chinese children in Australia have a lower prevalence of myopia than in East Asia.[5] This suggests that environmental factors, such as the amount of time spent indoors or performing tasks with high near-vision demands, may be environmental factors contributing to the rise of myopia.[6] Further studies may be able to explain why children who spend more time outdoors (performing tasks with high distance-vision demands) have a lower rate of myopia development.[7] Perhaps high-intensity outdoor light leads to higher retinal dopamine secretion or focusing on distant objects "trains" patients to avoid using excessive accommodation required for near-vision tasks?

[1]Dirani M, Shekar SN, Baird PN. Adult-onset myopia: the Genes in Myopia (GEM) twin study. Invest Ophthalmol Vis Sci. 2008 Aug;49(8):3324–7.

[2]Lyhne N, Sjølie AK, Kyvik KO, Green A. The importance of genes and environment for ocular refraction and its determiners: a population based study among 20–45 year old twins. Br J Ophthalmol. 2001 Dec;85(12):1470–6.

[3]Mutti DO, Mitchell GL, Moeschberger ML, Jones LA, Zadnik K. Parental myopia, near work, school achievement, and children's refractive error. Invest Ophthalmol Vis Sci. 2002 Dec;43(12):3633–40.

[4]Kleinstein RN, Sinnott LT, Jones-Jordan LA, Sims J, Zadnik K; Collaborative Longitudinal Evaluation of Ethnicity and Refractive Error Study Group. New cases of myopia in children. Arch Ophthalmol. 2012 Oct;130(10):1274–9.

[5]French AN, Morgan IG, Burlutsky G, Mitchell P, Rose KA. Prevalence and 5- to 6-year incidence and progression of myopia and hyperopia in Australian schoolchildren. Ophthalmology. 2013 Jul;120(7):1482–91.

[6]Guo Y, Liu LJ, Tang P, Lv YY, Feng Y, Xu L, Jonas JB. Outdoor activity and myopia progression in 4-year follow-up of Chinese primary school children: The Beijing Children Eye Study. PLoS One. 2017 Apr 27;12(4):e0175921

[7]Tasks with high near-vision demands include use of hand-held electronic devices, video games, etc. Perhaps your mom was right after all: too much TV will ruin your eyes and you should go play outside more!

G. V. Vicente (✉)
Clinical Pediatrics and Ophthalmology Georgetown University Hospital, Washington, DC, USA

Eye Doctors of Washington, Chevy Chase, MD, USA
e-mail: vvicente@edow.com

K. M. Riaz et al. (eds.), *Optics for the New Millennium*, https://doi.org/10.1007/978-3-030-95251-8_24

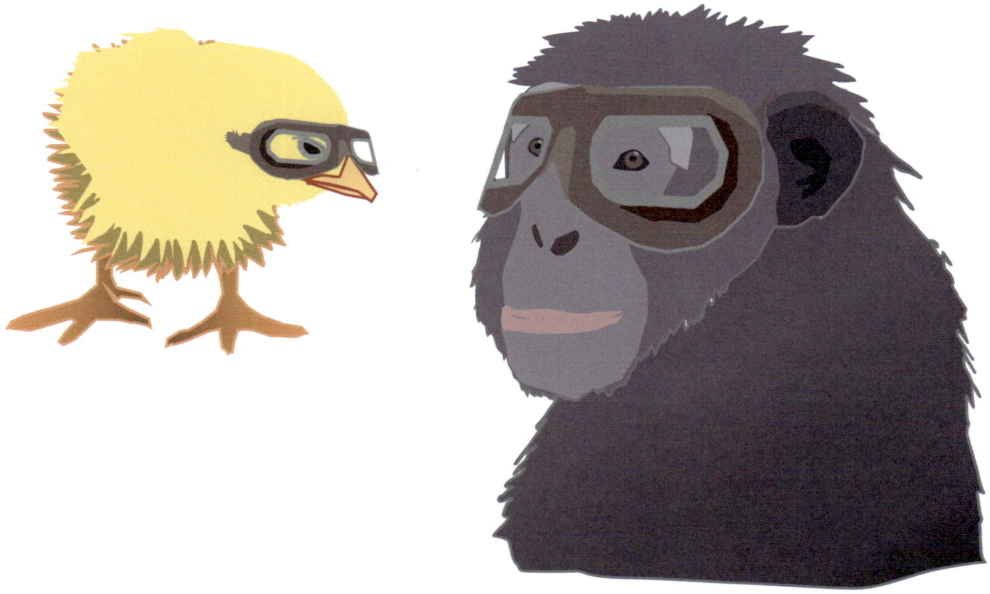

Fig. 1 The emmetropization mechanism is present in many animals. Infantile hyperopia will stimulate axial length growth; myopia will slow down axial length growth. This is why you may not see many baby chickens or baby monkeys wearing glasses other than the figure above

At present, our current understanding of myopia can be simplified to the following: A significant number of patients have a genetic predisposition towards myopia, but environmental factors accelerate or attenuate development of disease severity.

Importance of Slowing Myopia Progression

High myopia is not a benign condition in the pediatric population. It is associated with increased risk for glaucoma, cataracts, retinal detachment, and myopic maculopathy in adults.[8,9,10,11] Therefore, it is important to explore ways in which high myopia and axial length elongation can be prevented or at least halted: not only can this help patients see better during childhood, but it can also prevent late-term, adult-onset visual pathology as well. Since the fastest myopic shifts in humans tend to occur in ages 8–12, most clinical studies are aimed at slowing the growth in this demographic.

The topic of slowing myopia progression ("myopia control") has garnered significant clinical and research interest in recent years. This topic also allows us to connect some previously discussed Optics principles with the hopes that you, dear reader, can further appreciate the relevance of these principles in our profession!

Optical Interventions

Non-pharmacological and non-surgical interventions are considered as first-line therapy for myopia control. Several "glasses" and "contacts" options include the following:

Emmetropization

Here is a fun fact: Cute little baby animals also have refractive errors, but since there are not a lot of pediatric veterinarian optometrists, nature has found a way to help these animals out. For example, studies in monkeys and chickens have shown that eye growth in these animals' eyes responds to the refractive error over time; for example, if the baby monkey or chicken is hyperopic (near images are consistently focused behind the retina), then a visual feedback loop causes the eye growth to adjust by increasing axial length proportionally such that there is emmetropization over time (Fig. 1).[12,13]

While this may make for unemployed pediatric veterinarian optometrists, it does raise a fascinating observation: kids'

[8] Wong TY, Klein BE, Klein R, Knudtson M, Lee KE. Refractive errors, intraocular pressure, and glaucoma in a white population. Ophthalmology 2003;110:211–7.

[9] Leske MC, Wu SY, Nemesure B, Hennis A. Risk factors for incident nuclear opacities. Ophthalmology 2002;109:1303–8.

[10] Saw SM, Gazzard G, Shih-Yen EC, Chua WH. Myopia and associated pathological complications. Ophthalmic Physiol Opt 2005;25: 381–91.

[11] Risk factors for idiopathic rhegmatogenous retinal detachment. The Eye Disease Case-Control Study Group. Am J Epidemiol 1993;137: 749–57.

[12] Schaeffel F, Howland HC. Properties of the feedback loops controlling eye growth and refractive state in the chicken. Vision Res 1991; 31:717–34. 66.

[13] Hung LF, Crawford ML, Smith EL, III. Spectacle lenses alter eye growth and the refractive status of young monkeys. Nat Med 1995; 1:761–5

eyes can also potentially respond and adjust to infantile refractive errors. Basically, there is plasticity in the eye such that the eye wants to move towards emmetropia by adjusting axial length, both increasing and decreasing it, to respond to infantile hyperopia and myopia, respectively.

These vision-dependent mechanisms can operate in a very regional manner. When a refractive error is created for only a portion of the visual field in animal studies, the vitreous axial length of the corresponding retina was most affected.[14] This effect was present even when the fovea was ablated with a laser. These animal studies would support the theory that affecting the peripheral refractive error can influence the shape of the eye independent of central vision.[15]

This entire discussion raises a more fundamental (and hopefully clinically relevant) question: *Can clinicians actively intervene to initiate or accelerate emmetropization in pediatric refractive errors?*

Peripheral Defocus

As the name suggests, the philosophy behind peripheral defocus is as follows: By correcting the central visual field (for distance), the clinician can *intentionally* cause peripheral defocus with the "noble" intention of slowing axial length elongation and halting progression of myopia. For example, in children with myopia, it is common to see myopic defocus centrally with a *hyperopic defocus peripherally*; this hyperopic defocus on the peripheral retina may be a risk factor for worsening myopia.[16] Therefore, therapeutic peripheral defocus strategies for the treatment of myopia aim to cause a peripheral myopic defocus in order to slow down (or reverse) myopia.

The idea behind this is elegantly simple: While continuing to provide the child with sufficient refractive correction centrally (for distance vision needs and preventing amblyopia), we can also maintain enough peripheral blur in the retina so that the brain can signal to the eye: *Dear Mr. Eyeball, I beseech thee to cease and desist all axial length growth. Do you know that the images you are sending me from the periphery are extremely blurry—bang up job with the central images, by the way old boy, but the peripheral images are quite lousy. This child needs to see these interesting peripheral images that are currently blurry, so thou must comply immediately.*[17]

We will discuss three strategies that hold some promise based on clinical trials below. In the past, several other strategies, including (1) rigid gas permeable lenses; (2) bifocal or progressive spectacles; and (3) under-correction of myopic spectacles have not shown consistent clinical benefits to reduce of myopic shift or prevent axial elongation.[18,19]

Multifocal Contact Lenses

A multifocal contact lens (MF-CL) can be used to create a therapeutic peripheral defocus. This type of MF-CL would involve an architecture design, in which the *central portion* was set for *distance* and a *peripheral portion* had an *add power*—again, this intentionally created peripheral myopic image could slow down axial length growth.

We can further explain this point using the concept of "image shells" (Fig. 2). In an uncorrected myope (Panel A), central rays fall in front of the retina while peripheral rays fall behind the retina. Suppose we have corrected this patient with a standard contact lens (Panel B): now the central rays are in focus on the fovea, but the peripheral rays continue to fall behind the retina—this is known as a peripheral hyperopic shell. In this situation, distance objects of interest are visualized with good clarity; therefore, there is no significant stimulus to arrest axial length growth. Now suppose, we fit this myopic child with a contact lens with full distance correction centrally, but intentionally added extra plus power in the periphery (Panel C). Peripheral light rays will now come to focus *in front of the retina* (peripheral "myopic shell"). By causing peripheral myopia, the brain may be able to signal to the eye to arrest additional axial length growth. Finally, as discussed in the next section, orthokeratology (Panel D) lenses can similarly be used to intentionally create a steeper peripheral cornea and a myopic peripheral image shell.

In 2019, the US Food and Drug Administration approved the use of the MiSight® soft contact lens (CooperVision, Inc., Pleasanton, CA) after prospective studies showed they reduced the rate of myopia progression and the rate of axial elongation in children 8–12-year-olds. These MF-CLs are a single use, disposable soft contact lens with concentric peripheral add power. The BLINK study (published in August 2020) was a randomized, prospective, and double masked, 3-year clinical trial that compared monovision distance soft contact lenses and soft multifocal contact lenses (Biofinity Multifocal D from Cooper Vision) in 7–11-year-

[14] Smith EL, III, Huang J, Hung LF, Blasdel TL, Humbird TL, Bockhorst KH. Hemiretinal form deprivation: evidence for local control of eye growth and refractive development in infant monkeys. Invest Ophthalmol Vis Sci 2009;50:5057–69.

[15] Smith EL, III, Hung LF, Huang J, Blasdel TL, Humbird TL, Bockhorst KH. Effects of optical defocus on refractive development in monkeys: evidence for local, regionally selective mechanisms. Invest Ophthalmol Vis Sci 2010;51:3864–73

[16] Hoogerheide J Rempt F Hoogenboom W. Acquired myopia in young pilots. *Ophthalmologica*. 1971; 163: 209–215.

[17] This is how we imagine the brain and the eye communicate, and we dare you to prove us wrong.

[18] WSPOS – World Society of Pediatric Ophthalmology and Strabismus WSPOS Myopia Consensus Statement –2019

[19] Walline JJ, Lindsley K, Vedula SS, Cotter SA, Mutti DO, Twelker JD. Interventions to slow progression of myopia in children. Cochrane Database Syst Rev.; 2011. CD004916

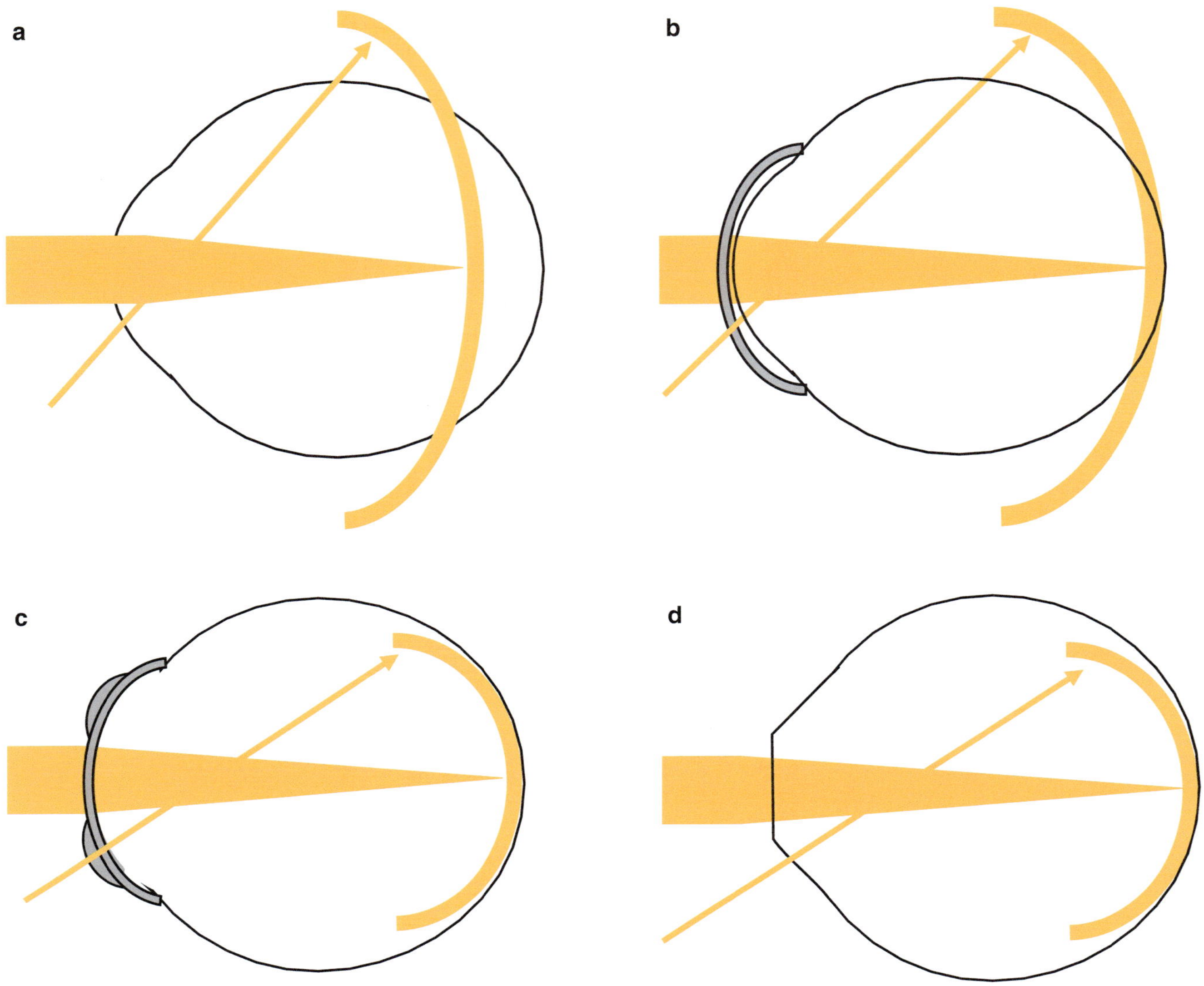

Fig. 2 Image shells. Panel A shows an image shell formed by light rays in an uncorrected myope with an oblate globe. Central rays fall in front of the retina but peripheral rays fall behind the peripheral retina. Panel B shows a myopic patient with a typical contact lens correction, central rays are in focus on the fovea but peripheral rays form a hyperopic shell in the periphery. Panel C shows a contact lens with an extra plus add power in the periphery, which would form a myopic image shell in the periphery while still maintaining the central rays in focus on the fovea. Panel D shows a cornea after orthokeratology with steeper peripheral cornea and a myopic peripheral image shell

old myopic children.[20] It showed a slower progression of myopia and axial elongation in patients with a + 2.50D peripheral add, compared to +1.5D or monovision (Biofinity) distance contact lenses.[21]

In this emerging field, every new clinical answer leads to additional questions such as:

- When should treatment be started and ended?
- How much do age, genetics, ethnicity, and amount of myopia affect the results?
- Which is the best demographic to treat?
- How much of a rebound effect will occur once treatment is stopped? (A second 3-year BLINK study is underway which includes a crossover and a wash out period).
- How many hours per day should a contact lens be worn to be effective?
- Will a contact lens with different peripheral add (increased depth of focus) work better than a contact lens with a single peripheral add?
- Would a stronger peripheral add (i.e., > +2.5D) work better?
- Does an add at different meridians work better?

[20] Walline JJ, Walker MK, Mutti DO, Jones-Jordan LA, Sinnott LT, Giannoni AG, Bickle KM, Schulle KL, Nixon A, Pierce GE, Berntsen DA; BLINK Study Group. Effect of High Add Power, Medium Add Power, or Single-Vision Contact Lenses on Myopia Progression in Children: The BLINK Randomized Clinical Trial. JAMA. 2020 Aug 11;324(6):571–580.

[21] Chamberlain P, Peixoto-de-Matos SC, Logan NS, Ngo C, Jones D, Young G. A 3-year randomized clinical trial of MiSight lenses for myopia control. Optom Vis Sci. 2019;96(8):556–567.

- How are patients with astigmatic myopia different?
- How can we help patients with smaller pupils?
- Would combining low dose atropine and peripheral defocus have an additive effect?
- Does a mild to moderate reduction in myopic progression in a child reduce the probability of developing retinal detachments, glaucoma in the future?

This is certainly a topic that will likely need to be updated in the future versions of this text. For now, the concept of peripheral focus should be appreciated.

Orthokeratology Contact Lenses

This is a somewhat controversial topic among ophthalmologists, but bears worth mentioning given recently published data. As introduced above (Fig. 1, Panel D), a peripheral hyperopic defocus can also be achieved with orthokeratology (Ortho-K) contact lenses. These specially designed lenses can be worn overnight to cause peripheral corneal steepening. A major convenience of Ortho-K is that the child does not have to wear glasses or contact lenses during the day, as the peripheral defocus created overnight can last for most (if not all) of the child's waking hours. Of course, infectious keratitis, especially in the pediatric population is a valid and significant concern.

Other factors to consider, include difficulty in evaluating the purported effect of the Ortho-K intervention: a cycloplegic refraction would not be useful in evaluating the effect of Ortho-K on patients as the goal is for patients to have uncorrected, central emmetropia during the day. Measurement of axial length has been suggested as a better indicator of success or failure, though this can also be temporarily affected by corneal flattening and anterior chamber shortening. Therefore, axial length must be measured after a washout period of no Ortho-K lens wear, similar to contact lens-wearing patients undergoing preoperative refractive or cataract surgery measurements. Furthermore, it is unknown how long Ortho-K lenses must be worn to be effective. In the general population, it is known that the cornea often resumes its pre-Ortho-K shape with recurrence of myopia.

A recent report in *Ophthalmology* reviewed the published evidence on this topic and concluded that this strategy may be cautiously considered in select patient populations.[22] Again, this remains a topic that will similarly need to be updated in the future versions of this text.

[22] VanderVeen DK, Kraker RT, Pineles SL, Hutchinson AK, Wilson LB, Galvin JA, Lambert SR. Use of Orthokeratology for the Prevention of Myopic Progression in Children: A Report by the American Academy of Ophthalmology. Ophthalmology. 2019 Apr;126(4):623–636.

Spectacles

Many different types of spectacles have been tried to reduce myopic progression without consistent effects. Bifocals, progressives, and under-correction lenses have been tested with the hope that reducing an accommodative lag during near tasks would help prevent emmetropization and axial elongation to no avail.

A full discussion as to why spectacles have failed is beyond the scope of this text. One potential reason is that peripheral defocus is difficult to achieve with glasses as compared to contact lenses. We encourage you, dear reader, to read about this in other texts to learn more about the various works that have been done on this topic.

Spherical Aberration

As introduced in Chap. 14 "Physical Optics and Advanced Optical Principles", spherical aberration (SA) plays an important role in various facets of Optics. For the purposes of myopia control, SA has recently gained attention as it has been suggested that SA can be intentionally manipulated to slow down axial length growth and myopia progression.

We previously discussed how the eye may grow in response to the hyperopic defocus present at birth: since incoming light rays fall behind the retina, the eye may increase its axial length to "catch" these posterior light rays. Since SA provides depth of focus, we can potentially increase positive SA by increasing the peripheral refractive power of the system to cause more peripheral light rays (which previously were landing behind the retina) to now land onto or even slightly anterior to the retina (while maintaining paraxial rays). In sophisticated terminology, we would say increasing the depth of focus helps to offset the problems of accommodation lag in a child's hyperopic eye. In more simpler terms, since the eye is sending both centrally focused and peripherally focused light rays to the brain, the brain is happy and does not feel the need to signal the eye to increase axial length.

As with all things in life, there is a balance in the perfect amount of SA for these cases. For example, much SA will degrade the quality of the central image and decrease the contrast sensitivity. At this time, no clear evidence exists to suggest that this is a standard therapy; indeed, we are not sure whether positive SA or peripheral myopia (peripheral defocus) is more important in slowing the progression of myopia. However, this is a topic that will likely continue to be studied and deserves attention for the future developments.

Pharmacologic Interventions: Low-Dose Atropine

Topical atropine has long been considered as a tool for myopia control since it can decrease accommodation and bind to scleral muscarinic receptors. Muscarinic receptors are found in the sclera but their influence on the scleral matrix is not understood.[23] Multiple studies have shown a positive clinical effect with low-dose topical atropine, but the mechanism of action is still unclear. Paradoxically, low dose atropine has little effect on accommodation, yet it can prevent myopic progression (and increased axial length).[24]

The ATOM2 study in 2012 reported that using 0.01% atropine drops once a day reduced the progression of myopia by 50% and did not have the rebound regression observed after cessation of 1% and 0.5%.[25] More recently, the LAMP phase 2 study in 2020 showed 0.05% atropine was more effective than 0.01%.[26]

As with peripheral defocus, multiple therapy questions remain for the future:

- What is the ideal demographic patient?
- At what age should atropine be stopped or tapered?
- Is it useful to combine low-dose atropine with other interventions, such as multifocal contacts or Ortho-K with atropine? Some early data suggest that Ortho-K with atropine may be effective in slowing axial elongation in children with low myopia.[27]

[23] Barathi VA, Beuerman RW. Molecular mechanisms of muscarinic receptors in mouse scleral fibroblasts: prior to and after induction of experimental myopia with atropine treatment. Mol Vis. 2011;17:680–692

[24] Pineles SL, Kraker RT, VanderVeen DK, Hutchinson AK, Galvin JA, Wilson LB, Lambert SR. Atropine for the Prevention of Myopia Progression in Children: A Report by the American Academy of Ophthalmology. Ophthalmology. 2017 Dec; 124(12):1857–1866.

[25] Chia A, Lu QS, Tan D. Five-Year Clinical Trial on **Atropine** for the Treatment of Myopia 2: Myopia Control with Atropine 0.01% Eyedrops. **(ATOM2)** Ophthalmology. 2016 Feb;123(2):391–9

[26] Yam JC, Li FF, Zhang X, Tang SM, Yip BHK, Kam KW, Ko ST, Young AL, Tham CC, Chen LJ, Pang CP. Two-Year Clinical Trial of the Low-Concentration Atropine for Myopia Progression (LAMP) Study: Phase 2 Report. Ophthalmology. 2020 Jul; 127(7):910–919.

[27] Kinoshita N, Konno Y, Hamada N, Kanda Y, Shimmura-Tomita M, Kaburaki T, Kakehashi A. Efficacy of combined orthokeratology and 0.01% atropine solution for slowing axial elongation in children with myopia: a 2-year randomised trial. Sci Rep. 2020 Jul 29; 10(1):12750.

Surgical Interventions

There are currently no proven surgical techniques to slow myopic progression. Future studies may involve scleral cross linking to stiffen the sclera or refractive corneal surgery to steepen the peripheral cornea.[28]

Practice Questions

1. A 10-year-old patient has been using Ortho-K at night time for myopia control for 2 years. She returns for a 12 month follow up. What is the most appropriate way to determine if a therapy is having any long term effect for myopia?
   A. Autorefractor.
   B. Manifest refraction.
   C. Cycloplegic refraction.
   D. Measurement of axial length.
   E. Answers A and C.
2. You wish to offer myopia control therapy to the family of a 10-year-old, avid daily swimmer, with a – 3.00 D refraction and strong family history of myopia. Which of the following myopia control therapies should be avoided?
   A. Multifocal contact lenses.
   B. Ortho-K.
   C. Atropine 0.01%.
   D. Atropine 0.05%.
   E. None of the above.
3. A 7-year-old patient started using one drop of Atropine 0.05% OU 1 week ago. He complains of having trouble reading since starting the drops. Examination of the patient with his distance glasses on reveals:
   Vision at distance 20/20 OU.
   Vision at near 20/50 OU.
   Dilated pupils and with motion at near during retinoscopy.
   What options can you offer this patient?
   A. Remove distance glasses while reading
   B. New bifocal glasses
   C. Switch to 0.01% atropine
   D. Consider multifocal contacts or Ortho-K if the patient is mature and responsible enough
   E. All of the above

[28] Zhang X, Tao XC, Zhang J, et al. A review of collagen crosslinking in cornea and sclera. J Ophthalmol. 2015; 2015: 289467.

Answers

1. **Answer: D.** In patients using Ortho-K, measuring axial length progression is the best way to determine how the patient's myopia may be changing since the corneal effects can last for weeks and affect the refraction.
2. **Answer A**. In a patient who is an avid swimmer, it may not be feasible to wear contacts during swim practice. This patient could wear Ortho-K lenses at night or use atropine drops.
3. **Answer E**. All options would help this patient have accommodation problems due to likely pharmacologic cycloplegia.

Acknowledgements The author would like to thank Dr. Gary Gerber, OD, Co-Founder, Chief Myopia Eradication Officer, Treehouse Eyes; Dr Rachel M. Caywood, OD, FAAO, Dean McGee Eye Institute / University of Oklahoma; and Dr. Ashley Wong, OD, Eye Doctors of Washington for their guidance in this subject.

Optics in Micro-Gravity and Zero-Gravity Conditions

Shehzad Y. Batliwala and Kamran M. Riaz

Objectives

- To review historical vision standards and criteria for astronaut selection and their evolution over time.
- To review various methods of vision correction in astronauts and potential candidates.
- To describe vision changes astronauts experience both during training and in microgravity.
- To describe terrestrial-based benefits stemming from NASA-led optics research.

Introduction

Imagine this: You have spent the last seven months traveling through space as the pilot of your three-member spacecraft, and the red glow of Mars emerges brighter, larger, and closer through your window. As your crew activates the Mars Landing System to enter the atmosphere and begin your descent, you realize something is different as you view the Red Planet. Your vision has gotten progressively blurrier over the past few months: You now have difficulty reading the landing checklist, and you are uncertain if you have the visual acuity to nail this landing! What do you do? Why is this happening?

If you thought Ophthalmic Optics only had relevance on planet Earth, remember we have warned you since the beginning: *You cannot escape Optics no matter where you go in the universe.*

Before we figure out how to land this multi-billion-dollar spaceship, let's first review current vision standards for astronaut selection and the various ways to correct vision in this unique patient population.

S. Y. Batliwala (✉)
Department of Ophthalmology, Dean McGee Eye Institute, Oklahoma City, OK, USA
e-mail: shehzad@drbatliwala.com

K. M. Riaz
Dean McGee Eye Institute, University of Oklahoma, Oklahoma City, OK, USA

Vision Standards and Criteria for Astronaut Selection

Historically, all NASA astronauts were military test pilots and thus were required to meet strict vision standards as determined by the military. These standards eventually were relaxed as the demand for astronauts increased in the post-Apollo era, and the effects of spaceflight on vision were better understood.[1]

Uncorrected distance visual acuity (UCDVA) requirement for pilot astronauts must be better than 20/100; for non-pilots, UCDVA must be better than 20/200. Best-corrected distance and near visual acuity (BCDVA and BCNVA) must reach 20/20 in each eye.[1]

However, these serve as historical trivia. NASA has now waived any UCDVA requirement for all astronaut selection categories and primarily set modern vision requirements based on the BCDVA and BCNVA. At present, astronaut candidates may not have a cycloplegic spherical refractive error that exceeds +5.50D or − 5.50D, while astigmatism cannot exceed 3 diopters in any meridian. These criteria are even more stringent for pilots, with cycloplegic spherical refractive error not to exceed +3.50 or − 4.50D, and astigmatism not to exceed 2 diopters in any meridian.

Does this mean that anyone with a mild refractive error has to wave goodbye to their astronaut dreams? Not exactly. NASA has approved laser refractive surgery (LASIK and PRK) for astronaut selection (meaning any individual applying for the selection process, including pilots and non-pilots) as of 2007. Pre-op cycloplegic refraction must be between +4.00D and − 8.00D sphere with 3.00D or less of (minus) cylinder.[1] This roughly aligns with criteria used for "safe" laser refractive surgery in the general population.

[1] Manuel, K, Mader, T.H. Ophthalmologic Concerns: Vision Standards and Selection Testing. Principles of Clinical Medicine for Space Flight, edited by Michael R. Barratt, Sam Pool, Springer, 2008, 535–545.

K. M. Riaz et al. (eds.), *Optics for the New Millennium*, https://doi.org/10.1007/978-3-030-95251-8_25

However, the upper limits for both myopia and hyperopia with current lasers for civilians are a bit higher.[2]

Regarding extraocular muscle function, testing must not reveal any evidence of microtropia, suppression, or diplopia.[3] Disqualifying factors include the presence of any tropia, 10PD or more of horizontal phoria, and 1.5PD or more of vertical phoria.

Stereopsis of less than 25 arc-seconds with Optec testing is disqualifying.[3] Color vision testing requires a score of at least 10 of 14 plates with the 14-plate Dvorine pseudoisochromatic test.[4]

In summary, visual assessment for astronaut candidacy includes measurement of refractive error, color vision, binocular vision, and stereopsis – obviously, there are all essential things for a potential astronaut!

Vision Correction Options

As stated in the previous section, a mild refractive error does not exclude a potential astronaut candidate. More than half of astronauts wear glasses and (even) contact lenses during flight missions. Furthermore, many astronauts may undergo surgical vision correction, including laser refractive surgery.

Spectacles

Several changes can be made to standard spectacles to make them more operational and safer in both the simulated and actual spaceflight environment. Given the close confines of spacecraft, astronauts must carry out a majority of their vision-intensive tasks in the near-to-intermediate range of vision. As such, modified executive-style trifocal spectacles with 11-mm (rather than the standard 7-mm) vertical separation between the bifocal and trifocal lines are well suited to this environment.

Additional modifications include using a slightly longer bifocal focal length calculation (optimized for a 51 cm focal distance) to accommodate the cockpit seating and instrument arrangements of the T-38 aircraft, which is used for astronaut training purposes. Interestingly, it is not uncommon to use spectacles with a vertical bifocal segment in the temporal aspect of the lens to allow the astronaut to see small nearby objects in the far periphery while wearing the extravehicular-activity helmet.[5]

It should be noted that "space glasses" must fit exceptionally well. Spectacles in space are especially prone to fogging; astronauts may also require a headband-type secure connection due to the effects of microgravity not being "strong" enough to secure the glasses to the nose and ears.

Contact Lenses

A 1989 study by NASA evaluated spherical soft, toric soft, and rigid gas-permeable contact lenses (RGPCLs) on simulated weightlessness parabolic flights and found that RGPCLs had a tendency to be displaced superiorly.[6] The official recommendation is to avoid RGPCLs, but nearly all other types of contact lenses are approved for spaceflight. There have been no reports to date of visual degradation or permanent corneal injury due to wearing contact lenses. Given the increasing prevalence of soft contact lenses among astronauts, extensive preflight training regarding the use of caution to remove contact lenses before sleep is provided.[7] Extended wear contact lenses are discouraged because the high concentration of carbonaceous particles in the spacecraft air leads to an increased risk of ocular foreign body injury and subsequent bacterial keratitis and conjunctivitis.

Refractive Surgery

Several refractive surgery procedures may be considered for astronauts:[1,3,4]

1. Radial keratotomy (RK) was a common procedure performed worldwide during the 1980s[8] to treat myopia. However, later research demonstrated a progressive hyperopic effect in most patients over time due to a weakened cornea.[9] This effect is exacerbated at altitudes above

[2] See Chap. 30, Optics for Refractive Surgery for a more detailed discussion on upper and lower limits of refractive error amenable to laser refractive surgery.

[3] Reschke, M, Clement, G, Thorson, S, Mader, T.H. Neurology: Visual Impairment. Space Physiology and Medicine, edited by Nicogossian, A.E, Williams, R.S., Huntoon, C, L., Doarn, C.R., Polk, J.D., Schneider, V.S. Springer, 2016, 245–283

[4] Wright, P, Scott, R.A.H, Ophthalmology. Ernsting's Aviation and Space Medicine, fifth Edition, edited by Gradwell, D.P, Rainford, D.J, 2016, CRC Press: Taylor and Francis Group.

[5] Recall the discussion for occupational/recreational bifocals in Chap. 16 Construction of Glasses

[6] Manuel, K, Mader, T.H. Ophthalmologic Concerns: Vision Standards and Selection Testing. Principles of Clinical Medicine for Space Flight, edited by Michael R. Barratt, Sam Pool, Springer, 2008, 535–545

[7] In other words, probably not a good idea to get a corneal ulcer due to overnight contact lens wear during your flight to Mars. However, microbial keratitis has occurred in space: https://www.escrs.org/Publications/Eurotimes/08Feb/NASAapprovesalllaser.pdf

[8] The 1980s were certainly a strange era… see Chap. 30 Optics for Refractive Surgery for more information regarding RK and other historical refractive procedures.

[9] Gwon A. Prospective Evaluation of Radial Keratotomy (PERK) Study 10 years after surgery. Arch Ophthalmol. 1995; 113(10):1225–1226.

9000 feet because the hypoxic cornea expands circumferentially in the periphery, leading to significant flattening of the corneal cornea and a hyperopic shift. This refractive shift is obviously a significant risk factor for spaceflight as even virgin eyes may develop a hyperopic shift. Therefore, any candidate with previous RK is not allowed by NASA for further consideration as an astronaut (disqualifying procedure).

2. Photorefractive keratectomy (PRK): As of 2007, NASA allows PRK for astronauts. Studies initially showed that a mismatch between optical zone diameters and the size of the entrance pupil could lead to significant glare and halos, leading some to believe that PRK would also be a potentially disqualifying procedure. However, this stance has been mitigated by modern wavefront-guided treatment modalities, which cause a lower incidence of glare, halos, and other higher-order aberrations. Studies have shown that individuals who have undergone PRK are not susceptible to altitude-related refractive shifts as those experienced by patients after RK surgery.

   Astronauts with previous PRK have successfully traveled to the International Space Station, suggesting that PRK is a well-tolerated procedure during space flight.[10] Interestingly in this patient, during the 12-day space flight, a hyperopic shift ≥1.00D did not occur during the flight. Ocular surface dryness, photophobia, and other symptoms were not significant throughout the flight, suggesting that PRK is stable for short space flights. After returning to earth, the refractive error and ocular exam were relatively the same as compared to the pre-space flight exam.
3. LASIK: NASA also allows LASIK for astronaut selection and retention as of 2007.[11] Findings from high-altitude studies of patients who have undergone LASIK have shown mixed stability results in one case and myopic shifts in other cases. This may affect aviators, but it is unknown how it may affect astronauts who are consistently exposed to normal atmospheric pressures and oxygen concentration during an extra-terrestrial flight but experience significant pressures (as described in the previous section) at the time of liftoff. To date, no astronaut has flown in space following LASIK.
4. IOL replacement: Interestingly, NASA considers prior cataract surgery a disqualifying procedure for astronaut *selection*, but *not retention*, even though a pseudophakic astronaut who had undergone bilateral cataract surgery was found to have stable vision during a 2-week spaceflight. Talk about a sweet grandfather deal (see what we did there).[12] More recently, an astronaut with an IOL in only one eye successfully completed a six-month mission to the International Space Station without any issues.[13] The NASA Study of Cataracts in Astronauts (NASCA) was a cross-sectional study that looked at the progression of nuclear, cortical, and posterior subcapsular cataracts in veteran astronauts. This 5-year study revealed a statistically significant and dose-dependent association between space radiation and posterior subcapsular cataracts.[14] An aging astronaut population and the association between space radiation and cataract formation will certainly increase the demand for cataract surgery in this special population of patients in the future!

Vision Changes during Space Travel

This topic brings us back to our scenario in the introduction, which is a genuine possibility in the near future, given NASA's recently announced plans of landing the first woman and second man on the surface of the Moon in 2024, and a potential Mars landing projected for 2033.[15] We are coming even closer to accomplishing such audacious goals thanks to the efficiencies and streamlined use of resources by private space companies such as SpaceX, which accomplished the first commercial crewed mission to the International Space Station on the Demo-2 Crew Dragon, launched on May 30, 2020.

When NASA began to conduct post-flight surveys of astronauts in 1989, they observed that 29% of astronauts on short missions (approximately two weeks) and 60% on long-duration missions experienced a degradation in distance and near visual acuity.[16] NASA escalated vision research activity in response, leading to additional data collection such as pre-

[10] Gibson CR, Mader TH, Schallhorn SC, Pesudovs K, Lipsky W, Raid E, Jennings RT, Fogarty JA, Garriott RA, Garriott OK, Johnston SL. Visual stability of laser vision correction in an astronaut on a Soyuz mission to the International Space Station. J Cataract Refract Surg. 2012 Aug; 38(8):1486–91.

[11] "NASA approves all-laser LASIK for astronauts." https://www.escrs.org/Publications/Eurotimes/08Feb/NASAapprovesalllaser.pdf. Accessed January 17, 2021

[12] Mader TH, Koch DD, Manuel K, Gibson CR, Effenhauser RK, Musgrave S. Stability of vision during space flight in an astronaut with bilateral intraocular lenses. Am J Ophthalmol 1999; 127:342–343

[13] Mader TH, Gibson CR, Schmid JF, Lipsky W, Sargsyan AE, Garcia K, Williams JN. Intraocular Lens Use in an Astronaut During Long Duration Spaceflight. Aerosp Med Hum Perform. 2018 Jan 1; 89(1):63–65.

[14] Chylack LT Jr., Feiveson AH, Peterson LE, Tung WH, Wear ML, Marak LJ, Hardy DS, Chappell LJ, Cucinotta FA. NASCA report 2: Longitudinal study of relationship of exposure to space radiation and risk of lens opacity. Radiat Res. 2012 Jul;178(1):25–32.

[15] https://www.space.com/spacex-crew-dragon-demo-2-test-flight-explained.html

[16] Nicogossian, A.E, Williams, R.S., Huntoon, C, L., Doarn, C.R. Living and Working in Space: An Overview of Physiological Adaptation, Performance, and Health Risks. Space Physiology and Medicine, edited by Nicogossian, A.E, Williams, R.S., Huntoon, C, L., Doarn, C.R., Polk, J.D., Schneider, V.S. Springer, 2016, 95–137.

and post-flight dilated fundus exams, MRIs, optical biometry, visual fields, and cycloplegic refractions.

During Lift-off and Initial Exposure to Micro-Gravity

Astronauts experience a variety of forces during space travel. For example, even during the initial lift-off, astronauts experience increased gravitational (G) forces that push the globe towards the optic nerve,[17] which stops as soon as the astronaut leaves Earth's atmosphere and now experiences microgravity. As blood rushes towards the head, this causes an increase in IOP upon exposure to microgravity, along with facial edema and increased sinus/periocular pressure.[18] Fascinatingly enough, the eye can quickly adapt to neutralize this initial IOP spike, causing glaucoma specialists everywhere to breathe a sigh of relief.[19]

During Space Flight (Micro-Gravity and Zero-Gravity Conditions)

In the introductory scenario, we assumed you were an emmetrope. A spaceflight-induced hyperopic refractive error most likely caused the blurry vision at near distance due to the flattening of the posterior aspect of the globe that has been described in long-duration fliers (at least six months duration). Interestingly enough, we may entertain the thought experiment that a myope may experience an improvement in UCDVA due to the hyperopic shift. This "favorable" refractive shift for myopes may create a new market in the future for space tourism combined with myopic vision correction (non)surgery!

Other considerations during actual space flight include increased reports of glare among astronauts and reduced contrast sensitivity.[20] Astronauts also experience lighting conditions ranging from extreme darkness to intense sunlight – astronauts experience much more solar radiation than their earth-bound friends.[21]

[17] Similar to a nervous first/second-year resident pushing down on the globe during cataract surgery, much to the chagrin of the teaching attending…

[18] Mader TH, Gibson CR, Caputo M, Hunter N, Taylor G, Charles J, Meehan RT. Intraocular pressure and retinal vascular changes during transient exposure to microgravity. Am J Ophthalmol 1993; 115:347–350

[19] Mader TH, Taylor GR, Hunter N, Caputo M, Meehan RT. Intraocular pressure, retinal vascular, and visual acuity changes during 48 hours of 10 degree head-down tilt. Aviat Space Environ Med 1990; 61:810–813

[20] Ginsburg AP, Vanderploeg J. Vision in space: near vision acuity and contrast sensitivity. NASA Interim Report: Space Shuttle Medical DSOs. Houston, TX, Johnson Space Center, 1986

[21] Parker DE, Reschke MF, Aldrich NA. Performance. In: Nicogossian AE, ed., Space Physiology and Medicine, second ed. Philadelphia, PA, Lea & Febiger, 1989 chapter "Accommodation and Presbyopia"

After Return to Earth and Spaceflight Associated Neuro-Ocular Syndrome (SANS)

Although the exact cause of vision changes is still unknown, current thinking suggests that the cephalad fluid shifts induced by microgravity lead to increased intracranial pressure. As NASA began to study vision and vision changes in astronauts meticulously, they identified seven astronauts who exhibited a "constellation" of unexplained findings including optic disc edema (5/7), globe flattening (5/7), choroidal folds (5/7), cotton wool spots (3/5), rNFL thickening on OCT (6/7), and decreased near visual acuity (6/7).[22] Collectively, these findings have been described as **Spaceflight Associated Neuro-ocular Syndrome (SANS)**. In response to decreased near visual acuity, astronauts over the age of 40 are prescribed "Space Anticipation Glasses" if they experience a hyperopic shift, which can be greater than +0.50D between pre- and post-mission spherical equivalent refraction in one or both eyes (range + 0.50D to +1.75D).[23]

Several hypotheses may be offered to explain the anatomical changes seen in SANS, but our focus here will be on the hyperopic shift. While posterior globe flattening can partially explain this refractive change, the etiology of flattening may be multifactorial. Increased intracranial pressure (ICP) with resultant increases in subarachnoid pressure could lead to various degrees of posterior globe flattening.[8] Alternatively, cephalad fluid shifts may elevate optic nerve sheath cerebrospinal fluid (CSF) pressure without an overall rise in CSF pressure. This causes the subarachnoid compartment to exert an anterior force that indents the posterior sclera resulting in posterior globe flattening.

Another mechanism leading to hyperopia may involve a weakened corneal refractive power after exposure to changes in atmospheric and oxygen partial pressure. However, research thus far has not revealed any definitive evidence supporting this mechanism. Indeed, our previous discussions regarding the stability of PRK in short-term space travel suggest that corneal refractive power is relatively stable during short-term flights; however, effects during long-term flights are still unknown.

Finally, choroidal expansion could theoretically lead to a hyperopic shift. The choroid is a highly vascular, spongy tissue that is usually approximately 0.3 mm in thickness, drained by the vortex veins, and thus could be congested as a

[22] Lee AG, Mader TH, Gibson CR, Tarver W, Rabiei P, Riascos RF, Galdamez LA, Brunstetter T. Spaceflight associated neuro-ocular syndrome (SANS) and the neuro-ophthalmologic effects of microgravity: a review and an update. NPJ Microgravity. 2020 Feb 7;6: 7.

[23] Bacal, K, Romano, J. Radiation Health and Protection. Space Physiology and Medicine, edited by Nicogossian, A.E, Williams, R.S., Huntoon, C, L., Doarn, C.R., Polk, J.D., Schneider, V.S. Springer, 2016, 197–227

result of cephalad fluid shifts. Stagnant choroidal blood volume can expand, resulting in a shortening of the distance between the macula and the lens by 0.3 mm, leading to an approximately 1D shift toward hyperopia.

Terrestrial-Based Benefits Stemming from NASA's Optics Research

Thus far, we have focused on how astronauts may undergo vision changes during space travel. However, in addition to the space-flight relevance of NASA's Optics research, we terrestrial bound folk have also benefited from these efforts in numerous areas. We will discuss a few of these contributions below:

A. Welding Industry[24]: Arc welding emits potentially harmful UV light and poses significant risks to the observer in terms of retinal damage, especially if viewed for long periods and from ultraviolet radiation and blue light. In the 1980s, NASA's Jet Propulsion Laboratory scientists James Stephens and Charles Miller began studying birds of prey whose eyes produced tiny oil droplets that filter out harmful radiation and transmit only specific visible wavelengths of light, protecting and enhancing vision. These brilliant NASA scientists used light filtering dyes and small zinc oxide particles to create a protective welding curtain, which has now been successfully commercialized and utilized in occupational welding glasses.
B. UV protection in sunglasses[25]: The same research process described above by Drs. Stephens and Miller also applied to a vast lineup of UV blocking sunglasses commercially marketed as Eagle Eyes Optics (Calabasas, California). The technology has now evolved into ski goggles and astronaut helmet visors applications. More recently, this technology has been inducted into the Space Foundation's Space Technology Hall of Fame.
C. LADAR technology[26]: The LADARVision 4000 (Alcon Laboratories, Fort Worth, TX, USA) was an early-generation laser that utilized a laser radar (LADAR) eye-tracking device to enhance accuracy during refractive surgery. The eye-tracking device was initially developed via contractual relationships between NASA and the U.S. Department of Defense's Ballistic Missile Defense Office (BMDO). The concept was to use LADAR technology for autonomous rendezvous and docking of space vehicles to service satellites. The science behind this work was later applied to aid in developing the LADARVision eye-tracking system. Alcon eventually acquired the technology via a series of mergers in 2000. LADAR technology was utilized in millions of excimer laser procedures in the early 2000s.
D. iDesign ® Advanced WaveScan Studio (Johnson and Johnson Vision, Santa Ana, CA, USA). This wavefront technology[27] is now used in mapping the cornea in preparation for laser vision correction and stems from investments made to develop the James Webb Space Telescope (JWST). This next-generation space telescope will replace the Hubble Space Telescope (HST) after its launch in March 2021.

As an aside, the JWST will offer infrared technology to allow it to observe the first galaxies that formed in the early universe. To allow for the viewing of such large distances, it requires extremely large mirrors.[28] The primary mirror is more than two stories in diameter and consists of 18 separate segments. Each segment must be perfect in terms of smooth contour, flatness, and completely scratch-free to cover astronomical viewing distances. To ensure high fidelity and quality, each mirror segment must be measured, ground, polished, and repeatedly tested. The grinding phase is one of the most time-consuming steps, so one wonders what kind of optical lab does this service and whether they can polish the author's glasses to be truly scratch resistant.

In order to save time, the infrared Hartmann-Shack Scanning System was developed to immediately test the mirrors after grinding and obtain a detailed map on how to do the next step of the grinding.[29] By introducing this new step of instantaneous feedback after grinding, the polishing and testing steps were optimized efficiently until the mirror was ground to the desired levels of near-perfect optical purity.

This same technology spun off into the Complete Ophthalmic Analysis System (COAS), which provided a

[24]NASA Technical Reports Server. Welding Curtains. 2002. ntrs.nasa.gov/archive/nasa/casi.ntrs.nasa.gov/20020091940.pdf. Accessed June 4, 2020.

[25]Bryan, William. NASA Spin-offs. Scratch-Resistant, UV-Reflecting Lenses. 2016. https://spinoff.nasa.gov/Spinoff2006/ch_6.html. Accessed June 6, 2020.

[26]NASA Technical Reports Server. The Right Track For Vision Correction. 2003. ntrs.nasa.gov/archive/nasa/casi.ntrs.nasa.gov/20030099657.pdf. Accessed June 5, 2020.

[27]See Chap. 14 "Physical Optics and Advanced Optical Principles", Physical Optics and Chap. 30 Optics for Refractive Surgery, for more information regarding wavefronts and their usage in refractive surgery.

[28]And you thought Mirrors were only there to make your life miserable on exams…

[29]See Chap. 14 "Physical Optics and Advanced Optical Principles", Physical Optics for a discussion about Hartmann-Shack technology

detailed map of the eye's front surface to detect pathology such as keratoconus.[30] COAS was later acquired by Advanced Medical Optics (now Johnson and Johnson Vision, Inc., Santa Ana, CA, USA), who incorporated this technology in their iDesign Advanced WaveScan Studio. The technology allows for accurate laser vision correction planning, working within 3 seconds to obtain four different measurements of the eye's refractive errors and higher-order aberrations. The technology initially used to optimize the JWST has led to increased efficiency in mapping the human eye for laser vision correction.

Future Considerations

Space is the final frontier.[31] While we have discussed some Optics related features of space travel and microgravity conditions, we are still scratching the surface of all the information and knowledge about future space travel.

As we have discussed thus far, the long-term consequences of microgravity-induced changes to ocular anatomy and vision before, during, and after spaceflight may be a significant barrier to future space travel. Perhaps, for this reason, NASA has specifically labeled SANS as one of the top five high-priority risks to mitigate to allow for further space exploration. In the near future, we hope to learn more information from currently ongoing research as the idea of long-term space flights is becoming more and more of a reality.

This discussion leads us to another reality: The need to address current limitations and barriers to much-needed research in space ophthalmology. Access to space is one of the primary limitations in conducting high-fidelity research for pathologies related to the microgravity environment. One of the best ways to conduct research in this realm is to do it in the appropriate environment, which currently exists on the International Space Station. Private space companies are crucial in helping NASA address the current stagnant status quo. Their efforts have led to the advent of highly cost-efficient reusable rocket launch systems, as demonstrated by the recent Demo-2 Crew Dragon launch. A collaboration between government and private industries appears to be the only way forward for more discoveries and applications. As such technologies evolve and the cost to launch is reduced, high-fidelity terrestrial equivalent research in microgravity will become more accessible to scientists, and opportunities for additional spin-offs that benefit life on Earth (as discussed in the previous section) will be numerous.

Finally, we can end this chapter with a more fundamental and slightly philosophical question: *Why bother with research in space? Don't we have more pressing needs, especially as ophthalmologists, right here on Earth*?

It is our opinion that, in addition to space ophthalmology research having the potential for creating technologies that can benefit humanity on Earth, another reason to continue learning about ophthalmic applications in microgravity is a philosophical one.

Since the advent of time, humanity's mandate has been to explore, push the boundaries of possibility, and discover the next frontier. This same spirit allowed unwavering explorers of the past to discover novel lands and resolute scientists to discover novel cures. Exploration is a mindset, and it is this mindset that clinicians and scientists must engage in collectively in order to solve humanity's most pressing challenges. It is not every day that physicians and other professionals who specialize in and study the human eye can contribute to the inspirational endeavors embodied by NASA and the spirit of exploration that it represents. By understanding the history of this unique niche within ophthalmology, we can learn from the past and aspire to impact future developments within the field. It is possible that in future editions of the book, we may have much more to share in this constantly evolving and seemingly-unknown super-subspecialty within ophthalmology.

Editors' Note This chapter was included in the textbook as it covers some exciting and recent developments in the field of Optics, including areas that likely will see even more research and findings in the near future. These novel concepts are not part of "standard" Optics curricula, so they are not likely to be tested on exams. We have intentionally not included any "Practice Questions" in this chapter. Interested readers may wish to consult other texts for additional reading or review questions, including some of the sources cited in this chapter.

[30] NASA Technical Reports Server. Telescope Innovations Improve Speed, Accuracy of Eye Surgery. 2013. https://ntrs.nasa.gov/api/citations/20130009008/downloads/20130009008.pdf. Accessed June 21, 2021

[31] What? You didn't think we'd finish the chapter without that reference, did you?

Part III

Optics for Surgical Practice

Preoperative Optics for Cataract Surgery

Kamran M. Riaz

Objectives

- To understand various methods of assessing vision potential before cataract surgery.
- To review introductory principles of optical biometry.
- To understand the role of angle alpha and angle kappa in cataract surgery.
- To compare and contrast the differences between spherical and aspheric IOLs.
- To discuss considerations for cataract surgery in special situations, such as patients with long axial length, silicone oil, and previous refractive surgery.
- To appreciate various strategies for correcting astigmatism at the time of cataract surgery, including advantages and disadvantages of currently available options.
- To review optical principles of advanced technology IOLs.

Introduction

Greetings and welcome to Part III: Hooray, you made it through the (boring) fundamental stuff so that we can finally discuss real-life applications of the Ophthalmic Optics that we have discussed so far. In Part III, we hope you will better appreciate our previous discussions when we see how it they relate to the most exciting part of ophthalmology: cataract surgery.[1]

This chapter will review important Optics principles that every cataract surgeon should know before surgery.

Assessing Visual Potential

While some may argue that the best way to assess visual potential in the presence of a cataract is first to take out the cataract and then figure out the vision… This is neither appropriate surgical practice nor the correct answer on board exams. Before performing cataract surgery, we should familiarize ourselves with the proper preoperative workup, including assessing a patient's visual potential after cataract surgery. In addition to good clinical practice, this also helps the surgeon and patient have reasonable (and similar) expectations for the upcoming cataract surgery.

This may not be of much concern in the presence of mild-moderate visually significant cataracts. Currently, there are no absolute requirements for determining a "visually significant cataract" for billing and documentation purposes. Patient complaints of decreased visual function, including glare/halos at nighttime, difficulty with night driving, impaired reading, and other subjective visual complaints, can be sufficient documentation, though this author wonders if health insurance companies will make us all fill out 1000-page forms for every cataract surgery in the future.

There is no one-method-fits-all strategy regarding *when* to do cataract surgery. We should tell our patients, barring any significant medical urgency (e.g., phacomorphic/phacolytic glaucoma), that the *correct time* to do surgery is when the patient feels the decrease in vision quality is *hindering* their ability to perform activities of daily living. Visually significant can mean different things to different people. An airline pilot may have different visual needs compared to

K. M. Riaz (✉)
Dean McGee Eye Institute, University of Oklahoma, Oklahoma City, OK, USA

[1] With due apologies to those of you who don't perform cataract surgery anymore…

K. M. Riaz et al. (eds.), *Optics for the New Millennium*, https://doi.org/10.1007/978-3-030-95251-8_26

someone who simply wants to pass the vision screening requirements for a driver's license.

Previously, a BCVA <20/40 was required for billing purposes; this requirement has changed. Some clinicians objectively score the cataract using classification systems such as the LOCS II grading system. Devices to measure glare, such as a straylight meter (C-Quant, Oculus, USA), may also be utilized. Recently, ray-tracing aberrometry devices such as the iTrace (Tracey Technologies, Houston, TX, USA) have incorporated features such as the dysfunctional lens index (DLI) to objectively "grade" light rays passing through the crystalline lens to determine cataract severity. The DLI may be helpful in situations when clinical examination of the cataract may suggest a visually insignificant cataract, but objective assessment of light rays passing through the cataract may indicate otherwise.

Assessing Vision Potential in Dense Cataracts

Several other principles must be kept in mind in the presence of long-standing, dense, and visually-incapacitating cataracts. We will focus our discussion on this type of patient.

History and Exam

A thorough history is the first step in the preoperative assessment of patients with dense cataracts. Important questions include the following:

- How long has the patient noted the visual decline? Is it in one or both eyes?
- Is there a known history of amblyopia?
- Is there a history of trauma, steroid use, or medications[2] associated with the development of cataracts?
- Any history of ocular surgery, especially laser refractive surgery?
- Did the patient wear glasses or contact lenses during their lifetime? Specifically, is there a high refractive error present, especially pathologic myopia and hyperopia?
- Does the patient have (or have access to) any old eye examination records?

During the preoperative exam, in addition to performing a detailed slit-lamp with dilated fundus exam, several areas should be given additional attention:

- Assessing pupillary function, including the presence or absence of an afferent pupillary defect.
- Extraocular motility exam, especially for the presence of exotropia that may indicate long-standing visual decline.
- Assessment of contrast sensitivity (see Chap. 18, "Visual Acuity Testing and Measurement"): decreased contrast sensitivity may be present even with good visual acuity.
- A thorough examination of the anterior segment and lens with attention given to the cataract type, density, subluxation presence, zonular integrity, etc.
- Dilated fundus exam with attention given to the macula and optic nerve.

In the presence of extremely dense cataracts that preclude examination of the fundus, a B-scan (ultrasound) is vital to ensure that there is no retinal detachment, retinal mass, or other posterior segment pathology that may preclude immediate cataract surgery or warrant referral to other specialties, both within and outside of ophthalmology.

Standard Techniques

We can now focus on some specific "standard" testing strategies and devices that can be used to assess a patient's vision potential. We previously discussed some of these in Chap. 14 "Physical Optics and Advanced Optical Principles".

- Pinhole testing (PHT): When a patient looks through the 1.2 mm pinhole, we have maximized the number of undeviated paraxial light rays that reach the retina while limiting diffraction. This increased depth of focus allows us to correct upto 3D of refractive error in the presence of lenticular pathology. If the lens opacity is minimal, PHT will improve the visual acuity. However, if the lens opacity is dense centrally (e.g., posterior subcapsular (PSC) cataract), then the visual acuity may not improve (or even worsen).
- The retinal acuity meter (RAM; AMA Optics Inc., Miami, FL, USA) is similar to PHT as it is also helpful in determining macular function.[3] It is beneficial to distinguish between cataractous and retinal causes of visual dysfunction. While it relies on a pinhole aperture similar to PHT, it has an *additional + 2.50D lens* allowing for testing at 40 cm from the patient. RAM can compensate for both spherical and astigmatic refractive errors and may predict postoperative visual acuity better than the potential acuity meter (see below).
- Potential Acuity Meter (PAM; Haag-Streit, Switzerland): This device can *project a visual acuity chart directly onto the retina* to allow an estimate of visual acuity. However, the PAM might be unwieldy for most patients as it has a learning curve and carries a larger physical footprint. In addition, PAM relies on a skilled examiner to accurately

[2]Cumming RG, Mitchell P. Medications and cataract. The Blue Mountains Eye Study. *Ophthalmology*. 1998;105(9):1751–1758

[3]Airiani S, Braunstein RE. "The Retinal Acuity Meter." *CRST Europe* 2007. https://crstodayeurope.com/articles/2007-oct/1007_08-php/. Accessed June 21, 2020

direct incoming light through the patient's pupil. Finally, the PAM only corrects for spherical refractive errors.

- Laser interferometry (aka retinometry): Two laser light beams (red helium-neon) can be used to create a *diffraction fringe pattern* on the patient's retina to assess retinal function. By varying the widths of the fringe patterns, visual acuity can be determined on a range (20/600 to 20/20).
- Projection of color or light through colored gel films: This can be used to create an *entoptic phenomenon* to estimate gross retinal function. This technique does not quantify potential visual acuity compared to the previously discussed tests.
- Maddox rod orientation: A gross evaluation of retinal function to detect a scotoma can be determined by asking the patient whether s/he can "see the red line" – inability to see the red line suggests macular pathology.
- ERG and VEP testing: These two tests can assess retinal function and optic nerve/brain function, respectively. These two tests are also a spectacular waste of time/money and are best used for extreme circumstances and research purposes...
- On mission trips without fancy technology and severe long-standing white cataracts, we can use a muscle light gently pressed and moved against the closed lid to similarly create an entoptic phenomenon. The retina is presumed to function if the patient sees a dark branch pattern with a red background. You can try this in the clinic or at social functions (though we cannot be held responsible for your declining popularity among your friends and associates if you choose to go full Optics Nerd in all aspects of your life).

Haidinger's Brush

Finally, the rite of passage test that merits its own section: *Haidinger's Brush*. Note, the authors fully confess that we have never used this test, nor do we ever plan on using this test, and we pray for the souls of those who have used this test.[4]

Haidinger's brush refers to a technique wherein the examiner can use a lens (such as a lens from a pair of polarized sunglasses) to rotate polarized light in front of a blue-white background to create an entoptic phenomenon that the patient may perceive as a yellow light (Fig. 1). The "spinning" nature of the yellow light creates a "brush" (rotating yellow and blue patterns perpendicular to each other) shape that can be better described as a propeller-like phenomenon that can be visualized by the patient as the brush is centered on the fovea.[5]

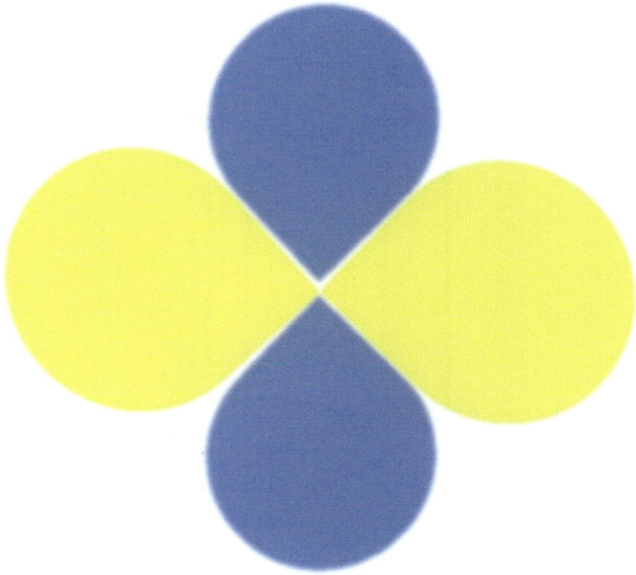

Fig. 1 Haidinger's brush appears as a propeller shape with blue and yellow "dumbbells" oriented 90 degrees from each other. The brush phenomenon can be best visualized against a white background or blue sky. Due to the dichroism of xanthophyll pigment in the macula, the observer perceives incoming polarized light with two distinct colors and locations. The size of the brush is approximately the size of the macula. A patient's ability to perceive the brush, even in the presence of dense media opacity, indicates gross macular function. The brush may also be used to aid patients undergoing eccentric fixation training

The perception of the "brush" of yellow light is thought to be due to the dichroism of xanthophyll pigment in the macula, as some pigment molecules are arranged circularly. Because the fovea is not flat, some nerves will run orthogonal to the central fovea while other nerves will run parallel. This creates different areas of the fovea that are sensitive to two different degrees of polarization. The size of the brush is approximately the size of the macula. Basically, this test can detect that the macula is functioning correctly to justify to the surgeon and patient that some visual function can be expected after surgery.

[4] See also Chap. 14 "Physical Optics and Advanced Optical Principles" for other uses of Haidinger's brush testing in clinical practice besides pre-cataract surgery.

[5] Note: the "brush" used to describe this entoptic phenomenon can be a misleading term since it more closely resembles a propeller. Nevertheless, since Haidinger described it as a brush, we will maintain the nomenclature, but it may be easier to understand this as a propeller shape instead.

Table 1 Optical biometry axial lengths versus immersion ultrasound biometry and 3 axial length adjustment formulas

Optical biometry	IUS (Recalc)	Wang-Koch modified Holladay 1_{2011}	Wang-Koch modified Holladay 1_{2018}	Sum-of-segments
20.00	20.00			20.14
25.00	24.89	24.91		24.95
26.50	26.35	26.23	26.35	26.40
30.00	29.78	29.31	29.21	29.76
34.00	33.69	32.84	32.48	33.61

Principles of Biometry

A full review of every detail regarding biometry is beyond the scope of this text. We will instead focus on several Optics-relevant principles of biometry.

Ultrasound Biometry (A-Scan Techniques)

Ultrasound biometry (USB) is the old-school, original method of determining the axial length (AXL). While optical biometry (OB) has become more popular (see next section), there may still be situations when USB is necessary, such as in the presence of dense cataracts, mission trips, and/or the need for intraoperative biometry due to patient inability to sit for preoperative biometry.

USB can be done in two ways: 1) contact applanation or 2) immersion. Contact applanation requires corneal contact: this can indent the cornea and artificially shorten the AXL. Immersion requires more examiner skill but is more accurate than contact applanation. In general, immersion is preferred over contact applanation despite the limitations of both methods. Several points about USB are as follows:

- USB is especially advantageous in the presence of dense cataracts. Since this technique relies on measuring the transit time of the ultrasound signal, it can measure AXL through an extremely dense cataract when OB may be unable to get a reliable measurement.
- The USB technique relies on certain assumptions, such as the presence of "normal" amounts of aqueous and vitreous, as each of these ocular structures has its own index of refraction. The device relies on the average velocity of the ultrasound signal to calculate AXL. This is not a significant problem in normal eyes. However, in the presence of silicone oil, for example, the signal will slow down, leading to an abnormally long AXL. We will discuss silicone oil in greater detail later in this chapter. Similarly, the AXL may be falsely skewed in a pseudophakic eye if the machine is not adjusted accordingly.
- USB is prone to measuring the AXL in a non-central line to the fovea. To ensure a coaxial reading, there must be good "spikes" from the retina and anterior/posterior lens surfaces. If USB measurements are misaligned, especially in long AXL eyes where perpendicularity may be more challenging to obtain, then the AXL may be falsely overestimated. Thus, the probe must be accurately placed on the patient's eye and relies on the presence of a skilled examiner.
- Sound waves travel through the various structures in the eye differently. For example, sound travels faster through the lens and cornea (approximately 1640 m/s) as compared to the aqueous and vitreous (approximately 1530 m/s).
- Sound waves will travel through short AXL eyes at a faster rate as compared to average AXL eyes, and at a slower rate for longer AXL eyes. One way to understand this concept is to realize that the longer AXL has "more vitreous" compared to the shorter AXL eye. This may further increase the inaccuracy in measured AXL in these eyes, further confounding accurate IOL power calculations.
- USB additionally relies on the examiner putting in the correct sound velocity at the time of obtaining measurements. If a wrong velocity is entered, the measurement will be inaccurate. While it is good clinical practice to ask the patient to return for a repeat measurement with the correct sound velocity, this may not always be possible logistically. Therefore, some authors recommend adjusting the AXL measurement using the following equation:

$$AXLc = AXLi \times \left(Vc / Vi\right)$$

where AXL_c is the "correct" (desired) AXL, AXL_i is the incorrect AXL, V_c is the correct sound velocity, and V_i is the incorrect sound velocity.

Several authors have reported that AXL measurements obtained by USB are consistently different from those obtained by OB; specifically, OB-AXL measurements are falsely longer-than-real in long AXL eyes and shorter-than-real in short AXL, when compared to USB-AXL measurements (Table 1).[6] This has significant implications: if we use OB-AXL measurements in long eyes, then the AXL is "too long" and we may end up inadvertently using a lower-than-needed IOL power and causing an undesirable more-than-intended hyperopic postoperative refractive error. You may think: "fine, let's just use USB-AXL measurement in all patients with long AXLs to avoid this problem with OB-AXLs". This sounds like a good idea, but lens constants for modern IOLs have been optimized for OB and not for USB. You may want to read the preceding paragraph few times because it is confusing on the first read! Table 1 lists AXL values obtained by OB when compared to immersion USB and three commonly used AXL adjustment formulas.

Currently, we are searching for methods to make the USB-AXL usable with current IOL constants (which are optimized

[6]Cooke DL, Waldron R, Savini G, Riaz KM, Taroni L, Murphy DA, Guaraldi F. Immersion ultrasound biometry vs optical biometry. J Cataract Refract Surg. 2022 Jul 1;48(7):819–825.

for OB, such as those found on online user-group databases[7]) for increased accuracy. Some authors suggest (1) either modifying the USB-AXL with an adjustment factor to calculate an "adjusted AXL" that can be entered into OB devices so that the OB-optimized lens constants can be used or (2) adjusting the lens constant and using the measured USB-AXL data as is. The latter option requires an easier calculation. This author recommends subtracting 0.23 from the lens constant so that the USB-AXL can be used.[6] For example, if the online lens constant for a given IOL is 119.0 and one is using USB-AXL measurements, then a "new" lens constant of 118.77 can be used in one's IOL formula of choice and no further adjustments to the USB-AXL are needed.

Optical Biometry (OB)

Optical biometry (OB) is the newer, most commonly used type of biometry in modern day cataract surgery. OB was developed as a more straightforward, non-contact method of obtaining measurements to yield results similar to USB.[8] One interesting modification is the measurement of AXL: When Haigis calibrated the original optical biometer, he calibrated OB AXL measurements to be equivalent to US AXL measurements with a necessary adjustment.[9] Since this original device could only locate two points on the eye (anterior corneal surface and retinal pigment epithelium), Haigis mathematically adjusted the image-side reference position from the retinal pigment epithelium (RPE) to the internal limiting membrane (ILM). Most biometers have since adjusted their devices to produce similar values.[10] Nonetheless, as discussed above and demonstrated in Table 1, if you perform a USB and OB on a given patient, the AXL measured by OB will likely be *slightly longer than the AXL measured by USB*.[11]

Since the USB-AXL is (usually) slightly shorter, the calculated IOL power may be slightly stronger-than-required, leading to a *potential myopic surprise* – not the end of the world, but something to keep in mind in these unique situations. Hence, an adjustment to the USB-AXL or the lens constant, as described in the previous section, can help overcome this potential limitation.

OB uses partial-coherence interferometry (PCI) (infrared laser light, wavelength 780 nm), optical low-coherence reflectometry (OLCR) (wavelength 820 nm), or swept source optical coherence tomography (SS-OCT) (wavelength 1300 nm) to measure reflected light from the tear film and the RPE.[12] One significant advantage of OB is that since it relies on patient fixation, it allows us to measure the true visual axis rather than the optical axis (we will discuss these concepts later in the chapter).[13] Additional advantages include increased measurement speed; less measurement error from the tear film; user-group optimized IOL constants for OB; and, perhaps most importantly, better corneal power measurement. Ancillary staff (or residents at the VA) performing biometry measurements usually find performing OB easier than USB.

OB not only measures the AXL, but also measures other biometric parameters such as keratometry, anterior chamber depth (ACD), lens thickness (LT), corneal thickness (CCT), and horizontal white-to-white diameter (HWTW); thus, it is a magical all-in-one device. With USB (and even some PCI OB devices), we may have to get these other measurements from other devices. As stated above, one limitation of OB is the presence of dense cataracts, corneal scars, or vitreous hemorrhage that may prevent the partial-coherence signal from accurately measuring the eye. Newer OB devices, such as the Lenstar LS 900 (Haag-Streit, Switzerland) and IOL Master 700 (Carl Zeiss Meditec, Dublin, CA) use strategies such as OLCR and SS-OCT, respectively, to further improve accuracy through dense lens opacities.

Studies have shown that while the AXL measured by OB and USB may be similar in normal AXL eyes, OB is better at

[7]For example, the User Group for Laser Interference Biometry (ULIB): http://ocusoft.de/ulib/c1.htm. Accessed January 19, 2021. More recently, IOLCon has replaced ULIB: https://iolcon.org/lensesTable.php. Accessed February 25, 2022

[8]Haigis W, Lege B, Miller N, Schneider B. Comparison of immersion ultrasound biometry and partial coherence interferometry for intraocular lens calculation according to Haigis. Graefes Arch Clin Exp Ophthalmol. 2000 Sep;238(9):765–73

[9]Haigis W, Lege B, Miller N, Schneider B. Comparison of immersion ultrasound biometry and partial coherence interferometry for intraocular lens calculation according to Haigis. Graefe's Arch Clin Exp Ophthalmol 2000; 238:765–73.

[10]A potentially more accurate method of measuring AXL has been proposed known as "sum-of-segments AXL" (SOS-AXL). In SOS-AXL, the individual segment lengths of each structure (cornea, aqueous, lens, vitreous, etc.) is measured according to both incoming wavelength of the device and the individual refractive index of the structure, rather than using an assumed index of refraction (e.g., 1.3375) for the entire eye. Using SOS-AXL may further improve the preciseness of AXL measurement, and therefore improve the function of many IOL formulas. See (1) Cooke DL, Cooke TL. Approximating sum-of-segments axial length from a traditional optical low-coherence reflectometry measurement. J Cataract Refract Surg. 2019 Mar; 45(3):351–354 and (2) Cooke DL, Cooke TL, Suheimat M, Atchison DA. Standardizing sum-of-segments axial length using refractive index models. Biomed Opt Express. 2020 Sep 25; 11(10):5860–5870.

[11]This is particularly true for long AXL eyes, where the OB-AXL may be ≥0.2 mm longer than the USB-AXL.

[12]This is why we spent all that time discussing interference and coherence in Chap. 14 "Physical Optics and Advanced Optical Principles"!

[13]Among the three types of OB, there are additional features/advantages to consider. For example, PCI is the "oldest" of these three methods, yet it gives an accuracy to the level of 0.02 mm. OLCR and SS-OCT have recently been introduced and each have their distinctive features. For example, SS-OCT uses lasers of variable wavelength to obtain multiple B-scans during the imaging process. The integrated OCT may also help assess retinal pathology – a rudimentary OCT can be done at the time of biometry!

predicting the final refractive outcome (likely due to its ability to better measure the corneal power).[14]

Biometry in Special Situations

While there are many situations where additional considerations have to be made (such as a physical handicap preventing the patient from sitting for biometry measurements), these are beyond the scope of our discussion. One critical situation has Optics relevance: the contact lens wearer who presents for cataract surgery.

If a patient uses contact lenses, the following should be kept in mind:

- Always measure both eyes, even if one eye is pseudophakic.[15]
- Patients who wear *soft contact lenses* should be out of their lenses for a *minimum of 3–7 days* (textbooks vary) before biometry. This is to avoid inaccuracies that may happen due to corneal warpage from the lenses that may falsely skew keratometry measurements.
- Patients who wear *rigid gas permeable contact lenses (RGPCLs)* should be out of their lenses for *at least 2–3 weeks* (again, textbooks vary) prior to biometry. Some authorities recommend a minimum of two weeks with an additional week for every 10 years of RGPCL use for a maximum of 6 weeks out of RGPCLs. For example, patients who have worn RGPCLs for 20 years should be out of their lenses for at least 4–5 weeks before biometry. Serial measurements may also be taken every two weeks after RGPCL removal to ensure the stability of corneal measurements, especially if planning for a toric or presbyopia-correcting IOL.

Principles of Keratometry

While a complete discussion of this topic merits a whole other textbook, several essential principles should be kept in mind when obtaining, assessing, and compensating for keratometry (K) measurements as an estimation of corneal power. Along with AXL, accurate K values are highly desirable and weighted heavily in all IOL formulas (see next section).

We have previously discussed how a traditional keratometer works.[16] Recall that this device primarily measures the anterior corneal curvature and assumes the power of the posterior cornea by using a fixed ratio between the anterior and posterior cornea. For example, if the device reads "43D" for an average K measurement, this is likely the combination of approximately +48.8D from the anterior cornea and – 5.8D from the posterior cornea. The measurement does **not** account for corneal thickness or variation of posterior corneal toricity.

The IOL Master 700 (Carl Zeiss Meditec) uses telecentric keratometry for anterior keratometry measurements and swept-source acquired pachymetry to define a toric posterior surface model (incorporating corneal thickness) for posterior corneal measurements. The resulting total keratometry (TK) value is constructed to work with established IOL formula lens constants and offers the surgeon a measurement of the anterior and posterior corneal radii that can potentially be used for more accurate IOL calculations. Large data sets evaluating the superiority of TK over K measurements have not been reported; however, TK values may be used in post-refractive surgery eyes to improve the accuracy of older formulas, such as Haigis, to be equal to the accuracy of other modern post-refractive IOL calculation formulas.[17] TK measurements (specifically posterior keratometry (PK) measurements) may also improve accuracy of KCN-specific formulas (e.g, Kane-KCN, Barrett True K KCN, etc.) in KCN corneas with K values > 50D.

In general, the anterior cornea acts like a plus lens (with either with-the-rule (WTR) or against-the-rule (ATR) astigmatism, while the posterior cornea acts more like a minus lens (usually steep in the vertical axis and having ATR astigmatism, ranging from −0.26 to −0.78D).[18] This means that depending on the anterior corneal astigmatism (ACA) measurement, the posterior corneal astigmatism (PCA) may neutralize, increase, or have no effect on ACA. In younger patients with WTR, the ATR of the posterior cornea will compensate for some of the WTR (of the anterior cornea); in older patients, the posterior cornea's ATR will increase the total corneal astigmatism.

As we age, total corneal astigmatism will shift toward ATR as *ACA shifts from WTR to ATR*. Since the PCA remains constant, it may seem that we are gaining ATR, but this is mainly due to the ACA changes. This relationship is even more skewed in post-refractive patients.

[14]Levison AL, Han Y, Chiu CY. Comparison of Refractive Results between IOL Master and Immersion A-scan Ultrasonography. *Invest. Ophthalmol. Vis. Sci.* 2011;52(14):5686

[15]This is a good rule for all patients, even those who do not wear contacts. For most patients, the measured AXL should be similar in both eyes (excluding patients with pathologies, such as amblyopia, or previous trauma/surgeries, such as scleral buckles). The authors are anecdotally aware of at least one lawsuit that resulted due to a -10D myopic surprise that occurred because the other (pseudophakic) eye was not measured. Further review led to the realization that the AXL measurement was inaccurate; had the other eye been also measured, then the discrepancy in AXL measurement would have (potentially) been detected before surgery.

[16]Please see Chap. 17, Optical Instruments and Machines

[17]Wang L, Spektor T, de Souza RG, Koch DD. Evaluation of total keratometry and its accuracy for intraocular lens power calculation in eyes after corneal refractive surgery. J Cataract Refract Surg. 2019 Oct; 45(10):1416–1421.

[18]Koch DD, Ali SF, Weikert MP, et al. Contribution of posterior corneal astigmatism to total corneal astigmatism. *Journal of Cataract and Refractive Surgery* 2012; 38: 2080–87.

Why is all of this (confusing) discussion so important? In addition to the inherent inaccuracy of K measurements, this understanding of ACA/PCA is essential when we consider surgical options, such as toric IOLs (discussed in the next chapter), to correct corneal astigmatism. If we only relied on ACA (and ignored the PCA) for a toric IOL, we would potentially end up over-correcting WTR and under-correcting ATR. For this reason, it is recommended to *intentionally under-correct WTR astigmatism in a young patient* (<60 years old) to allow the increased ATR (that will happen in the future) to correct the residual WTR astigmatism remaining after toric IOL surgery.[19]

Various devices and methods have been employed to measure the true corneal power (i.e., measure PCA). We can broadly group them into direct methods and indirect methods:

- Direct methods to measure PCA: Scheimpflug devices, SS-OCT biometry (e.g., the previously discussed TK), and slit-scanning devices.
- Prediction methods (formulas) to estimate PCA: Modern IOL formulas and toric calculators (available online) use complex algorithms to estimate the PCA. Examples of these include the Baylor nomogram, Abulafia-Koch regression transformations, and the Barrett toric IOL calculator.

However, no single instrument, device, method, or formula is considered the be-all/end-all accuracy method. This field remains rapidly evolving (and confusing!) for cataract surgeons.

Intraocular Lens Formulas

A complete discussion of all available IOL formulas, including the history, applications, and limitations of each formula, is beyond the scope of this text. Advanced level Optics nerds may wish to consult several texts on this subject.[20] For the rest of us mere mortals, we will focus on a few key principles under this topic.

In general, all IOL formulas are essentially trying to accurately capture the "D" value from our good old friend "U + D = V"![21]

For example, the Fyodorov formula, upon which many modern IOL power calculation formulas are based on, sought to calculate the "D" as such:

$$D = V - U$$

$$D = \left(1336/[AL - ELP]\right) - \left(1336/\left[1336/\left\{1000/\left([1000/DPostRx] - V\right) + K\right\} - ELP\right]\right)$$

where *K* is net corneal power, *AL* is Axial length, *ELP* is effective lens position (*ELP*), *DPostRx* is desired refraction, and *V* is vertex distance.

Don't be scared by the above formula. You will never have to calculate this on an exam. We have included it above so you can (1) appreciate the complexity of IOL calculation and (2) appreciate how U + D = V impacts so many things in ophthalmology!

Theoretical and Regression Formulas

Theoretical formulas (e.g., Binkhorst, Colenbrander, Fyodorov) are IOL formulas derived by applying geometric optics to the reduced schematic eye.[22] Many of our "old friends" we met in Part I were used historically: thin-lens formulas, thick-lens formulas, and ray-tracing models. In modern surgical practice, these formulas have been essentially abandoned due to their inaccuracy, especially at extreme AXL and K measurements.

Regression formulas (empirical or statistical formulas) were based on actual measurements rather than assumptions made by the theoretical formulas. The grand-daddy of these formulas is the SRK Formula. Even though we do not use this anymore, this formula must be committed to memory and serves as a useful model to understand advanced concepts that we will discuss later. Why is this formula still important? For example, you may wonder why some cataract surgeons are always freaking about the "correct" lens constant for a new IOL: we can see that a higher or lower "A" will lead to a higher- or lower-than-needed IOL power, causing myopic or hyperopic surprise, respectively.

The SRK Formula is:

$$IOL\ Power\ for\ emmetropia\ (Po) = A - 2.5L - 0.9K$$

where *A* is the a-constant according to the *IOL* (determined by the manufacturer usually by ultrasonic measurement)[23]; *L*

[19] This intentional under-correction of WTR is slightly controversial. Some authorities recommend leaving behind approximately 0.3–0.5D residual WTR in these patients, which this author favors. Other surgeons recommend correcting as much astigmatism as possible, even if it involves a small flip in the axis.

[20] An excellent resource is Bissen-Miyajima, H, Weikert M, Koch DD (eds). Cataract Surgery: Maximizing Outcomes Through Research (2014). Springer Publishing.

[21] A good nerdy mathematics review of this can be found here: Olsen, T. Calculation of intraocular lens power: a review. *Acta Ophthalmologica Scandinavica* 2007; 85: 472–485.

[22] Yet another old friend (enemy) returns! See Chap. 7, "Schematic Eye".

[23] This is why we must ensure the correct a-constant is being used for a given IOL if we use optical biometry since the manufacturer a-constant (i.e., what is written on the box) is usually for ultrasound biometry, unless specified otherwise.

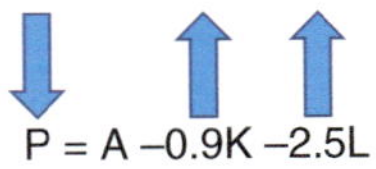

Fig. 2 Understanding the SRK formula is helpful for understanding commonly encountered advanced topics. For example, both falsely elevated keratometry measurements (e.g., post-myopic PRK/LASIK) and falsely elongated AXL measurements (e.g., long AXL and silicone oil) will call for a lower-than-required IOL power, leading to potential postoperative hyperopic surprise

is the *AXL* (as measured by ultrasound); and *K* is the average keratometry readings (using an index of 1.3375).

The SRK formula has several limitations. First, it is not recommended for extreme AXLs because the formula assumes a linear relationship between IOL power and AXL. This relationship is not linear in short and long AXL eyes. A similar assumption is made with corneal power causing a limitations when dealing with flat/steep corneas. Second, the A-constant itself is an "estimate" made by the manufacturer that needs to be adjusted if OB is used, for example. To overcome these limitations, surgeons ideally need to back-calculate postoperative results to personalize their individual A-constants.

What else do you need to know about the SRK formula? A favorite question that you may encounter about this formula is: *Which measurement error is more devastating when using the SRK formula: keratometry or AXL?*

This is relatively simple to understand when we see that the formula "weighs" the AXL by a factor of 2.5 and the keratometry measurements by a factor of 0.9. Therefore, a 1 mm AXL error will affect IOL power by approximately 2.5D (especially in short AXL eyes, up to 3D error), whereas a 1D keratometry error will affect IOL power only by about 1D.

Understanding the SRK formula is also helpful for understanding some of the advanced topics later on (Fig. 2). For example, in **post-myopic LASIK/PRK eyes**, the measured K values are falsely higher than real even though the cornea has undergone flattening from the refractive surgery.[24] This causes the formula to suggest a *lower power IOL than needed*, leading to the dreaded hyperopic surprise. Similarly, in patients with **long AXL or SO** in the vitreous cavity, the *measured AXL is falsely longer*; this again causes the formula to suggest a *lower power IOL* leading to the dreaded hyperopic surprise.

While most biometry devices can measure AXL accurately, the real challenge lies in obtaining accurate K measurements. The cornea accounts for about 2/3rd of the total refractive power of the eye. Thus, while an error in AXL is certainly impactful numerically, an error in corneal power measurements is more commonly encountered clinically. As discussed previously, K measurements are indirect measurements of true corneal power since we are actually measuring the size of the image reflected by the tear film (which is a convex mirror, another old friend!).[25] These measurements also make assumptions about the index of refraction, posterior corneal power, and corneal spherical aberration, further causing additional potential errors.[26]

After these "first-generation" formulas, several "second-generation" formulas (such as SRK II and Binkhorst II) were introduced. These formulas mainly sought to estimate the postoperative IOL position based on the AXL measurements in long and short eyes. Unfortunately, while they performed slightly better, they too faced the same limitations as the first-generation formulas.

As a result, newer formulas have been developed to ameliorate the deficiencies of older-generation IOL formulas.

Estimated (Effective) Lens Position

The estimated (effective) lens position (ELP) is simply a way of asking: Where does the IOL eventually sit in the eye so that we can use this position as the principal plane of refraction. Historically, the ELP was also called the anterior chamber depth (ACD) when ACIOLs were standard practice. Since we now place IOLs in the posterior chamber, the term ELP is used instead. When we perform biometry, we are attempting to use preoperative measurements to estimate the postoperative (pseudophakic) state of the eye, including a prediction of the ELP.

Third-generation formulas (discussed below) sought to calculate a more accurate ELP. For example, the Holladay I formula uses the AXL and K measurements to calculate an ELP value, termed the "surgeon factor" (SF). As another example, the Haigis formula uses the preoperative ACD measurement (and does not include K measurements at all) to calculate the ELP. A complete discussion of the "nuts and bolts" in each formula is beyond the scope of our discussion. We should appreciate the concept of ELP and understand how emerging IOL formulas seek to improve their accuracy by primarily improving the ELP value (either directly or indirectly).

In the next section, we will discuss how the newer-generation formulas account for this ELP. By accounting for

[24]For example, if keratometry readings from the optical biometer suggest 40/41 (at a given axis), it is likely that the real K values are *even flatter* than these measurements.

[25]See Chap. 17, Optical Instruments/Machines for a discussion regarding keratometry.

[26]An additional comment can be made about the index of refraction (1.3375) used by most biometry devices. If one uses online calculators (e.g., online multivariable IOL formulas or online toric IOL formulas), it is important to make sure that the formula is using the index of refraction used by the biometer. For example, the popularly used Barrett Toric Calculator has two options for index of refraction: 1.3375 and 1.332. If we accidently clicked on 1.332, it can create 0.5–1.0D hyperopic error by calling for a lower-than-needed IOL power. Thus, it is important to make sure that the formula(s) used has the correct index of refraction entered.

(or calculating) the ELP, third-generation formulas seek to improve the accuracy of previous-generation formulas, especially in long/short AXL and steep/flat K eyes. While we may think that the ELP is basically the ACD, it turns out that this is not an accurate assumption. Remember the old saying about what happens when you assume…

Third-Generation and Multivariable Formulas

These formulas represent a return to the theoretical formulas (first generation) with additional modifications made to account for the previously discussed limitations.

Third-generation formulas (Holladay I, Hoffer Q, and SRK/T) still primarily rely on AXL and K measurements. However, they also attempt to predict ELP (as it relates to AXL) using the original datasets from which the formulas have been derived. The actual "secret recipe" of each formula is beyond the scope of this text. The take-home message is that these formulas are much more accurate than previous-generation formulas, especially for eyes with unique biometric data. However, when dealing with extreme AXLs, these formulas too suffer from the limitations of their predecessors.

The Ladas Super Surface Formula (LSSF) was recently introduced to combine the strengths of these third-generation IOL formulas to improve refractive accuracy. Think of the LSSF like a Megazord-formula that combines all these third-generation formulas (the power rangers, in this analogy) into a real-time AI-influenced formula that adjusts based on surgeons' data via crowdsourcing.[27] While LSSF seeks to improve the results of third-generation formulas, it has not proved to be superior to multivariable formulas, especially for extreme AXL eyes.

Multivariable formulas (aka "fourth-generation formulas") primarily seek to better calculate the ELP by including other biometric measurements such as ACD, LT, CCT, HWTW, age, refraction, and retinal thickness.[28] For example:

- The Haigis formula attempts to measure ELP by including ACD and three different IOL constants (a0, a1, and a2).
- The Holladay 2 formula uses seven different measurements to predict ELP, including HWTW, refraction, and patient age.
- The Olsen formula uses thick-lens geometric optics and ray-tracing, and factors in preoperative ACD, corneal diameter (WTW), and LT. A key feature is the "C-constant," which can be conceptualized as a ratio by which the empty capsular bag will encapsulate and fixate an IOL following in-the-bag implantation. This formula primarily predicts ELP as a function of ACD and LT.
- The recently popular Barrett Universal II formula accounts for ELP by relating ACD to AXL/K and a relationship between the A-constant and a separate "lens factor." This formula also utilizes LT and WTW values when available to improve accuracy further, though it can be run solely off of AXL, K, and ACD measurements.[29]
- The Hill RBF is like a Tesla ®: Technically, there is no math in the formula as it relies on pattern recognition AI to review the inputted biometry measurements and determine the IOL power needed.[30]
- The Kane formula uses theoretical optics, regression, and AI components to calculate the IOL power.[31]

Several of these formulas have been integrated into commonly used biometry devices, while others are freely available online. You may wish to keep your eyes on several other formulas as authors publish their results, including the K6,[32] EVO 2.0, Pearl DGS, VRF, Castrop, Næser, and OKULIX formulas.

To date, when considering eyes with relatively average AXL and K values, there is no clear evidence that a single formula is leaps and bounds superior to other formulas. This author recommends that each surgeon uses several multivariable formulas with optimized lens constants for your preferred IOL in a comparative fashion, with the inclusion of your surgeon-induced astigmatism (SIA), to ensure relative agreement and similarity for the calculated IOL power. In other words, if 3–4 multivariable formulas all agree that a given IOL power will cause similar postoperative refraction, then go with that IOL power and hope for the best.

For eyes with unique biometric data (e.g., long/short AXL and flat/steep K's), this author strongly recommends that surgeons avoid using "traditional teaching" methods that favor third-generation formulas (e.g., SRK/T for long eyes and Hoffer Q for short eyes). Instead, surgeons should utilize *multivariable formulas whenever possible*. In addition, simultaneous comparison of several multivariable formulas should be strongly considered. Though it may require time and effort (for which you can't bill for, unfortunately), this author recommends using online multivariable formulas for eyes with unique measurements. In the future, a centralized online repository for multiple formula calculations with simultaneous comparison, similar to the ASCRS IOL power calculator in eyes with previous refractive surgery may

[27] Ladas Super Surface Formula available at www.IOLcalc.com. Accessed June 21, 2020

[28] "IOL Calculation Formulas Explained." https://cataract-community.zeiss.com/iol-calculation-formulas-explained. Accessed June 21, 2020

[29] "Barrett Universal II Formula." http://calc.apacrs.org/barrett_universal2105/. Accessed June 21, 2020

[30] "Hill-RBF Calculator Version 2.0." https://rbfcalculator.com/. Accessed June 21, 2020

[31] "Kane Formula" https://www.iolformula.com/about/. Accessed June 21, 2020

[32] Cooke Formula (K6). https://cookeformula.com/. Accessed January 9, 2021

further help surgeons to effectively and efficiently select an appropriate IOL power in short and long AL eyes. Ideally, a collaborative, multinational effort to amalgamate formulas for extreme AL eyes is needed to create a resource that is freely available to all surgeons. There is no one-size-fits-all, Swiss-army-knife type of formula that can be used for every single eye at this time. Future studies may shed further light on ideal formulas for a given biometry device and a given IOL platform.

It seems there is a new IOL formula released every few months – in future versions of this book, we may have to add much more information about each. It is beyond the scope of this text to say which IOL formula is best for which situation.[33] We have mainly included the previous discussion for you, dear reader, to appreciate how Optics plays a role in your life as a cataract surgeon and how all the "boring" stuff we discussed earlier actually has relevance!

Optical Angles and Axes

We may assume that when we look at an object in the distance, we can draw a straight line from the center of the fovea that goes through the center of the pupil and leads to the object of interest. However, this is not the whole story… there are **three axes** and **two angles** relevant to cataract surgery, especially when considering advanced technology IOLs (ATIOLs) for presbyopia correction.

Optical Axis, Pupillary Axis, and Visual Axis

A theoretical scenario can serve as an introduction to what is arguably a confusing topic: suppose you just performed perfect LASIK surgery on a + 3.50D OU hyperopic patient. You centered your treatment zone in the center of the pupil and pat yourself on the back for a job well done. You are imagining that she will return in a few days thrilled with your expertise and will name her first child after you.

Instead, the patient returns a week later, furious that she has disabling glare, halos, and starbursts that worsen with low-light conditions. Her objective visual acuity is 20/25, but she is bitterly angry.

What may have happened? Everything should be perfect, right? We centered our treatment in the exact center of the pupil and that's the spot that all patients look through… right?

Well, the answer to this question is a bit more complicated and requires us first to understand the various "axes" relevant for cataract and refractive surgery.

Note: the following discussion of the various axes intentionally does not use the term "line of sight", which other authors have discussed extensively as a distinct entity from the visual axis. As most cataract and refractive surgeons today use the term "visual axis", we will use this term in place of, but also inclusive of, the "line of sight". While we will briefly introduce the "line of sight", interested readers may wish to consult other texts on this topic.[34]

The three most important axes are as follows (Fig. 3):

- **Optical Axis**: The optical axis (OA) is an imaginary line that connects the optical center of the cornea and the optical center of the lens. We may additionally draw an extended imaginary line to the optical center of the retina for visualization purposes only. In optical biometry, the midpoint of the HWTW is used as a presumed location of the OA.
- **Pupillary Axis**: The pupillary axis (PA) is an imaginary line perpendicular to the corneal surface that passes through the midpoint of the pupil, similarly extended to the retina. The PA has no relationship to the visualized object or the foveal center.
- **Visual Axis**: The visual axis (VA) is an imaginary line that connects the visualized target and the foveal center. It has no relationship (necessarily) to the cornea, pupil, or lens. As stated previously, we will refer to the VA as inclusive of the "line of sight" as well.

In addition, some authorities defined OA as a line that connects the four Purkinje images that originate from a coaxial light source.[35] They have added the term (also referred to as the "line of sight") to refer to the line formed from the fixation point to the center of the entrance of the pupil. Therefore, by this classification, the line of sight can be considered the previously discussed OA, making the OA a separately defined axis altogether. Hopefully, you can see now why we have tried to minimize our discussions on the "line of sight".

Getting back to our hyperopic patient: In our good-intentioned efforts to center the ablation on the center of the pupil (PA), we may not have centered it on the VA. Though the objective visual acuity is good, the decentration is causing significant higher order aberrations (such as coma). Especially since this patient was a hyperope, there may have been a difference between the PA and VA, creating a *visual angle*. We will discuss these two angles in the next section.

[33]This is currently an area of significant interest among researchers, with many new formulas and papers being introduced every few months. The reader is directed to https://www.doctor-hill.com/iol-main/formulas.htm for a useful summary overview of when to use each formula.

[34]For example, see Azar DT (ed.), Refractive Surgery, third Edition. Elsevier Publishing, 2019.

[35]In addition to the below discussion on Purkinje images, see Chap. 28 Intraoperative Optics, for a more detailed discussion on the 4 Purkinje images seen through an operating microscope

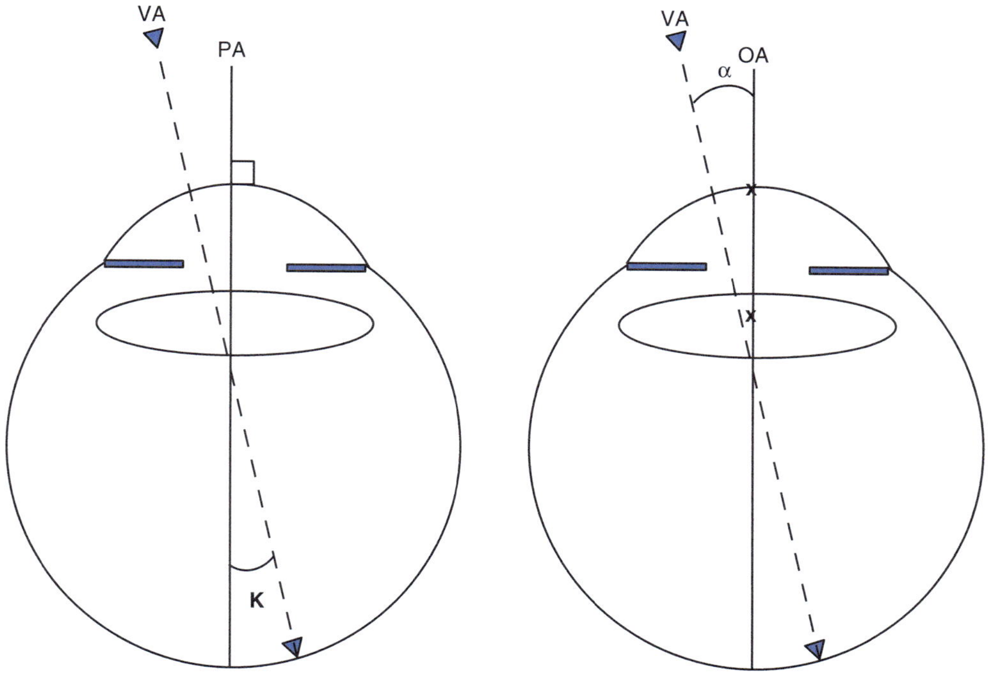

Fig. 3 Three axes (optical axis, pupillary axis, and visual axis) are relevant for cataract and refractive surgery. The optical axis (OA) is an imaginary line that connects the optical center of the cornea and the optical center of the lens. The pupillary axis (PA) is an imaginary line perpendicular to the corneal surface that passes through the midpoint of the pupil. The visual axis (VA) is an imaginary line that connects the visualized target and the foveal center. These three axes create two important angles: (1) Angle Alpha (α): this is the angle formed by the OA and the VA and (2) Angle Kappa (κ) (aka chord mu): this is the angle formed by the PA and the VA

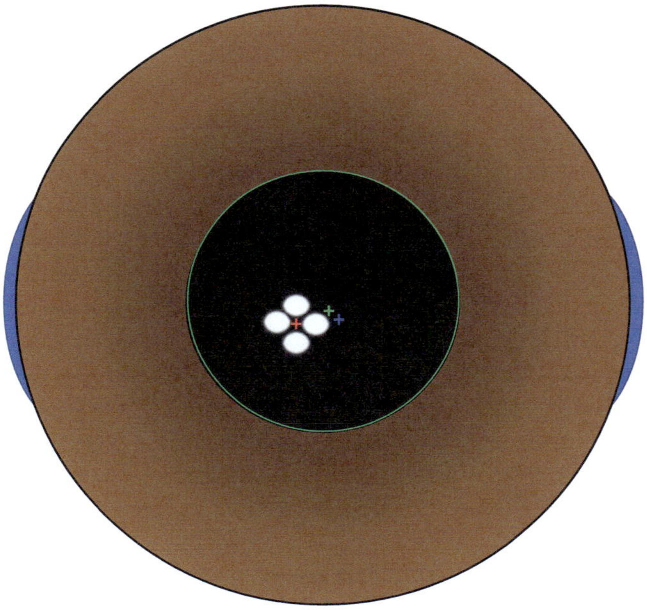

Fig. 4 Angle alpha and angle kappa are of significant interest when considering MFIOL/EDOF-IOLs. The first Purkinje image (red cross) represents the visual axis. The optical center (blue cross) is the center of the HWTW and is where the IOL will center. The pupillary axis (green cross) is the pupil center. In this example, the patient has a significant discrepancy between the visual axis (red cross) and the optical axis (blue cross), causing a significant angle alpha (>0.5 mm). The patient also has a large difference between the visual axis (red cross) and pupillary axis (green cross), indicating a large angle kappa as well. This patient is a poor candidate for an MFIOL or EDOF-IOL. Of note, the green circle represents the pupil (used to measure the pupillary axis), and the blue half-circles represent the horizontal white-to-white (used to measure the optical axis)

Angle Alpha and Angle Kappa

The VA would be the same as the OA and PA in a perfect eye. However, since this is not the case, we can use these three surgically relevant axes above to establish two additional surgically relevant angles (formed by these axes) (Fig. 4):

- **Angle Alpha**: This is the angle formed by the OA and the VA. The normal eye has about 5.2° horizontal and 1° vertical tilt of angle alpha. Angle alpha is *especially important for refractive IOL surgery* as it measures the degree of anatomical tilt of the eye relative to the optical axis. If there is a significant (>0.5 mm) angle alpha, the OA (which is the center of the capsular bag where the IOL will usually center) may not match the VA. This may not be an issue for a monofocal IOL, but when considering an MFIOL/EDOF-IOL, a patient with significant angle alpha may end up looking through the "rings" (through which the VA passes through) rather than the center of the IOL optic, despite a well-centered IOL (Fig. 4).[36]
- **Angle Kappa (aka chord mu)**: This is the angle formed by the PA and the VA.[37] It is supposed to represent the two-dimensional displacement of the entrance of the

[36] Some authors believe that the ideal location for a MFIOL/EDOF-IOL is halfway between the VA and PA. Usually, the VA is slightly nasal to the PA. When placing a MFIOL/EDOF-IOL, gently nudging the IOL nasally may help better land the IOL in this "sweet spot." See "Hidden Figures," https://crstodayeurope.com/articles/2018-apr/hidden-figures/. Accessed June 21, 2020

[37] A (questionably) useful mnemonic is "**AOV**" (alpha, optical, visual) and "**KPV**" (kappa, pupillary, visual)

pupil center from the subject-fixated, coaxially-sighted corneal light reflex. The normal eye has about a 2.6° tilt of angle kappa. Large angle kappa is commonly seen in hyperopes, indicating that the center of the pupil is not the true visual axis.[38] Angle kappa is especially important in excimer *laser refractive surgery.* The pupil-tracker will use iris landmarks to center the ablation, assuming that the pupillary axis is essentially the visual axis. Since this is not the case with hyperopes, ablation performed with pupil-tracking may inadvertently cause a decentered ablation since the patient's VA is not the same as the PA. In these situations, it may be helpful to align the ablation with the VA (as per the Purkinje image) rather than the PA. For ATIOL surgery, a patient with large angle kappa (>0.6 mm) may experience a central light ray to similarly hit the edge of the ring outside the central optic, thus increasing the unwanted effects of glare and optical aberrations. With modern biometry devices, the pupil barycenter values can be added together (ignoring positive or minus values) as a proxy for the angle kappa; *this measurement should be less than 0.6 mm.*[39]

Getting back to our clinical vignette, we can tie this all together by the following: Because the patient was a hyperope, she likely had a significant angle kappa. When we centered the ablation on the PA, we did not center it on the actual VA. As a result, the patient is looking "off-axis" from the ablation and likely has significant higher-order aberrations, including coma and irregular astigmatism.[40]

Overall, patients with abnormal angle alpha and/or angle kappa would also be poor candidates for diffractive ATIOLs (MFIOLs, EDOF-IOLs, and TF-IOLs). These patients would be better off with an aspheric, monofocal IOL. If they are interested in presbyopia correction, monovision, or an accommodating IOL would be better choices.

As a final aside: Recently, there has been significant discussion among refractive cataract surgeons regarding angle kappa and chord mu. Again, angle kappa is the angle formed between the pupillary axis and the visual axis; chord mu is defined as the distance between the pupil center and the subject-fixated, coaxially-sighted corneal light reflex. Modern IOL biometry devices, such as the IOL Master 700 (Carl Zeiss Meditec, Jena AG, Germany), can generate a chord mu value which serves as a proxy for angle kappa. Other biometers, such as the Lenstar (Haag-Streit, Switzerland), can show the x and y coordinates of the pupillary axis. By applying the Pythagorean formula, the chord mu (C) can be calculated as: $C = (x2 + y2)$. To simplify matters, one can simply add the absolute values of x and y and yield a "close enough" measurement of chord mu. Before you do your next cataract surgery, take a minute to look at the biometry printouts (which we cannot include due to copyrights) to see if you can find the chord mu. Again, this number should be less than 0.6 mm if one plans to implant an IOL with diffractive optics.

[38]There are many other conditions besides hyperopia that are associated with large angle kappa, such as cicatricial ROP, toxocariasis, and congenital retinal folds. These patients may present to the pediatric ophthalmologist for evaluation of (pseudo)strabismus and exotropia.

[39]These are the PCX/PCY and Px/Py values on the Lenstar® and IOL Master®, respectively.

[40]Some of you may wonder, what should be done for this patient? Therapeutic options now include a RGPCL/scleral contact lens or topography-guided ablation.

Considerations for Special Situations

Long and Short Axial Length Eyes

Third-generation formulas may calculate a lower-than-required IOL power in patients with long AXL (>25.5 mm). In these eyes, compared to normal AXL eyes, there is "more vitreous"; as a result, the optical signal spends more "time" traveling through the vitreous in a long AXL compared to a normal AXL. As the index of refraction of vitreous is slightly higher than aqueous (1.337 vs. 1.336, which we previously ignored), this plays a role in long AXL eyes. As a result, the measured AXL is **falsely long**, leading to **hyperopic surprise**. This would be devastating for any patient, especially those with long AXL, as they have presumably been myopic their whole lives and would be extremely unhappy if they became hyperopic after surgery. As always, being a hyperope stinks…

A landmark paper in 2011 was the first to describe a method for adjusting the AXL (popularly known as the "Wang-Koch" modification) if working with third-generation formulas (Holladay I, Hoffer Q, and SRK/T) and the Haigis formula.[41] Basically, the measured AXL (by OB) would need to be adjusted and re-entered as a modified AXL back into the biometry device for a more accurate calculation of the required IOL power. A follow-up paper from the same authors in 2018 included updated AXL factors for each formula.[42] This AXL modification improved the outcomes of these four popularly used formulas. In recent times, as surgeons have shifted toward favoring multivariable formulas, this modification has become unnecessary as the formulas have a built-in mathematical mechanism to compensate for long AXL. In other words, if you use Barrett, Hill RBF, Kane, etc., you do not have to worry about manually making this adjustment. Additionally, the Wang-Koch modification should not be used in patients with a history of laser refractive surgery.

[41]Wang L, Shirayama M, Ma XJ, et al. Optimizing intraocular lens power calculations in eyes with axial lengths above 25.0 mm. *J Cataract Refract Surg*. 2011;37(11):2018–2027.

[42]Wang L, Koch DD. Modified axial length adjustment formulas in long eyes. J Cataract Refract Surg. 2018 Nov; 44(11):1396–1397.

There is an even greater risk for inaccurate AXL measurements for short AXL eyes – again, it stinks to be a hyperope. Due to the math involved in the available IOL formulas, inaccurate AXL measurements in short AXL eyes will more profoundly affect the calculated IOL power than long AXL eyes. One reason may be that the IOL is "closer" to the retina in these eyes (as compared to normal AXL eyes), and even a small change in ELP may cause more of a refractive effect – we also know that these eyes are prone to significant variation in post-operative ELP. In addition, current IOL manufacturing standards for tolerance in higher powers (>30D) allow for greater variability: in other words, it may be that a +32D IOL is not really +32D. Finally, the ACD in these eyes is also quite shallow, either due to anatomical variation or thickness of the cataract; this also skews the calculated IOL power.

Thankfully, the most commonly encountered refractive error in short AXL eyes is a *postoperative myopic surprise*, likely due to a more anterior ELP of the IOL than predicted, especially in patients with shallow ACDs. As most of these patients are usually hyperopes prior to cataract surgery, they actually may be quite happy with a myopic outcome as they may be able to finally read without reading glasses!

As mentioned previously, this author recommends that surgeons utilize multivariable formulas (either biometry-integrated or online calculators) in a side-by-side comparison for formula agreement when calculating the desired IOL power in these extreme AXL eyes.

Silicone Oil

This is the one section that drives many trainees crazy – it is no surprise that it is also a topic that senior attendings may love to quiz you on. This is a confusing yet high-yield discussion.

Silicone Oil and Biometry

A foundational rule for this discussion is that any signal (USB more than OB) that travels through silicone oil (SO) (index of refraction: 1.40–1.52, depending on the type and weight of the SO) will be slowed down compared to the signal traveling through vitreous (index of refraction: 1.337). As a result, it will take *longer* for the signal to return, leading to an *erroneously high AXL* measurement (often >30 mm!).

If we are using USB, we can adjust the machine settings (from 1532 m/s to 980 m/s) so that the measurement taken through SO will be as if taken through vitreous. For example, if we measured an eye with USB without signal adjustment, we may measure an AXL of 33.85 mm (falsely long). However, when we measure that same eye with the adjusted velocity (980 m/s through SO of 1,000 cSt), we may get a more accurate measurement of 25.07 mm - this is a huge difference!. In this scenario, we are assuming that the SO <u>will be removed in the future</u> (more on this below).

When we use a modern OB device, we can select the "phakic silicone oil" mode, which similarly attempts to correct the potential error in AXL measurement. This setting again assumes that the SO <u>will be removed in the future</u> and will calculate an IOL power accordingly. Suppose we used this setting, but then the SO permanently stays in the eye; this will cause a 4–6D more-than-desired hyperopic refractive error because the SO will mold to the posterior surface of the biconvex IOL (recall the discussion in the previous section), thereby decreasing the effective power of IOL. Of course, we can reduce this effect by using a convex-plano IOL, but this type of IOL is no longer available in the USA.

If the patient was emmetropic before retina surgery, the AXL of the eye without SO can be used by those of us who forgot all the other pearls.

To summarize: If the SO **<u>will never be removed</u>**, then use non-adjusted measurements because the SO is the new vitreous. Even then, because the SO may mold to the back of the IOL, we will have to increase the power of the IOL by 4–6D to account for this hyperopic shift. If the SO **<u>can be removed in the future</u>**, then use the "phakic silicone oil" setting on the biometry device to calculate the needed IOL power.

Of course, this is all a moot point since most of these eyes have lousy vision potential anyway, but we digress.

Silicone Oil and IOL Choices

As discussed previously, a convex-plano IOL would be ideal for these eyes. Since we do not have this type of IOL, we are forced to use a biconvex IOL (unless we planned for intentional convex-plano ACIOL implantation, which is not recommended). A biconvex IOL can lose up to one-third its refractive power due to SO molding; if the SO can never be removed and biometry calls for a + 20.0D IOL, one may go ahead and place a + 25–26.0D IOL to account for this loss of IOL power.

In terms of IOL material, acrylic, collamer, or PMMA IOLs are reasonable choices. Silicone IOLs should be avoided in these eyes due to the risk of silicone IOL-SO interaction leading to visually significant opacities. As light passes through the IOL (which has a higher index of refraction; for example, acrylic IOLs have an index of refraction 1.47–1.55) into the vitreous (1.337), it is refracted to a certain degree. However, if it now passes through SO (1.40), it will be refracted much less, thanks to our good old friend Snell's Law(!). Therefore, the IOL must be strong by approximately 4–5D if the SO remains in the eye.

Silicone Oil and Cataract Surgery: Hi-Yield Summary

If one has to ever explain this, the following summary may suffice and should be committed to memory:

- First, we must understand that the optical issue with SO in the eye is the potential inaccuracy in IOL calculation, leading to a *high risk of hyperopic surprise*.
- The million-dollar question: *does the SO need to remain in the eye*? There are three possible scenarios:
- First Possibility: The SO can be removed immediately. If so, remove the SO, perform routine biometry, perform cataract surgery, and move along: nothing more to see here.
- Second Possibility: The SO can be removed in the distant future, but the cataract needs to be removed now. This itself has three potential answers:
  - Measure the SO filled eye and aim for -5D myopia to account for potential postoperative hyperopia.
  - Use a biometry machine with SO settings, but remember that the suggested IOL is for an eye with no SO. Therefore, if we use this SO setting and place an IOL aiming for emmetropia, we will end up with approximately 5D of hyperopia if the SO is not removed.
  - Assuming that the refraction and keratometry of the two eyes are similar (before placement of SO), we can consider using the measurements of the non-SO-filled eye to calculate the IOL.
- Third Possibility: The SO will never be removed. In this case, use the non-adjusted measurements because the SO is the new "vitreous." However, we should still aim for an additional +5.0D in the calculated IOL power to account for SO molding to the posterior surface of the IOL. For example, if the non-adjusted measurement calls for a 22D IOL for target plano, use a 27D instead.

If you can rattle this off coherently, please take a bow before moving to the next section.

Previous History of Refractive Surgery

When determining accurate IOL power in patients with a previous history of refractive surgery, there are two main issues: corneal power measurement inaccuracy and spherical aberration issues.

Corneal Power Measurement Inaccuracy: Corneal power measurements after refractive surgery may be inaccurate due to (a combination of) three reasons:

- Instrument errors: Keratometers only measure the central zone (3.2 mm) of the cornea, which is smaller than the effective central zone. This is especially important in patients with a previous history of high myopia. These corneas tend to be much flatter than virgin corneas, thus causing even more of a measurement error.
- Index of refraction: The corneal index of refraction (1.3375) used by most keratometry devices assumes a fixed ratio between the anterior and posterior corneal surfaces. Remember, the posterior surface of the cornea is like the dark side of the moon: We do not have a good way to measure it, so we measure the anterior surface and make assumptions about the posterior surface. This works (usually) well in virgin corneas, but this anterior-posterior relationship is no longer the same after refractive surgery. As a rule of thumb, the corneal power is over-estimated by approximately 1D for every 6D of treated refractive error.
- Limitation of IOL formulas: Older-generation formulas primarily rely on AXL and keratometry measurements to calculate the ELP. If the keratometry measurements are inaccurate (and not adjusted), the formula will call for a lower-than-required IOL power, and the patient will have a hyperopic surprise. Therefore, we have to use "modified" formulas to adjust for the keratometry measurement inaccuracies.

In normal corneas, we assume a constant ratio (called the Gullstrand ratio from the Gullstrand schematic eye[43]) between the posterior and anterior curvatures, which is approximately 0.883 (6.8/7.7, respectively, or 88.3%) or, as more recently suggested, 0.813 (81.3%).[44] Do not get too bogged down by these numbers. After refractive surgery, the anterior curvature will change (e.g., become flatter after myopic correction), and the Gullstrand ratio will increase. In addition to looking at the front surface K values, one pearl to determine whether a patient has had refractive surgery is to use Scheimpflug tomography to measure the posterior and anterior corneal curvatures (in mm). If the posterior-anterior cornea ratio is higher than 0.82, there is a high likelihood that the patient has undergone myopic laser vision correction.

In summary, the keratometry measurements are inherently inaccurate because refractive surgery alters the corneal curvature. Therefore:

- In *post-myopic* laser refractive surgery patients, the **keratometry measurements are falsely steeper-than-real**. This causes an **underestimation of the IOL power**, leading to potential **hyperopic surprise**. For example, we can see from Fig. 1 that if we falsely increase the value of "K," we will decrease the value of the calculated IOL.
- In *post-hyperopic* laser refractive surgery patients, the **keratometry measurements are falsely flatter-than-real**. This causes an **overestimation of the IOL power**, leading to potential **myopic surprise** (which is not a terrible outcome, one may argue).

[43] An old friend (enemy) returns! See Chap. 7, "Schematic Eye"

[44] Dubbelman M Van der Heijde GL Weeber HA Vrensen GF . Radius and asphericity of the posterior corneal surface determined by corrected Scheimpflug photography. Acta Ophthalmol Scand. 2002; 80:379–383. The anterior and posterior corneal radii can be used to calculate the APR (**a**nterior corneal radius/**p**osterior corneal radius **r**atio) or P/A (**p**osterior/**a**nterior corneal radii) ratio. Previous authors have reported the APR ratio (range 1.19–1. 23) and P/A ratio (approximately 0.83) in a normal population is significantly different from the ratio in post laser vision correction (LVC) patients. As the APR and P/A values are inversely related, post-myopic LVC eyes will have lower APR and higher P/A values, respectively.

Several methods have been proposed to measure corneal power more accurately (both via indirect and direct methods).[45] Modern OB machines may include formulas (e.g., Haigis-L) that make specific adjustments for more accurate keratometry measurements for post-refractive surgery eyes.[46] As mentioned previously, TK values can be used with an older formula, such as the Haigis formula. Most surgeons currently use a free online calculator hosted by the American Society of Cataract and Refractive Surgery (ASCRS) that offers multiple formulas that can be used in a side-by-side comparison fashion; each of these formulas, such as the Wang-Koch-Maloney, Shammas, Potvin-Hill, and Barrett True K formulas, attempt to calculate the true corneal power depending on available data to calculate the required IOL.[47] Notably, some of these formulas require additional measurements, such as corneal power from topography, tomography, or AS-OCT devices.

Spherical Aberration Issues: If you thought we were done with spherical aberration, guess again!

- Traditional myopic laser treatments (i.e., prior to wavefront-guided (WG) and wavefront-optimized (WO) treatments) primarily treated the central cornea and left the peripheral cornea relatively untouched. As a result, these traditional myopic laser treatments typically increased corneal spherical aberration.
- In contrast, traditional hyperopic laser treatments decreased the corneal spherical aberration due to mainly treating the peripheral cornea and leaving the central cornea relatively untouched. With WG/WO treatments, the SA theoretically remains relatively unchanged because of peripheral blend zone treatment.

The two most common types of post-refractive patients presenting for cataract surgery are patients with previous history of PRK/LASIK and previous history of radial keratotomy (RK).

Previous Laser Refractive Surgery: PRK and LASIK

We can summarize our strategy for these patients as follows:

For post-myopic refractive surgery patients:

- Use available post-refractive IOL formulas, including the ASCRS online calculator, to calculate the needed IOL and err on the side of additional myopia (i.e., aim for −0.50 or − 0.75 instead of emmetropia).
- An **aspheric** IOL with **negative spherical aberration** may be advantageous due to these eyes' increased positive spherical aberration. An aberration-free IOL is also be a good choice, especially if the patient desires some additional near vision (i.e., leaving behind some positive spherical aberration). A <u>spherical IOL</u> would be the <u>worst</u> choice.
- Thoroughly discuss with the patient the potential for postoperative refractive error (especially hyperopic surprise) and the need for potential postoperative adjustment(s) of these errors (e.g., glasses, contact lenses, piggyback IOL, IOL exchange, or additional excimer laser surgery).

For post-hyperopic refractive surgery patients:

- Use available post-refractive IOL formulas, including the ASCRS online calculator, to calculate the IOL power. Given the increased risk of myopic surprise, we can safely target close to emmetropia.
- A **spherical IOL** with **positive spherical aberration** or an aberration-free IOL is a good choice. An <u>aspheric IOL</u> with negative spherical aberration would be the <u>worst</u> choice.

Previous Radial Keratotomy (RK) Surgery

In retrospect, it remains unclear who was the bigger idiot: the fool under the microscope or the fool behind the microscope (source unknown).

Radial keratotomy (RK) was introduced in the late 1970s as an incisional procedure to correct myopia. A guarded blade was used to make radial cuts (approximately 90% corneal thickness) to cause secondary corneal flattening based on the number of incisions. For a while, RK worked; however, complications such as progressive hyperopia, irregular astigmatism, and corneal scarring rendered this procedure in modern times as an abandoned and obsolete surgery.[48] Please see Chap. 30, "Optics for Refractive Surgery", for more information about RK.

Cataract surgeons must know about RK because these post-RK patients may now require cataract surgery. There are several considerations for these patients:

Preoperative Considerations

- Corneal measurements are even *more inaccurate* in post-RK eyes than post-PRK/LASIK eyes. Again, the keratometry measurements are falsely steeper-than-real (similar to post-myopic laser refractive surgery), leading to an inaccurately low IOL power and increased risk of hyperopic surprise. The current post-RK IOL formulas

[45] A good summary of these strategies may be found at: https://eyewiki.aao.org/Biometry_for_Intra-Ocular_Lens_(IOL)_power_calculation#After_Refractive_Surgery. Accessed June 21, 2020.

[46] Recall from our previous discussions above that the Haigis formula does not rely on the K values to determine the ELP, and instead relies on ACD measurements and 3 constants (a0, a1, and a2). The Haigis-L is a modification of this Haigis formula.

[47] "IOL power calculation in eyes that have undergone LASIK/PRK/RK." https://iolcalc.ascrs.org/. Accessed June 21, 2020.

[48] For example, the PERK Study (1982–83) evaluated the safety and efficacy of RK. Ten-year results showed that 53% of patients ≥20/20 vision. However, the biggest finding was the instability of the procedure: a hyperopic shift (≥1 D) was seen in 43% of the study patients. See Waring GO third, Lynn MJ, McDonnell PJ. Results of the prospective evaluation of radial keratotomy (PERK) study 10 years after surgery. *Arch Ophthalmol.* 1994; 112(10):1298–1308.

are even less accurate than post-PRK/LASIK IOL formulas. As such, surgeons should target more myopia (-1D or more) to account for a postoperative hyperopic surprise. Post-RK formulas can be found on the ASCRS website like the post-LASIK formulas.
- Patients should be strongly counseled regarding the challenges associated with accurate biometry measurements and should have reasonable expectations. They should not expect perfect vision immediately after cataract surgery.

Intraoperative Considerations

- Depending on the number of wounds (usually 8 RK incisions were made, though up to 50 incisions have been seen!), the old RK incisions may splay open with a standard clear corneal incision. If the RK cuts are minimal, using a smaller blade (≤2.2 mm) with strategic placement of the incision may be sufficient; otherwise, a scleral tunnel may be the safest option.
- Surgeons should have suture available in case the RK incisions splay open during surgery. Use low flow settings to minimize stress to the incisions. Move slowly but efficiently during every step of the procedure. This should not be a 10-minute cataract!
- Avoid any diffractive ATIOLs (MFIOLs, EDOF-IOL, and TF-IOLs). Stick with aspheric monofocal IOLs as the safest option. This is somewhat controversial as some surgeons maintain that EDOF-IOLs can be used in these patients without difficulty. For exam purposes, a conservative approach is recommended; thus, aspheric monofocal IOLs are the safest option. An accommodating IOL or monovision may be considered if that patient desires presbyopia correction.

Postoperative Considerations

- The RK incisions may swell after cataract surgery, causing corneal flattening and immediate postoperative (transient) hyperopia. Do not panic! Wait at least 6–8 weeks with serial refraction and examination before jumping into doing additional piggyback IOL or IOL exchange surgery.
- Patients should be counseled that the postoperative refraction may vary considerably. These patients should **not** expect immediate 20/20 vision like routine cataract surgery patients – they have to atone for their past sins by being patient postoperatively. Some patients may require up to 3 months to allow for stabilization of the refractive error.
- Patients may require glasses or contact lenses (including RGPCLs for irregular astigmatism) to manage postoperative errors. Surgical intervention may include piggyback IOL (especially for confirmed, persistent hyperopic surprise), IOL exchange, or cautious PRK. LASIK is highly discouraged(!) in these patients as flap creation would be extremely challenging and risky.

Phakic IOL

A few Optics related considerations should be kept in mind when performing cataract surgery in patients with existing phakic IOLs:

- The phakic IOL does **not** have to be removed before performing preoperative biometry measurements. It can be removed (obviously) at the time of cataract surgery.
- When using OB for preoperative measurements, we do not have to make any additional adjustments because the phakic IOL's effect on low-coherence light is minimal, especially for collamer phakic IOLs, which are the most commonly implanted phakic IOLs in the United States.[49]
- If we have to use USB, we should keep in mind that the AXL measurement will likely be inaccurate. The least amount of inaccuracy is with collamer phakic IOLs. If the patient has a silicone phakic IOL (especially a hyperopic one, which is not available in the United States), there is a greater chance of inaccurate AXL measurement.
- To calculate the "correct" AXL, the following formula can be used[50]:

$$AL\left(corrected\right) = AL\left(1555\right) + \left(X \times T\right)$$

- where $X = +0.42$ (0.41–0.42) for poly (methyl methacrylate), −0.59 (0.56–0.59) for silicone, +0.11 (0.10–0.12) for collamer, and + 0.23 (0.23–0.24) for acrylic; and T is the central thickness of the phakic IOL.

Biometry in Undilated Versus Dilated States

Performing biometry on patients without dilation (and other diagnostic drops, such as topical anesthetics) is ideal clinical practice. Multivariable formulas factor in other biometric measurements, such as ACD, in calculating the IOL power. It is also well known that ACD increases after dilation, and multivariable IOL formulas incorporate ACD measurements differently.[51]

In real-world clinical settings, patients with visually significant cataracts may be examined by a clinician after dilation, and the decision for surgery may follow. In this setting, while it is ideal for the patient to return and undergo undilated biometry measurements, it may be convenient to perform post-dilation biometry so that the patient does not have to return for an additional visit for biometry testing. If using first- to third-generation formulas, post-dilation biometry

[49] Sanders DR, Bernitsky DA, Harton PJ Jr., Rivera RR. The Visian myopic implantable collamer lens does not significantly affect axial length measurement with the IOLMaster. J Refract Surg. 2008 Nov; 24(9):957–9.

[50] Hoffer KJ. Ultrasound axial length measurement in biphakic eyes. J Cataract Refract Surg. 2003 May; 29(5):961–5.

[51] Rodriguez-Raton A, Jimenez-Alvarez M, Arteche-Limousin L, et al. Effect of pupil dilation on biometry measurements with partial coherence interferometry and its effect on IOL power formula calculation. Eur J Ophthalmol. 2015;25:309–14

measurements are essentially the same as undilated biometry measurements. However, if using multivariable IOL formulas, post-dilation biometry measurements may favor a higher-power IOL in a significant portion of cases, increasing the likelihood of a myopic surprise.[52] Again, not the end of the world, but not an ideal situation, nonetheless.

Combined Cataract and Corneal Surgery

For some patients, combined cataract and corneal transplant surgery may be needed. While there is seemingly an alphabet soup of corneal transplant surgeries these days, we will focus on two types of combined cataract-corneal surgeries. Again, the common theme is the risk of the dreaded hyperopic surprise…

Penetrating Keratoplasty (PKP)

As expected, the major drawback to combined cataract/PKP surgery ("the old triple procedure") is the inaccuracy of IOL power prediction given the unpredictable power of the cornea after PKP. Unless one is a superhero corneal surgeon who can consistently predict "x" keratometry readings (and astigmatism) after PKP, inaccuracies in IOL selection are likely.

Therefore, some authorities recommend performing the PKP first, waiting at least a year for the cornea to stabilize (including astigmatism management with suture removal), and then performing cataract surgery using the post-PKP corneal measurements (that presumably have stabilized and are accurate). While this is an ideal approach, it may not always be possible to delay the cataract surgery, especially in trauma or rapid progression cases. Others recommend performing the PKP with cataract removal only, waiting until the keratometry measurements have stabilized, and placing a secondary IOL 6–12 months later. This also may be less-than-deal, as the capsular bag may fibrose, preventing in-the-bag IOL placement. This also requires an additional surgical procedure with potential risks and setbacks.

There may be various postoperative refractive errors, especially high/irregular astigmatism and the dreaded hyperopic surprise. For exam purposes, if one has to do combined cataract/PKP, several strategies for keratometry readings may be considered, including but not limited to the following:

- Reviewing his/her previous historical post-PKP astigmatism values (at least 10 cases), a surgeon may use the average of these K-readings as a reasonable estimate for postoperative K-readings.
- Use an assumed K-reading of 44-45D, aim −1 to −2D myopic, and proceed with cataract surgery.
- Use the K-readings from the fellow eye (if available), especially in cases of unilateral disease (e.g., corneal scar from infection). This may not work well if the other eye also may soon need PKP (e.g., bilateral advanced keratoconus).
- Multiple-regression analysis with surgeon-specific values and individualized a-constants can also be applied – this also requires a lot of historical data and meticulous effort.

For real-world purposes, one should aim for additional myopia; this author routinely uses a -2D target in these situations. Alternatively, you may consider referring these cases to a corneal surgeon with experience dealing with this scenario.

Endothelial Keratoplasty (EK)

The field of EK has undergone significant advancements, with a variety of new procedures now being routinely performed, including Descemet's stripping (automated) endothelial keratoplasty (DSEK/DSAEK), Descemet's membrane endothelial keratoplasty (DMEK), and Pre-Descemet's endothelial keratoplasty (PDEK). EK procedures are much more amenable to being combined with cataract surgery. While some surgeons advocate staging procedures whenever possible, combined cataract and EK surgery may be necessary given the clinical scenario and patient expectations.

DSAEK is a tissue additive procedure (40–150 μm of tissue, including endothelium, Descemet's membrane, and some stroma. This leads to changes in posterior corneal curvature as well as corneal deturgescence. The net result of this magical symphony is a *hyperopic shift after DSAEK*, ranging from 0.5 to 2.0D. As a result, the refractive target should be about −1 to −1.5D with combined cataract/DSAEK to compensate for potential hyperopic shit.

DMEK is a 1:1 tissue replacement surgery. Since there is significantly less transplanted tissue, the amount of *postoperative hyperopic shift is less than DSAEK*. As a result, the refractive target should be about –0.5 to –1D to compensate for potential hyperopic shifts. Alternatively, using an IOL power +1D higher than the biometry print out values can also help achieve emmetropia. For example, if a given IOL formula predicts that a +19.0D will get a –0.50D final refraction, surgeons can instead use a +20.0D IOL to obtain the desired –0.50D refraction in such a scenario.

Preoperative considerations include the presence of significant corneal edema that may confound biometry measurements. To obtain better keratometry measurements, one may consider using topical glycerin before biometry or performing a superficial keratectomy to "debulk" astigmatism. Intraoperatively, surgeons should avoid placing a hydrophilic IOL as the concurrent use of air or gas may

[52] Simon NC, Farooq AV, Zhang MH, et al. The Effect of Pharmacological Dilation on Calculation of Targeted and Ideal IOL Power Using Multivariable Formulas [published online ahead of print, 2020 May 27]. *Ophthalmol Ther.* 2020; https://doi.org/10.1007/s40123-020-00261-x

cause opacification of the IOL. A smaller (4.5–5.0 mm) capsulorrhexis is also useful, to ensure that the IOL remains in the bag during the EK procedure, especially during moments of iatrogenic anterior chamber flattening for graft manipulation. Finally, patients should be counseled about the risk of refractive error after cataract/EK surgery, including hyperopic surprise and the need for glasses.

Cataract Surgery in Pediatric Patients

Biometry measurements in kids have a potential for inaccuracy for a variety of reasons. For example, USB is usually performed after induction of general anesthesia in the OR rather than OB in the clinic. There are also increased errors in AXL measurement (due to the short AXL). Finally, the biggest question: *What IOL power should be selected to balance good vision and allow the child to "grow"?*

This is a controversial topic. At present, fewer surgeons are placing primary IOLs in infants since the 5-year results of the Infant Aphakia Treatment Study were published.[53] This study reported that infants who received an IOL had the same vision as those left aphakic and used contact lenses.[54] The patients with an IOL tended to need more follow-up surgeries than those who were aphakic.

However, placing an IOL at the time of the cataract surgery may be preferred for patients who cannot afford the contact lenses. Pediatric cataract surgeons will place an IOL that causes initial hyperopia (under-correction) to allow the child to "grow into" the IOL and avoid potential later myopic shift. This makes sense because kids can usually wear glasses or even contact lenses for low hyperopia. Recently, several tables for postoperative refractive targets based on age have been published, with a range from +5D at age 2yrs to +1D at age 10. For older kids, emmetropia may be targeted. Age of the child, compliance with patching and spectacles, and unilateral vs. bilateral cataracts are also factors that should be considered in deciding which refractive goal is best.

Uncorrected postoperative hyperopia is more amblyogenic than uncorrected myopia. Patients with the latter will at least be able to see at near uncorrected. In other words, if post-op spectacle and patching compliance are expected to be poor, then a goal of post-op emmetropia (and increasing myopia later in life) may be preferable than +5D uncorrected hyperopia and long-term BCVA 20/200 due to dense amblyopia.

A published model in the literature recommends using axial length and age to predict a long term postoperative axial length[55]:

Postoperative AXL = 1.93 + 0.91 x (baseline AXL) – 0.07 x (baseline age) + 0.14 x (age at follow-up) – 0.005 x (baseline age) x (age at follow-up).

For example: A 3-year-old child with an AXL of 21.95 mm may be expected to have an axial length of 24.19 mm at age 20 years.

Postoperative AXL = 1.93 + 0.91 x (21.95) - 0.07 x (3) + 0.14 x (20) - 0.05 X (3) X (20) = 24.19 mm.

This predicted AXL can then be used in the surgeon's IOL formula of choice to plan for emmetropia at age 20.

The takeaway from this discussion is not to debate the merits of whether or not you should place an IOL in a pediatric patient. Instead, keep in mind the Optics-related details, especially due to changing refractive errors in this patient population.

Cataract Surgery in Keratoconus Patients

Many keratoconus (KCN) patients may require cataract surgery without concurrent or future corneal transplant surgery. Recall that KCN progression tends to plateau in middle-age years, and these patients may have good vision with glasses or contact lenses until they develop visually significant cataracts.

As a simplification, we can classify KCN patients into two groups:

- KCN patients who are accustomed to wearing glasses only
- KCN patients who are accustomed to primarily wearing contact lenses (e.g., soft toric contact lenses (STCLs), rigid gas permeable (hard) contact lenses (RGPCLs), and scleral contact lenses (ScCLs))

We can further divide these groups into subgroups: patients who desire astigmatism correction at the time of cataract surgery and those who do not. Since many of these patients are significantly myopic their entire lives, the last thing we want is to make them hyperopic after cataract surgery. The crux of the problem in KCN corneas is *that the steeper the cornea, the greater the risk for postoperative hyperopia.*

Measurement of corneal power remains challenging in KCN patients. One area of confusion for many surgeons is that given the numerous devices to obtain keratometry (K)

[53] VanderVeen DK, Drews-Botsch CD, Nizam A, Bothun ED, Wilson LB, Wilson ME, Lambert SR; Infant Aphakia Treatment Study. Outcomes of Secondary Intraocular Lens Implantation in the Infant Aphakia Treatment Study. J Cataract Refract Surg. 2020 Sep 7.

[54] Infant Aphakia Treatment Study Group, Lambert SR, Lynn MJ, Hartmann EE, DuBois L, Drews-Botsch C, Freedman SF, Plager DA, Buckley EG, Wilson ME. Comparison of contact lens and intraocular lens correction of monocular aphakia during infancy: a randomized clinical trial of HOTV optotype acuity at age 4.5 years and clinical findings at age 5 years. JAMA Ophthalmol. 2014 Jun; 132(6):676–82.

[55] Trivedi RH, Barnwell E, Wolf B, Wilson ME. A Model to Predict Postoperative Axial Length in Children Undergoing Bilateral Cataract Surgery with Primary Intraocular Lens Implantation. Am J Ophthalmol. 2019 Oct; 206:228–234.

measurements, which K values should we use if different devices give us different K measurements? In addition, should one device's K values be given preference over another?

As a broad simplification, we can classify devices that give K measurements into the following categories:

- Biometry devices: e.g., IOL Master, Lenstar, etc. These are usually preferred because IOL formulas are primarily based on K measurements from biometry devices.
- Topography devices: e.g., Atlas, Antares, etc. These devices are helpful to check for irregular astigmatism and axis skew.
- Ray-tracing devices: e.g., iTrace.
- Tomography devices: e.g., Pentacam, Galilei. These devices are helpful to assess anterior and posterior elevation changes. The Pentacam can generate two maps that may be of interest: (1) Holladay EKR Detail Report (which has the EKR65 mean at 4.0 mm values) and (2) Power Distribution Map (which has the True Net Power (TNP) at 4.0 mm values). We should avoid using the SimK values for IOL calculations, such as those shown on the default 4 Maps Refractive screen, because these values were *not* designed for IOL calculation purposes! This is a common mistake made by many well-intentioned surgeons.

Some surgeons have suggested that the *mean of five values* obtained on different devices give sufficient accuracy to predict the appropriate IOL power. Alternatively, to derive this "synthesized keratometry," one can average the K1, K2, and axis values to derive this "synthesized keratometry." Still, five or more values seem to be the magic number if one has access to this many devices(!).

After obtaining K measurements, we can choose which IOL formula(s) to use. Most formulas tend to produce *more-than-intended hyperopic* postoperative refractive errors.

Older-generation IOL formulas tend to be inadequate for eyes with unique biometric measurements. However, and somewhat fortuitously, good old SRK/T can work well in KCN eyes because it produces myopic errors in non-KCN eyes with steep K measurements (Melles RB, Holladay JT, Chang WJ. Accuracy of intraocular lens calculation formulas. Ophthalmology. 2018;125(2):169–78). If we use SRK/T, we can aim for approximately −2D myopia and expect some "hyperopic shift" such that we end up with a close-to-plano refractive error. We can also use the Holladay I formula with the mean ERK65 values taken from the Pentacam for both the flat and steep K in a given IOL formula. Remember to use the WK adjustment for AXL in both formulas since many KCN eyes are longer than 26 mm.

When we examine currently available multivariable IOL formulas, we have several options:

1. Barrett True K KC: make sure to choose the *keratoconus* option and aim for approx. -0.75 to −1 D. This formula can be found at: http://calc.apacrs.org/Barrett_True_K_Universal_2105
   (a) Use the regular K values from the biometry device.
   (b) Do not use the TK values from the IOL Master 700 or the EKR65 values on the main page. Why not? Since this formula inherently adjusts for the posterior cornea, using either the TK or EKR65 will cause us to inadvertently "double-dip" in the posterior cornea adjustment. However, the website offers surgeons the option to use the "predicted PCA", which means the formula does the "hard work" of calculating the posterior corneal power; or "measured PCA", which requires us to separately input the posterior Pentacam or posterior keratometry (PK) values (NOT the TK values!) and central corneal thickness. The measured PCA may give better outcomes, especially in KCN eyes with K values > 50 D.
   (c) Current results indicate that this formula gives slightly more than-intended myopic results, which may not be bad for KCN patients who are likely accustomed to myopia.
2. Kane KC: make sure to choose the *keratoconus* option and aim for approx. -0.75 to −1 D. This formula can be found at: https://www.iolformula.com
   (a) Like the previous formula, use the regular K values from the biometry device.
   (b) Current results indicate that this formula gives slightly more than-intended myopic results, which may not be bad for KCN patients who are likely accustomed to myopia.
3. Barrett Toric Calculator (note this is different from the first Barrett formula in this list). This formula can be found at: https://calc.apacrs.org/toric_calculator20/Toric%20Calculator.aspx
   (a) This formula can use modified K values. Therefore, use TK or the ERK65K values for this formula.
   (b) This formula is beneficial if you want to put in a toric IOL in KCN patients (more on this below).
4. Other multivariable formulas such as Barrett Universal 2, Olsen, and Hill RBF have internal mechanisms to account for posterior corneal power. However, in KCN eyes (especially if both K's are < 50D), one may cautiously use the TK or EKR65 values instead of the K values. As mentioned previously, some surgeons prefer using the EKR65 Km value (for both K1 and K2) with the Holladay I formula (with AXL adjustment, if needed).

When considering IOL options in KCN patients, we should avoid diffractive-optics IOLs for presbyopia correction (see Chap. 27 What's on the Menu: An Overview of Currently Available IOLs and Relevant Optics, for more information on IOL options). Our two IOL options are as follows:

Monofocal IOLs: Recall that many KCN corneas have serendipitous multifocality and significant HOAs. Paradoxically, many KCN patients may be accustomed to these higher amounts of HOAs, especially spherical aberration (SA), which confers some depth of focus and enhanced intermediate-near vision. Thus, while it may be tempting to use a monofocal, aspheric IOL with high amounts of negative SA correction (e.g., ZCB00 platform (Johnson and Johnson Vision, Jacksonville, FL, USA) and AcrySof platform (Alcon Laboratories, Inc., Fort Worth, TX, USA)), it may be advisable to use an aberration-free IOL (e.g., Envista IOL (Bausch and Lomb, Tampa, FL, USA)) so that these patients can maintain their "favorable" HOAs for intermediate and near vision tasks.

Toric IOLs: Most KCN patients presenting for cataract surgery will have already "cross-linked" themselves as a result of aging – it is unlikely that their KCN will progress. Thus, we can consider astigmatism correction with toric IOLs in a select group of KCN patients with central, regularly symmetrical, and bowtie-shaped keratometric astigmatism with a non-skewed axis in the central 3 mm. During the preoperative examination, we should also consider the following:

- The patient's refraction should demonstrate stability over the past 18–24 months. The refractive astigmatism axis should also be within 10 degrees of the keratometric astigmatism axis.
- The ideal KCN patient should have keratometric astigmatism that can be mostly corrected with the toric IOL alone. Avoid any corneal incisions (such as limbal relaxing incisions or femtosecond laser-assisted arcuate keratotomies) in these corneas!
- While we will primarily rely on the K measurements obtained by optical biometry to calculate the toric IOL power, it is imperative to get topography, and ideally, tomography, to ensure no irregular astigmatism is present. Topography and tomography maps can also help ensure the astigmatism shape is symmetrical without axis skew. The "pencil test" can be used on the topography map to ensure that one can draw a straight line within the steep meridian of the cornea such that the superior and inferior corneal meridians can be connected with a line within the central 3-4 mm. If there is any break or skew, irregular astigmatism is present, and a toric IOL should be avoided.
- During the preoperative exam, we must ask the patient if a) they wear contact lenses (of any kind) and b) they wish to wear contact lenses after surgery. If a patient is happy wearing contact lenses postoperatively, avoid a toric IOL and place a monofocal IOL so that the patient can continue contact lens wear.
- Be very cautious (and probably avoid altogether!) when considering a toric IOL in a patient who wears RGPCLs or ScCLs. Suppose we place a toric IOL and pat ourselves on the back for doing a good job correcting the patient's astigmatism. In that case, we may be dismayed to realize that the patient is angry postoperatively, especially if they have paid for the toric IOL when they attempt to wear their contact lenses. Why? When the patient wears their contact lens (which corrects keratometric astigmatism), the toric IOL will essentially serve as unmasked iatrogenic lenticular astigmatism. This is a critical discussion to have before surgery. You will have an upset patient if they have paid out-of-pocket fees for a toric IOL only to have worse vision postoperatively. In other words, to paraphrase a famous rapping DJ, congratulations, you just played yourself.

Some under-correction of WTR astigmatism may be desirable. See Chap. 27, What's on the Menu: An Overview of Currently Available IOLs and Relevant Optics, for more information regarding toric IOLs in the general population that can also be used for KCN patients.

Astigmatism Correction and Cataract Surgery

Upto 50% of patients may have visually significant keratometric astigmatism at the time of cataract surgery. The full discussion of this rapidly changing topic is beyond the scope of this text, but a brief summary follows.

Incisional Procedures

Incisional options to correct astigmatism include the following:

- Operating on the steep meridian: This was a popular strategy in older times when surgeons routinely made large incisions (>3.0 mm) that caused flattening in the meridian of the incision and steepening 90 degrees away. Historically, most surgeons sat superiorly so it was quite easy to use this strategy to correct low amounts of WTR astigmatism. In recent times, as more surgeons are sitting temporally and shifting toward smaller incisions (≤2.4 mm), the astigmatism impact of the main wound (surgically induced astigmatism) has become less (≤0.5D). This may still be considered for patients with <1D astigmatism (especially ATR, allowing for surgeons to sit temporally).
- Opposite clear corneal incision (OCCI): Some authors have discussed using an OCCI along with operating on the steep meridian to correct astigmatism. The most significant disadvantage of this technique is the (unnecessary) creation of an additional full-thickness corneal wound.
- Limbal relaxing incision (LRI) (manual): A guarded blade targeted for 80–90% depth of the peripheral cornea may be used to cause corneal flattening in the steep meridian (along with steepening of the flat meridian 90 degrees away). Advantages of LRIs include effectiveness for mild-moderate astigmatism (1-2D), low cost, and the availability of nomograms (published and online) to plan the LRI. The most significant disadvantage of LRIs is the inevitable regression (up to 50% or more of the intended correction) that occurs over time, along with perforation, bleeding, and induction of irregular astigmatism. Please see Chap. 29, "Postoperative Optics for Cataract Surgery", for further discussions regarding the use of LRIs outside of cataract surgery.

- Femtosecond laser-assisted arcuate incisions: This is a highly controversial topic as no large data sets have been published at the time of this writing to demonstrate sustained effectiveness of this approach.[56] Based on the published papers thus far, we can say that this technique is, at best, similar to manual LRIs at this time in terms of effectively correcting astigmatism. They are definitely inferior to toric IOLs. These incisions have several disadvantages, such as cost to the patient and potential for irregular astigmatism because they are placed much closer to the corneal center. Many post-surgical complications have been reported from poorly placed incisions of this type. Extrapolating the lessons learned from the days of incisional refractive procedures close to the corneal center (AK, RK, Hex-K), it seems unwise to stir the sleeping giant known as the corneal center. Further published studies are needed to validate this technique.

Calculating Surgically Induced Astigmatism

Surgically induced astigmatism (SIA) is the amount of keratometric astigmatism (and secondarily refractive astigmatism) caused by you, the wonderful cataract surgeon, either intentionally or unintentionally. This is not necessarily the same as the amount of astigmatism that one intends to correct at the time of cataract surgery, either with the main incision or LRIs; this is known as target-induced astigmatism (TIA). In an ideal situation, the TIA and SIA are equal; for example, if the surgeon wanted to correct 0.75D of keratometric astigmatism at the time of cataract surgery with a combination of a main incision at the steep meridian and a limbal relaxing incision 180-degrees away, and the net result was the patient postoperatively had 0.0 D of keratometric astigmatism, then the TIA will equal the SIA. Of course, this never happens in real life, so the SIA is nearly always different from the actual TIA.[57]

Most toric IOL calculators and even LRI nomograms require the surgeon to input his/her habitual SIA. Many trainees are taught to put in an arbitrary value, ranging from 0.25D–0.50D (or more), rather than actually calculating it based on their individual surgical outcomes. Accurately calculating one's SIA can be done, but it requires a bit of effort, planning, and postoperative vigilance (and additional testing).

Fortunately, several online tools and spreadsheets can make this seemingly arduous task more manageable. This author recommends downloading the freely-available Surgically Induced Astigmatism Calculator developed by Warren Hill, MD,[58] which allows surgeons to input their individual data and generate accurate SIA values, even down to SIA for right eye vs. left eye surgeries; temporal vs. superior incisions; incision size; and even incision style (such as clear corneal, near-clear corneal, and scleral). This tool requires not only preoperative keratometry measurements (e.g., manual or automated keratometry values) but also postoperative keratometry values. Many surgeons do not routinely obtain the latter, so interested surgeons must ensure that additional keratometry measurements are taken at least one month after the surgery, ideally after the patient's refraction has stabilized and they are eternally grateful for the wonderful cataract surgery you performed.

For surgeons who genuinely wish to master refractive cataract surgery, especially those who want to use premium IOLs, assessing one's unique SIA is essential. As should be evident by now, there is more to cataract surgery than simply being able to finish a case in 10 minutes!

Toric IOLs

See Chap. 27, "What's on the Menu: An Overview of Currently-Available IOLs and Relevant Optics", for more information regarding toric IOLs.

Practice Question

1. Which of the following statements is TRUE?
   A. Visual acuity will typically improve when performing pinhole testing in a patient with PSC cataract.
   B. The retinal acuity meter (RAM) has a built-in +3.00D lens allowing for testing at 33 cm.
   C. The potential acuity meter (PAM) is especially useful because it can account for both spherical and astigmatic refractive errors.
   D. When performing Maddox rod test, a patient who is unable to discern a red line may have macular pathology.

[56] For example, the Roberts et al. paper only reported 1-month data after femtosecond laser arcuate incisions. Roberts HW, Wagh VK, Sullivan DL, et al. Refractive outcomes after limbal relaxing incisions or femtosecond laser arcuate keratotomy to manage corneal astigmatism at the time of cataract surgery. *J Cataract Refract Surg*. 2018;44(8):955–963

[57] For those readers interested in a more advanced, mathematical analysis of astigmatism, the Alpins Method, developed by Noel Alpins, is recommended for additional information. This approach further breaks down success of astigmatism correction by metrics such as the correction index (CI): how much astigmatism was actually corrected as compared to the intended correction (basically the SIA/TIA); the magnitude of error (intended correction (D) - actual correction (D) and the index of success. See (1) Alpins NA, Goggin M. Practical astigmatism analysis for refractive outcomes in cataract and refractive surgery. Surv Ophthalmol. 2004 Jan-Feb; 49(1):109–22. and (2) Alpins NA. Practical Astigmatism: Planning and Analysis, Slack Incorporated; New Jersey, 2018.

[58] Available at https://www.doctor-hill.com/iol-main/toric_sia_calculator.htm. Also available as an online-only database at: https://sia-calculator.com/. Accessed March 21, 2021.

2. Which of the following statements regarding the Haidinger's brush test is TRUE?
   A. The test involves rotating polarized light to assess whether the patient can detect an entoptic phenomenon as a proxy for visual potential.
   B. The perception of the brush/propeller of yellow light is due to the parallel arrangement of xanthophyll pigment in the macula, allowing for light to interact with photoreceptors equally.
   C. This test can be used to test the gross retinal function of both the central and peripheral retina.
   D. When performing this test, the optical principle of diffraction is employed to improve depth of field by limiting negative effects of diffraction.
3. Which of the following statements regarding biometry is TRUE?
   A. Immersion biometry has a major limitation due to potential indentation of the cornea by the immersion shell device.
   B. Optical biometry (OB) AXL is typically longer than USB AXL.
   C. OB is more effective at assessing AXL in the presence of dense cataracts as compared to USB AXL.
   D. OB uses ultraviolet wavelengths of light (193 nm) to penetrate lens opacities better, allowing for more accurate measurement of AXL.
4. Which of the following statements regarding corneal astigmatism is TRUE?
   A. The majority of patients <40 years of age will have much more ATR as compared to WTR.
   B. Consideration should be given for intentional undercorrection of WTR in a 45-year-old patient.
   C. Consideration should be given for intentional undercorrection of ATR in an 80-year-old patient.
   D. Direct measurements of posterior corneal astigmatism (PCA) will usually yield better refractive outcomes than estimated measurements of PCA.
5. Which of the following statements regarding IOL formulas is TRUE?
   A. The SRK formula weighs the K measurements much more significantly than the AXL measurements.
   B. Third-generation IOL formulas incorporate other biometric measurements such as WTW, CCT, LT, and HWTW to measure the ELP better.
   C. Multivariable formulas have internal mechanisms to compensate for long/short AXL and steep/flat Ks.
   D. Third-generation IOL formulas are as accurate as multivariable IOL formulas for long AXL eyes.
6. Which of the following statements concerning IOL calculation in patients with a previous history of LASIK surgery to correct myopia is TRUE?
   A. Optical biometry tends to overestimate axial length because of the corneal changes after LASIK.
   B. Optical biometry tends to underestimate axial length because of the corneal changes after LASIK.
   C. Corneal topography underestimates true central corneal curvature and power in corneas with previous LASIK surgery.
   D. Corneal topography overestimates true central corneal curvature and power in corneas with previous LASIK surgery.
7. Which of the following statements concerning optical angles and axes is TRUE?
   A. Angle kappa is the angle formed between the optical axis and the visual axis.
   B. Angle alpha is the angle formed between the pupillary axis and the visual axis.
   C. Angle kappa is an important consideration for laser refractive surgery in a hyperope.
   D. A patient with high angle kappa would not be a good candidate for an accommodating IOL.
   E. Modern biometry devices can calculate angle alpha with good accuracy.

Answers

1. D. Maddox rod testing can be performed as a gross evaluation of retinal function to detect a scotoma. If a patient cannot see the "red line," this suggests macular pathology. Visual acuity will typically worsen with pinhole testing in the presence of a PSC cataract as the lens opacity primarily involves the (central) visual axis. The RAM has a built-in +2.50D lens to allow for testing at the given reading distance of 40 cm. The PAM only corrects for spherical refractive errors and thus may feel to improve vision in patients with additional astigmatic errors.
2. A. In this technique, the examiner uses a polarized lens to rotate (polarized) light in front of a blue-white background to create an entoptic phenomenon – perceived as "spinning yellow light" by the patient (in the shape of a "brush"). Dichroism of xanthophyll pigment means that some molecules are parallel while others are circular; similarly, some nerves will run parallel to the fovea while others will run orthogonal. Hence, two different orientations of nerves and molecules in the fovea will be sensitive to two different degrees of polarization. This test only assesses the central retina. Diffraction is not employed in this test.
3. B. USB measures the AXL from the anterior corneal surface to the ILM (neurosensory retina), whereas OB measures the AXL from the anterior cornea to the RPE. This means that OB measurements may be slightly longer as compared to USB. Suppose USB measurements are used in an OB device (without adjustment). In that case, there is a risk of (slight) myopic surprise, which is typically

not that devastating for patients with dense lens opacities. Contact biometry utilizes a probe to contact the cornea physically; this potentially may indent the cornea (especially if done by an inexperienced practitioner), falsely yielding a shorter-than-real AXL. USB is more effective than OB in the presence of dense media such as infrared laser light (wavelength 780).

4. B. As we age, the total corneal astigmatism will shift towards ATR. Therefore, leaving younger patients with some WTR may be advantageous to compensate for the inevitable shift towards ATR with aging. In older patients, it is best to correct the ATR fully. At present (June 2021), there is no consensus regarding the superior accuracy of using directly measured PCA vs. estimated PCA.
5. ANSWER: C. Multivariable formulas improve the errors made by older-generation formulas that assumed a fixed, linear relationship between IOL power and AXL values. When using third-generation formulas (without the Wang-Koch adjustment) in long AXL eyes, the risk of hyperopic surprise is much more significant than using multivariable IOL formulas, which have internal mechanisms to adjust for long (and short) AXL measurements. The SRK formula weighs the AXL measurements by a factor of 2.5 vs. the K measurements (factor of 0.9); thus, inaccuracy in AXL measurements is much more "devastating" than inaccuracy in K measurements. Third-generation formulas primarily rely on the AXL and K values to estimate the ELP and do not consider the biometric variables.
6. D. Optical biometry measurements of AXL are not significantly affected by LASIK (choice A or B). However, the true central curvature tends to be overestimated (choice D) in these patients, leading to a lower-than-required IOL power and potential hyperopic surprise.
7. C. Angle kappa is a critical consideration for laser refractive surgery. If the treatment is centered on the pupil, it may not be centered on the visual axis, leading to a decentered ablation and higher-order aberrations. Angle kappa is the angle formed between the pupillary and visual axes; angle alpha is the angle formed between the optical and visual axes. Patients with high angle kappas may inadvertently look through the rings of a diffractive MFIOL/EDOF-IOL/TF-IOL; if these patients desire presbyopia correction, monovision and/or an accommodating IOL may be a better choice. Modern biometry devices can measure chord mu, an approximation for angle kappa.

Acknowledgments The author is very grateful to David L. Cooke, MD (Great Lakes Eye Care, St. Joseph, MI), for his editorial assistance and critical review of the material presented in this chapter.

What's on the Menu: An Overview of Currently Available IOLs and Relevant Optics

Kamran M. Riaz

Objectives

- To discuss clinically relevant information regarding IOL materials, architecture, shape design, and structure
- To provide a brief overview of currently accepted IOL power standards
- To discuss optical properties of the most-commonly implanted single- and three-piece IOLs in the United States
- To present options for surgeons encountering eyes requiring extreme IOL powers
- To review optical properties of toric IOLs
- To survey currently available advanced technology IOLs, including relevant technology and features
- To provide the reader with an understanding of modular transfer function curves as a method of assessing IOL performance

Introduction

Modern cataract surgery is a combined therapeutic and refractive procedure, as many patients are increasingly motivated to decrease dependence on glasses after surgery. Even for standard cataract surgery cases with monofocal intraocular lenses (IOLs), patients may have certain vision goals that may or may not be achieved when using a given IOL as compared to another. Recent years have also seen a significant number of advanced technology IOLs (ATIOLs) that can correct astigmatism and presbyopia.

The "menu" of IOLs is quite large, seemingly larger than even the menu of a popular chain restaurant that is a "factory" for cheesecakes but makes a hundred other items as well. The abundance of IOL choices seems to have created a "paradox of choice": with so many IOLs on the menu, which IOL should be used in a given situation?[1] In some ways, the cataract surgery itself has become the easy part. Determining which IOL to use in a given situation, especially to meet a given patient's visual goals after surgery, has now become the hard part.

This chapter is intended to provide the novice surgeon with an overview of all currently available IOLs in the United States. Knowledge of these IOLs, and their advantages and disadvantages, is useful for surgeons to provide their patients with the best possible outcomes. While we have intentionally glossed over some super-nerdy Optics details, we have kept the essential details in the chapter.

Disclaimer: This chapter is meant to highlight the features of commonly used IOLs as a singular compendium reference, especially for trainees. It is not our intent to promote or disparage a given IOL. None of the authors have any financial interests in any of the IOLs discussed in this chapter.

Optics of IOLs

IOL Materials

The material used to make an IOL will have optical and clinical implications. Old-school, first-generation IOLs were made of polymethylmethacrylate (PMMA) and hydrogels. While they had excellent optical quality, these IOLs required

[1] This may be especially difficult for trainees to keep up with. After finishing training in 2013, this author himself has seen the introduction of multiple monofocal IOLs; two new toric IOLs; three new diffractive multifocal IOLs; two extended depth of focus IOLs (one using diffractive optics and the other using wave front modification optics); one trifocal IOL; and one monofocal-plus IOL.

K. M. Riaz (✉)
Dean McGee Eye Institute, University of Oklahoma, Oklahoma City, OK, USA

K. M. Riaz et al. (eds.), *Optics for the New Millennium*, https://doi.org/10.1007/978-3-030-95251-8_27

large incisions as they could not be folded (think of modern-day ACIOLs).[2]

Acrylic, Silicone, and Collamer IOLs

In modern times, a variety of materials are utilized in IOLs. Some of the more popular choices include *acrylic* (index of refraction range: 1.47–1.55), *silicone* (index of refraction: 1.43), and *collamer* (index of refraction: 1.44). The index of refraction chosen for the IOL involves a bit of a trade-off: A higher index of refraction means that the IOL optic can be thinner (especially for higher diopter powers), which allows for easier folding and insertion at the time of cataract surgery. However, a higher index of refraction may also lead to higher rates of both positive and negative dysphotopsias.[3]

Acrylic IOLs became popular not only for their relative ease of insertion through smaller incisions but also for the decreased rates of posterior capsular opacification (PCO) noted with these IOLs (more on this below). Studies have shown that acrylic is a "stickier" material that adheres to the capsular bag. A "sandwich" like structure accumulates between the IOL surface and the capsule, further hindering the growth and proliferation of PCO.[4] While single-piece acrylic (SPA) IOLs are currently the most commonly implanted IOLs in the United States, the other two IOL materials have their unique advantages as well. For example, silicone IOLs are often preferred for IOL exchanges in patients with intractable dysphotopsias. In addition to having a low incidence of dysphotopsia, collamer is the preferred material for phakic IOLs.

Hydrophobic Versus Hydrophilic Acrylic IOLs

We can further subclassify acrylic IOLs into their biomaterial properties: *hydrophobic* and *hydrophilic* variants. Both are associated with lower PCO rates than other IOL materials, though hydrophobic IOLs have lower PCO and YAG rates compared to hydrophilic IOLs.[5] One reason may be that hydrophobic IOLs can adhere to collagen membranes better, resulting in better apposition of the IOL to the posterior capsule.[6] Another reason may be that hydrophilic IOLs have "less sharp" edges than hydrophobic IOLs, thereby allowing lens epithelial cell migration.[7] Finally, the hydrophilic surface itself may promote epithelial cell migration and increased PCO.[8]

Hydrophobic IOLs are more popularly implanted in the United States at the time of this writing. Most of the monofocal IOLs that discussed in the next sections are hydrophobic acrylic IOLs. Most sources define hydrophobic IOLs as having less than 1% water content.[9]

Hydrophilic IOLs have their unique advantages. For example, because of the "slippery" material, the IOL can be folded and inserted into a very small incision (<2 mm) with rapid opening once inside the eye. Additionally, hydrophilic IOLs are gentler to the uvea/angle structures as they may induce less inflammation in the eye. Hence, some surgeons prefer using a hydrophilic IOL like the Akreos AO60 (Bausch and Lomb, Inc., Tampa, FL, USA) for four-point scleral fixation with sutures for the treatment of aphakia. Hydrophilic IOLs are very popular outside the United States.[10]

Hydrophilic IOLs have a water content ranging from 18% to 38%, depending on the particular manufacturer and model. For example, the aforementioned Akreos IOL has a water content of 26%. Hydrophilic IOLs have several limitations that may explain why many US surgeons prefer hydrophobic IOLs. First, because the square edge of these IOLs is made via a lathe-cut or drill-cut in a dry state, when exposed to aqueous, the IOL will swell and the square edge becomes much rounder—this may explain why the square edge of a hydrophilic IOL is less effective than the square edge of a hydrophobic IOL in preventing PCO. Second, while controversial, some reports have suggested that bacterial biofilms may more easily form on these IOLs than their hydrophobic counterparts.[11] Finally, and perhaps of most relevance,

[2]It is said the idea of implanting an intraocular lens came to Harold Ridley after an intern asked him why he was not replacing the lens he had removed during cataract surgery. The acrylic plastic material was chosen because Ridley noticed it was inert after seeing RAF (Royal Air Force) pilots of World War II with pieces of shattered canopies in their eyes. See Williams HP. Sir Harold Ridley's vision. Br J Ophthalmol. 2001 Sep;85(9):1022-3.

[3]See Chap. 1, Geometric Optics for a discussion of how the index of refraction (and good ole Snell's Law) may affect the incidence and severity of dysphotopsias. Dysphotopsias are additionally discussed in Chap. 29, Postoperative Optics for Cataract Surgery

[4]Linnola RJ, Werner L, Pandey SK, et al. Adhesion of fibronectin, vitronectin, laminin and collagen type IV to intraocular lens materials in human autopsy eyes. Part I: histological sections. J Cataract Refract Surg 2000; 26:1792-180

[5]Zhao Y, Yang K, Li J, Huang Y, Zhu S. Comparison of hydrophobic and hydrophilic intraocular lens in preventing posterior capsule opacification after cataract surgery: An updated meta-analysis. Medicine (Baltimore). 2017 Nov;96(44):e8301.

[6]Heatley CJ, Spalton DJ, Kumar A, Jose R, Boyce J, Bender LE. Comparison of posterior capsule opacification rates between hydrophilic and hydrophobic single-piece acrylic intraocular lenses. J Cataract Refract Surg. 2005 Apr;31(4):718-24.

[7]Iwase T, Nishi Y, Oveson BC, Jo YJ. Hydrophobic versus double-square-edged hydrophilic foldable acrylic intraocular lens: effect on posterior capsule opacification. J Cataract Refract Surg. 2011 Jun;37(6):1060-8.

[8]Dorey MW, Brownstein S, Hill VE, Mathew B, Botton G, Kertes PJ, El-Defrawy S. Proposed pathogenesis for the delayed postoperative opacification of the hydroview hydrogel intraocular lens. Am J Ophthalmol. 2003 May;135(5):591-8.

[9]Of note, the Envista MX60/MX60E (Bausch and Lomb, Tampa, FL, USA) has approximately 5% water content.

[10]For example, the Rayner C-flex and Superflex (Rayner Intraocular Lenses, Ltd., West Sussex, United Kingdom)

[11]Qiu X, Wu Y, Jiang Y, Ji Y, Zhu X, Yang J, Lu Y. Management and Microbiological Characteristics of Membrane Formation on a

hydrophilic IOLs may undergo opacification when exposed to intraocular air or gas. Thus, patients who may subsequently undergo retinal surgery or endothelial keratoplasty (DSAEK/DMEK) requiring air or gas may develop vision-limiting opacification on the IOL optic that may require IOL exchange. Therefore, these IOLs should therefore be cautiously used in patients with increased risk for these future surgeries (e.g., Fuchs endothelial dystrophy).

There is no perfect IOL material. All currently available materials have their optical and clinical advantages and disadvantages. The surgeon ultimately determines the final choice of IOL. While most trainees are primarily exposed to acrylic IOLs, it is important to be aware of other IOL material choices as well.

IOL Architecture: Edge Design

The edge of the IOL optic also has interesting optical and clinical implications. The two broad classifications of edge design are *rounded edge* and *square edge* (also known as a ridged or truncated edge). While a rounded lens edge more closely approximates the shape of the natural crystalline lens, the "lens edge barrier" theory proposes that a square-edge design creates a better mechanical barrier at the capsular bag equator, decreasing the risk of PCO formation.[12]

This should mean that square-edged IOLs are great, right? Well, it is not that simple. In the valiant efforts to decrease PCO, several authors have noted that the square edge may create an additional plane of refraction and reflection, which may contribute to unwanted positive and negative dysphotopsias.[13] This may explain why in the "old days" of non-square edge IOLs, dysphotopsias were rarely ever a problem.

Some manufacturers have attempted to combine the best of both worlds in edge design. For example, the Sensar AR40 series (three-piece) IOL platform (Johnson and Johnson, Jacksonville, FL, USA) utilizes a *rounded anterior edge* and a *square posterior edge*. The IOL is designed to maintain the favorable optics of the rounded edge at the anterior optic surface (where most of the incoming light undergoes refraction), while also maintaining the benefits of a square edge at the posterior optic edge to reduce PCO formation.

IOL Architecture: Optic Design

While the optic design options and variations of modern IOLs are quite lengthy, we will focus on a few salient issues with Optics relevance.

Haptic-Optic Planarity

While you may not have scrutinized it during your cataract surgeries at the time of IOL insertion, as you were undoubtedly more focused on getting the IOL into the eye safely before anything went wrong, there are subtle variances in the design of SPA IOLs, especially in regards to the plane in which the haptics and optic are located. In broad terms, the haptics and optic can be in the *same plane*, or the *haptics may be slightly anterior to the optic* (Fig. 1). The planarity of an IOL should minimally affect its optics, but it may affect its functionality inside the eye. For example, an offset planar design may theoretically reduce the risk of PCO formation by creating additional contact between the IOL and the posterior capsule. The Tecnis platform (Johnson and Johnson, Jacksonville, FL, USA) is an example of a SPA with offset planar design; the Acrysof platform (Alcon Laboratories, Fort Worth, TX, USA) is an example of a SPA with "uni-planar" haptics-optic design.

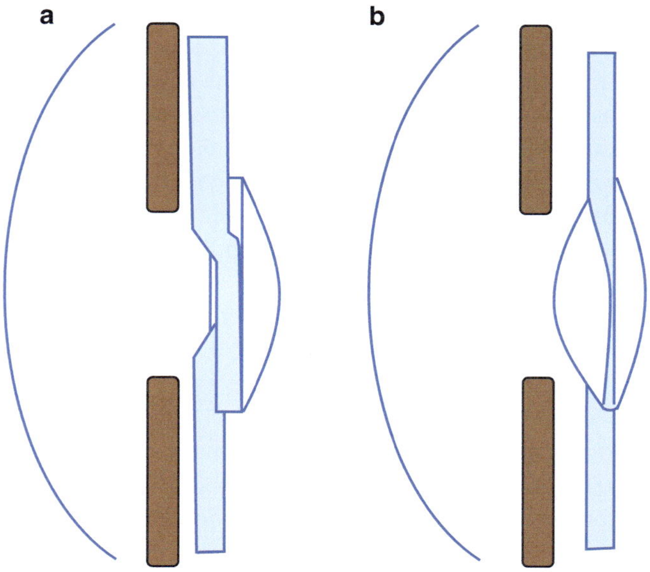

Fig. 1 Haptic-optic planarity can vary among commonly used SPA IOLs. Panel **a** shows an offset planar design in which the haptics are located slightly anterior to the optic. This design potentially allows for more contact between the posterior aspect of the optic and the posterior capsule and may reduce PCO formation. Panel **b** shows a uniplanar design in which the haptics and optic are located in the same plane

Hydrophilic Acrylic Intraocular Lens: A Clinical Case Series and Material Comparative Study of Different IOLs. J Ophthalmol. 2019 Feb 3;2019:5746186.

[12] Some may argue that PCO formation is a good thing because it allows you to do another billable procedure. Don't be that guy or gal!

[13] See Chap. 29, Postoperative Optics for Cataract Surgery, for a detailed discussion on dysphotopsias

Edge-to-Edge Power and Inert Carriers

Another thought that you may not have given much consideration during the stresses of cataract surgery: When we place a SPA IOL, how much of the IOL contains refractive power? In other words, does the entire optic (usually 6 mm for most SPA IOLs) have refractive power, or do some portions not have any power?

The Acrysof IOL platform is a SPA with full edge-to-edge power. The Envista platform (Bausch and Lomb, Tampa, FL, USA) has a minimal inert carrier ring that increases in size with higher diopter powers. Notably, the Tecnis platform has a peripheral 0.5 mm inert carrier ring, essentially giving it a 5.0–5.25 mm functional optic. This inert carrier makes it easier to fold the IOL, allowing it to go through a smaller incision. The peripheral carrier is also slightly depressed compared to the central optic when viewed in cross-section, making it easier to remove in cases of IOL exchange. One drawback of an inert carrier is that it renders peripheral retinal examination a bit more difficult, as the optics of the inert carrier affect visualization. In patients with large pupils and complex retinal history, using an IOL with full edge-to-edge power may be a better choice. Another reported drawback is a unique combination of positive-negative dysphotopsia and "night halos" when incoming light passes through the inert carrier portion of the optic.

Biconvex IOLs

Most modern-day SPA IOLs are biconvex lenses, meaning they have dioptric power on the front and back surfaces. One advantage of using a biconvex configuration is minimizing unwanted spherical aberration caused by the IOL. The net result of this configuration means the effective power is actually "inside" the IOL rather than either of the optic surfaces. Historically, biconvex IOLs were designed with a 1:2 curvature (not power) distribution. The posterior optic had a larger curvature, but this is no longer valid as there is significant variation in modern IOLs. Each IOL's specification sheet may have information regarding the type of biconvex curvature configuration (e.g., 1:2, 1:1, or 2:1), but this is only for average IOL powers (between 15-25D). When considering lower and higher power IOLs, the shape configuration may change.[14]

Note that the above ratios refer to the *radius of curvature*, not the actual power. For most modern SPA IOLs, the majority of the power is *on the front surface of the IOL optic*. If we place a + 21.0 D IOL in the capsular bag in its correct orientation, we can safely assume it will behave like a + 21.0D IOL. However, if we inadvertently place the IOL *backward* (assume it has an offset haptic-optic design with more power on the anterior optic surface), in addition to getting yelled at by your supervising attending and causing him/her gray hairs, what is the net refractive effect of this backward IOL?

Since the front surface (which has more plus power) is now on the back surface, the +21.0D IOL will lose some plus power, it may now act like a ~ +20.0D IOL and cause a *hyperopic surprise*. If the optic and haptics are in the same plane and/or utilize a 1:1 curvature design, this should cause a minimal refractive effect, even if the IOL is placed upside down.

The situation with three-piece IOLs is slightly different. While they also utilize a biconvex design, historically, three-piece IOLs had a 5- or 10-degree slant from where the haptics inserted into the optic; this led to *more effective power* on the *posterior surface* of the IOL. If these IOLs were placed backward, they would cause a *myopic surprise*. Since three-piece IOLs were routinely used, older texts (and attendings) may state that if an IOL is placed backward, it will cause a myopic surprise. Many popularly used 3-piece IOLs continue to utilize a "slant" design in modern practice. The Tecnis ZA9003 (Johnson and Johnson, Jacksonville, FL, USA) and AcrySof MA60AC/MA60BM/MA60MA (Alcon Laboratories, Fort Worth, TX, USA) are examples of three-piece IOLs with slant design optic.

Suppose a senior attending asks you, "What is the refractive effect of placing an IOL backward?" In that case, you should first inquire whether he/she is referring to a SPA or 3-piece IOL before giving your answer for both types of IOLs. Hopefully, this will win you some bonus points for the day.

As stated previously, a biconvex configuration with a more rounded posterior surface allows the optic to have better contact with the posterior capsule. Thus, a backward placed biconvex IOL may also increase the risk of posterior capsule opacification.

You can avoid this problem if you check to make sure that the *leading haptic* of the C-haptic IOL (one-piece or three-piece) is *facing to the left*; if the IOL looks like an "S" with the leading haptic *facing to the right, then you should STOP* because the IOL is backward (Fig. 2).[15]

Convex-Plano IOLs

This type of IOL is somewhat of a relic to days gone by since there is no currently available one-piece posterior chamber convex-plano IOL in the United States at the time of this writing (September 2021).[16] Older texts may mention this IOL, including recommending using this IOL for eyes with

[14] Personal communication, Thomas Olsen, MD and David L. Cooke, MD, March 7, 2021.

[15] Another, more memorable mnemonic is if you see the "S", then "you need to fix it, stupid."

[16] The last of this type of IOLs was the MC70CM 3 piece convex-plano PMMA IOL (Alcon Laboratories, Fort Worth, TX, USA) with a 7.0 mm optic. Currently available anterior chamber IOLs, such as the MTAXUO series, are convex-plano IOLs.

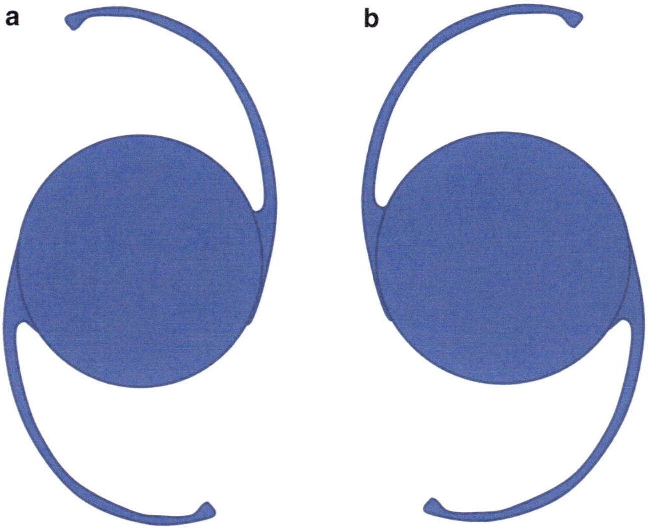

Fig. 2 The leading haptic of a C-haptic IOL (one-piece or three-piece) should be facing to the left (Panel **a**) so that the IOL looks like a backward letter "S." If the leading haptic is facing to the right (Panel **b**), the IOL will look like the letter "S," indicating that you should *stop* immediately and adjust the IOL orientation

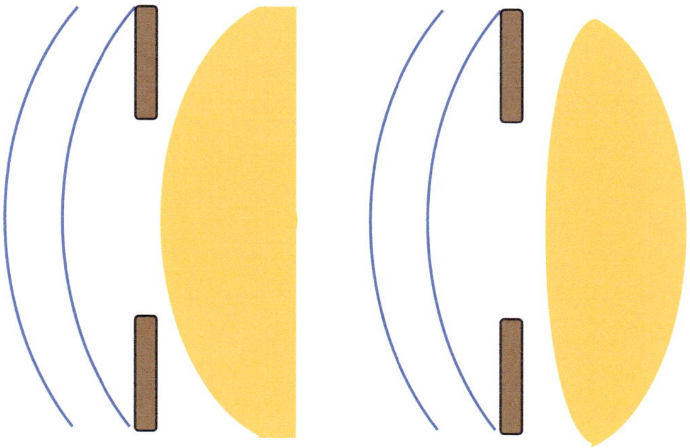

Fig. 3 Convex-plano IOLs compared with biconvex IOLs. Convex-plano IOLs contain all the effective refractive power in the front surface of the optic. These IOLs induce significantly higher amounts of spherical aberration

silicone oil. This inevitably creates confusion among trainees because no such mythical IOL exists at this time (at least available for on-label use in the United States)!

A convex-plano IOL is configured such that all the refractive power is on the front surface of the optic, and the back surface has no dioptric power (Fig. 3). One advantage of this configuration is that if placed in an eye with silicone oil, there is minimal effect on the IOL power because the silicone oil does not have a "curve" to mold itself upon and cause a refractive change. However, one major disadvantage is the significant spherical aberration caused by this type of IOL shape.

IOL Sphericity

IOLs can be either spherical or aspheric; each of these shapes has its advantages and disadvantages. At present, most of the commonly implanted SPA IOLs are aspheric IOLs.

Spherical IOLs

Recall our previous discussion regarding spherical aberration in Chap. 14, "Physical Optics and Advanced Optical Principles". As a quick review, the cornea has positive spherical aberration, the crystalline lens has negative spherical aberration, and the net result of the visual system is slightly positive spherical aberration, wherein peripheral light rays fall slightly in front of the retina. We gain more positive spherical aberration with age.

Spherical IOLs are older-generation IOLs that do not correct for spherical aberration.[17] As a result, patients with spherical IOLs will have increased (positive) spherical aberration (due to loss of negative spherical aberration from removing the crystalline lens and the positive spherical aberration of the IOL added to the already-existing positive spherical aberration of the cornea) after cataract surgery. Comparatively, spherical IOLs have similar objective distance visual acuity to aspheric IOLs.

Advantages of spherical IOLs include an increased depth of focus secondary to increased spherical aberration (pseudo-accommodation). It is not uncommon to see these patients read well uncorrected at near without any reading glasses. Two situations in which spherical IOLs are especially advantageous include the following:

- Cataract surgery in the setting of high decentration risk (e.g., pseudoexfoliation syndrome, loose zonules, eccentric pupils): Even if the IOL shifts slightly, the effective power of the IOL remains the same.
- Post hyperopic laser refractive surgery: These eyes tend to have increased negative spherical aberration, so using an IOL with positive spherical aberration can help "shift" the eye's spherical aberration back toward zero.

Spherical IOLs sound great, right? Well, not exactly. Their numerous disadvantages are why we have shifted towards aspheric IOLs. The biggest disadvantage is significantly decreased contrast sensitivity due to increased spherical aberration. While patients may objectively have good distance/near visual acuity, the subjective visual quality, especially in low-light conditions, may be suboptimal. Remember that spherical aberration is ultimately an imper-

[17]Currently available models of spherical IOLs include the SN60AT/SA60AT (SPA) (Alcon Laboratories, Fort Worth, TX USA) and Sensar AAB00 (SPA) and AR40 (three-piece) series (both from Johnson and Johnson Vision, Jacksonville, FL, USA)

Table 1 Increasing the spherical aberration will correspondingly increase the effective power of the IOL

For SA of 20 µm, this corresponds to an A-constant change of 0.3. This equals a refraction change of ΔRef = 1.3375*ΔA-constant; ΔRef = 0.4 D more myopic ΔRef ≈ 0.75*ΔIOL Power 0.4/0.75 = 0.54 D ≈ increase in IOL Power caused by SA of 20 µm.
For SA of 26 µm, this corresponds to an A-constant change of 0.41. This equals a refraction change of: ΔRef = 1.3375*ΔA-constant ΔRef = 0.55 D more myopic ΔRef ≈ 0.75*ΔIOL Power 0.55/0.75 = 0.73 D ≈ increase in IOL Power caused by SA of 20 µm.

Special thanks to David L. Cooke, MD, for his assistance with the calculations displayed in the examples

Table 2 Comparison of spherical and aspheric IOLs

	Spherical IOLs	Aspheric IOLs
Potential objective visual acuity	20/20	20/20
Near (reading) vision ability	Good uncorrected reading acuity (~J4/J5)	Poor uncorrected reading acuity
Decentration	Minimally affected	Visual acuity may be mildly to severely affected
Contrast sensitivity	Poor	Good
Spherical aberration	Increased; proportionally more with higher power IOL (e.g., +30D spherical IOL will increase spherical aberration much more than a + 10D IOL)	Neutral to decreased (better subjective visual acuity)
Example of patient wherein this IOL may be especially preferred	Post-hyperopic laser refractive surgery; pseudoexfoliation; post-trauma (zonular instability)	Routine patients; post-myopic laser refractive surgery; mild-moderate glaucoma
For patients with large pupils	Discouraged due to worsening of spherical aberration	Preferred
True power of the IOL	Slightly higher than labeled	As labeled

fection in the visual system; therefore, whenever possible, reducing spherical aberration is preferable to upholding it for its purported advantages. In addition, glaucoma patients may artificially test worse on visual field testing with a spherical IOL due to this decreased contrast sensitivity. Another disadvantage is the amount of spherical aberration induced due to the power of the IOL. For example, a + 30D spherical IOL will cause much more spherical aberration than a + 10D spherical IOL. Furthermore, the negative effects of spherical aberration are amplified by pupil size: patients with large pupils (or in low-light conditions) will experience much more spherical aberration than patients with small pupils.

Finally, due to spherical aberration effects, the *"true" power* of a given *spherical IOL* is *higher than its "labeled" power* and *higher than the same power aspheric IOL with negative spherical aberration*. Thus, a + 21.0D spherical IOL (labeled) may have the same effective power as a + 21.50 or + 21.75D (labeled) aspheric IOL, depending on the amount of asphericity. The math involved is a bit advanced (yet fascinating), and is shown in the following table (Table 1).

While not exhaustive, Table 2 can be used to compare monofocal spherical IOLs with aspheric IOLs as you read the next section.

Aspheric IOLs

Aspheric IOLs are currently the most popular type of IOL implanted in the United States at the time of this writing. As the name suggests, an aspheric IOL optic has a different peripheral curvature than the central curvature. Furthermore, these IOLs are designed to avoid adding any positive spherical aberration to the patient's optical system. Most aspheric IOLs have negative spherical aberration built into the IOL (range − 0.18 to −0.27 µm).[18] Table 3 lists the amount of negative spherical aberration present in some of the more popularly implanted IOLs—we should emphasize that this table should not be committed to memory and is not inclusive of all available IOLs.

Each manufacturer has a different strategy toward spherical aberration correction, ranging from no correction to (attempted) full correction. These differences lead to a philosophical discussion that enraptures many optics nerds: What is the ideal spherical aberration for a pseudophakic patient? What is the "perfect" amount of "imperfection" to leave in a pseudophakic eye?

As with many things in life, the answer is quite complicated. We discussed some of these principles in Chap. 14, Physical Optics. While the full scope of this particular discussion is beyond the scope of this book, to give you an idea of the complexity of this question, we have to consider multiple factors. For example, the refractive error can compensate for residual spherical aberration. Again, recall that positive spherical aberration causes a myopic shift while negative spherical aberration causes a hyperopic shift. For example, refractive myopia may be assisted by some negative spherical aberration (which causes a hyperopic shift). We also know that pupil size should not affect the refractive error, but it does affect the spherical aberration, especially for larger pupils. Putting these three factors together (refractive error, pupil size, and spherical aberration), we can see that refractive error may compensate for induced spherical

[18] An exception to this is the Envista MX60(E) series (Bausch and Lomb, Tampa, FL, USA) which is a zero-aberration (aberration-free) aspheric IOL.

Table 3 Spherical aberration correction profile of commonly used aspheric IOLs in the United States

	Acrysof	Tecnis	Envista and Akreos	Lenstec	Nanoflex	Hoya
Aberration correction of IOL	−0.20 μm	−0.27 μm	0 μm	0 μm	−0.019 μm	−0.18 μm
Targeted residual spherical aberration of the pseudophakic eye	+0.07 μm	0 μm	+0.27 μm	+0.27 μm	+0.251 μm	+0.09 μm

Note: This assumes that the crystalline lens (cataract) had approximately +0.27 μm before cataract surgery

aberration due to larger pupil sizes but may worsen defocus due to smaller sizes.[19]

The biggest advantage of aspheric IOLs is the "restoration" of the spherical aberration equilibrium previously present in the "youthful" crystalline lens. Correction of spherical aberration leads to better contrast sensitivity[20] (especially in low-light conditions), better subjective visual acuity, and avoidance of artificially worsening visual field testing in glaucoma patients. In addition, most younger cataract surgeons, including those of you in training, likely have more experience with these IOLs.

As can be expected, there are disadvantages with these IOLs as well. The biggest disadvantage is its single focal point (usually distance vision) with loss of depth of focus; most patients with aspheric IOLs set for distance vision cannot read well at near. In addition, decentration of an aspheric IOL (>0.8 mm) and tilt (>10°) will degrade visual acuity.

IOL Power Standards

When we place a SPA IOL of a given power, we assume that the true power of the IOL is the same as what is written on the box. For example, we assume (and should hope!) that a + 22.0D IOL should behave like a + 22.0D IOL inside the eye. However, some "acceptable" inaccuracy is allowed by the American National Standards Institute (ANSI). In general, IOL powers <25D are supposed to be within ±0.4D; IOL powers 25-30D are supposed to be within ±0.5D; and IOL powers >30D are supposed to be within ±1.0D.

The manufacturing process of IOLs is too detailed for this text, but one key point is that after production, the actual power of a given IOL is measured down to the decimal point of power. Each IOL is placed in a "bin" closest to the corresponding "box label" power. For example, suppose we measured two IOLs targeted for 24D of power immediately as they emerged from the magical IOL-making machine. One IOL is measured as 23.7D of power, and the other is measured as 24.1D. Assuming 0.5D power steps, the first IOL will be placed in the 23.5D bin and the second in the 24.0D bin.

This example may help provide an additional explanation for why IOL calculation in short AXL eyes is challenging. Recall that IOL powers in higher power ranges are usually produced in 1.0D steps. Thus, if you use a + 33.0D IOL, for example, there is a chance it may be closer to 32.5D or 33.5D! This may be another reason why refractive outcomes in hyperopic and short axial length eyes may be inaccurate. Even if we have the most accurate measurements, the "true" IOL power for these high-diopter power IOLs may be different than labeled. Most manufacturers usually keep track of the "true" IOL power for every IOL produced based on the serial number. Suppose you ever encounter a situation wherein your postoperative refraction is strangely and totally different from what you expected. In that case, you may want to put on your detective hat and contact the manufacturer and ask what that IOL's power was based on its serial number. This task may be a quality improvement type of project for a trainee if such a situation arises.

See Chap. 26, "Preoperative Optics for Cataract Surgery" for more information regarding other challenges in obtaining accurate IOL calculations in short axial length eyes.

Monofocal IOLs

A detailed discussion of every available monofocal IOL is beyond the scope of this book. We will limit our discussion to the most popularly implanted monofocal IOLs.

Before we proceed further, we would like to *strongly emphasize* that this section is meant to serve as an overview about monofocal IOLs. While we will highlight certain features of a given IOL, we *do not intend* to promote or disparage a given IOL; as educators, it is not our intent to influence your IOL choices.

All of the IOLs discussed below have a good track record of optical performance. We are assuming that you, as the reader, are an adult and can conscientiously choose the IOL that works best for you and your patients using your best clinical judgment.

Single-Piece Acrylic IOLs

AcrySof Platform

The AcrySof platform (Alcon Laboratories, Fort Worth, TX, USA) includes the SN60WF (yellow), SA60WF (clear), and AU00T0 (preloaded) models. This same platform is used in this manufacturer's toric and presbyopia-correcting IOLs

[19] Don't worry if you don't understand this paragraph on the first read. It takes several readings to fully digest this material.

[20] Recall the inverse relationship between spherical aberration and contrast sensitivity: reduction of spherical aberration will improve contrast sensitivity. See Chap. 14, "Physical Optics and Advanced Optical Principles" for more information.

(discussed later). At present, it is the most popularly implanted IOL in the United States.

This single-piece IOL is a hydrophobic, acrylic, biconvex, aspheric, square-edged, C-haptic IOL. The optic contains a copolymer of phenylethyl acrylate and phenylethyl methacrylate, cross-linked with butanediol diacrylate, which leads to the highest fibronectin adhesion among SPA IOLs. In English, this means that this IOL "sticks" well to the capsular bag with minimal rotation and low rates of PCO formation.

The optic size is 6.0 mm and features a square-edge design with full edge-to-edge power. Available powers are +6 to +30D in 0.5D steps. The SN60AT features an anterior asymmetric biconvex design goes from +31.0 to +40.0D in 1.0D increments. The index of refraction is 1.55, which is the highest among its fellow SPA IOLs. In late 2021, the Clareon platform was introduced as an updated hydrophobic acrylic material in the USA.

Advantages of this IOL include low rates of PCO, excellent in-the-bag stability, UV light blocking (SN60WF) and filtering (SA60WF), and familiarity among most surgeons.

Disadvantages of this IOL include the cosmetic yellow glint (cat's eye reflex noticed by observers), glistenings, subsurface nanoglistenings, anterior optic membranes,[21] and high rates of dysphotopsias.

Tecnis Platform

The Tecnis platform (Johnson and Johnson, Jacksonville, FL, USA) includes the ZCB00 PCB00, and DCB00 (preloaded) models. This same platform is used in this manufacturer's toric, monofocal "plus" (Eyhance), and presbyopia-correcting IOLs.

This single-piece IOL is a hydrophobic, acrylic, biconvex, anterior aspheric with square optic edge C-haptic IOL. As mentioned previously, the haptics have a slightly anterior offset from the optic plane.

The optic size is 6.0 mm with an inert carrier ring of approximately 0.5 mm, yielding a functional 5–5.25 mm optic. The inert carrier ring allows for a higher power range. Available powers are +5 to +34D in 0.5D steps. The index of refraction is 1.47, which is the lowest among its fellow hydrophobic SPA IOLs.

Advantages of this IOL include the offset haptics-optic design, which causes low rates of PCO. The optic is a relatively "clean" optic with minimal glistenings. The inert carrier ring makes IOL exchange easier as the anterior rhexis does not adhere tightly to the anterior optic.

Disadvantages of this IOL include the previously discussed issues with the inert carrier ring, as well as a relatively slow IOL unfolding time intraoperatively.

In February 2021, the Eyhance (DIB00) was introduced as a "monofocal plus" IOL. It is difficult to accurately classify this IOL as it is neither a pure monofocal nor an ATIOL (discussed in the later sections). However, its indications for use designate this IOL as a monofocal IOL. While it utilizes the same Tecnis platform as the ZCB00, the Eyhance features a continuous change in power from the periphery to the center of the IOL. In other words, by using a higher-order asphere, additional plus power is located in the central portion of the lens, allowing for a modest improvement in intermediate vision while maintaining distance vision quality comparable to an aspheric monofocal IOL. The IOL optic has no "architectural" modifications, such as diffractive rings. Under the microscope, the IOL appears to be similar to a standard monofocal IOL, though a subtle donut-ring can be seen under certain light conditions intraoperatively.

Data from clinical trials report MTF values in low-light conditions superior to other monofocals; in addition, defocus curves comparing the Eyhance to the ZCB00 suggest a slight improvement (1–2 lines) in intermediate and near vision. Thus, while it is not a true ATIOL in terms of its intermediate/near vision, it also avoids the unwanted glare and halos associated with diffractive-optics ATIOLs. This IOL may be a suitable option for patients who desire improved intermediate vision but may not be ideal candidates for an ATIOL with out-of-pocket fees. Given the modest improvements in intermediate and near vision, we can think of this as a "pseudo-ATIOL", as awkward as that term sounds. A toric version of this IOL (DIUxxx) is also available. As this is a relatively new IOL to the US market, long-term clinical performance is unknown at the time of this writing.

Envista Platform

The Envista platform (Bausch and Lomb, Tampa, FL, USA) includes the MX60 and MX60E models. The optical function of both IOL models is the same; however, the MX60E features a modification in the IOL material that allows for faster unfolding than the MX60. Recently, a preloaded model (MX60PL) has been introduced to market. This same platform is used in this manufacturer's toric IOL models.

This single-piece IOL is a hydrophobic, acrylic, biconvex, aspheric, square-edged, C-haptic IOL. The haptics are notable for prominent eyelets ("loops" or "holes") at the haptic-optic junction, which facilitate IOL rotation within the bag at the time of insertion.

The optic size is 6.0 mm with edge-to-edge power. The optic has slight posterior vaulting, but the haptics and optic are located within the same plane. Available powers are the highest among the IOLs discussed thus far in this section: 0 to +34D, with +10 to +30D in 0.5D steps and 0 to +10D and +30 to +34D in 1 D steps. The index of refraction is 1.53. As noted in the previous section, while this is an aspheric IOL, no spherical aberration correction (aberration-neutral) is built into this IOL.

Advantages of this IOL include an optic without glistenings and low rates of PCO. Additionally, the angulation of the haptics (55-degrees) is higher than the previous two IOLs,

[21] Riaz KM, Williams BL, Safran SG, Gallardo MJ. Proliferative Anterior Optic Membranes in Hydrophobic Acrylic Intraocular Lenses. Clin Ophthalmol. 2020 Oct 22;14:3451-3455.

Table 4 Summary of commonly used monofocal IOL features

IOL model	AcrySof	Tecnis	Envista	Softec	iSert	Nanoflex
Architecture shape	Biconvex aspheric with C-shaped haptics	Biconvex aspheric with C-shaped haptics	Biconvex aspheric with C-shaped haptics	Biconvex aspheric with C-shaped haptics	Biconvex aspheric with C-shaped haptics	Plate haptic
Material	Acrylic	Acrylic	Acrylic	Acrylic	Acrylic	Collamer
Hydrophobic / hydrophilic	Hydrophobic	Hydrophobic	Hydrophobic	Hydrophilic	Hydrophobic	Hydrophilic
Index of refraction	1.55	1.47	1.53	1.43	1.52	1.442
Power range	6–30D in 0.5D steps	5–34 in 0.5D steps	0–34D: 10–30 in 0.5D steps, 0–10 and 30–34 in 1D steps	5–36D, see text for additional details	6-30D in 0.5D steps	10.5–30.5D in 0.5D steps
Optic size	6.0 mm	6.0 mm with inert carrier	6.0 mm	5.75 mm	6.0 mm	6.0 mm
Diameter	13.0 mm	13.0 mm	12.5 mm	12.0 mm	12.5 mm	10.8 mm
Spherical aberration correction	−0.20 μm	−0.27 μm	0 μm	0 μm	−0.18 μm	−0.019 μm

which allows for more capsular bag contact and potential stability as it has a pseudo-capsular tension ring effect. This may be advantageous when using the toric version of this IOL.

Disadvantages include a relatively high index of refraction with associated dysphotopsias. The MX60 model unfolds the slowest among these three IOLs.

Softec Platform

The Softec platform (Lenstec, Inc., St. Petersburg, FL, USA) includes the Softec HD, Softec HDM, and Softec HDO models.

This single-piece IOL is a hydrophilic, acrylic, bi-aspheric, C-haptic IOL. The optic size is 5.75 mm with edge-to-edge power. Available powers include +5.0 to +36.0D, with +15.0 to +25.0D in 0.25D steps; +10.5-14.5 and +25.5-29.5D in 0.5D steps; and +5 to +10D/+30 to +36D in 1.0D steps. This IOL is available in 0.25D steps in the most commonly used IOL power ranges. Among SPA IOLs, this has the lowest index of refraction at 1.43.

The main difference between the HD and HDM models is that the latter can be inserted through a sub-2.2 mm incision. Interestingly, while the HD and HDM models are "circular," the HDO features an "oval" shaped optic that can be placed with the haptics in the horizontal position to decrease the incidence of dysphotopsia.

iSert Platform

The iSert platform (Hoya Surgical Optics, Inc., Chino Hills, CA, USA) includes the iSert 250 (clear) and iSert 251 (yellow) models.

This single-piece IOL is a preloaded, hydrophobic, acrylic, bi-aspheric C-haptic IOL. The optic is 6.0 mm with edge-to-edge power. The index of refraction is 1.520. Available powers include +6 to +30D in 0.5D steps. One interesting feature about this IOL is that the haptics have a mixture of PMMA added to increase adhesion to the capsular bag.

In 2013, an older version of this IOL was recalled due to high rates of inflammation.

Table 4 summarizes the highlights of these commonly used monofocal IOLs.

Three-Piece IOLs

Knowledge of three-piece IOLs remains an invaluable tool for any cataract surgeon, despite many surgeons favoring the use of SPA IOLs. First, no matter how "excellent" a cataract surgeon you may be, there will come a day when you encounter our dear friend Mr. Vitreous, and you may have to forego a SPA IOL in favor of a three-piece IOL. Second, recall that you must never place an SPA IOL in the sulcus (despite some surgeons saying otherwise), due to the risk of postoperative complications such as UGH syndrome.[22] In addition, there are certain situations in which a three-piece IOL is favored, such as:

- Patients with moderate-high risk of late-term dislocation due to zonular weakness or instability (e.g., pseudoexfoliation syndrome), wherein a three-piece IOL (with or without a capsular tension ring and/or capsular tension segment), might be a safer option
- Patients requiring high or low IOLs powers that are not available in SPA IOLs (e.g., high myopia)
- Patients requiring piggyback IOLs for correction of refractive surprise (see Chap. 29, "Postoperative Optics for Cataract Surgery" for more information)
- Patients requiring iris or scleral-fixation of IOL in cases of aphakia

[22] See Chap. 28, Intraoperative Optics for Cataract Surgery, for additional information regarding sulcus IOLs (e.g., sulcus IOL power calculations, types of placement, etc.)

While you may not use these IOLs often, you should be comfortable with using them when the situation demands. Remember that many of these IOLs usually will require a larger (≥2.8 mm) incision than SPA IOLs.

For situations requiring common IOL powers, available acrylic choices include the following:

- AcrySof MA60AC (clear)/MN60AC (yellow) (Alcon Laboratories, Fort Worth, TX USA): Both of these acrylic IOLs are available from +6 to +30.0D in 0.5D steps. The MA50BM (clear) is similar but features a larger 6.5 mm optic, making it useful for large eyes or suture fixation as it offers a bit more forgiveness in terms of decentration.
- Tecnis ZA9003 and Sensar AR40e models (Johnson and Johnson, Jacksonville, FL, USA): The ZA9003 is available from +10 to +30.0D in 0.5D steps, and the Sensar AR40e is available from +6 to +30.0D in 0.5D steps. These acrylic IOLs have PMMA haptics with a *rounded anterior edge* optic and *square posterior edge* optic.
- CT Lucia 602 (formerly EC3-PAL) (Carl Zeiss Meditec Inc., Dublin, CA): This hydrophobic acrylic IOL has recently gained significant attention among surgeons who perform scleral fixation IOL surgery. The polyvinylidene fluoride (PVDF) haptics are robust, nearly indestructible, and useful for intraocular gymnastics, making this IOL an ideal choice for transconjunctival intrascleral haptic fixation (Yamane technique) in cases of aphakia. This IOL is available from +4 to +34.0D in 0.5D steps. The refractive index (1.49) is similar to PMMA. The optic has an inert carrier which may contribute to dysphotopsias.

Silicone IOLs are mainly available as three-piece IOL models. The two most popularly used are as follows:

- SofPort Li61AO (Bausch and Lomb, Tampa, FL, USA): This silicone optic IOL is available from 0 to +4D in 1.0D steps, +5.0 to +30.0D in 0.5D steps, and + 31 to +34D in 1.0D steps. This zero-aberration IOL has PMMA haptics attached to the silicone optic with a rounded anterior edge and square posterior edge. It has a very low index of refraction (1.429), which is the lowest among all available IOLs, and thus has the lowest reported incidence of dysphotopsia. This IOL can be inserted in incisions as small as 2.4 mm in its dedicated cartridge and inserter.
- Tecnis Z9002 (Johnson and Johnson, Jacksonville, FL, USA): This silicone optic IOL is available from +5.0 to +30.0D in 0.5D steps. The IOL has PMMA haptics with a rounded anterior edge and square posterior edge. It has an index of refraction of 1.46. This IOL requires a 3.0 mm incision in its dedicated cartridge and inserter.

Caution should be exercised when considering silicone IOLs for patients who may need silicone oil in the future. In addition, a "bimanual" insertion is required as the IOL unfolds quite suddenly inside the eye compared to commonly used SPA IOLs.

Extended Range IOLs

Occasionally, you may encounter a patient (such as a high hyperope or pathologic myope) who requires an IOL power that you did not think existed. It is helpful to know what IOL options are available for these unique patients in these situations. We hope this section will make IOL selection a bit easier—of course, surgery in these patients can be an adventure, so we wish you good luck in advance on that!

Extreme Low Power IOLs

A few options exist for these extremely myopic, insanely long axial length eyes. Recall that one of the SPA IOLs (Envista) goes down to 0D, as does the Akreos IOL (Bausch and Lomb, Tampa, FL, USA).

The following options are three-piece, hydrophobic acrylic IOLs:

- AcrySof MA60MA (clear) and MN60MA (yellow) (Alcon Laboratories, Fort Worth, TX, USA): Available in *minus 5.0 to plus 5.0D* in 1D steps.
- Sensar AR40M and AR40e (Johnson and Johnson, Jacksonville, FL, USA). The AR40M is available in *minus 10 to + 1.5D*, and the AR40E is available in *+2 to + 5.5D* powers; both models are available in 0.5D steps.
- MZ60PD and MZ60MD (Alcon Laboratories, Fort Worth, TX, USA): These obscure PMMA IOLs are available in *minus 10 to minus 4D* in 1.0D steps (MZ60PD) and *minus 3 to + 3.0D* in 1.0D steps (MZ60MD). The 6.0 mm optic size will require an extremely large incision as this is a non-foldable IOL.

In addition, some surgeons have discussed using the phakic collamer IOL (Staar Surgical, Monrovia, CA, USA) as an off-label IOL. This IOL goes from −3 to −20.0D. The cost of this IOL may also make it prohibitive for routine use. Again, we cannot endorse this as an on-label use for this IOL in this situation.

Extreme High Power IOLs

Similarly, a few options exist for these extremely hyperopic, very short axial length eyes:

- AcrySof SA60AT (clear) and SN60AT (yellow) (Alcon Laboratories, Fort Worth, TX, USA): This SPA IOL is available in commonly used powers but is also available from *+31 to + 40.0D* in 1D steps. Recall that this is a spherical IOL.

- P359UV (Bausch and Lomb, Tampa, FL, USA): This PMMA IOL is a spherical IOL with a 5.5 mm optic. It is available from *0 to + 45.0D* in 1.0D increments. Note that it cannot be folded and will require a large incision.

Additionally, some surgeons recommend a "double" IOL approach in these eyes. With this strategy, the highest available power SPA is placed in the capsular bag, and the remaining needed IOL power (usually a three-piece IOL of a different material, such as silicone) is placed in the sulcus or even in the capsular bag. Some additional IOL calculations are required, such as calculating the resulting hyperopia with the SPA IOL and then using the piggyback IOL calculation for a hyperopic surprise (Piggyback IOL power = 1.5 × hyperopic refractive error) to place the second IOL, either at the time of the initial surgery or as a staged procedure for piggyback IOL (secondary IOL) placement.

Anterior Chamber IOLs

In the United States, at the time of this writing, there are two main ACIOL model types available, both made of PMMA and with equally comparable long-term visual outcomes[23]:

- The Kelman Multiflex III ACIOL (MTA2UO-MTA7U0 models; Alcon Laboratories, Inc., Fort Worth, TX, USA) features a 5.5 mm optic. The model numbers (2–7) increase in 0.5 mm overall length sizes, corresponding to a range of 12.0–14.5 mm. This ACIOL has a *convex-plano* design.
- The S122UV/L122 UV (Bausch and Lomb, Tampa, FL, USA) types (12.5/13.5 mm lengths) feature a 6.0 mm optic and a *biconvex* design.

See Chap. 28, "Intraoperative Optics for Cataract Surgery", for more discussion on ACIOLs, including calculating the needed IOL power in unplanned situations.

Miscellaneous IOLs

Several other IOLs may be significant in certain situations:

- Nanoflex CC4204A (Staar Surgical, Monrovia, CA, USA): This hydrophilic plate-haptic IOL is made of collamer, which has a high water content (40%). Collamer is a highly biocompatible material with a very low index of refraction (1.442). This material is also used for the phakic IOL (Visian ® ICL). Collamer's unique properties allow for good adherence to the lens capsule, incite minimal inflammation and reduce the risk of calcification. The optic is 6.0 mm with edge-to-edge power. Nanoflex IOLs are available from +10.5 to +30.5D in 0.5D steps. One unique feature of this IOL is its ability to "mend itself" if damaged during the course of a YAG capsulotomy (such as when done by a first-year resident). The IOL has approximately −0.019 microns of negative spherical aberration. Unlike previous-generation plate-haptic IOLs, there have not been reports of late-term dislocations, including after YAG capsulotomy.
- CZ70BD (Alcon Laboratories, Fort Worth, TX, USA): This UV-absorbing, single-piece PMMA IOL is popularly used in secondary IOL surgery due to its uniquely designed haptics that facilitate suture passing for scleral fixation. It has a low index of refraction (1.49) and is available from +4.0 to +34.0D in 0.5D steps. The less commonly used MZ60MD/PD models go down to −3.0D and −10.0D, respectively. This is the only IOL available in the USA with a 7.0 mm optic, making it ideal for scleral fixation by allowing some "wiggle-room" for decentration. Because of its size and material, a large (≥7 mm) incision (e.g., scleral tunnel) is required.

Toric IOLs

Most trainees are familiar with toric IOLs and usually have gratis-access to these IOLs during residency. All three major IOL manufacturers in the United States make monofocal toric IOLs that can correct up to 4.5D of corneal astigmatism.[24] The terminology for a given toric IOL power varies slightly among manufacturers, but the range of correctable corneal astigmatism is the same. The cylinder power is mainly in the posterior aspect of the toric IOL. The meridian of the correcting cylinder is usually denoted by circular marks or a dashed line that helps the surgeon place the IOL in the correct meridian (steep meridian, aka the axis meridian); recall that the cylinder power will then act at the (power) meridian 90-degrees away.

A full discussion of the pros/cons and variations of each toric IOL model is beyond the scope of this text. Overall, they are quite similar to their monofocal counterparts in terms of material, index of refraction, etc. Reports in the literature vary regarding the superiority of one type of toric IOL over another.

[23] Suelves AM, Siddique SS, Schurko B, et al. Anterior chamber intraocular lens implantation in patients with a history of chronic uveitis: five-year follow-up. *J Cataract Refract Surg*. 2014;40(1):77-81.

[24] IOLs that combine presbyopia- and astigmatism-correction are discussed in the next section.

Advantages of toric IOLs include superior accuracy in astigmatism correction, avoiding additional corneal incisions, improving UCVA/BCVA, and sustained reduction of astigmatism, as shown in numerous studies. Disadvantages include cost, inability to correct high(>4.5D)/irregular astigmatism, late-term rotation, and inadvertent undercorrection/overcorrection of astigmatism.

This last point merits some additional discussion. Recall our discussions in the previous chapter on total corneal astigmatism, including anterior and posterior corneal astigmatism. For example, if we have a young patient (40-50 years) with WTR astigmatism and we fully correct the WTR astigmatism, then as the patient gets older, s/he may gain additional ATR. For these patients, it may be prudent to leave some residual WTR astigmatism (approximately 0.5D) so that they can "grow into" their ATR astigmatism. We can safely correct the full WTR astigmatism in older patients because they may not have much time left to "grow into" their ATR astigmatism.[25] For ATR patients, most surgeons would feel comfortable correcting the full astigmatism, regardless of age.

Finally, it may be preferable to avoid "flipping the axis" as much as possible when correcting astigmatism, especially for WTR astigmatism. However, some surgeons argue that reducing astigmatism to the lowest possible quantitative amount, even if one has to flip the axis, is preferable for all types of preoperative astigmatism. We suggest that undercorrection of WTR astigmatism has two unique advantages. First, residual WTR allows patients to "grow" into their ATR astigmatism with age. Second, residual WTR confers an optical advantage for viewing letters with vertical strokes at a distance. Additionally, we recommend that surgeons aggressively correct ATR astigmatism regardless of patient age. Patients with preoperative ATR astigmatism who have mild postoperative WTR astigmatism are better able to tolerate this "axis flip" than their WTR counterparts.

Advanced Technology IOLs

If you have made it this far, now comes the real fun stuff. Please take a minute to stop and play Abba's "*Money, Money, Money*" (1976) in the background before continuing.[26]

Advanced technology IOLs (ATIOLs), aka presbyopia-correcting IOLs, allow surgeons to correct distance, intermediate, and near vision (presbyopia correction) for patients who are motivated to decrease the need for spectacles postoperatively. We will focus our discussion on diffractive multifocal IOLs (MFIOLs), extended depth of focus IOLs (EDOF-IOLs), trifocal IOLs (TF-IOLs), and accommodative IOLs (AIOLs). One key point: All MFIOLs, EDOF-IOLs, and TF-IOLs "purchase" this greater range of vision by paying the currency of contrast sensitivity. In other words, especially when compared to monofocal IOLs, patients with MFIOLs/EDOF-IOLs/TF-IOLs will experience reduced contrast sensitivity. In addition, patients may have visually significant glare, haloes, starbursts, and other subjective visual disturbances. AIOLs do not incur these subjective visual disturbances but tend to not perform well for near vision needs.

Furthermore, this is an area that is rapidly changing and evolving with new ATIOLs available seemingly every few months like smartphones. We will limit our discussion to ATIOL models and technologies available in the United States at this writing (September 2021). Technologies on the horizon, such as newer EDOF IOLs and light-adjustable IOLs, are topics to watch for in the peer-reviewed literature.

Again, before we proceed further, we would like to *strongly emphasize* that this section is serves as an overview of ATIOLs. While we will highlight certain features of a given ATIOL, we *do not intend* to promote or disparage a given ATIOL. We are assuming that you, as the reader, are an adult and can conscientiously choose the ATIOL that works best for your patients using your best clinical judgment.

Diffractive Multifocal IOLs

Diffractive MFIOLs rely on the principle of *diffraction* to correct intermediate and near vision. Recall that in the principle of diffraction, light waves slow down and change direction when they encounter an obstacle (aka the "diffractive zone"). MFIOLs utilize a combination of microscopic steps (diffractive zones) to split light toward distance and near focal points.

Incoming light rays will be directed towards a near and distance focal point depending on the step height they encounter. If the step height is the same wavelength as the incoming light, all the particles are directed towards the near focal point. If the step height is a small fraction of the incoming light wavelength, more light particles are directed towards the distance focal point. Therefore, MFIOLs utilize a combination of step heights to split incoming light into "distance," "intermediate," and "near" focal points.

Apodized Diffractive MFIOLs

Do not be scared by the word "apodized." It simply means that there is a gradual reduction (apodization) in step height from the center to the periphery. Apodization allows incoming light to be directed toward far and near points in a gradual pattern, rather than an abrupt split between far and near.

[25]Yes, that sounds morbid so apologies in advance!

[26]Remember how we spent time discussing *refraction* and *diffraction* back in Chap. 1, "Geometric Optics?" It may be worthwhile to review these definitions before proceeding further.

An example of an apodized diffractive MFIOL is the Restor (+3.00 add (SN6AD1) and + 2.50 add (SVT25T0); custom order +4.00 add available (Alcon Laboratories, Fort Worth, TX USA). Technically, this lens combines a refractive (monofocal) and diffractive MFIOL. The central 3.6 mm of the optic contains an *anterior apodized diffractive region* and a *refractive (monofocal) peripheral portion*. When the patient's pupil size increases (e.g., distance vision), more diffractive zones with small step heights (and the peripheral refractive zone) are exposed, thereby directing more incoming light towards the distance focal point. This combination of a "central" apodized diffractive region with a peripheral "donut" of a refractive region allows for good near and distant vision, respectively.

The *SV25T0* (+2.50D add) is a MFIOL model with 7 rings and is better suited for distance vision (due to an extra distance and intermediate vision zone). The SN6AD1 (+3.00D add) model features 9 rings and has more rings dedicated for near vision; it is better suited for distance and near vision. Patients who desire good distance and intermediate vision (computer vision) may prefer the +2.50D add, whereas patients who desire good distance and near may prefer the +3.00 D add in both eyes. Surgeons should consider patients' height and preferred reading distance as well. For example, taller patients or patients who like to hold reading material farther away may be happier with a lower add power than shorter patients. Finally, "mix and match" options have also been used, such as placing a +2.50 add in the dominant eye and a +3.00 add in the non-dominant eye. This combination allows the patient to utilize the dominant eye for distance-intermediate vision and the non-dominant eye for distance-near vision. The idea is that with both eyes open, the "gaps" created by one MFIOL model can be filled in by its counterpart MFIOL model.

Toric versions of both models (SV25Tx and SND1Tx) can correct up to 2.5–3.0D corneal cylinder.

One potential disadvantage of this MFIOL is the 3.6 mm diffractive zone: patients with large pupils, especially those who enjoy reading in low-light conditions, may have reduced near vision since more incoming light is directed towards the refractive distance zones as compared to the central diffractive zones.

Non-apodized Diffractive MFIOLs

As you may have guessed, non-apodized diffractive MFIOLs utilize rings of *uniform step height (1 wavelength)* to direct a significant percentage of incoming light toward the near point.

The Tecnis MFIOL is available in three versions: ZKB00 (+2.75D add), ZLB00 (+3.25D add), and ZMB00 (+4.00D add) (Johnson and Johnson Vision, Jacksonville, FL USA). This MFIOL features 18 rings on the posterior aspect of the optic extending to the periphery. The non-apodized rings direct an equal amount of incoming light to the near and distance focal points. As a result, this MFIOL performs better for distance and near vision with some compromise of intermediate vision. Patients who desire good distance/intermediate vision with some compromise of near vision may be good candidates for a lower add power model. As a corollary, patients who desire good distance/near vision with some compromise of intermediate vision may be good candidates for a higher add power model. Since the rings encompass the entire optic, patients with large scotopic pupils and/or patients who enjoy reading in low-light conditions may be well-suited for this MFIOL.

Given the three models with varying add power options, patient height and reading distance preference can similarly be considered as discussed in the previous section. Remember, using a lower add power may be advantageous in patients who naturally read at a longer distance when holding reading material. For example, a retired professional basketball player may prefer +2.75D add power in both eyes, while a 4′11″ grandmother may prefer +4.00D adds in both eyes. A similar "mix and match" strategy has been advocated by some surgeons, such as using a +3.25D add in the dominant eye and a +4.00D add in the non-dominant eye. As discussed with apodized MFIOLs, the strategy to utilize the strengths of the lower add MFIOL to compensate for the weaknesses of the higher add MFIOL and vice versa.

In September 2020, toric versions (ZKUxxx with +2.75 add and ZLUxxx with +3.25 add) that can correct 2.5–3D of corneal astigmatism were made available.

Refractive IOLs (Historical)

Refractive IOLs are no longer available in the USA and are mainly of historical interest. The ReZoom (Abbott Medical Optics, Santa Anna, CA, USA) refractive IOL was an example of this technology.

These ATIOLs were constructed by incorporating two different powers into multiple circular refractive zones. Because each "donut" of the IOL has a different effective power, distance/near vision primarily depended on the patient's pupillary response to light. The ReZoom featured five refractive zones to provide a range of vision: Zones 1(central zone), 3, and 5 (far peripheral) were set for distance while Zones 2 and 4 were set for near vision. The "transition" lines between each zone offered intermediate vision.

Theoretically, this sounded like a great idea for an ATIOL. However, due to the extremely high rates of glare, halos, and subjective visual dysfunction, it was discontinued in 2011.

Extended Depth of Focus (EDOF) IOLs

One optics nerd note: Diffractive optics (Symfony IOL; Johnson and Johnson Vision, Jacksonville, FL USA and AT LARA 829 MP IOL; Carl Zeiss Meditec, Dublin, CA, USA) is one method to create an EDOF-IOL. Other EDOF-IOL strategies include stretching the wavefront (as used in the Vivity IOL (Alcon Laboratories, Fort Worth, TX USA), pinhole optics (IC-8 IOL; Acufocus, Irvine, CA, USA), and opposite spherical aberrations (Mini Well IOL; SIFI S.p.A., Catania, Italy). As the name suggests, the goal with EDOF is to shift or extend the focal point (rather than split incoming light into distinct focal points) to increase intermediate and near visual function. We will focus primarily on the two EDOF-IOLs available in the United States at the time of this writing.

Diffractive Optics Extended Depth of Focus IOLs

Diffractive EDOF-IOLs contain ring structures in the optic termed as "echelettes."[27] Instead of arriving at two distinct focal points, incoming light is redirected towards an elongated focal point shaped like a cylindrical column of light ("the depth of focus"). The Symfony EDOF-IOL (ZXR00) and a toric option (ZXTxxx) were approved in the USA in August 2016. The Symfony has a posterior achromatic diffractive surface with 9 echelettes.

In addition to correcting spherical aberration, this EDOF-IOL also corrects chromatic aberration. Theoretically, if we corrected both spherical aberration and chromatic aberration, we could get 20/12 or 20/10 vision at distance. However, using echelettes means we are still relying on diffractive optics, so this slightly reduces the range of vision correction to the level of 20/20. Again, we are paying for presbyopic correction with the currency of enhanced distance vision.

Benefits of this ATIOL include better subjective vision and better intermediate vision. However, glare/halos are similar to MFIOLs (despite initial claims to the contrary), and patients may lose some near vision while gaining more intermediate vision.

Some surgeons have described using an EDOF-IOL set for emmetropia in the dominant eye and an EDOF-IOL set for –0.50D in the non-dominant eye to improve binocular near vision. "Mix and match" strategies to use an EDOF-IOL in the dominant eye (distance/intermediate) and an MFIOL in the non-dominant eye (distance/near) have also been reported.

[27] A useful rule in life: whenever you want to sound intelligent, use a French-origin word and people will think you are a genius.

Modified Wavefront Extended Depth of Focus IOLs

Wavefront modification is used in the "new kid on the block" EDOF IOL; the Vivity IOL (DFT015/DAT015) was released in January 2021 and included a toric option (DFT315/415/515 and DAT315/415/515 models).

Compared to diffractive IOLs, this EDOF IOL contains a modification of the central aspect of the anterior optic to "stretch and shift" the wavefront of incoming light to give depth of focus.[28] In layman's terms, this essentially allows the IOL to have a + 1.5D reading add with similar distance visual acuity as a monofocal IOL, but with better MTF values than diffractive IOLs (both diffractive MFIOLs and diffractive EDOF IOLs). Furthermore, the absence of rings allows this EDOF-IOL to be pupil independent for scotopic and mesopic vision needs.

Surgeons may still choose to do a modified mini-monovision (dominant eye plano, nondominant eye approximately −0.5 to −0.75D) to allow for improved near vision. This IOL also has negative spherical aberration to compensate for corneal spherical aberration. Patients can expect good distance and intermediate vision, but near visual tasks may still require reading glasses. Due to the stretched and shifted wavefront, there are minimal "gaps" between distance, intermediate, and near vision. Since there are no "rings", some surgeons have suggested that this ATIOL may be used effectively in post-refractive surgery patients.

Subjective visual disturbances, including glare and halos, have been reported in the FDA clinical trials.[29] As with many things in life, we have to lose something to gain something. With this IOL, there is approximately 50% MTF reduction at distance, but better MTF at near. In other words, we are sacrificing contrast sensitivity at distance to gain near vision. There have been reports of subjectively blurry vision at all distances due to loss of contrast sensitivity. Long-term real-world results of this IOL remain to be seen at the time of this writing. However, this IOL offers a different philosophical and technological approach to previous generations of presbyopia-correcting IOLs.

Combined EDOF-MFIOLs

The Tecnis Synergy (Johnson and Johnson Vision, Jacksonville, FL, USA) was launched in June 2021 as a combined EDOF-MFIOL. The EDOF portion of this ATIOL is in

[28] One way to understand "stretching and shifting" is to understand that a transition element in the central part of this IOL stretches the incoming wavefront in the X-Y direction; a second transition element shifts the incoming wavefront in the Z direction. The combination of this "stretch and shift" creates EDOF optics.

[29] "Patient Information Brochure". https://www.accessdata.fda.gov/cdrh_docs/pdf/P930014S126D.pdf. Accessed January 9, 2021.

the near to intermediate range (approximately 33 to 80 cm). The MFIOL portion has two distinct focal points at approximately 33 cm (near) and infinity (distance). This ATIOL is basically a combined Symfony and Tecnis MFIOL; it has 15 rings (compared to the 9 echeleettes of the Symfony and the 18 rings of the Tecnis MFIOL). By using the strengths of one, the limitations of the other can potentially be mitigated.

The Synergy is available in both a spherical (DFR00V) and toric models (DFWxxx). Like the Symfony, this ATIOL corrects both spherical and chromatic aberration. One distinguishing feature is its champagne-like color, which confers both UV and violet-light filtering. In addition, surgeons should target closest to plano in their refractive target, even if that incurs slight hyperopia (less than +0.25D). A 0.5D myopic "miss" with this IOL can cause a 1-line vision drop compared to a 0.5D hyperopic miss, which only causes a half-line vision drop.

When looking at the defocus curve for the Synergy (as compared to a monofocal Tecnis IOL), patients can expect ≥ 20/25 vision until 33 cm. Similarly, MTF values are only modestly decreased compared to a monofocal IOL and much higher when compared to other diffractive ATIOLs. Given its relatively recent introduction to the market, long-term real-world data are needed to determine other advantages and limitations of this ATIOL.

Trifocal IOLs

TF-IOLs are the "old new kid on the block." Approved in August 2019, they represent a variant of MFIOLs as they have distinct zones for distance, intermediate, and near vision.

In the United States, the PanOptix TFNT00/TFAT00 (Alcon Laboratories, Fort Worth, TX, USA) is the only currently available TF-IOL. The PanOptix is an upgraded SN6AD1 with several changes. First, the apodized platform has been replaced with a non-apodized platform that basically contains a + 3.25D add and a + 2.17D add for near and intermediate vision, respectively (corresponding to a + 1.65D and + 2.35D add power at the corneal plane). Second, the 3.6 mm diffractive zone of rings has been expanded to 4.5 mm, thereby limiting the monofocal refractive zone to an outer 1.5 mm peripheral "donut." Third, this ATIOL contains 14 rings, as compared to the SV25T0 (7 rings) and SN6AD1 (9 rings). Finally, the peripheral monofocal "donut" and central "button" within the rings are maintained for good distance vision.

The construction of the TF-IOL creates three distinct focal points: distance, intermediate (60 cm), and near (40 cm). The intermediate diffractive split allows for light to incoming light to be split into the dedicated intermediate focal point. Toric versions of this IOL (T3-T6) are available.

Advantages of this ATIOL include a good range of vision with dedicated zones for all three distances. Potential disadvantages include compromise of near vision, worse halos/photic phenomena (even compared to older-generation MFIOLs), and reduced MTF (20%) at distance and near.[30]

Accommodative IOLs (AIOLs)

While AIOLs allow for presbyopia correction, their mechanism of action is totally different from the previously discussed ATIOLs. There is no use of diffractive optics, so there are no rings/echelettes in an AIOL.

We can think of AIOLs as monofocal IOLs with elongated haptics on hinges that allow the IOL to move (to simulate accommodation) forwards and backward, allowing for the full range of vision. For example, when the patient wants to read, ciliary muscle contraction will move the optic forward, inducing a myopic shift and allowing for near vision.

The Crystalens AO1UV/AO2UV (Bausch and Lomb, Inc., Tampa, FL, USA) is the only AIOL available in the United States. A toric option (TruLign; BL1UT125/200/275) is also available.

Advantages of this AIOL include no glare/halos, good range of vision at distance and intermediate, and a zero-aberration profile. It may be especially useful in post-refractive cataract surgery patients who desire presbyopia correction but want to avoid glare/halos.

Disadvantages of this AIOL primarily include a "locking" of the IOL after some time that prevents good near vision, though patients still maintain good distance and fair intermediate vision. Patients may also have to do "eye training" exercises after cataract surgery to enhance their near vision. Finally, a rare complication known as "Z-syndrome" may occur. Due to exuberant capsular fibrosis and contraction, haptic-hinge issues can cause an asymmetric vaulting of the AIOL so that it looks like a "Z" (one portion tilted anteriorly, the other portion tilted posteriorly), usually requiring laser or surgical intervention. This author has anecdotally noted that placing a capsular tension ring at the time of surgery may help reduce the incidence of Z-syndrome.

Several additional AIOL designs are awaiting FDA approval at the time of this writing.

[30]Lee S, Choi M, Xu Z, et al. Optical bench performance of a novel trifocal intraocular lens compared with a multifocal intraocular lens. *Clin Ophthalmol*. 2016;10:1031-1038.

Additional Comments About ATIOLs

As stated previously in the chapter, no single ATIOL has demonstrated consistent superiority over its counterparts or can be thought of as a "one ATIOL to rule them all" type of option. The ultimate choice of which ATIOL to use for a given patient is for the surgeon to decide after a meticulous preoperative exam, including appropriate diagnostic testing, and lengthy preoperative discussion about vision goals after cataract surgery. While tempting, it is crucial to not promise patients "complete independence" from glasses. It is better to under-promise and (hopefully) over-deliver. It is also important to carefully parse through the bravado of "refractive IOL" surgeons who speak on behalf of a given company that regale audiences with tales of their patients who are "universally happy 20/15 vision at all distances." Peer-reviewed clinical studies, rather than hype and showmanship, is the ultimate arbiter. Be wary of the surgeon who boasts an "80 percent premium IOL practice!" Also, be wary of the surgeon who implants "tons of ATIOLs" but cannot explain the optics involved in each of the ATIOLs.

As previously discussed in Chap. 18, "Visual Acuity Testing and Assessment", optical systems, including IOLs, are incapable of full 100% transmission of the object's details. The modular transfer function (MTF) is a mathematical graphic representation of how we perceive contrast based on the spatial frequency emanating from an object. A perfect IOL would have an MTF of 1. this means that every single detail of the object is faithfully captured and transmitted.

Since we live in a world with intricate details, the MTF is a way to measure the accuracy of image transmission based on how much modulation (contrast) is present in the transmitted image. Thus, the MTF is a way to assess how well the IOL performs: a more desirable IOL will have a higher MTF value at the measured distance.

When we look at MTF curves for a monofocal IOL, for distance visual acuity, the monofocal IOL will have a very high peak for distance (test distance infinity) and very low peaks for intermediate and near vision. This makes sense as it confirms what we already know: Monofocals do well for distance vision and not-so-good for intermediate and near vision, so patients will have to use reading glasses for these tasks.

When it comes to ATIOLs, the MTF and defocus curves are one way to assess how well a given ATIOL performs at the various test distances. Recall that ATIOLs redistribute incoming light to various target distances to give the patient better intermediate and near vision. One analogy may be useful: Imagine that the ATIOL is like the federal government. The government initially collects taxes and then distributes the revenue to various projects in varying amounts.

The ATIOL similarly collects incoming light but cannot distribute all of it.[31] Since it only has a fraction of the incoming light, it must now decide how much to allocate toward its three biggest projects: distance, intermediate, and near vision. Imagine that the ATIOL has $100 (after the squandered incoming revenue). It must now distribute that $100 to these three areas. Most ATIOLs will spend most of that $100 toward distance vision. After all, patients still prioritize good distance vision. Therefore, when we look at the MTF and defocus curves for ATIOLs, we notice that the highest peak (highest area of spending) is for distance vision. Thus, when compared to monofocal IOLs, the distance peak is lower, but that is because monofocals spend the entire $100 toward distance vision.

The MTF curves for ATIOLS become more interesting for intermediate (40–75 cm) and near vision (<40 cm). When we look at the literature on ATIOLs that report MTF values, we should focus on where the secondary high peaks for each are located; this is where the ATIOL is spending the remainder of the $100 budget. For example, we can observe that low-add power diffractive MFIOLs and EDOF-IOLs spend most of the budget on distance and intermediate vision; thus, these ATIOLs may not function well for near vision. One the other hand, high-add power diffractive MFIOLs spend most of the budget on distance and near vision; thus, these ATIOLs may not function well for intermediate vision. Trifocal IOLs seem to have three prominent peaks for distance, intermediate, and near vision as they spend the budget a bit more equally in these three areas compared to other ATIOLs. However, there are significant gaps in between these three areas that patients may report as "dead zones" in their vision.

In summary, there is no perfect ATIOL. However, understanding MTF curves may give the surgeon additional insight on which ATIOL functions better for a given visual distance and what compromises are made. It will also allow trainees to critically read literature regarding ATIOLs, rather than blindly follow a (paid) speaker on the platform, and understand the pros/cons with each IOL. This knowledge will allow the surgeon to set reasonable expectations with the patient and hopefully achieve a favorable surgical outcome for all parties involved.

[31] A certain percentage of incoming light is lost with an ATIOL due to absorption and destructive interference: think of this as "wasteful" government spending in the above analogy. This should not be interpreted as a political statement of any kind.

Practice Questions

1. Which of the following patient examples represents the best candidate for ATIOL surgery?
   A. 65-year-old patient with refractive error plano in the dominant eye and – 1.75D sphere in the nondominant eye
   B. A 65-year-old patient with refractive error of –16.00D in both eyes
   C. A 65-year-old patient who desires to see at 20/15 vision across all distances and fervently desires to not use glasses for any visual activities
   D. A 65-year-old patient who is +1.50D sphere in both eyes
   E. A 65-year-old patient with extra money in their flex spending account who wants to use it before the end of the calendar year
2. Which of the following is TRUE in regards to spherical IOLs?
   A. Spherical IOLs will yield a much lower objective best corrected visual acuity when compared to aspheric IOLs
   B. The amount of spherical aberration induced by a spherical IOL is independent of the dioptric power of the spherical IOL
   C. Spherical IOLs are a poor IOL choice in patients with a history of pseudoexfoliation syndrome
   D. Spherical IOLs may confer better near vision to patients when compared to aspheric IOLs
3. Which of the following statements about multifocal intraocular lenses (MFIOLs) is TRUE:
   A. MFIOLs can correct higher-order aberrations of the cornea
   B. An apodized diffractive MFIOL is an IOL, wherein the optic has abrupt, discrete steps from the center to the periphery, allowing for splitting light into distinct focal points
   C. A non-apodized diffractive MFIOL has diffractive steps of uniform height, located on the posterior aspect of the optic that encompass the entire optic
   D. A refractive MFIOL has significantly less glare and haloes as compared to a diffractive MFIOL
4. Which of the following statements about modular transfer function curves is TRUE?
   A. A monofocal IOL has an MTF of 1.0
   B. The highest MTF peaks for a diffractive MFIOL are at intermediate (40 cm) and near (25-33 cm) distances
   C. TF-IOLs have the highest peak at distance with nearly similar peaks at near and intermediate ranges
   D. Higher add MFIOLs will have better MTF peaks at intermediate as compared to near ranges
5. Which of the following patients is comparatively the *worst* candidate for a toric IOL?
   A. A 65-year-old mild hyperope with ATR astigmatism
   B. A 40-year-old patient with scarring from severe keratoconus
   C. A 55-year-old moderate myope with WTR astigmatism
   D. A 75-year-old patient with forme-fruste keratoconus
6. Which of the following statements regarding IOL materials and design is TRUE:
   A. Square-edge IOLs are associated with lower rates of PCO formation
   B. Square-edge IOLs are associated with lower rates of dysphotopsias after cataract surgery
   C. Square-edge IOLs are associated with late-term dislocation
   D. Square-edge IOLs have fallen out of favor as rounded-edge IOL designs are primarily used in the construction of single-piece acrylic IOLs
7. Which of the following statements regarding hydrophobic and hydrophilic IOLs is TRUE?
   A. Hydrophilic IOLs have sharper optic edges as compared to hydrophobic IOLs
   B. Hydrophilic IOLs require a larger incision for insertion as compared to hydrophobic IOLs
   C. Hydrophilic IOLs may undergo opacification if exposed to intraocular gas or air
   D. Hydrophilic IOLs confer better visual acuity as compared to hydrophobic IOLs
   E. Hydrophilic IOLs are only available in limited power ranges as compared to hydrophobic IOLs

Answers

1. D. Among the options, a low hyperope may be the best candidate for ATIOL surgery. In choice A, the patient has naturally occurring monovision and may be best left with postoperative monovision, especially to avoid potential glare/halos with an ATIOL. In choice B, an ATIOL power may not be available in the power needed for a pathological myope; in addition, these patients may not do well with an ATIOL due to demands for reading and potential movement of the ATIOL (due to large capsular bag). In choice C, a patient with unreasonable expectations ("type A personality") may not be best suited for ATIOL as all current ATIOLs involve some compromise of visual acuity and contrast sensitivity for increased range of vision. In choice E, do not be greedy: no information was given regarding the clinical candidacy.
2. D. Spherical and aspheric IOLs both confer similar objective visual acuity. However, the subjective visual acuity with an aspheric IOL is usually much better due to

improved (retained) contrast sensitivity. Higher powers of spherical IOLs (e.g., +30D) will induce much more spherical aberration than their lower power counterparts (e.g., +10D). Spherical IOLs may be advantageous in patients prone to IOL decentration, such as patients with pseudoexfoliation syndrome, traumatic cataract, etc., because of the consistent power throughout the IOL. Because of increased depth of focus, spherical IOLs will usually confer better near vision than aspheric IOLs.

3. C. Choice C is the definition of a non-apodized diffractive MFIOL. An apodized diffractive MFIOL (choice B) has a *gradual* reduction of steps from the center to the mid-periphery (3.6 mm). MFIOLs cannot correct any higher-order aberrations. A refractive IOL (no longer available) has much higher rates of glare/halos compared to MFIOLs.
4. C. As there is no perfect lens system, there is no IOL that has an MTF of 1.0 (100 percent transmission of contrast). All monofocal IOLs will have a higher MTF than ATIOLs. Regardless of technology, the highest MTF peaks for all ATIOLs will be at distance. Peaks for near and intermediate vision will vary, depending on the technology and add power in the ATIOL. TF-IOLs have the highest peak at distance with comparatively equal peaks at near and intermediate to yield three focal points of vision. Higher add MFIOLs will have better MTF peaks at near; lower add MFIOLs will have better MTF peaks at intermediate ranges.
5. B. The other three patients are all good candidates for a toric IOL. Elderly patients with forme-fruste keratoconus may benefit from a toric IOL to reduce refractive astigmatism. However, they should be counseled that glasses and/or contact lenses may still be needed. As their corneal disease is unlikely to progress at this age, a toric IOL is a reasonable option. The 40-year-old patient with corneal scarring is the worst candidate as there is likely irregular astigmatism present that cannot be corrected with a toric IOL. The patient may eventually need corneal transplant surgery in the future as well. If the patient needs to undergo cataract surgery, a monofocal IOL is the safest option. In this scenario, the patient may benefit from specialty contact lenses (e.g., scleral contact lenses) for additional vision correction.ANSWER: A. Square-edge IOLs have been shown to decrease lens epithelial cell migration and development of PCO, regardless of the IOL material used. However, they are also associated with higher rates of dysphotopsia (both positive and negative) compared to rounded-edge IOLs. There is no evidence to suggest that square-edge IOLs can dislocate in the long-term, in the absence of exacerbating factors such as pseudoexfoliation syndrome or trauma. Square-edge IOLs are the most popular design for SPA IOLs.
6. C. Hydrophilic IOLs may undergo opacification if exposed to intraocular air or gas, making them a poor choice in patients who may need endothelial keratoplasty and/or retinal surgery in the future. Hydrophilic IOLs have smoother optic edges than hydrophobic IOLs, which may be why they are associated with slightly higher PCO formation rates than hydrophobic IOLs. Hydrophilic IOLs may be inserted via smaller surgical incisions (1.8–2.2 mm) compared to hydrophobic IOLs. Both hydrophobic and hydrophilic IOLs confer equal visual acuity and are available in similar power ranges.

Acknowledgments The author is very grateful to David L. Cooke, MD (Great Lakes Eye Care, St. Joseph, MI) for his editorial assistance and critical review of the material presented in this chapter.

Intraoperative Optics for Cataract Surgery

Kamran M. Riaz

Objectives

- To understand to adjust the power of sulcus and/or anterior chamber IOLs, and why this adjustment is necessary
- To understand the potential usefulness of intraoperative Purkinje images, especially when placing diffractive ATIOLs
- To discuss potential advantages and current limitations of intraoperative aberrometry
- To review intraoperative aspects of toric IOLs and ATIOLs

Introduction

In the previous chapters, we discussed the considerable thought processes and planning a good cataract surgeon must perform *before* to the day of surgery. As for the actual day of surgery, we may have (false) ideas of surgery day being a time to turn our brains off, fire the phaco machine and crank out a bunch of ten-minute cataracts. Alas, it is never that simple.

Careful preoperative planning should make the actual intraoperative process fun. In some ways, modern cataract surgery, especially when using advanced technology intraocular lenses (ATIOLs), requires cataract surgeons to spend more time planning and designing the surgery than it takes to perform the actual surgery. However, there are certain situations and considerations we should keep in mind intraoperatively.

This chapter will discuss a few optics-related things a surgeon should keep in mind as he/she performs cataract surgery.

K. M. Riaz (✉)
Dean McGee Eye Institute, University of Oklahoma, Oklahoma City, OK, USA

Optics of Sulcus and Anterior Chamber IOLs

Congratulations, you just broke the posterior capsule. While you may feel awful in the immediate moment, you can take solace that you have now joined a fellowship of elite cataract surgeons (read: every cataract surgeon alive) who have done the exact same thing.[1] While the usual steps of vitreous management are important, we will focus our discussion on the optics involved with intraocular lenses (IOLs) not placed in the capsular bag.

First, it is important to follow the Boy Scouts' motto: *be prepared*. Surgical planning should include having biometry printouts available for review (e.g., by a circulating nurse) and ensuring that one has access to backup IOLs at the surgical facility.

Remember that single-piece IOLs are one-trick ponies: they can only be placed in the capsular bag. On the other hand, 3-piece IOLs are the Swiss army knives of IOLs: they can be placed in multiple locations and fixated in various techniques: in the capsular bag, in the sulcus, via optic capture, iris-fixated, and/or scleral fixated. Remember that placing a 3-piece IOL requires additional maneuvers, such as ensuring proper injector style, enlarging the surgical incision, and taking care during injection to unfold the IOL properly. Some residents never experience injecting a 3-piece IOL during training because of the regular use of single-piece IOLs; if so, please spend some time in a wet-lab setting learning how to load and insert 3-piece IOLs. Politely asking your surgical facility manager for expired IOLs is a great place to start.

[1] Some people argue that if you do not have complications, you are not operating enough. The authors know of a fellow trainee who went through all of residency without breaking a capsule. He then went into private practice and immediately broke a capsule and had no idea what to do. He tried calling his former attendings during surgery. Do not be that guy/gal.

K. M. Riaz et al. (eds.), *Optics for the New Millennium*, https://doi.org/10.1007/978-3-030-95251-8_28

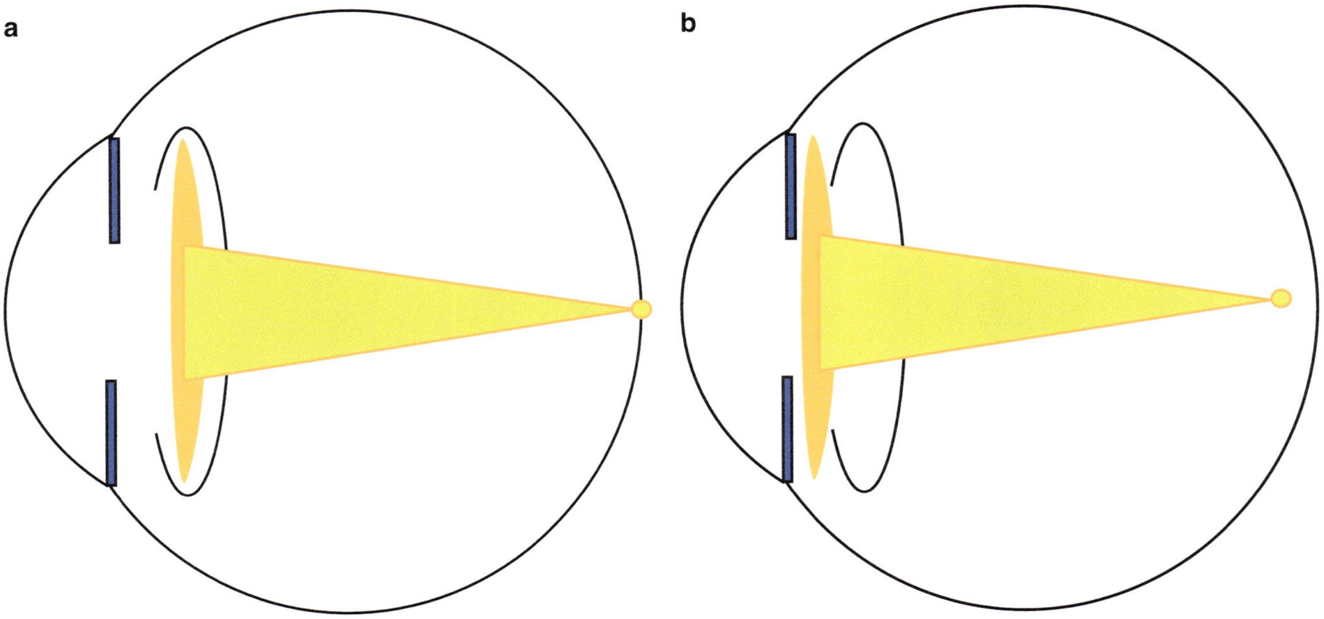

Fig. 1 If a 3-piece IOLs optic is placed in the capsular bag (Panel **a**), then no adjustment to the planned IOL power is necessary. If a 3-piece IOLs optic is placed in the sulcus (Panel **b**), then the planned IOL power will need to be reduced accordingly, depending on the power of the intended IOL

Depending on where we place a 3-piece IOL, we may need to make certain adjustments to the power of the IOL. The following principles should be applied:

- A 3-piece IOL may be placed safely in the bag (Fig. 1) if the capsular defect is minor, either entirely or via optic capture (where the optic is placed in the capsular bag and the haptics are placed in the sulcus). In this case, no IOL power adjustment is necessary compared to the biometry printout because the IOL optic has been placed in the capsular bag. For example, if the biometry sheet calculated a + 18.0D 3-piece IOL, an +18.0D IOL can be placed without additional adjustments.
- A 3-piece IOL may be placed in the sulcus (Fig. 1) for various reasons. Sulcus placement can involve either placing the entire IOL in the sulcus (more common) or via reverse-optic capture, wherein the haptics are placed in the capsular bag and the optic is placed in the sulcus.[2] In either case, we have to adjust the calculated IOL power: because the IOL will now sit more anterior to the retina, we have to *decrease* the power of the 3-piece IOL. If we did not do this, we would have a myopic surprise—which some may argue is not that bad of an outcome, and we would not argue too much either. However, for the sake of accuracy, the following adjustment to the calculated IOL power should be made if placing a 3-piece IOL in the sulcus:
  - For IOL powers >26D: decrease the IOL power by 1.5D.
  - For IOL powers 17-26D: decrease the IOL power by 1.0D.
  - For IOL powers <17D: decrease the IOL power by 0.5D.

What happens if we, ruh-roh, destroy the capsular bag and cannot place a 3-piece IOL?[3] In this case, we may have to place an ACIOL. Several considerations must be made when using these ACIOLs—it is worthwhile to review these periodically, even though the need for them should be (hopefully!) very infrequent:

- When placing ACIOLs, the horizontal white to white (WTW) measurement is crucial to ensure that the ACIOL

[2]Reverse optic capture has been advocated by some surgeons as a technique to alleviate pseudophakic dysphotopsia, either as a primary technique or postoperative adjustment of an already-placed IOL.

[3]It is this author's opinion that whenever possible, an ACIOL should be avoided due to the increased risks of UGH and corneal edema/bullous keratopathy. It would be better to close the eye at this point and return for a planned scleral fixation IOL procedure (e.g., Yamane technique, Aggarwal glued IOL technique, or Gore-Tex® fixation of IOL) or iris-fixation of 3-piece IOL (less-preferred) along with a thorough pars plana vitrectomy. However, reports in the literature have found that there are no-long term differences in the visual outcomes and complications when comparing ACIOL and secondary scleral-fixated IOL eyes. See Chan TC, Lam JK, Jhanji V, Li EY. Comparison of outcomes of primary anterior chamber versus secondary scleral-fixated intraocular lens implantation in complicated cataract surgeries. Am J Ophthalmol. 2015 Feb;159(2):221–6.e2.

is appropriately sized. The biggest reason for problems with ACIOLs is not due to the proximity of the ACIOL to the cornea but due to the ACIOL movement (pseudophacodonesis) that causes chronic, low-grade mechanical irritation of the iris and anterior chamber angle structures. This leads to glaucoma, recurrent hyphema, and corneal edema (bullous keratopathy). As a rule of thumb, we must size the ACIOL *1.0 mm larger than the measured WTW.*

- When placing an ACIOL, we must ensure that the ACIOL is correctly oriented with the haptic resting in the scleral spur, away from any iris defects/iridectomy, and away from any vitreous. The wound size will need to be enlarged (approximately 6 mm) and closed accordingly with sutures.
- Some surgeons will recommend placing an intraoperative peripheral iridectomy to reduce the risk of pupillary block.
- In the United States, there are two main ACIOL model types available, both made of PMMA and with equally comparable long-term visual outcomes[4]:
  - The Kelman Multiflex III (MTAXUO models; Alcon Laboratories, Inc., Fort Worth, TX, USA) features a 5.5 mm optic and is available in 12.0–14.5 mm lengths. This ACIOL is a *convex-plano* design.[5]
  - The S122UV/L122 UV (Bausch and Lomb, Tampa, FL, USA) types (12.5/13.5 mm lengths) feature a 6.0 mm optic and a *biconvex* design.
- When adjusting the power of the ACIOL, the following calculation is used:
  Power of planned PCIOL – (PCIOL A-constant – ACIOL A-constant).
  - For example, if we had planned to place a + 23.0D PCIOL with A-constant 119.0 and our ACIOL (e.g., L122UV) has A-constant 116.0:
    Power of ACIOL = 23 – (119–116) = +20.0D.
  - During surgery, if we panic and forget the above calculation, we can simply decrease the ACIOL power by 2.5–3.0D as compared to the planned PCIOL.
  - You may wish to have the ACIOL power calculated in advance of the surgery day using your biometry device, especially for trainee surgeons or if planning high-risk cataract surgery.

[4]Suelves AM, Siddique SS, Schurko B, et al. Anterior chamber intraocular lens implantation in patients with a history of chronic uveitis: five-year follow-up. *J Cataract Refract Surg*. 2014;40(1):77–81.

[5]See Chap. 27, "What Is on the Menu: An Overview of Currently Available IOLs and Relevant Optics" for more information regarding IOL optic shape and architecture.

Purkinje Images and IOLs

You may wish to review the previously introduced concept of Purkinje images and their application in keratometry in Chap. 17, "Optical Instruments and Machines".

As we have shifted into the era of aspheric IOLs, even a 0.4 mm decentration of a monofocal aspheric IOL may decrease visual performance.[6] When using diffractive ATIOLs (MFIOLs, EDOF-IOLs, and TF-IOLs), the centration of the IOL becomes even more critical. A decentered ATIOL may lead to higher rates of glare, halos, and decreased subjective visual acuity postoperatively. Intraoperatively, centration relying on the pupil alone may be challenging as studies have shown that the pupil may shift ≥0.5 mm after dilation.[7]

Only the P1, P3 and P4 Purkinje images are seen during surgery (remember that P2 is "hidden" within P1 and does not relevance to our discussion).[8] We can begin with how these images appear on the slit-lamp exam in the clinic as a starting frame of reference (Fig. 2, Panel a). Notice that we primarily see "two" Purkinje images easily (P1 and P4, blue arrow and red arrow, respectively). Notice the "inversion" of the P4 image. During surgery (Fig. 2, Panel b), three Purkinje images are present. Starting from anterior to posterior, we will (ironically enough) first see P4 (inverted pyramid-shaped red dots) form on the cornea, even though this reflex originates from the posterior surface of the lens (or IOL) (more on this in the next section). Next, we will see P1 (upright pyramid-shaped blue dots),[9] which originates from the anterior cornea. Finally, we will see P3 (upright pyramid-shaped green dots), which originates from the anterior surface of the lens (or IOL).

Additional intraoperative features of each image are described below. You may wish to refer to Fig. 3, which represents a graphical illustration in the cross-section of each of these Purkinje images. Specifically, note each image's struc-

[6]Wang L, Koch DD. Effect of decentration of wavefront-corrected intraocular lenses on the higher-order aberrations of the eye. *Arch Ophthalmol*. 2005;123(9):1226–1230.

[7]Yang Y, Thompson K, Burns SA. Pupil location under mesopic, photopic, and pharmacologically dilated conditions. *Invest Ophthalmol Vis Sci*. 2002; 43:2508–2512.

[8]One weird thing about the Purkinje images is that the numbering system has no relationship with where the image is actually located. For example, one would think P1 is located most anteriorly and P4 is located most posteriorly. In reality, even though the source of P4 is the posterior lens/IOL, it is located on the corneal surface

[9]Note that P2 is "contained" within P1, thus making P1 the brightest intraoperative Purkinje image.

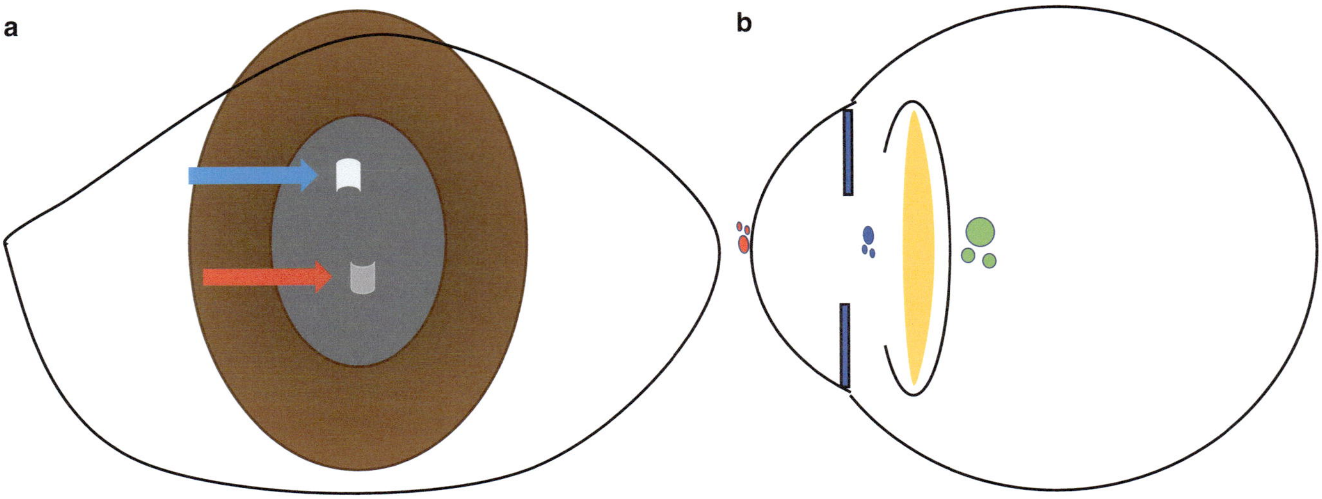

Fig. 2 During routine slit lamp exam (Panel **a**), two Purkinje images (P1 and P4, blue arrow and red arrow, respectively) are easily recognizable. Note the inverted light reflex caused by P4. Intraoperatively (Panel **b**), three distinct Purkinje images are seen and depicted in cross-section. From anterior to posterior, these are P4, P1, and P3. See the text for additional details regarding the origin and location of each image

tural origin and location as this is somewhat counterintuitive, especially for P4![10]

- P1 is formed by the *anterior corneal surface* and is located on the *anterior aspect of the crystalline lens* (or IOL). It is the *smallest yet brightest image* seen on the anterior lens/IOL (even though the source is the anterior cornea). During cataract surgery, it has an upright orientation (see Fig. 4, blue dots) of three dots forming an upright pyramid shape (i.e., two dots at the bottom, one dot at the top). The main illumination light forms the larger top dot while the bottom two dots are coaxial to the surgeon's oculars. It is particularly appreciable in an aphakic eye (Fig. 5). *When centering a diffractive ATIOL, P1 is the most critical image* because of the characteristics mentioned above and serves as a proxy for the visual axis. In addition, it moves minimally with patient eye movement.
- P3 is formed by the *anterior surface of the crystalline lens/IOL* and is located in the *vitreous*. It is the *largest image,* has an upright pyramid shape, and can vary in brightness (Fig. 4, green dots).
- P4 is formed by the *posterior surface of the crystalline lens/IOL* and, oddly enough, is actually *located on the corneal surface*. It has a medium size but has an *inverted* pyramid shape orientation (Fig. 4, red dots) (i.e., two dots at the top, one dot at the bottom; the bottom dot is hidden with the brighter dot of P3). It is located very close to P1 and may be hidden in certain fixation positions.
- In cases where the patient does not fixate on the microscope light, P1 may not be helpful. If this occurs, P3 and P4 can also be used to determine fixation. Ideally, P3/P4 can be used to "capture" P1 into a superbright, solitary image (Fig. 6, Left Panel). P3 can also be placed at the nasal edge of the IOL and P4 at the temporal mid-periphery of the IOL to generate P1 and approximate the patient's fixation (Fig. 6, Right Panel).

Figure 7 provides a summary diagram that shows the cross-section location of the three most important Purkinje images (without inclusion of their structural origin).

A few additional, advanced optical principles may be further discussed in regards to the surgical Purkinje images as the IOL index of refraction and power changes:

- When considering IOLs with a high index of refraction (e.g., acrylic IOLs), a more intense P3 and P4 image may be seen compared to IOLs with lower indices of refraction (e.g., silicone IOLs). The AcrySof IQ IOL (Alcon Laboratories, Inc., Fort Worth, TX, USA) has an index of refraction of 1.55; the intensity of the P3 image seen with this IOL helps to explain the "cat's eye glimmer" that is seen by observers.
- Recall that as IOL power increases, the anterior surface of the IOL will become more convex as well. As a result, as IOL power increases, the P3 usually becomes smaller while the P4 size remains the same (for example, while the anterior portion of a biconvex IOL increases in power when going from a + 21.0D to a + 31.0D IOL, the posterior power of the biconvex IOL is minimally changed).
- Similarly, as the IOL power decreases, the P3 becomes larger; the P4 also becomes larger depending on the IOL

[10] In order to maintain consistency, we have attempted to "color-code" the images in both the figure diagrams as well as the intraoperative images: P1 = blue, P3 = green, and P4 = red

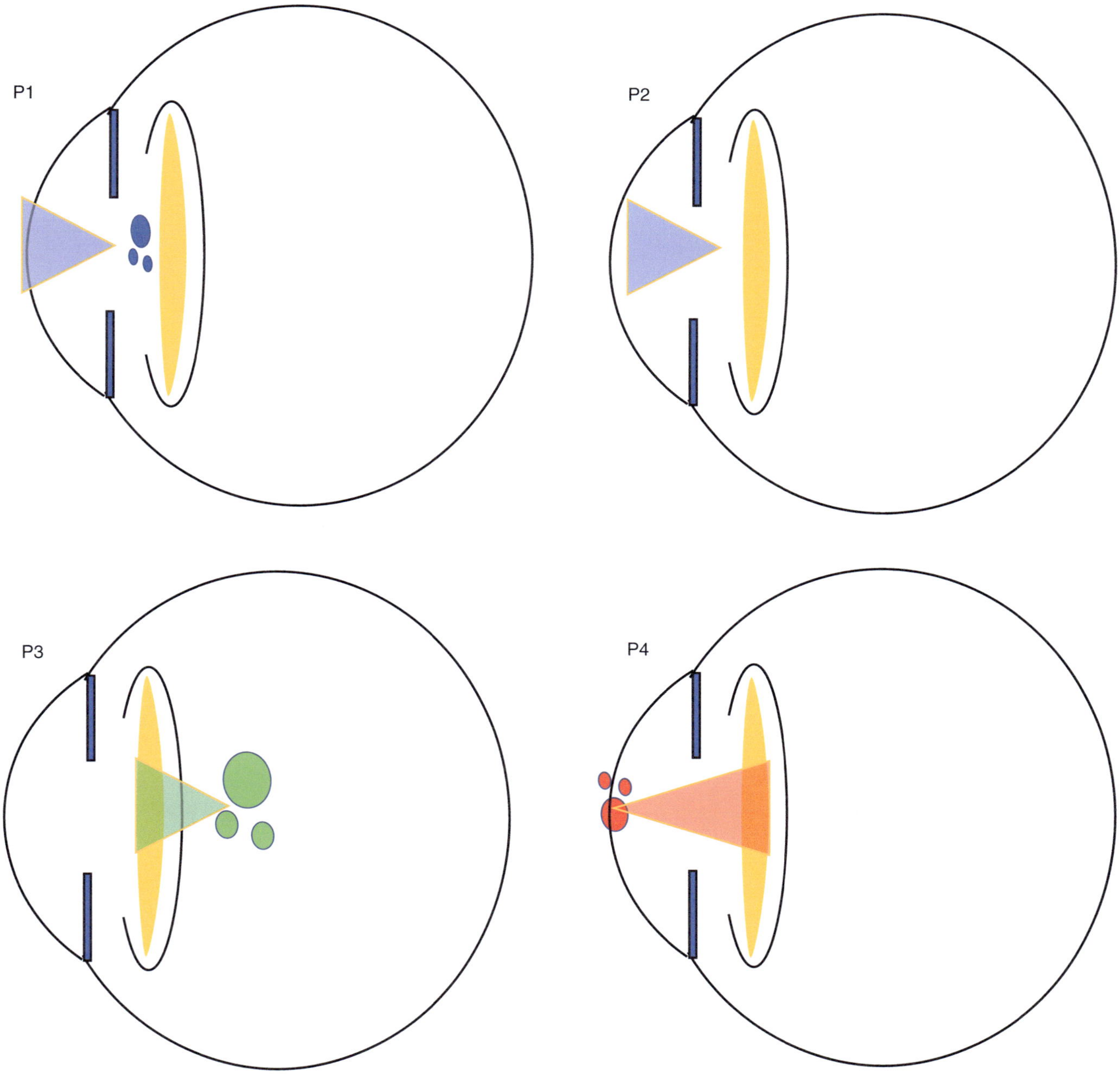

Fig. 3 Cross-section diagram representing the structural origin and image location for the four Purkinje images. P1 (blue) originates from the anterior corneal surface and forms on the anterior aspect of the lens (or IOL). P2 (yellow) originates from the posterior corneal surface, and while it also forms on the anterior aspect of the lens, its image is hidden within the P1 image. P3 (green) originates from the anterior lens capsule and forms the "deepest" image behind the lens. P4 (red) originates from the posterior lens capsule and forms on the anterior corneal surface. It is the only image to have an inverted image orientation

brand (Fig. 8). As the IOL power decreases to ≤10.0D, the P3 may actually invert and appear like an inverse pyramid shape, similar to P4 (Fig. 9).

- The IOL shape becomes a meniscus in the minus IOL power range (rather than a biconvex shape). As a result, the P4 will also invert (i.e., become upright) in minus power ranges while the P3 remains like an inverted pyramid.
- A fun surgical "parlor" game is to predict the power of the IOL by looking at the size and orientation of the P3 and P4 IOL, similar to guessing the power of a patient's eyeglasses by looking at the amount of indentation (or distortion) of the patient's temporal face/cheek through the edge of the spectacle lens. Optics nerds are the epitome of nerds.

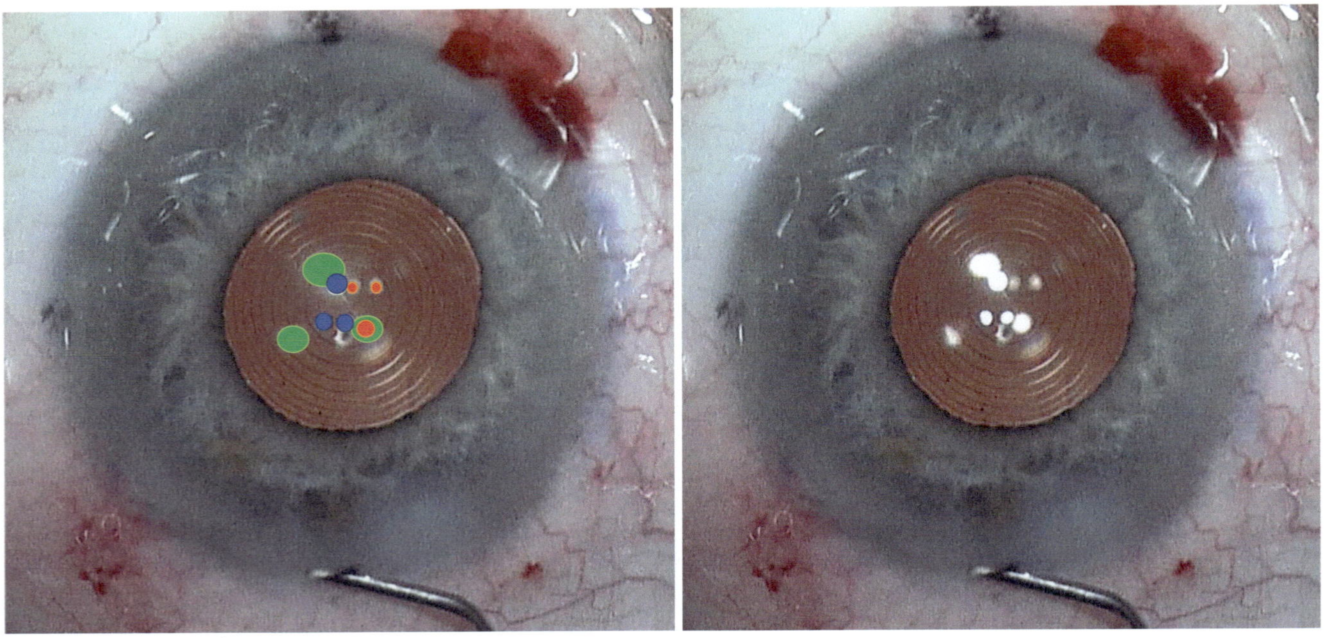

Fig. 4 Intraoperative view of Purkinje images during cataract surgery using a diffractive ATIOL. P1 (blue circle) is seen as an upright pyramid; P3 (green circles) is also an upright pyramid but much larger; P4 (red circles) is seen as an inverted pyramid located close to P1. Note that the lowermost dot of P4 is hidden by the bottom-right dot of P3. In this image, the P1 is used to center an EDOF-IOL effectively

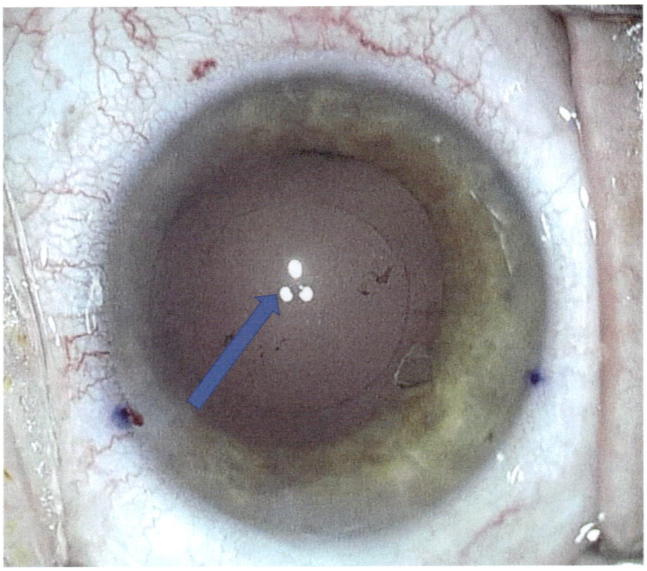

Fig. 5 P1 (blue arrow) is easily observed in the aphakic eye. P4 may also be seen as a dim light behind P1

Finally, here are a few more fun facts regarding Purkinje images in toric and diffractive MFIOLs:

- For toric IOLs, recall that the cylindrical power is mainly in the posterior aspect of the toric IOL.[11] In non-toric IOLs, P4 will be located relatively close to P1. With low cylinder power toric IOLs, P4 will be slightly further apart from the P1 image (Fig. 9). P4 will be extremely far from the P1 image as the cylinder power increases.
- Diffractive MFIOLs may have unique P3 and P4 image quality patterns. Recall that non-apodized MFIOLs (e.g., Tecnis multifocal IOL; Johnson and Johnson Vision, Tampa, FL, USA) have diffractive rings on the posterior surface of the MFIOL; as a result, the P4 image may have a "banded (ringed)" pattern. Apodized MFIOLs (e.g., ReStor; Alcon Laboratories, Fort Worth, TX, USA) have diffractive rings on the anterior surface of the MFIOL; as a result, the P3 image may have a "banded" pattern (Fig. 10).

Intraoperative Aberrometry

Please refer to Chap. 14, "Physical Optics", for basic principles regarding the usage of wavefront analysis and aberrometry in ophthalmology.

Intraoperative aberrometry (IOA) refers to the intraoperative use of wavefront aberrometry to measure the refractive state of the aphakic and pseudophakic eye. Surgeons can use this tool to refine the preoperatively calculated IOL power further. Currently, a "whole-eye" assessment of the eye's refractive power can be done for a range of -5D to +20D in the aphakic state. Measurements are performed in under a minute. Corneal data is limited to the central 4 mm, and the results are extrapolated to calculate an IOL power.

[11] See Chap. 27, "What Is on the Menu: An Overview of Currently Available IOLs and Relevant Optics" for more information regarding toric IOLs.

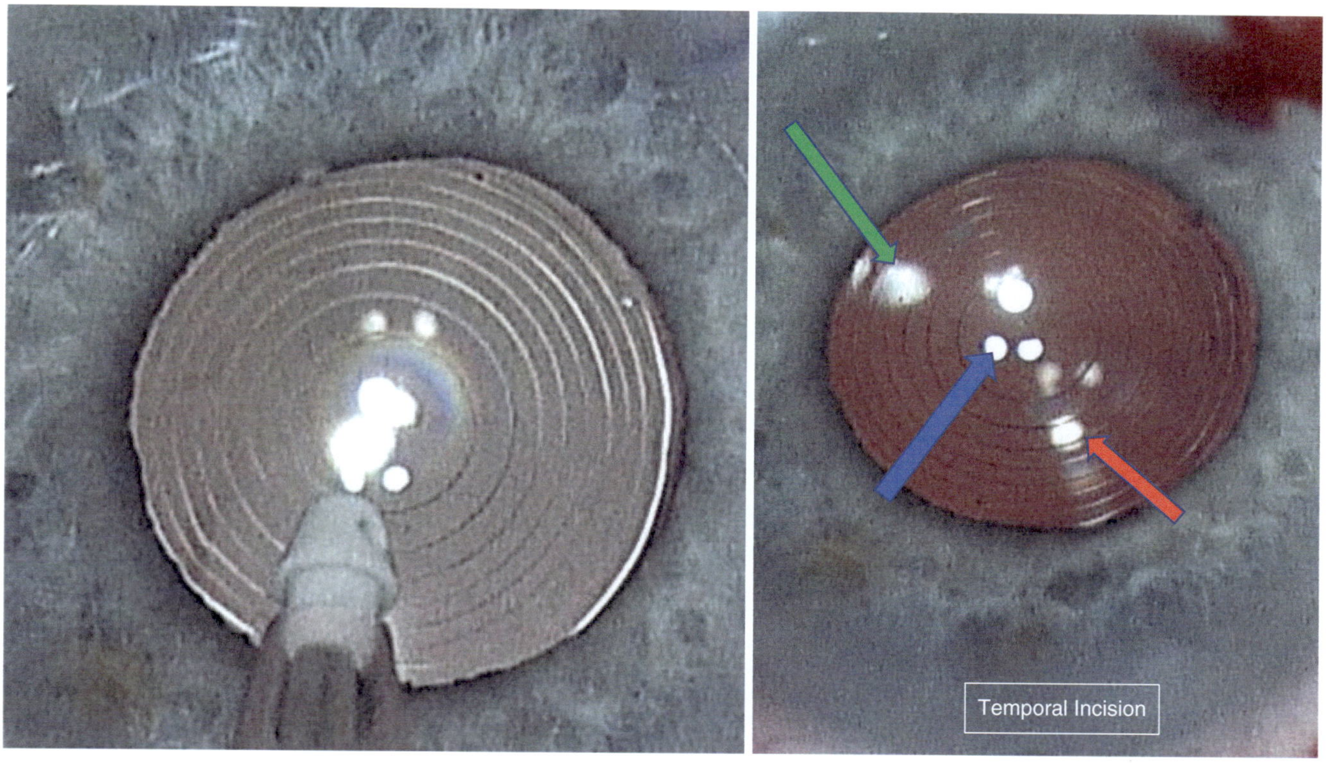

Fig. 6 Left Panel: P3 and P4 can be superimposed upon P1 to create an extremely bright reflex that can further help centration, especially when placing a diffractive ATIOL. Right Panel: P3 (red arrow) can be placed at the nasal edge of the IOL and P4 (green arrow) at the temporal mid-periphery to further approximate the patient's fixation (P1, blue arrow)

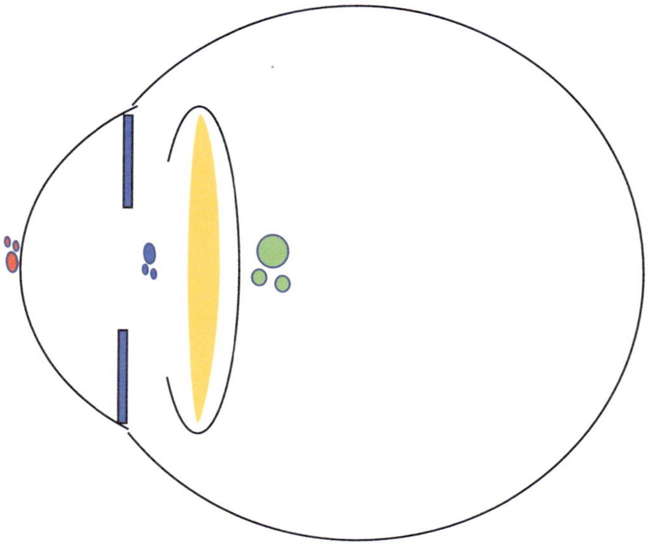

Fig. 7 Cross-section diagram of the eye showing the intraocular locations of the three most important Purkinje images; P1 is blue, P3 is green, and P4 is red

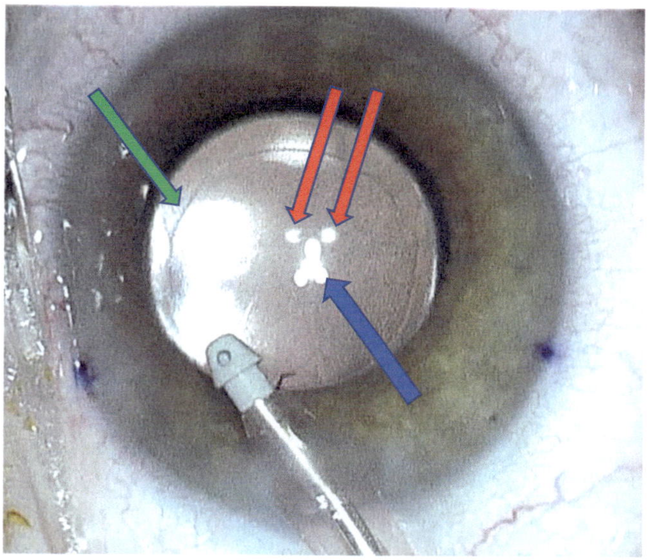

Fig. 8 As the IOL power decreases, the P3 (green arrow) becomes much larger than P1 (blue arrow). P4 also slightly increases in size while remaining relatively close to P1. The top two spots (red arrows) of P4 can also be seen in this image

This technology may be beneficial in cases wherein preoperative IOL calculations are potentially inaccurate, such as in post-refractive surgery and patients with a wide range of preoperative corneal astigmatism. Note that IOA *should not* replace meticulous and thoughtful preoperative planning, including optimal measurements, treatment of ocular surface disease, and other good surgical measures. Just because the technology exists does not mean that surgeons should switch off their brains and let the technology do the work—

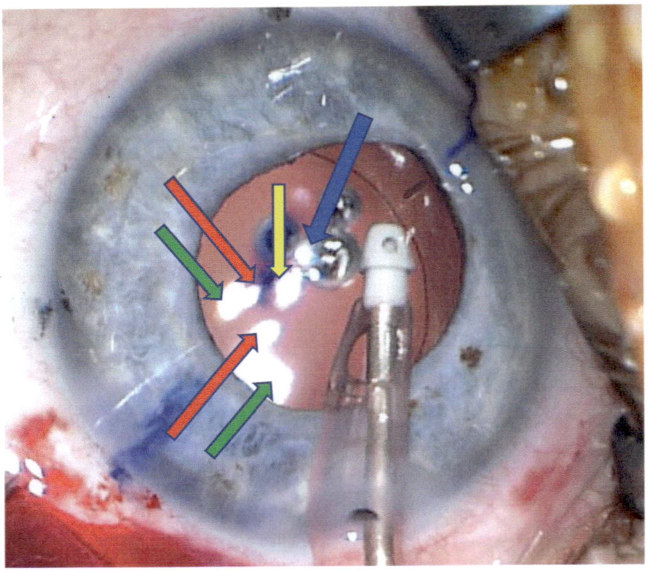

Fig. 9 In a low-power IOL, the appearance of P3 may invert (green arrows) and look similar to P4 (red arrows). In this intraoperative picture of a + 6.0D (Toric) IOL placement, notice P1 (blue arrow) maintains its upright pyramid shape. P3 and P4 are nearly superimposed in an inverse pyramid shape; the P3 light spots are larger than the P4 light spots. The yellow arrow indicates a light spot wherein P3 and P4 are overlapped, and it is difficult to distinguish the two. Author's note: apologies for the air bubbles that may make it challenging to appreciate P1 clearly

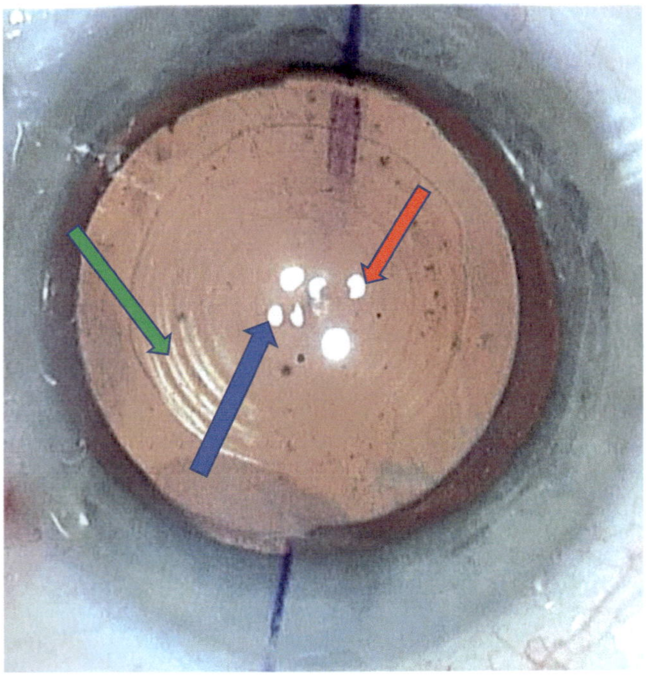

Fig. 10 Toric IOLs have cylindrical power on the posterior surface of the IOL. A low-power toric will have a P4 image (red arrow) relatively close to the P1 image (blue arrow). In this apodized toric diffractive MFIOL, the rings are located on the anterior surface of the optic. As a result, the P3 image may appear as a "banded (ringed)" pattern (green arrow) instead of the usual pyramidal shape

this is how Skynet may one day come to power and wage war on the human race.[12]

IOA is primarily performed after cataract removal and prior to placement of the IOL. The technology is dependent on patient fixation to obtain a line-of-sight aphakic refraction, in addition to physiological IOP and a clear ocular surface. Thus far (June 2021), there have been no definitive reports in the literature proving the superiority of IOA in routine cataract surgery or post-refractive surgery when compared to modern preoperative biometry, use of multivariable formulas, and meticulous surgical technique.

IOA may also be performed after placing a toric IOL to confirm the correct axis meridian location. The aphakic reading will give a potential meridian of placement, whereas post-IOL placement IOA can confirm alignment, including real-time information to the surgeon for the need to rotate the toric IOL intraoperatively. The implementation of good preoperative measurements, surgical planning, and usage of multivariable formulas for toric IOLs have been reported to be as good or better than results obtained with IOA.[13]

IOA is an evolving technology. In addition to the limitations mentioned above, other factors such as globe changes secondary to tight speculum placement; accuracy of "supine" refraction with likely cyclotorsion (as compared to seated refractions which are customary clinical practice); suboptimal ocular surface (post-dilation drops, viscoelastic, corneal edema from phacoemulsification, etc.) and other limiting factors must also be further studied. Finally, IOA does not incorporate multivariable formulas at this time.

Intraoperative Considerations for Toric IOLs and ATIOLs

Several intraoperative considerations for toric IOLs and ATIOLs include:

- It is essential to place the toric IOL on the intended meridian (or as close to humanly possible) due to decreased astigmatism correction due to wrong-meridian placement. It has become a commonly accepted teaching that 1-degree misalignment of a toric IOL leads to a 3.3% reduction in cylinder correction effect.[14] However, recent

[12] Shame on you if you did not get the *Terminator 2: Judgment Day* (1992) reference.

[13] Solomon KD, Sandoval HP, Potvin R. Evaluating the relative value of intraoperative aberrometry versus current formulas for toric IOL sphere, cylinder, and orientation planning. *J Cataract Refract Surg*. 2019;45(10):1430–1435.

[14] The source of this claim, which has in turn been repeated by many authorities, is this paper from 1994(!): Shimizu K, Misawa A, Suzuki Y. Toric intraocular lenses: correcting astigmatism while controlling axis shift. *J Cataract Refract Surg* 1994; 20: 523–26. In this paper, the

findings suggest that the amount of toric IOL rotation and effect on visual acuity is nonlinear.[15] For example, a rotation ≤10 degrees is far more tolerable than a rotation ≥10 degrees. The most significant "devastation" happens between 10 and 20 degrees; if there is a ≥ 45-degree rotation, the toric IOL essentially has no correction. In other words, instead of 30 degrees, it seems that only a ≥ 45-degree rotation leads to the total effect-loss of cylindrical correction.[16]

- Toric IOLs usually have a marking (three dots or a line) to indicate the meridian of the corrective cylinder to help alignment with the intended marked corneal location.
- There is an increased risk of toric IOL rotation in patients with large capsular bags (e.g., high myopes). Placing a capsule tension ring/segment may help stabilize the IOL-capsular bag complex and reduce the risk of future rotation.
- There is no sulcus-toric IOL available in the United States at the time of this writing.
- The ideal placement of an IOL is centration on the visual axis and pupillary axis, which is not possible unless angle kappa (chord) is zero. However, every eye has some amount of chord. While we discussed the usefulness of centering an IOL on the P1 image previously, recent reports suggest that the optimal centration of a diffractive ATIOL is to place it at the midpoint of the pupillary center (pupillary axis) and visual axis (P1).[17] In other words, after centering the ATIOL upon P1, surgeons may consider nudging the haptics so that they are closer together nasally; simply pushing the optic nasally is inadequate.
- Several additional surgical steps are essential for surgical success with accommodating IOLs: careful polishing of anterior capsule and removal of lens epithelial cells; positioning the IOL with posterior vault intraoperatively (anterior vault may cause unintended myopic surprise); meticulous wound closure; and appropriately sized capsulorrhexis.

authors only studied 47 patients, used 5.7 mm incisions (with sutures), only corrected ATR astigmatism, and used an early model 3-piece toric IOL.

[15] Tognetto D, Perrotta AA, Bauci F, et al. Quality of images with toric intraocular lenses. *J Cataract Refract Surg*2018; 44: 376–81.

[16] Németh G. One degree of misalignment does not lead to a 3.3% effect decrease after implantation of a toric intraocular lens. *J Cataract Refract Surg*. 2020;46(3):482

[17] "Multifocal IOLs: Patient selection and optical performance". https://www.healio.com/news/ophthalmology/20170125/multifocal-iols-patient-selection-and-optical-performance. Accessed June 29, 2020

Practice Questions

1. During cataract surgery, posterior capsule rupture occurs so that the intended single-piece +20.0D IOL cannot be placed in the bag. Assuming the A-constant of the 3-piece IOL is similar to the planned IOL, which of the following IOL powers is *the best choice* for sulcus placement?
   A. +19.0D
   B. +19.5D
   C. +20.0D
   D. +20.5D
   E. +21.0D
2. During cataract surgery, the surgeon experiences a severe case of indigestion in the middle of lens removal. The entire bag-zonule complex is lost and a thorough vitrectomy is performed. A + 17.0D single-piece IOL (A-constant: 119.0) was planned for the capsular bag. Which of the following anterior chamber IOL powers should be placed, assuming the ACIOL A-constant is 115.5?
   A. 15.0D
   B. 14.5D
   C. 14.0D
   D. 13.5D
   E. 13.0D
3. Which of the following statements is TRUE?
   A. P1 is the brightest and largest of the four Purkinje images
   B. P2 is best seen in an aphakic state
   C. The size of P3 increases as the IOL power decreases
   D. P4 will always have an inverted pyramid shape
4. Which of the following statements regarding Purkinje images in toric and diffractive optics ATIOLs is TRUE?
   A. For high cylinder power toric IOLs, P4 will be extremely close to P1, and the brightness of P1 may obscure P4
   B. For all toric IOLs, the Purkinje images appear similar to Purkinje images of a non-toric model of that same IOL platform
   C. In non-apodized diffractive MFIOLs, P3 may appear to have a banded (ridged) pattern
   D. In apodized diffractive MFIOLs, P3 may appear to have a banded pattern

Answers

1. ANSWER: A. For IOL powers between 17 and 26D, the 3-piece IOL power for sulcus placement should be decreased by 1.0D. If this IOL is placed via the optic-capture method, the planned +20.0D IOL can be safely placed.
2. ANSWER: D. The formula for calculating the power of the needed ACIOL is as follows: ACIOL power = power of planned PCIOL – (PCIOL A-constant – ACIOL A constant) = 17.0 – (119.0–115.5) = 13.5D
3. ANSWER: C. The size of P3 increases as the IOL power decreases; conversely, the size of P3 will decrease as the IOL power increases. While P1 is the brightest of the 4 Purkinje images, it is not the largest—P3 is the largest Purkinje image. P2 is rarely, if ever seen, as it is usually hidden in the brightness of P1. While P4 usually has an inverted pyramid shape, it can appear as an upright pyramid shape when using minus-powered IOLs.
4. ANSWER: D. In non-toric IOLs, P4 will be located relatively close to P1. With low cylinder power toric IOLs, P4 will be slightly further apart from the P1 image (Fig. 9). P4 will be extremely far from the P1 image as the cylinder power increases. The Purkinje images of a toric IOL will differ from non-toric IOLs based on the amount of cylinder power present. In non-apodized diffractive MFIOLs, the P4 image may have a banded (ridged) pattern.

Postoperative Optics for Cataract Surgery

Kamran M. Riaz

Objectives

- To understand potential optics-relevant problems after cataract surgery, including myopic surprise, hyperopic surprise, and issues related to astigmatism.
- To identify reasons contributing to patients' subjective complaints after cataract surgery, including issues related to dysphotopsias.
- To appreciate various non-surgical and surgical options for correcting problems after cataract surgery.

Introduction

Imagine the following scenario: you have just completed second-eye cataract surgery on Mr. C.M. Burns and are examining him at his one-week post-op visit. In all of your previous interactions, he has been an extremely grouchy curmudgeon, criticizing you, your staff, and his meek assistant as being "incompetent peasants." Today, however, he is delighted: he can see 20/20 at all distances and even has a smile on his face. He tells you that you have done an "excellent" job with his cataract surgery. He tells you that he is so happy with your work that he henceforth names you the sole inheritor of his multibillion-dollar fortune. You exit the room similarly happy, wondering what tropical island you should purchase and how soon you can retire from ophthalmology.

Despite our best efforts, not every patient ends up this happy in real life. This chapter deals with troubleshooting and managing various optics-related postoperative issues that may arise after cataract surgery.

Postoperative Myopic Surprise

If we had to select between two options, postoperative hyperopia or postoperative myopia, one might argue that the latter is not necessarily a bad thing. A patient might be quite happy with −1.00D postsurgical refractive error as they may be able to read, use their cellphone, and read from their tablet device with minimal need for glasses.[1]

Nonetheless, we should understand common reasons for unexpected myopic errors after cataract surgery. Some of these reasons, such as short axial length (AXL) and using post-dilation biometry measurements with multivariable formulas, were previously discussed in Chap. 1, Preoperative Optics for Cataract Surgery.

Commonly Encountered Scenarios

Among the various reasons for an unexpected myopic surprise after cataract surgery, some of the most commonly encountered (and important for exams) reasons include the following:

- Error in IOL power placed (too strong of an IOL power placed): For example, if a + 24.0D of a given IOL model was inadvertently placed instead of a + 22.0D IOL)
- Backward placement of 3-piece IOL IOL: Recall from Chap. 26, Preoperative Optics for Cataract Surgery, that most 3-piece IOLs have a biconvex design with slant haptics insertion, meaning that there is slightly more power on the posterior aspect of the optic as compared to the

[1]The least amount of summated blur that exists through the range of object distance 0.5–6 m is approximately −1.00 + 0.75 (SE: −0.63) with WTR astigmatism, followed by −0.75 + 0.50 (SE: −0.50). In other words, having some myopic sphere and cylinder power is potentially a good thing! See: Sawusch MR, Guyton DL. Optimal astigmatism to enhance the depth of focus after cataract surgery. *Ophthalmology*. 1991;98(7):1025–1029.

K. M. Riaz (✉)
Dean McGee Eye Institute, University of Oklahoma, Oklahoma City, OK, USA

K. M. Riaz et al. (eds.), *Optics for the New Millennium*, https://doi.org/10.1007/978-3-030-95251-8_29

anterior aspect. If such an IOL was inadvertently placed backward in the capsular bag, then the effective power of the IOL will increase, causing a myopic surprise. Single-piece IOLs wherein the haptics and optic are in the same plane should have minimal change if the IOL is accidentally placed upside down.

- Error in biometry measurements and/or A-constant: Recall from our discussions with the SRK formula, a myopic surprise may occur in any of the three following errors: (1) use of a (falsely) higher A-constant; (2) use of flatter-than-actual keratometry (K) measurements; and (3) use of shorter-than-actual axial length (AXL) measurements. In all three scenarios, a higher-than-required IOL power may be falsely calculated.
- (Inadvertent) sulcus placement of IOL: If a given power IOL was meant to be placed in the capsular bag but ends up in the sulcus, the effective lens position (ELP) will be more anterior-than-expected, thus causing a myopic shift. Depending on the IOL that was implanted, surgical intervention may be necessary. If a single-piece IOL intended for in-the-bag placement ends up in the sulcus, then surgical intervention to either reposition the IOL in the bag (if safe) or remove the single-piece for a 3-piece IOL should be undertaken promptly. Recall that if a single-piece IOL is in the sulcus, the thick haptic edges may cause mechanical iris chafing, leading to chronic inflammation or a uveitis-glaucoma-hyphema (UGH) syndrome. Nearly all authorities maintain that a single-piece IOL should *not* be left in the sulcus. If a 3-piece IOL that was intended for in-the-bag placement ends up in the sulcus, it may be managed with nonsurgical options.
- Anterior dislocation of IOL: This may occur in cases of postoperative hypotony, large rhexis, and anterior capsule compromise, to name a few common scenarios. Similar to the previous example, the ELP will be more anterior-than-expected, similarly causing a myopic shift. Management options are essentially the same as the previous example. Of note, assuming the same distance of displacement, anterior IOL displacement will require a greater magnitude of (minus) sphere correction as compared to the (plus) sphere correction required for posterior IOL displacement.[2]
- IOL labeling error: Recall from the previous discussions in Chap. 26, Preoperative Optics for Cataract Surgery, some "acceptable" inaccuracy is allowed by the American National Standards Institute (ANSI). IOL powers <25D are supposed to be within ±0.4D; 25–30D are supposed to be within ±0.5D; >30D are supposed to be within ±1.0D. The latter helps to provide an additional explanation for why IOL calculation in short AXL eyes is challenging: Even if you put in a + 33.0D IOL, for example, there is a chance it may actually behave like a + 32.5D or + 33.5D IOL!

[2]For example, when comparing a 2 mm IOL anterior vs. posterior displacement, the former may require up to −5D sphere to correct, whereas the latter may only require +0.5D sphere correction. See: Lakshminarayanan V, Enoch JM, Raasch T, Crawford B, Nygaard RW. Refractive changes induced by intraocular lens tilt and longitudinal displacement. Arch Ophthalmol. 1986 Jan;104(1):90–2

Capsular Block Syndrome (CBS)

Though a favorite for exam scenarios, this complication is thankfully a rare complication in modern practice. Capsular Block Syndrome (CBS), also known as Capsular Bag Distension Syndrome, is thought to occur in the setting of uncomplicated cataract surgery with a relatively small (<4 mm) capsulorrhexis combined with incomplete removal of viscoelastic, especially behind the IOL (Fig. 1). Clinical examination characteristically shows a small rhexis such that the edge(s) may be visible even in the undilated state. Using a thin slit technique, one may be able to appreciate a "milky" fluid behind IOL, along with a notable gap between the posterior optic border and the posterior capsule. The IOL may appear extremely bright with white-yellowish material behind the IOL causing distension of the capsular bag (Fig. 2). Anterior segment imaging (such as AS-OCT) may be additionally helpful to visualize the turbid fluid-IOL complex in cross-section view (Fig. 3).

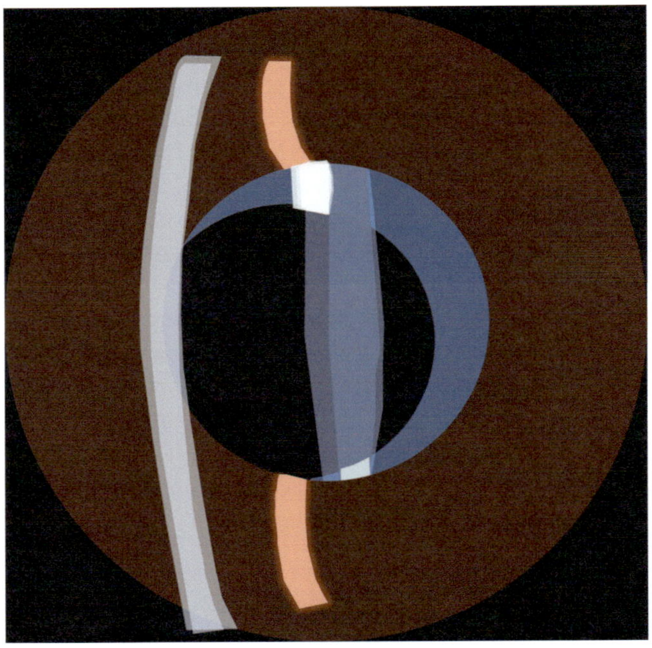

Fig. 1 Capsular block syndrome (CBS) may occur in the presence of a small, intact capsulorrhexis (<4 m) and retained viscoelastic material behind the IOL. This creates an osmotic gradient drawing fluid into the space between the IOL and the posterior capsule, eventually causing a forward shift of the IOL and myopic refractive error

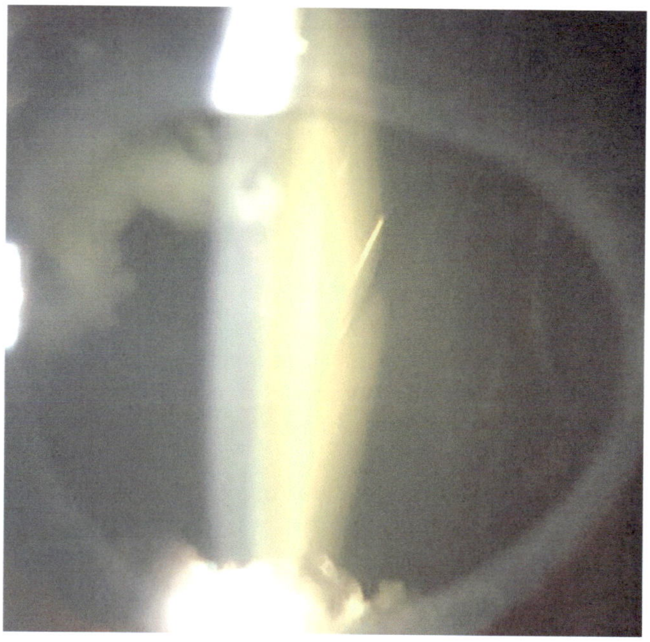

Fig. 2 CBS may cause the IOL to appear extremely bright on examination. Whitish-turbid material can be seen behind the IOL causing fluid to accumulate between the IOL and the posterior capsule. Image Credit: William Trattler, MD, Miami, FL

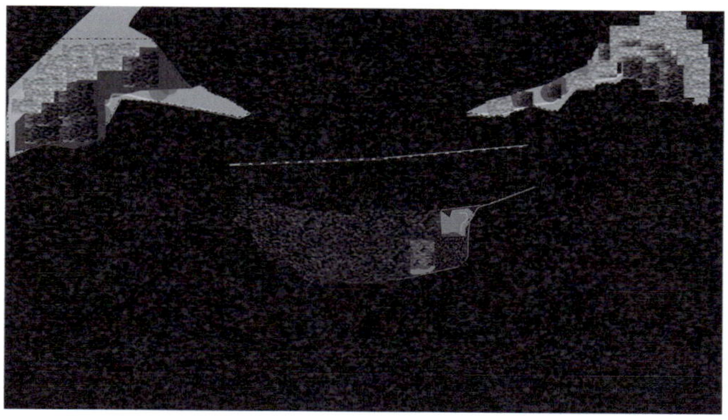

Fig. 3 Anterior segment imaging (AS-OCT or UBM) may be extremely helpful to visualize the anterior shift of the IOL caused by milky/turbid fluid behind the IOL causing the posterior capsule distension

The small capsulorhexis and retained viscoelastic combination create an osmotic gradient drawing fluid into the space posterior to the IOL optic and anterior to the posterior capsule. The fluid gradient causes a circumferential adherence between the anterior capsule opening and the anterior optic of the IOL. As the capsular bag behind the IOL distends, the IOL is pushed forward, causing a myopic shift. In addition, there may be increased IOP and low-grade inflammation.

If CBS is seen in the early-postoperative phases (1–4 days), it may be acceptable to cautiously observe to see if a spontaneous resolution occurs. Of course, this assumes the IOP and inflammation are acceptable, and daily examination (and parking validation for their visits to your fancy downtown office) of these patients may be required.

If CBS is seen after 7 days, further interventions may be necessary. If there is excess inflammation and increased IOP, then topical steroids/NSAIDs and hypotensive medications, respectively, may be utilized. Otherwise, YAG capsulotomy or surgical disruption of the posterior capsule can be both diagnostic and therapeutic. A posterior capsule opening will allow the retained fluid to fall back into the vitreous and (hopefully) shift the IOL back into its intended position.

Treatment Options

Depending on the etiology of myopic surprise, various treatment options may be considered. Conservative options such as glasses and contact lenses (including monovision and/or multifocal options) may be considered for cases that are not surgical emergencies. Surgical interventions include IOL exchange (with the new IOL placed in the capsular bag, if possible, or in the sulcus, with appropriate power modification) and excimer laser refractive surgery (LASIK/PRK).

Another approach that may be considered is the placement of a secondary IOL ("piggyback" IOL) on top of the already existing IOL. This latter approach involves placing a *minus-powered* 3-piece IOL in the sulcus, assuming that the in-the-bag IOL is left in place or too dangerous to remove (e.g., capsular compromise and post-YAG capsulotomy). For example, if a single-piece acrylic (SPA) IOL is placed in the bag, a 3-piece non-acrylic IOL (such as silicone or collamer IOL) is preferred for the sulcus to treat the residual refractive error. While there are several nomograms available to calculate the power of the piggyback IOL a simple rule of thumb is that a 1:1 ratio of IOL power: refractive error can be used to correct a myopic refractive error. For example, if a patient has an unintended −2.00D sphere after cataract surgery with a SPA IOL placed in-the-bag but post-YAG capsulotomy, then one acceptable approach may be to place a – 2.0D 3-piece IOL in the sulcus to treat the refractive error.

In the previous paragraph, we stated that a non-acrylic 3-piece IOL is preferred. A 3-piece acrylic IOL can be cautiously placed in the sulcus as well, though there is a small risk for *intralenticular opacification (ILO)*. While ILO has been previously reported for acrylic-on-acrylic IOLs placed in the capsular bag, it has not been reported for 3-piece acrylic placed in the sulcus with a SPA acrylic IOL in the bag.[3] ILO may cause a visually significant loss of vision (similar to corneal scarring) that cannot be treated with additional YAG capsulotomy. Surgical removal of both IOLs may be required for cases of visually significant ILO.[4]

While the above discussion about using piggyback IOLs to treat postoperative myopic refractive errors sounds lovely, in the United States, surgeons have limited options when considering this technique. At this time, there are no minus-powered silicone or collamer IOLs available in the United States; only minus-powered *acrylic* IOLs are currently available.[5]

Finally, for the sake of completion, a collamer phakic IOL (Visian ICL; Staar Surgical, Monrovia, CA, USA) may technically be used in this setting as a piggyback IOL (range −3.00 to −20.0 D); however, the cost for this IOL may be prohibitive for most patients. In addition, this is an off-label use of this IOL.

Postoperative Hyperopic Surprise

In contrast to our previous discussions on postoperative myopic surprise, overall, a postoperative hyperopic surprise is far less tolerated by patients, especially for myopic patients prior to cataract surgery. Remember that while postoperative myopia may help with some near-intermediate vision tasks, postoperative hyperopia is good for absolutely nothing other than an angry patient who may decide to "release the hounds" on you.

In addition to embarking upon the walk of shame, we should also understand common reasons for unexpected hyperopic error after cataract surgery. Some of these reasons, such as long axial length and post-refractive surgery, were previously discussed in Chap. 26, Preoperative Optics for Cataract Surgery.

Commonly Encountered Scenarios

Among various reasons for an unexpected hyperopic surprise after cataract surgery, some of the most commonly encountered (and important for exams) reasons include the following:

- Error in IOL power (too weak of an IOL power placed): For example, if a + 20.0D IOL was inadvertently placed instead of a + 22.0D IOL.
- Error in biometry measurements and/or A-constant: Recall from our discussions with the SRK formula, a hyperopic surprise may occur in any of the three following errors: (1) use of a (falsely) lower A-constant; (2) use of steeper-than-actual keratometry (K) measurements (as in post-myopic refractive surgery); and (3) use of longer-than-actual axial length (AXL) measurements (as in long AXL eyes and eyes with silicone oil). A lower-than-required IOL power may be falsely calculated in all these scenarios causing the unwanted hyperopic surprise.
- Backward placement of a SPA IOL: This only applies to SPA IOL models with offset haptic-optic designs, as discussed in Chap. 26, Preoperative Optics for Cataract Surgery.
- Corneal ectasia: The measured K values may be extremely high (often >50D) for patients with stable corneal ectasia not requiring corneal transplant surgery. Most IOL formulas, especially third-generation formulas, do not account for the nonlinearity of higher K measurements in the formulas.[6] As a result, the high K values may lead to a lower-than-required IOL power and increase the risk of hyperopic surprise.
- Outlier biometry measurements such as increased lens thickness (LT) (>5 mm) and decreased anterior chamber depth (ACD) (<3 mm) when using multivariable formulas. Recall that multivariable formulas incorporate ACD and LT measurements when calculating the IOL. When these values are abnormal, the calculated ELP may be significantly different from the actual postoperative ELP. While a complete discussion of this math is beyond the scope of

[3]There is considerable debate on this point. Some surgeons argue that ILO has been reported only in the context of acrylic-on-acrylic IOLs both placed in the capsular bag, and the risk of ILO with a three-piece acrylic IOL in the sulcus and a single-piece acrylic IOL in the capsular bag is extremely low. For hyperopic surprises, this author advises using three-piece silicone IOLs as piggyback IOL options and avoiding acrylic IOLs as much as possible. For myopic surprises, a three-piece acrylic IOL may be placed as a piggyback option after thorough discussion with the patient. However, laser refractive surgery (PRK or LASIK) might be a better option in these cases to avoid additional intraocular surgery. Financially, piggyback IOL for myopic surprise would likely incur out-of-pocket costs for the patient anyway, so they might as well pay for a more predictable and safer refractive procedure.

[4]In this case, if both IOLs are removed with preservation of the capsular bag, then a "correctly-powered" IOL can be placed, either a one-piece or three-piece IOL. The latter can be placed in the bag or sulcus (including optic capture). More often than not, these cases will involve significant scarring of the IOLs to the capsular bag, and therefore amputation of the embedded haptics or removal of the entire bag-IOL complex may be necessary. This may require additional vitreous management and subsequent placement of an iris- or scleral-fixated IOL

[5]The last available minus-powered silicone IOL in the United States was the AQ5010V (Staar Surgical, Monrovia, CA USA), and it was discontinued in August 2016. At present, the two most commonly available minus-powered acrylic IOLs are the MN60MA (Alcon Laboratories, Fort Worth, TX USA) and AR40m models (Sensar; Johnson & Johnson Vision, Sarasota, FL USA)

[6]More recently, the online Barrett true K and online Kane formulas have a "keratoconus" option that makes internal adjustments for high K values to minimize the risk of postoperative hyperopic surprise. Still most surgeons will aim for additional myopia to adjust for a hyperopic surprise.

the text, suffice it to say that this may increase the risk of hyperopic surprise. In such scenarios, it may be helpful to look at "older" generation formulas (such as Holladay I or SRK/T) side-by-side with newer formulas (such as Barrett) to see if there is agreement. Alternatively, one may choose to aim extra myopic (−0.75 or −1.00D) to compensate for the likely postoperative hyperopic surprise.

Treatment Options

Depending on the etiology for hyperopic surprise, several treatments may be considered. Conservative options, such as glasses and contact lenses (including monovision and/or multifocal options), may be considered for cases that are not surgical emergencies. Surgical interventions include IOL exchange (with the new IOL placed in the capsular bag, if possible, or in the sulcus, with appropriate power modification) and excimer laser refractive surgery (LASIK/PRK). It should be noted that hyperopic excimer laser correction is *significantly less effective* than myopic excimer laser correction. For example, treating a −2.50D refractive error with laser refractive surgery is much easier than a +2.50D refractive error.

In contrast to treating myopic errors, placing a secondary IOL ("piggyback" IOL) on top of the already existing IOL is a much more viable option. Silicone and collamer IOLs, such as the Li61AO (SofPort; Bausch and Lomb Inc., Tampa, FL USA) and CQ2015 (Staar Surgical, Tampa, FL USA), can be employed, especially when removing the original IOL may be challenging or risky. The Li61AO, in particular, is a useful option as it is available in a wide range of powers (full range: 0 to +34.0D).

While several nomograms can be used accurately calculate the power of the IOL to correct the postoperative refractive error, a simple rule of thumb is that a 1.5:1 ratio of IOL power: hyperopia can be used for the piggyback IOL power. For example, suppose a patient's refractive error is +2.00D sphere after cataract surgery with a SPA placed in-the-bag (additionally, assume the enterprising referral surgeon has already performed a YAG capsulotomy!). In that case, one acceptable approach may be to place a +3.0D 3-piece silicone IOL in the sulcus to treat the refractive error.

IOL Decentration

There are three types of IOL position errors:

- IOL displacement (or IOL shift): A *longitudinal shift* of the IOL either toward or away from the retina. This shift is the most important IOL position error, and is also the simplest one to understand as it mainly causes a hyperopic or myopic shift, respectively.
- IOL decentration: A *lateral shift* of the IOL, perpendicular to the visual axis.
- IOL tilt: A rotational tilt of the IOL, not perpendicular to the visual axis.

Both IOL decentration and IOL tilt will negatively impact visual acuity postoperatively as they both will induce myopic sphere and astigmatism to the clinician's refraction. IOL tilt, defined as an increased angle between the IOL axis (i.e., the axis in which the optic is oriented) and the reference axis (which can be either the optical axis or the visual axis), is discussed in the next section. As a rule of thumb, approximately 1 mm IOL decentration is equivalent to 7° IOL tilt.

IOL decentration is defined as an increased distance in the lateral direction between the center of the IOL and the reference axis. Several risk factors, such as long axial length, thicker lens, capsule fibrosis, an incomplete overlap of the optic by the rhexis, and large/poorly constructed capsulorrhexis have been shown to increase the risk of IOL decentration. Aspheric IOLs are much more negatively affected by IOL decentration than spherical IOLs. Similarly, the efficacy of toric IOLs is affected both by decentration and by tilt. ATIOLs using diffractive optics are severely affected by even minute amounts of IOL decentration. Patients who have paid a small fortune for these IOLs will be extremely unhappy with IOL position errors. IOL decentration and tilt happen more frequently than we realize; thankfully, these shifts are minimal. Clinical studies have shown that 2–3° tilt and 0.2–0.3 mm decentration are common and clinically insignificant for most IOL types.[7] However, >1 mm decentration and ≥ 5° tilt may be visually significant.[8]

Lateral IOL decentration, in the absence of the other two IOL position errors, nearly always adds myopic astigmatism to the eye's refractive error. IOL decentration negatively impacts visual function more than IOL tilt, especially when evaluating aspheric IOLs, toric IOLs, and diffractive optics ATIOLs. In one study, the best-corrected visual acuity (BCVA) decreased from approximately 20/15 with perfect centration to approximately 20/25 with 0.4mm decentration.[9]

Treatment of IOL decentration includes nonsurgical options such as glasses and contact lenses. Surgical options, such as IOL repositioning, placement of capsule tension ring, capsule tension segments, IOL exchange, and/or laser refractive surgery, can be considered if clinically necessary. If the IOL decentration happened because you made a lousy capsulorrhexis, then an apology letter (along with a box of candy) may be required.

[7] Ale JB. Intraocular lens tilt and decentration: a concern for contemporary IOL designs. Nepal J Ophthalmol. 2011 Jan-Jun;3(1):68–77.

[8] Korynta J, Bok J, Cendelin J, Michalova K. Computer modeling of visual impairment caused by intraocular lens misalignment. J Cataract Refract Surg. 1999 Jan;25(1):100–5.

[9] Madrid-Costa D, Pérez-Vives C, Ruiz-Alcocer J, Albarrán-Diego C, Montés-Micó R. Visual simulation through different intraocular lenses in patients with previous myopic corneal ablation using adaptive optics: effect of tilt and decentration. J Cataract Refract Surg. 2012 May;38(5):774–86.

Postoperative Astigmatism Issues

Astigmatism issues arising after cataract surgery can be divided into two broad categories: expected postoperative astigmatism and unexpected postoperative astigmatism.

Expected Astigmatism

The first category is straightforward: A typical scenario would include a patient with moderate astigmatism (1.5-2D of keratometric astigmatism) measured before cataract surgery who opts for a monofocal IOL due to financial limitations.[10] Dealing with this situation is quite simple: prescribe the patient glasses and/or contact lenses and move on with life. Both the surgeon and the patient are usually quite happy with this situation because this possibility was discussed and managed appropriately after surgery.

While we may be trained to think that astigmatism is "bad," there are some optics-related merits of residual astigmatism after cataract surgery, especially when comparing pseudophakic with-the-rule (WTR) and against-the-rule (ATR) astigmatism types. We previously discussed some of these concepts in the previous two chapters, but we can expand that discussion here.

Residual pseudophakic WTR (greater plus power at the 90-degree meridian) will bring in vertical stroke letters (such as b, d, h, k, p, t,) at a *distance* into better focus.[11] WTR astigmatism also helps reading languages (such as English) that have less "space" in-between individual letters as compared to the "space" between lines of text on a page (such as this engrossingly entertaining optics book you are reading right now). Furthermore, according to Javal's Rule, WTR astigmatism requires less cylinder correction in glasses than ATR. As mentioned previously, the Sawusch and Guyton model suggests that 0.50–0.75D WTR astigmatism allows for the least amount of summated blur from 50 cm to 6 meters, which is where most distance vision occurs. Finally, recall that we "gain" ATR as we get older, so having some residual WTR astigmatism allows us to "grow into" our eventual ATR later in life.

Residual pseudophakic ATR (greater plus power at the 180-degree meridian) will bring vertical strokes at *near* into better focus. Thus, it may be beneficial to leave intentional ATR in a patient with high demands for near work, such as a jeweler and coin collector, especially if the patient wants to perform these activities without glasses. Additionally, patients whose primary language revolves around a horizontally oriented alphabet (e.g., Arabic, Russian, and Hindi) may use ATR astigmatism advantageously for distance vision (in such patients, residual WTR astigmatism may help with near vision tasks).

The takeaway from this entire discussion is this: the human eye is imperfectly perfect. Astigmatism is an "imperfection" that we attempt to treat and reduce whenever possible, but it may not be necessary (or even beneficial) to fully treat this "imperfection." Some "imperfection" may actually lead to a subjectively happy patient. Do not be hasty to treat low amounts of pseudophakic astigmatism with additional surgery (especially laser refractive surgery): you may end up causing more harm than good!

Unexpected Astigmatism

The second category (unexpected postoperative astigmatism) is more complex and requires a detailed discussion with specific examples.

Three potentially common examples of this scenario include the following:

IOL Tilt

Continuing our previous discussions on IOL displacement and IOL decentration, IOL tilt primarily causes induced astigmatism. Risk factors for IOL tilt include short AXL eyes, previous history of PPV, and exuberant capsule fibrosis.

As previously discussed in Chap. 11, Astigmatism, if a + 20.0D monofocal IOL undergoes tilting around the 180-degree axis (e.g., suppose that the superior part of the optic is now closer to the cornea, the inferior part of the optic is now closer to the retina), then the IOL may no longer function as a + 20.0D IOL. The IOL will gain some plus sphere power and plus cylinder power in the 180-degree (axis) meridian.

This next part is slightly confusing, so it may take several readings to comprehend this concept fully. The amount of "gained" sphere and cylinder depends on both the power of the IOL and the degree of tilt.[12] We previously stated that 1 mm of decentration is equivalent to 7° tilt; to make the math easier, let's assume we are dealing with a + 19.0D IOL with a 15° tilt. Assuming no longitudinal displacement, this IOL

[10] Perhaps we should have asked Mr. CM Burns to donate the costs of a toric IOL for this fictional patient prior to cataract surgery.

[11] Morlet N, et al. Astigmatism and the analysis of its surgical correction. *Br J Ophthalmol* 2001; 85:1127–38.

[12] Specifically, we can think of IOL tilt in lower power IOLs as more "devastating" in terms of their equivalence to 1 mm of IOL decentration as compared to higher power IOLs. The previous sentence is understandably awkwardly worded and counterintuitive. For example, a + 15.0D IOL only requires 5.55 degrees of tilt to equal 1 mm of decentration, whereas a + 21.0D requires 7.79 degrees of tilt to equal 1 mm of decentration. An elegant article that discusses this in more detail: Erickson P. Effects of intraocular lens position errors on postoperative refractive error. J Cataract Refract Surg. 1990 May;16(3):305–11.

will function like a + 19.50 + 1.00 × 180. On clinical refraction, assuming the patient's refraction was previously plano, we may now obtain a − 1.50 + 1.00 × 90 (corresponding to −0.50 − 1.00 × 180). Note that because the IOL has gained plus sphere power, the clinician will note increased minus sphere power in the refraction. However, though the IOL has gained more plus cylinder power in the 180-degree (axis) meridian, the clinician will either note a refraction of increased minus cylinder power in the 180-degree (axis) meridian, or because we are ophthalmologists and prefer plus cylinder, a refraction of increased plus cylinder power in the 90-degree (axis) meridian.

Depending on the stability of the IOL, single-piece vs. 3-piece, presence of vitreous, etc., this may be managed conservatively (glasses or contact lenses) or require surgical intervention (IOL repositioning/fixation or IOL exchange with or without vitreous management).

Unmasked Corneal Astigmatism

Suppose a patient presents to your office 2 months after uneventful cataract surgery in both eyes by a provider in another state. She reports ghosting and blurred vision when she does not wear the glasses prescribed after surgery. As your curiosity is piqued, you ask her if the ghosts ever talk to her. She says "No," but is concerned because she was told after surgery that she has "astigmatism" in her glasses, which she reports she never had before surgery.

Exam:	Distance visual acuity without correction: 20/40 OD, 20/40 OS
	Today's Manifest Refraction:
	OD : − 1.50 + 2.00 × 170 (20/20)
	OS : − 1.00 + 2.00 × 10 (20/20)
	Slit lamp exam: WNL, including PCIOL well-centered OU. DFE normal.

She then shows you her old (presurgery) glasses: −1.00D sphere in both eyes.

What happened? Did the surgery go wrong? Did our patient magically develop astigmatism after cataract surgery?

This vignette is a classic scenario of favorable preoperative lenticular astigmatism counteracting the (significant) corneal astigmatism. Hence, the patient only needed to wear glasses with spherical correction.

After cataract surgery, the outside provider likely placed a monofocal IOL in both eyes. Since the cataracts (and the favorable lenticular astigmatism) were removed, she now has prominent corneal astigmatism, aka unmasked corneal astigmatism, that requires glasses correction.

We can confirm this by obtaining keratometry measurements today:

Keratometry measurements
OD : 43.00 / 45.00 @ 170
OS : 43.25 / 45.25 @ 10

Treatment options at this time include first educating the patient about what has happened and informing her that she does not have any ophthalmic disease. We can reassure her that she can still see very well with glasses at this time and overall has had an acceptable surgical result. Contact lenses, including a soft toric, rigid gas permeable (RGPCL), and/or scleral lens (ScCL), may also be offered. Surgical options include limbal relaxing incisions (which can be done in the office or minor operating room), IOL exchange (replacing both monofocals with toric IOLs, if safe and the patient is financially able), and/or excimer laser refractive surgery.

As an aside, this vignette also highlights the importance of a thorough preoperative discussion with patients prior to cataract surgery. Patients at risk for unmasked corneal astigmatism after cataract surgery should be counseled about options for astigmatism correction *before* deciding to proceed with cataract surgery. The surgeon should document that astigmatism correction options were offered to the patient. They should also be informed about the need for glasses/contact lenses after surgery to correct unmasked astigmatism; most importantly, they should understand that the cataract surgery did not cause the astigmatism.

Toric IOL Rotation

Suppose a 68-year-old male patient presents for his postoperative one-week visit to your office. You had previously performed cataract surgery in his left eye and placed a toric IOL. At his postoperative one-day visit, he saw 20/25 and was quite happy with this vision. Today, he reports decreased vision, especially noting "ghosting" around images. He fears that something terrible has happened and will lose his vision.

Exam (today) Visual acuity without correction OS : 20 / 60
Manifest refraction OS : $-1.50 + 4.00 \times 95$ (20 / 25, slow)

Preoperative keratometry : $42.25 \times 44.25@94$

A review of your operative report reveals that you placed a toric IOL at the 94-degree meridian.

Slit-lamp exam today reveals the following (Fig. 4).

What happened? Will our patient lose his vision?

Unfortunately, it appears that the toric IOL was initially placed at the correct meridian (approximately 95 degrees) but has since rotated approximately 70 degrees in the past few days. This undesirable rotation has worsened the preexisting

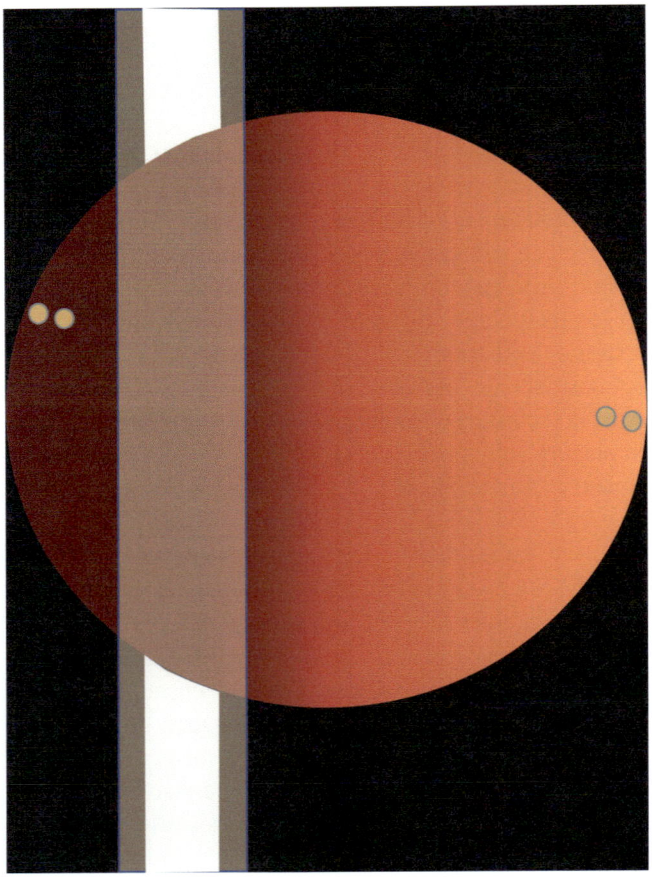

Fig. 4 Slit-lamp exam today showing a toric IOL with markings located at approximately 165 degrees

corneal astigmatism from 2D to approximately 4D (refractive cylinder).

When placing a toric IOL, surgeons should make every attempt to place the IOL in the correct meridian. Recall that if a toric IOL rotates away from its appropriate location, there is a reduction in its effect. The classic teaching (which has recently been called into question, see next paragraph) is that a 1-degree rotation causes a 3.3% reduction in astigmatism correction effect. Extending this, we can see that if the IOL rotates 30 degrees, there is a 100% reduction of effect. Finally, if the IOL rotates more than 30 degrees, it can worsen astigmatism, which happened in our example.

As discussed in the previous chapter, this 1-degree rotation equaling a 3% reduction rule has become a commonly accepted fact. The source of this claim, which in turn has been repeated by many authorities is a paper from 1994(!) which reported the results of 47 patients with ATR astigmatism, used a 5.7 mm incision (with sutures), and used an older-generation 3-piece toric IOL with an oval optic.[13] Of course, much has (thankfully) changed with cataract surgery since that time. Recent findings suggest that the amount of toric IOL rotation and effect on visual acuity is nonlinear.[14] For example, a rotation of ≤10 degrees is far more tolerable than a rotation of ≥10 degrees. The largest loss-of-effect (proportionally) occurs between 10 and 20 degrees; only if there is a ≥ 45-degree rotation, then the toric IOL has a total effect-loss of astigmatism correction.[15]

Getting back to our patient, we can begin by validating his concerns with reassurance and explaining what has happened. Thankfully, refraction improves his vision (albeit with more cylinder than he would have liked), so the vision potential remains quite good. Nonsurgical options at this time would include glasses and/or contact lenses (soft toric, RGPCL, and/or ScCL) to manage the astigmatism. Since it is still early in the postoperative period, a reasonable option would be to return to the operating room and rotate the IOL back into its intended location with meticulous surgical technique to remove viscoelastic and ensure IOL stability. A capsular tension ring can be placed to stabilize the IOL-bag complex. A sutured capsular tension segment may also be required if there is any zonular compromise. If the toric IOL is defective or compromised, replacing it with a new toric IOL may also be necessary.

Suppose our patient had surgery performed by another surgeon 18 months ago and presents with the same findings. At this time, it may be difficult to rotate the IOL due to fibrosis and scarring that have likely occurred postoperatively. Rotating the IOL may cause additional damage to the IOL-bag complex, including potential vitreous loss. Similarly, an IOL exchange may be difficult, especially if a YAG capsulotomy was performed after surgery. For these situations, glasses/contact lenses remain a good option. Finally, excimer laser refractive surgery can be offered to treat the refractive error and may be the safest surgical option for these late-term rotation situations.

Correcting Postoperative Astigmatism

We have discussed some of these options before, but for the sake of completion and a compiled source of options, the following are potential strategies to manage and correct postoperative refractive astigmatism.

Nonsurgical Options

- Glasses
- Contact Lenses, including toric, RGPCL and ScCLs

[13]Shimizu K, Misawa A, Suzuki Y. Toric intraocular lenses: correcting astigmatism while controlling axis shift. *J Cataract Refract Surg* 1994; 20: 523–26.

[14]Tognetto D, Perrotta AA, Bauci F, et al. Quality of images with toric intraocular lenses. *J Cataract Refract Surg* 2018; 44: 376–81.

[15]Németh G. One degree of misalignment does not lead to a 3.3% effect decrease after implantation of a toric intraocular lens. *J Cataract Refract Surg*. 2020;46(3):482

Surgical Options

- Exchanging a monofocal IOL for a toric IOL or a wrongly-powered toric IOL for a correctly-powered toric IOL
- Rotation and stabilization of a previously placed toric IOL
- Incisional procedure(s) in the office or operating room, such as limbal relaxing incision and manual/femtosecond laser-assisted arcuate keratotomy
- Laser refractive surgery

Troubleshooting Other Postsurgical Issues

Several other problems may also present after cataract surgery as a combination of objective and subjective refractive issues.

Magnification and Minification Issues

One would think that patients with high myopia and/or hyperopia who become emmetropic after cataract surgery should be delighted to get rid of their glasses. Usually, that is the case with most of these patients, especially with high myopes, though they may complain about needing reading glasses as they previously may have been able to read without correction – though they likely had to hold the reading material extremely close!

However, a minority of these patients may complain about subjective size distortions with their new emmetropia.[16] Recall that high myopes experience minification effects as they view the world through a reverse Galilean telescope; conversely, high hyperopes experience magnification effects as they view the world through a Galilean telescope. For these high myopes and high hyperopes, emmetropia may now cause them to view the world as much larger or much smaller, respectively, compared to their perception prior to cataract surgery. Myopes usually tolerate this postoperative "magnification" quite well: they probably are so happy to get rid of their glasses that they may not want to complain any further!

However, our high hyperope friends may complain about postoperative "minification" or a "Lilliputian" perception of the world: they may subjectively feel that everything around them looks much smaller. When performing cataract surgery in a high hyperope, it is vital to discuss postoperative "minification" with emmetropia prior to cataract surgery. Thankfully, most patients will eventually learn to adjust over time, so in the immediate postoperative period, one can employ the magical treatment of "MICLO": mindful inaction with cat-like observation. If the patient is persistently unhappy, then a myopic overcorrection with contact lenses (e.g., a −5D CL would make the patient effectively a + 5D hyperope) with glasses (+5D) can give them back their preoperative hyperopia. Surgically, if a patient continues to be unhappy, an IOL exchange for restoring hyperopia may be considered. This author has had to resort to this option for one memorable patient who insisted on going back to her preoperative hyperopia.

[16]See Chap. 8, Magnification and Telescopes to review this concept.

Unmasked Tropia

As much as we pride ourselves in making a patient objectively see 20/20 after cataract surgery, we should be cognizant of certain patients who may have been dependent on glasses for correcting both refractive error and tropias.

For example, suppose a 67-year-old male patient presents to your office for an unscheduled visit 2 months after uncomplicated surgery in both eyes. At his postoperative 1-month surgery, he was 20/20 in both eyes with a plano refractive error. You advised him to use +2.50 OTC readers and patted yourself on your back so much that you pulled a neck muscle. Today, he bitterly complains that while he would read with glasses prior to surgery, now he cannot read for more than a few seconds before his eyes feel extremely tired and the words "seem to move all over the page."

Suppose that a repeat exam today shows 20/20 vision uncorrected in both eyes with plano refractive error in both eyes. When each eye is tested individually with a + 2.50D lens, he can read the J1 line without any problems. However, binocularly, he cannot read for more than a few seconds.

What happened? Is he malingering? What if he is a friend of Mr. Burns and tells him to remove you from his will?

At this time, we should suspect that the old glasses may have been helping more than the refractive error. Suppose when we test his old glasses, we note the following prescription:

$$OD: -1.50 + 0.75 \times 95, +2.50 \text{ add, } 3\,PD\,BD$$

$$\text{OS}: -1.25 + 0.75 \times 85, +2\,50 \text{ add}$$

Suppose we test his motility and note a 3 PD RHT (comitant).

By now, we should realize that this patient had a significant RHT that was successfully treated with his old glasses that had a 3 PD BD in the right lens. Now that he does not need glasses for distance (or near vision, when each eye is tested individually), he was not given his previous prism correction. In other words, he may objectively read 20/20 with each eye, but when trying to read (looking down) with both eyes, he experiences diplopia and adverse effects of the RHT. We can simply prescribe glasses with the required prism correction for this patient.

We can also ask him not to tell Mr. Burns about this unfortunate oversight. The learning point here is to ensure that preoperative correction of tropia is documented and maintained postoperatively.[17]

Dysphotopsias

Suppose a meek, mild-mannered, constantly fearful fellow named Mr. W.J. Smithers comes in for a second opinion after cataract surgery in both eyes with another provider. He reports a shimmering crescent-shaped light seen in the temporal field of his right eye and a banana-shaped temporal shadow in his left eye. What's going on?

This clinical scenario may be one of the more fascinating (and frustrating) recent developments in postoperative issues after cataract surgery. A full review of this condition, including etiology and treatment, is beyond the scope of this text.[18]

Dysphotopsias are aberrant, unwanted, and frustrating optical phenomena subjectively experienced by patients after uncomplicated cataract surgery that may affect nearly 20% of patients, with varying symptoms intensity and duration levels. There are two main types of dysphotopsias: positive dysphotopsia (PD) and negative dysphotopsia (ND) (Fig. 5).

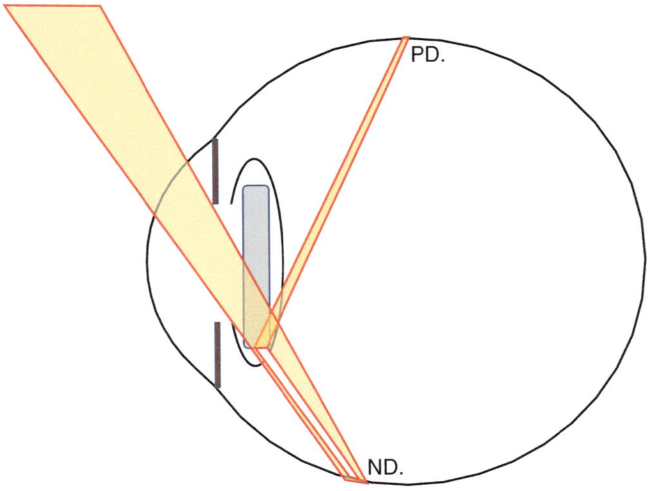

Fig. 5 Simplified schematic diagram representing etiology of positive and negative dysphotopsia (PD and ND). Both involve incoming temporal light creating either an edge reflection (PD) or edge scotoma (ND)

We still do not fully have a grand unified theory that explains the etiology of dysphotopsias. However, some theories and observations include the following:

- There is a higher incidence of PD and ND with high-refractive index acrylic IOLs with square-edge optics (the most common type of 1-piece IOLs implanted in the USA today, regardless of manufacturer).[19]
- The nasal retina extends more anteriorly than the temporal retina. If areas of the nasal retina are stimulated by light postoperatively that were previously not, this may contribute to PD. Similarly, if areas of the nasal retina are no longer stimulated by light postoperatively (whereas they were receiving light preoperatively), this may contribute to ND.
- Small pupil size: This is somewhat counterintuitive as one may think that a larger pupil size would be more of a culprit. However, studies have shown that the ND shadow may be easier seen with smaller pupils as this leads to increased contrast between the ND shadow and adjacent rays, similar to the pinhole effect. In other words, with a larger pupil, enough rays that get through may "hide" the ND, but the ND becomes more noticeable with a smaller pupil.[20]
- Positive angle-kappa
- Smaller axial distance of the IOL behind the iris
- Nasal anterior capsule overlying the anterior nasal aspect of the IOL (controversial)
- High dioptric power of a biconvex IOL
- Hydrophilic IOLs
- History of previous refractive surgery
- FLACS corneal incision
- Smaller IOL optic (<6.0mm)
- Type A personality

As we can see, that is quite the laundry list and can theoretically include a significant number of patients. We should understand PD and ND further before delving into potential treatment options.

Positive Dysphotopsia (PD)

PD is usually reported as a temporal light streak, hazy glare, or arc induced in *bright light* conditions from an oblique light source; this distinguishes it from retinal pathology (e.g., vitreous traction) that usually occurs in dark light conditions. While many etiologies and risk factors may cause PD, the likeliest reason is that incoming, oblique light rays strike the

[17] Another example of "new" diplopia may occur in a patient who developed a sensory exotropia due to a long-standing white cataract; fittingly enough, the patient may not have complained about the double vision because he could not see out of the affected eye. After the cataract is removed, the patient may now "see" the exotropia as the pseudophakic eye still deviates.

[18] An excellent and comprehensive review article may be found here: Masket S, Fram NR. Pseudophakic Dysphotopsia: A Review of Incidence, Etiology and Treatment of Positive and Negative Dysphotopsia [published online ahead of print, 2020 Aug 12]. *Ophthalmology*. 2020;S0161–6420(20)30787–9.

[19] See Chap. 27, What's on the Menu: An Overview of Currently-Available IOLs.

[20] Hong X, Liu Y, Karakelle M, Masket S, Fram NR. Ray-tracing optical modeling of negative dysphotopsia. J Biomed Opt. 2011 Dec;16(12):125001

nasal edge of the optic-anterior capsule-pupil complex and undergo a combination of refraction, scattered and internal reflections, striking portions of the nasal retina, especially those regions not previously stimulated by light in the phakic state, and creating a PD in the patient's temporal field.

For example, one major contributing factor is the popularity of square-edge acrylic IOLs with a high refractive index. While a square-edge IOL may reduce the incidence of PCO, it may also create unwanted refractions and reflections at the anterior optic edge, redirecting incoming light onto a smaller area of the retina; this is typically not seen with a round-edge IOL, which spreads incoming light onto a larger area of the retina. Therefore, a theoretically "ideal" IOL may have a rounded anterior edge and a squared posterior edge to both reduce PD and PCO.[21] Similarly, a high refractive index may contribute to PD as well.[22]

Other factors contributing specifically to PD include a lenticular design optic (which allows for a consistent optic thickness across a range of IOL powers), thickness of the square edge, and placement of more IOL "power" in the posterior optic versus the anterior optic. For this last factor, it has been reported that high-index IOLs with a flat anterior radius of curvature cause central light flashes from backward reflections of the optic.[23]

Negative Dysphotopsia (ND)

ND is usually reported as a dark, temporal crescentic shadow seen in *bright light* conditions. ND may occur slightly more frequently than PD (15–20% of patients) and may be seen much earlier in the postoperative period. However, compared to PD, patients may be much less bothered by ND through neuro-adaptation at 1 year after surgery, though this is controversial as others believe ND is worse than PD.[24] The etiology of ND is slightly more hallenging to understand than PD.[25] There are some similar inciting factors as PD and as some different ones as well.

For example, similar to PD, ND symptoms are due to incoming temporal light and can be reduced if the temporal light is blocked. On the other hand, unlike PD, ND symptoms are worse with pupil constriction. ND may occur more frequently in women and in the left eye. ND may occur with non-acrylic and non-square edge IOL as well.

At present, the likely explanation for the "enigmatic penumbra" of ND is that incoming light rays that previously illuminated the nasal retina no longer do so after cataract surgery. This "illumination gap" can be eliminated by restoring illumination to the dark band of the nasal retina, or at least shifting this gap beyond the noticeable areas of the nasal retina. Other factors contributing to ND include high angle kappa, high hyperopia, short axial length, overlying nasal anterior capsule, increased posterior chamber depth of the pseudophakic eye, and position of in-the-bag 1-piece IOL haptics. The latter factor is somewhat controversial as evidence for placing the haptics in a horizontal inferotemporal position showed benefit for transient ND rather than late-term ND; in this study, the treatment group actually had a *higher rate* of ND at 1-month when compared to the control group (silicone IOLs).[26] Further complicating these factors is the recent proposition that CNS components may also contribute to ND.[27]

If you are confused after reading the previous paragraphs, join the club: it includes most cataract surgeons in the world, indicating that there is still much to learn about ND. ND is a topic that we will hopefully learn more about in the coming years, including practical strategies to prevent and treat this unwanted temporal shadow.

Treatment Strategies

Numerous treatment strategies have been described for PD and ND. When too many treatment options exist, it usually indicates that no single option is perfect or effective in every situation. The following is a list of the most commonly employed options, with notation given for whether an option may be more effective for PD, ND, or both (B).

Nonsurgical Options

- Validation/reassurance until neuroadaptation occurs (B): this is probably the strategy most cataract surgeons use.[28] Thankfully, most PD/ND eventually resolves: whether it truly goes away or whether patients learn to deal with it is subject to debate.

[21] For example, the ZA9002 (silicone IOL; Johnson and Johnson, Sarasota, FL USA), AR40 platform (acrylic IOL; Johnson and Johnson, Jacksonville, FL, USA), and the CQ2015A (collamer IOL; Staar Surgical, Monrovia, CA USA) have a rounded anterior edge and squared posterior edge optic.

[22] See the discussion in Chap. 1, Geometric Optics

[23] Erie JC, Bandhauer MH, McLaren JW. Analysis of postoperative glare and intraocular lens design. J Cataract Refract Surg. 2001;27(4):614–621.

[24] Osher RH. Negative dysphotopsia: long-term study and possible explanation for transient symptoms. *J Cataract Refract Surg.* 2008;34(10):1699–1707.

[25] An appropriately titled paper that deals with this concept: Holladay JT, Zhao H, Reisin CR. Negative dysphotopsia: the enigmatic penumbra. *J Cataract Refract Surg*. 2012;38(7):1251–1265.

[26] Henderson BA, Yi DH, Constantine JB, Geneva II. New preventative approach for negative dysphotopsia. *J Cataract Refract Surg.* 2016;42(10):1449–1455.

[27] Masket S, Rupnik Z, Fram N, Vikesland R. Binocular Goldmann Visual Field Testing of Negative Dysphotopsia. J Cataract Refract Surg. 2020;46(1):147–148.

[28] This option may/may not include another strategy: wait until the patient becomes mad at you and then refer them to your across-town competition. Please do not refer such patients to the authors! What did we ever do to you, other than try to teach you optics?

- Treatment of refractive error (B): Glasses, especially frames with thick edges, may help reduce symptoms, especially with PD.
- Treatment of ocular surface disease (B): As with many problems in ophthalmology, give them the magical potion known as preservative-free artificial tears.
- Pupillary dilation (ND).

Non-incisional Surgical Options

- YAG capsulotomy to remove the nasal aspect of the anterior capsule (ND)
- Not polishing the nasal anterior capsule at the time of cataract surgery to promote early nasal capsular clouding and contraction (ND > PD)

Incisional Surgery Options

- Repositioning vertically oriented haptics horizontally while keeping the IOL in the capsular bag (ND).
- Placing the IOL in the bag such that the haptic-optic junction is horizontally inferotemporal (useful for short term, no evidence for post 1-month symptoms) (ND). See above for why this may not truly be an effective strategy.
- Reverse optic capture (ND > PD): This strategy involves placing the haptics of the IOL in the bag and then lifting the optic out of the bag such that it is anterior to the capsulorrhexis edge. This maneuver can be combined with a horizontal haptic orientation.
- Truncation of the nasal-edge of the IOL haptic has been reported. However, this may create a sharp optic edge that can secondarily damage critical capsule structures.
- IOL exchange: Exchanging a square-edge acrylic IOL for rounded-edge and/or non-acrylic (silicone, collamer) IOL (both, but especially PD).
- Implanting a secondary non-acrylic plano-power piggyback IOL (ND > PD): this may be particularly useful post-YAG capsulotomy and/or in situations where an IOL exchange may be risky.
- Primary sulcus placement of 3-piece IOL (ND > PD): This can be done at the time of original cataract surgery (i.e., not placing an IOL in the bag at all and instead placing a 3-piece in the sulcus) or at the time of IOL exchange (i.e., removing the in-the-bag IOL and placing a 3-piece IOL in the sulcus). This is a similar strategy to reverse optic capture in that the IOL optic is anterior to the capsulorrhexis edge.
- Primary placement of an IOL with frosted edges (ND): currently in clinical trials.
- Primary placement of an IOL with grooves within the optic to allow for "tucking" of the capsulorrhexis edges "behind" the edge of the anterior optic while keeping the IOL in the capsular bag (ND): currently in clinical trials.

Photic Phenomena with ATIOLs

Photic phenomena (glare, halos, starburst, streaks of lights) can cause frustration for patients who receive ATIOLs with diffractive optics (e.g., MFIOLs, EDOF-IOLs, and trifocal IOLs). While there is some overlap with the previous PD/ND discussion,[29] these phenomena are due to the more central portion of the optic rather than the optic edge causing multiple focal points. The subjective glare/halos are due to the forward light scattering (Mie scattering) and other higher-order aberrations. Some risk factors, such as ocular surface disease, IOL decentration, and type A personality, have been previously well described in the literature. More recently, there has been an understanding that aberrant angle-kappa and angle-alpha may contribute to these issues as well.[30]

Ideally, with good screening, diagnostic imaging, application of optical principles, meticulous surgical technique, and appropriate patient selection, we can minimize the number of unhappy ATIOL patients.[31]

Postoperatively, there are not a lot of good options for these patients. In the immediate postoperative period, the best strategy may be a healthy dose of reassuring the patient that surgery went well and writing a prescription for observation/hand-holding. If there is any residual refractive error, it may be tempting to treat with excimer laser surgery as ATIOLs rely on minimal refractive error. However, photic phenomena may worsen with overaggressive treatment. Therefore, temporary treatment of refractive error with glasses and contact lenses may be helpful to see if that resolves the photic phenomena. If so, laser refractive surgery may be employed; if these do not work, then laser refractive surgery may not help or worsen the symptoms. If intractable glare/halos remain even after a period of observation, an IOL exchange with a monofocal or accommodating IOL may be offered, which usually fixes the problem definitively. IOL exchange surgery must be carefully considered in general, but even more so in the presence of an open capsule (post-YAG capsulotomy), as the IOL exchange may necessitate concurrent vitrectomy. It can be frustrating for the ATIOL patient to undergo additional incisional surgery, especially if he/she has previously spent a significant amount of out-of-pocket money for the "upgraded" IOL.

[29] In fact, some authorities refer to these as "diffractive dysphotopsias" are they are seen only in ATIOLs that use diffractive optics to create multiple focal points; this is compounded by the glare that results from forward light-scatter (Mie-scattering) from the diffractive optics elements (rings or echelettes)

[30] See Chap. 26, Preoperative Optics for Cataract Surgery, for a review of these topics.

[31] In other words, be wary of the surgeons that boast of a >50% ATIOL surgical practice…

Postoperative Refraction: Room Lengths and Optimizing Lens Constants

Author's Note: A special thanks to David L. Cooke, MD (Great Lakes Eye Care, St. Joseph, MI), for his assistance and instruction in the material presented in this section.

We can comment on one last point for postoperative refraction that is slightly technical and definitely nerdy. When we perform postoperative refractions, we simply measure the patient's visual acuity on the screen in the room, become very happy if the patient is 20/20, and move on with life. However, as with many things in Optics, this is not entirely accurate for the actual refractive error, which may be necessary for some clinically-relevant things, such as optimizing one's unique lens constant(s) so that one can have an even higher percentage of 20/20 patients.

We must refer to a common reference point for our final refraction. And no, that reference point does not mean referring to an optometry colleague to finalize the refraction. When we finish our perfect manifest refraction in whatever room we are using, we must adjust the final refraction to give the "perfect" correction at some distance, either at optical infinity (for perfect distance vision) or 20 feet (6 meters) - the latter is the standard refraction distance for IOL clinical studies.

When testing at room lengths less than 20 feet/6 meters (most ophthalmology offices), we have to account for non-parallel (overly divergent) light rays. For example, suppose our room was 4 meters: a person without accommodation (e.g., a dilated patient or your pseudophakic 80-year-old) will be slightly "over-plussed" in the manifest refraction at this distance. Remember that at 4 meters, incoming light has a divergence of approximately −1/4D; to account for this extra −1/4D, our refraction has an "extra" +1/4D sphere (compared to what we would get if we refracted at optical infinity). Therefore, we have to add approximately −0.25D to the final refraction to adjust for the room distance.

We can use an example to make this point a bit clearer. Suppose that our patient's refraction after cataract surgery was −1.00 + 0.50 × 90 (20/15) when refracted at 4 meters. However, we have inadvertently included an "extra +0.25 D" in this measurement, so the manifest refraction at infinity should actually be −1.25 + 0.50 × 90. Remember that optical infinity requires a room of at least 8 meters (26.25 feet) - who among us can afford to renovate all of our exam lanes to have this distance?!

Therefore, we have to find a happy medium between optical infinity and a typical ophthalmology exam lane (usually ranging from 8 to 10 feet for most offices, as measured as the distance from the phoropter to the visual acuity chart). One option is to make the reference distance for IOL studies (i.e., for developing lens constants) 6 meters (20 feet) instead of infinity. This standard reference distance has merits for several reasons. First, we can generally get the lens constants with this distance as in the ULIB database.[32] Second, if we get the room distance to 20 feet, the refraction is "close enough" that we do not need to further extend it to 26.25 feet.

The second option is an elegant proposal by Simpson et al. to move the refraction reference distance, regardless of one's exam lanes, to equal 6 meters[33]; in other words, use some math instead of renovating your entire office:

$$\text{Refraction at } 6\,\text{m} = \left(1/6\,\text{D} - 1/4\,\text{D}\right) = -0.08333\text{D} \approx -0.08\text{D}$$

Returning to our previous fictional refraction of −1.00 + 0.50 × 90, we would need to add an additional minus sphere power (−0.08D) for the final refraction of −1.08 + 0.50 × 90. Note that this is obviously theoretical because we cannot write this as an eyeglass prescription unless you are trying to pull an April Fool's joke on your optician friends. Moreover, only a few refractions will be wrong because we cannot dial-in 0.08D into the phoropter. However, *on average,* the refraction of one's surgical patients, when looked at as a group, will be overplussed by 0.08D. This adjusted refraction value will be significant when calculating one's own unique lens constant.

If one has shorter rooms, this will be even more important. Suppose the testing distance between the phoropter and the chart/screen was 9.5 feet (2.9 meters). Using the ideal IOL power prescription adjustment:

$$\left(1/6 - \left(1/2.9\right)\right) = -0.18\text{D}$$

This means that our patient's refraction for infinity is actually −1.18 + 0.50 × 90. We can see how this can skew the data set's average refraction and, in turn, affect the calculated value of one's unique, surgeon-optimized lens constant.

In conclusion, it is obviously very difficult and nearly impractical to do this adjusted refraction for every single patient in a busy surgical practice. However, if one is genuinely interested in determining one's individual lens constant, then taking the time to perform this in 50–100 eyes with one's preferred IOL platform will be invaluable to finding an individualized lens constant to achieve even more precise surgical outcomes.

[32] ULIB User Group for Laser Interference Biometry. http://ocusoft.de/ulib/c1.htm. Accessed January 10, 2021.

[33] Simpson MJ, Charman WN. The effect of testing distance on intraocular lens power calculation [letter]. J Refract Surg 2014; 30:726

Practice Questions

1. Which of the following statements concerning myopic surprise is TRUE?
   A. A myopic surprise can occur if the surgeon planned to place a + 23.0D IOL in the capsular bag but accidentally placed a + 20.0D in the capsular bag
   B. A myopic surprise can occur if the planned 1-piece IOL is inadvertently placed inverted down in the capsular bag
   C. A myopic surprise can occur if a lower-than-actual A-constant is used
   D. A myopic surprise can occur if the IOL-bag complex shifts posteriorly after cataract surgery
2. All of the following treatment strategies may be used to treat myopic surprise EXCEPT:
   A. IOL exchange: replacing the existing in-the-bag IOL with a lower power in-the-bag IOL
   B. Placement of a plus-powered 3-piece silicone/collamer IOL in the sulcus
   C. Laser refractive surgery (LASIK or PRK)
   D. Repositioning an anteriorly dislocated 1-piece IOL from the sulcus back into the capsular bag
3. Which of the following statements about capsular block syndrome (CBS) is TRUE?
   A. AS-OCT and/or UBM will typically show a posterior shift of the IOL-bag complex
   B. Risk factors for CBS include a small diameter optic (<6 mm) and a large capsulorrhexis
   C. CBS seen in the first few days after surgery may be observed if IOP and inflammation are acceptable
   D. A YAG capsulotomy is often ineffective at treating CBS
4. All of the following patients are at risk for postoperative refractive error more hyperopic-than-intended EXCEPT:
   A. Patients with a previous history of myopic LASIK/PRK surgery
   B. Patients with ACD < 3 mm and LT > 5 mm when using the Barrett formula
   C. Patients with corneal ectasia
   D. Patients who receive IOLs based on a higher-than-actual A constant
5. Which of the following treatment options is LEAST effective for a hyperopic surprise?
   A. Excimer laser refractive surgery
   B. Placement of plus-powered 3-piece sulcus ("piggy-back") IOL
   C. IOL exchange with a higher-powered IOL
   D. Glasses and/or contact lenses

Answers

1. B. Most 1-piece IOLs have a biconvex design with the posterior aspect of the optic having more power than the anterior aspect. A myopic shift may occur if the IOL is inadvertently placed upside down in the capsular bag. If a lower IOL power is accidentally placed (choice A), a lower-than-actual A constant is used (choice C), or if the IOL-bag complex shifts posteriorly (choice D), then a hyperopic surprise may occur.
2. B. Placing a plus-powered 3-piece IOL as a piggyback IOL in the sulcus will worsen the refractive error. All of the other options can treat postoperative myopia to varying degrees.
3. C. CBS seen immediately after surgery may be carefully monitored with topical hypotensive and/or steroids with the hopes that it may self-resolve. Imaging of the IOL-bag complex will show an anteriorly shifted IOL (choice A) within the capsular bag with posterior distension of the posterior capsule due to the built-up fluid. A large IOL optic and small capsulorrhexis (choice B) are risk factors for CBS. A YAG capsulotomy may be both diagnostic and therapeutic for this condition (choice D)
4. D. Patients who receive IOLs based on a higher-than-actual A constant may end up with a higher-than-required IOL power causing a myopic surprise, not a hyperopic surprise. All of the other patients (choices A, B, and C) are at risk for a more hyperopic-than-intended refractive error. This does not mean a hyperopic refractive error necessarily (e.g., +1.00D) but may mean that if −1.00D was targeted with the surgery, the patient may end up −0.25D instead.
5. A. PRK/LASIK for hyperopic refractive errors tends to be less predictable and less effective than myopic treatments; in other words, it is far easier to treat a patient with −2.00D refractive error as compared to a patient with +2.00D refractive error. All of the other treatments (B, C, and D) may be effectively used in this setting.

Optics for Refractive Surgery

Kamran M. Riaz

Objectives

- To understand optics concepts previously discussed concerning modern refractive surgery.
- To identify refractive reasons and concepts important in determining suitable laser refractive surgery (LRS) candidates.
- To diagnose and troubleshoot postoperative problems after LRS in the context of previously discussed optics principles.
- To survey other types of incisional refractive surgeries currently in practice.

Introduction

Before we start this chapter, let's get something important out of the way: *by no means should this chapter be considered a primer, replacement, or even supplement for a textbook on refractive surgery, especially excimer laser refractive surgery (LRS)*. The purpose of this chapter is not to make the reader a refractive surgeon. Ideally, a fellowship in cornea/refractive surgery and tutelage under experienced, skilled refractive surgeons should be completed before embarking on refractive surgery in actual patients.[1]

Instead, the purpose of this chapter is to primarily serve as an introduction for the reader to understand how some of the previously discussed optics principles are used in refractive surgery, especially in preoperative screening and postoperative management. This chapter is intentionally designed to present the basics of what a comprehensive ophthalmologist *who does not perform refractive surgery* needs to know for community-based practice and/or exam preparation.

The other purpose of this chapter is to hopefully string together some of the previous optical concepts we have discussed, especially advanced topics such as higher-order aberrations (HOAs) (Chap. 14, Physical Optics), which may have initially overwhelmed a first-time reader with its seemingly irrelevant nature. Instead, we hope to show how these concepts are clinically and surgically relevant and reinforce their understanding and appreciation.

For this chapter, we will assume that the reader knows the fundamental procedural aspects of LRS. If you are unfamiliar with how photorefractive keratectomy (PRK), laser in situ keratomileusis (LASIK), and small incision lenticule extraction (SMILE) are performed, please consult other resources for this information.[2]

Review of Relevant Corneal Anatomy, Biomechanics, and Function

In a simplified model of relevant anatomy, the cornea has 5 main layers; for the purposes of refractive surgery, the majority of these procedures occur in the corneal stroma.[3] The stroma primarily consists of collagen fibrils arranged in approximately 200 parallel lamellae; each fibril is oriented angularly to fibrils in adjacent lamellae, leading to increased

[1]Please also see the recommended reading list for Refractive Surgery resources for those who wish to understand this subject further, including advanced preoperative, postoperative management, and intraoperative principles.

[2]For the purposes of this chapter, we will use the term "PRK" to refer to any type of surface ablation procedure, including variations of PRK such as epi-LASIK, LASEK, and anterior surface ablation (ASA). The full discussion of the nuances and differences of these procedures is beyond the scope of this text.

[3]Recently, a sixth layer, known as the pre-Descemet's layer (Dua's Layer), has been introduced.

K. M. Riaz (✉)
Dean McGee Eye Institute, University of Oklahoma, Oklahoma City, OK, USA

K. M. Riaz et al. (eds.), *Optics for the New Millennium*, https://doi.org/10.1007/978-3-030-95251-8_30

biomechanical strength of the cornea. Fibrils are densely packed in the anterior two-thirds of the cornea; this means that there is less likely to be swelling within the anterior two-thirds of the stroma than the posterior one-third. When the cornea is *healthy or edematous*, the *anterior* lamellae take up most of the strain; when the cornea is *dehydrated*, the posterior lamellae take up more. Strain is also related to intraocular pressure and other external mechanical factors.

Why should we care about all of this? The lack of uniformity in the biomechanics of the cornea explains the variation in corneal response to various refractive procedures. For example, LASIK and SMILE both have a more significant effect on the total corneal biomechanical load because of the flap (with LASIK) as well as ablation in the "deeper" areas of the stroma (LASIK and SMILE) as compared to PRK. As another example, procedures that weaken the cornea, such as radial keratotomy (RK) or limbal relaxing incisions (LRIs), have different refractive effects than a procedure wherein tissue is removed, such as LASIK or PRK.

Recall that the air-tear film interface is the most important refractive surface of the eye.[4] Therefore, any refractive surgery will require a healthy and optimized air-tear film interface to optimize surgical results.

The eye's optical power derives primarily from the anterior surface of the cornea (+48.0 D). The posterior surface contributes a NEGATIVE power (−6 D), yielding an overall corneal power of ~ +42.0 D. Even though the posterior cornea is a convex surface, since light rays travel from a medium of higher refractive index (stroma) into a medium of lower refractive index (aqueous humor), the posterior cornea can be assumed to function as a minus lens.

The normal cornea flattens from the center to the periphery (by approximately 4D); the nasal cornea is flatter than the temporal cornea.[5] A *prolate* cornea is one wherein the central cornea is *steeper* than the peripheral cornea; this type of cornea is usually found in patients with myopic refractive errors.[6] An *oblate* cornea is one wherein the central cornea is *flatter* than the peripheral cornea; this type of cornea is usually found in patients with hyperopic refractive errors. We can use this foundation to understand how LRS can advantageously change the shape of a prolate or oblate cornea and correct refractive errors. For example, by flattening a prolate cornea, we can make it more oblate-like and treat myopic refractive errors.

[4]See Chap. 1, Geometric Optics and Chap. 5, Power of Lenses in Different Media for a more detailed explanation of the air-tear film interface.

[5]The mnemonic "flat nasal bridge" may help to remember that the nasal cornea is flatter than the temporal cornea.

[6]A useful mnemonic is to think of a prolate cornea as being "too professional" of a cornea: it does such a professional job of refracting incoming light rays that they don't reach the retina.

As a vastly simplified principle, most refractive surgical procedures on the cornea involve altering the corneal curvature to alter the eye's refraction favorably.

Finally, a rudimentary knowledge of higher order aberrations (HOAs) is vital for refractive surgery.[7] Among HOAs, spherical aberration (SA) is perhaps the most important one to keep in mind, especially regarding the effects of LRS on SA. Prolate corneas usually have positive SA; oblate corneas usually have negative SA. Since most emmetropes and myopes have prolate corneas, most patients usually have low amounts of positive SA. While the crystalline lens has negative SA, the cornea has a greater positive SA magnitude, leading to a mean net value of approximately +0.36 μm (SD = 0.31 μm). As we get older, we typically develop more positive SA.

In regards to LRS, the following considerations can be kept in mind:

- Patients who undergo *standard (i.e., not wavefront guided (WFG) or wavefront optimized (WFO))* ablations for *myopia* will develop an oblate corneal pattern (central flattening with a relatively steep untreated peripheral cornea). These patients' postsurgical wavefronts will show a significant *increase* in positive spherical aberration. A typical wavefront pattern for these patients may demonstrate emmetropia centrally (green) with "annular myopia" in the periphery (red) (Fig. 1a).
- Patients who undergo *standard* ablations for *hyperopia* will develop a more prolate corneal pattern (steeper centrally). These patients' postsurgical wavefronts will show a significant decrease in spherical aberration (they may even have net negative spherical aberration), and the wavefront-shaped pattern may become inverted (Fig. 1b).

Preoperative Considerations for Excimer Laser Refractive Surgery

Selected Ophthalmic Considerations

Laser refractive surgery (LRS) is performed on healthy eyes in patients with excellent vision potential. LRS is primarily used for myopes to flatten the central cornea with minimal treatment of the periphera cornea. For hyperopes, LRS is used to primarily flatten the peripheral cornea to steepen the central cornea secondarily. This summary is a gross simplification but is a primary concept that can be kept in mind as we discuss LRS procedures such as PRK and LASIK.

Remember that any refractive surgery will not "improve" a patient's vision potential; the primary goal of LRS is to achieve vision comparable to a level with glasses and/or contact lenses. If a patient cannot achieve 20/20 vision prior to

[7]See Chap. 14, Physical Optics, for a more detailed explanation and review of higher-order aberrations.

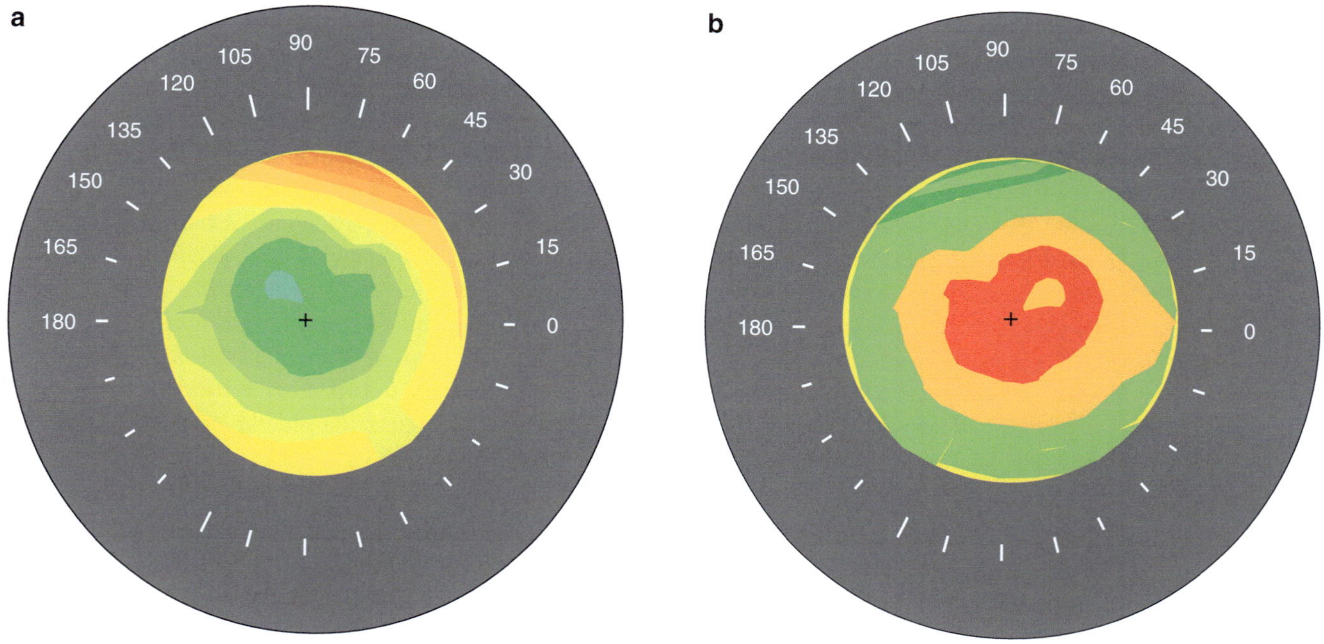

Fig. 1 Typical wavefront appearances of post-LRS corneas. In Panel a, a typical post-myopic LRS cornea shows a flat surface centrally (green) and ring-shaped steeper area peripherally (red). In Panel b, a typical post-hyperopic LRS cornea shows a steep surface centrally (red) and ring-shaped flatter area peripherally (green)

LRS, this must be conveyed to avoid creating unrealistic expectations. Even if a patient gives you a briefcase of cash, it's not worth it.

Patient History

In order to select appropriate candidates for LRS, refractive surgeons must carefully evaluate preoperative data (such as keratometry measurements to exclude steep and flat corneas, etc.) and anatomical considerations, such as unusual orbit and lid anatomy, severe ocular surface disease, and corneal sensation.

There are several *absolute contraindications* for LRS that can be elicited in the patient history that should be committed to memory:

- Systemic Conditions
  - Pregnancy
  - Collagen vascular diseases
  - *Uncontrolled* diabetes
- Ocular Conditions
  - Corneal ectasia (keratoconus, pellucid marginal degeneration, etc.)
  - *Severe* ocular surface disease/dry eye syndrome

Additionally, there are a few *relative contraindications* for LRS that may be helpful to know:

- Systemic Conditions
  - Diabetes (even if controlled): these patients are at increased risk for poor epithelial healing, so photorefractive keratectomy (PRK) may be less desirable than laser in-situ keratomileusis (LASIK)
- Ocular Conditions
  - Mild-moderate ocular surface disease/dry eye syndrome
  - Controlled glaucoma: LASIK requires increased intraocular pressure for suction during flap creation, so PRK may be preferable
  - Epithelial basement membrane dystrophy (EBMD) and recurrent corneal erosion syndrome (for LASIK; PRK may serendipitously help improve these patients' pathology and refraction simultaneously since the "PTK" portion is part of the PRK)
  - Presence of cataract

From an optics perspective, several important considerations from the patient's history and medical records that can help determine whether a patient is a good candidate for LRS include:

- Age of Patient: Unless part of a clinical study, LRS can only be performed on 18 years of age or older patients in the United States. Many surgeons may wait until a patient is at least 21 years of age to ensure refractive stability and reduce the risk of exacerbating subclinical corneal ectasia.[8]
- Stability of Refractive Error: A patient's manifest refraction should be stable for at least *12 months* before LRS. Every refractive surgeon and/or a given laser platform may have different cutoff rules. Most surgeons

[8] A useful resource for patients written in non-technical language can be found at: https://www.aao.org/eye-health/treatments/lasik. Accessed February 15, 2021.

would agree that a sphere or cylinder change of >0.50D should warrant repeat examination in 4–6 months until the refractive error is reproducibly stable.

- Magnitude of Refractive Error: while there are many available laser platforms available in the United States, a complete discussion of the parameters of each manufacturer's laser is beyond the scope of this text. Currently, excimer lasers in the USA can correct up to −11/−12D myopia, +5/6D hyperopia, and + 5/6D astigmatism.[9]
- Contact Lens History: patients should be out of SCLs 3–7 days and out RGPCLs 3 weeks with an additional one week for every decade of wear prior to any exam for LRS candidacy. Suppose the initial candidacy exam reveals abnormal topography (also known as "corneal warpage") due to contact lens wear. In that case, the patient should be advised to remain out of contact lenses for an additional 1–2 months until repeat examination is consistently stable, especially with reproducibly acceptable corneal topographies.[10]

As an aside, in the early days of LRS, sequential treatment of both eyes was the norm. As a result, patients often had considerable, temporary anisometropia (and aniseikonia) between the two procedures requiring short-term contact lens use. If sequential LRS is performed and a contact lens is needed after the first procedure, the patient should be out of contact lenses at least one week prior to any (first or second) laser treatment.

Examination Considerations

While a full discussion of the preoperative exam is beyond the scope of this chapter, there are a few important candidacy considerations related to optics. First, both manifest refraction and cycloplegic refraction are essential parts of the preoperative exam. An autorefraction or streak refraction may be useful starting points, but neither can replace subjective manifest refraction. If you want to do refractive surgery, you should be an expert at manifest refraction. The sharpest visual acuity with the least amount of minus ("pushing plus") should be the final endpoint, especially in young myopic patients; the Duochrome test and/or cycloplegic refraction can be especially useful to ensure we are not inadvertently overminusing these patients.

Second, most refractive surgeons also obtain a wavefront assessment preoperatively to assess pre-existing higher order aberrations and assist with custom treatments (wavefront guided/wavefront optimized treatments). Aberrometry can further identify whether a patient's refractive error has corneal (or indirectly, lenticular) causes for aberrations. However, the importance of a skilled examiner, ideally the refractive surgeon him/herself, performing a meticulous manifest refraction cannot be overstated. Hence the previous discussions in Chap. 15, (Glasses in Clinical Practice) and Chap. 18, (Visual Acuity Testing and Assessment) are relevant for all you aspiring LASIK surgeons.

Important preoperative candidacy exam considerations include the following guidelines. If a patient does not meet these requirements, the measurements can be repeated in 3–4 months until stability or normalcy is noted.

- Reproducibility and agreement of refractive error: For myopic candidates, the sphere and cylinder components of the manifest refraction should not differ from the cycloplegic refraction by more than 0.5D. The astigmatism axis should be within 15 degrees as well. For hyperopes, the sphere and cylinder components of the manifest and cycloplegic refraction should differ no more than 0.75D, whereas the astigmatism axis should be within 15 degrees.
- Keratometric (corneal) astigmatism and refractive astigmatism: for an ideal LRS candidate, the keratometric astigmatism should approximate the refractive astigmatism. For example, if a patient has keratometry of 43.50/45.00 @ 90 in the candidate eye, a reassuring manifest refraction would be −3.00 + 1.50 × 90 (20/15). However, if the keratometric astigmatism significantly differs from the refractive astigmatism (and the patient still achieves good vision), there is likely lenticular astigmatism. Using the previous example, if the patient's refraction was instead −3.00D sphere (20/15), there is likely lenticular astigmatism that neutralizes keratometric astigmatism. Therefore, as a general rule for all LRS patients, the laser treatment should be based on refractive astigmatism rather than keratometric astigmatism; otherwise, we may inadvertently unmask lenticular astigmatism to an undesirable post LRS refractive outcome (and probably a very unhappy patient!).
- Corneal measurement values: Corneal topography is an absolute requirement for any LRS candidacy examination. Modern topography devices can give additional information regarding irregular astigmatism and potential ectasia. As a general rule, *approximately 0.75-8D of corneal flattening occurs for every 1D of myopic ablation.* For example, if we had a patient with a preoperative −4D sphere refractive error, then LRS would cause approximately 3–3.25D of corneal flattening. Similarly, if we had a patient with a preoperative +3D sphere refractive error with average K's of 42D, then the postoperative K's would be: 42D + (1*3D) = 45D. While different surgeons have different cutoff parameters, most would agree that *excessive flattening of the cornea (<35D) is undesirable* as it may cause issues such as decreased corneal integrity,

[9] A mnemonic to remember this is the "10/5/5" or "12/6/6" rule.

[10] These same principles apply to biometry in contact lens wearers prior to cataract surgery

irregular astigmatism, and higher order aberrations (HOAs). Conversely, *approximately 1D of central corneal steepening occurs for every 1D of hyperopic ablation*. Most would agree that *excessive steepening of the cornea (>50D) is undesirable* with a similar risk of inducing irregular astigmatism and HOAs.

- Flat and steep corneas: In addition to calculating postoperative corneal shape, preoperative corneal measurements can be used to determine potential intraoperative risks, especially with LASIK. For example, a flat cornea (<40D) increases the risk of small flaps and free caps (especially in the days of microkeratome-based LASIK). Similarly, a steep cornea (>48D) increases the risk of a buttonhole flap (especially in the days of microkeratome-based LASIK).[11] Such patients may be better candidates for PRK or no LRS at all.
- Pupil size: It is crucial to measure pupil size in both light and dark conditions. Patients with light-colored irises, especially women, are more likely to have significantly large pupil sizes (>7 mm) under mesopic, low light conditions. Remember from our previous discussions that larger pupil sizes will incur more glare and HOAs. In the previous days of LRS, myopic treatment patterns were limited to the central 6–6.5 mm of the cornea. Therefore, these patients had a "donut-shaped" untreated peripheral cornea that increased the severity of HOAs, especially spherical aberration, leading to unhappy patients. We have learned from these early days as newer lasers, primarily wavefront guided/optimized treatment strategies will treat ("smoothen") additional portions of the peripheral cornea to limit the severity of HOAs. Therefore, patients with large mesopic pupils may benefit from customized laser treatments to minimize these subjective postoperative causes of unhappiness and poor online reviews.
- Ocular motility: Who would have thought that refractive surgeons had to remember some skills from their residency days doing neuro-ophthalmology and pediatrics? Preoperative examination for both tropias and phorias is necessary as some patients may have controlled motility problems when wearing their glasses.[12] If we simply treat the refractive error and pat ourselves on the back for making a patient glasses-free, we may inadvertently unmask a compensated phoria and create an unhappy patient.[13] For example, suppose we have a young myopic patient with exophoria who wears glasses; when the patient wants to read, the eye will converge nasally, and he will enjoy some base-in help with the glasses (Fig. 2a). If we treat the patient with LRS, the favorable base-in effect is lost and the patient may be unhappy with the decompensated exophoria. Similarly, a hyperope with an esophoria may be happy in glasses because of the base-out effect of the glasses enjoyed by the patient during convergence (Fig. 2b). These patients can still undergo LRS but must understand they may need strabismus surgery or prisms post LRS. Another situation to avoid in patients with intermittent strabismus is prolonged monocular blurred vision from corneal haze or uncorrected refractive error after LRS as this can break their fusion and worsen their strabismus.

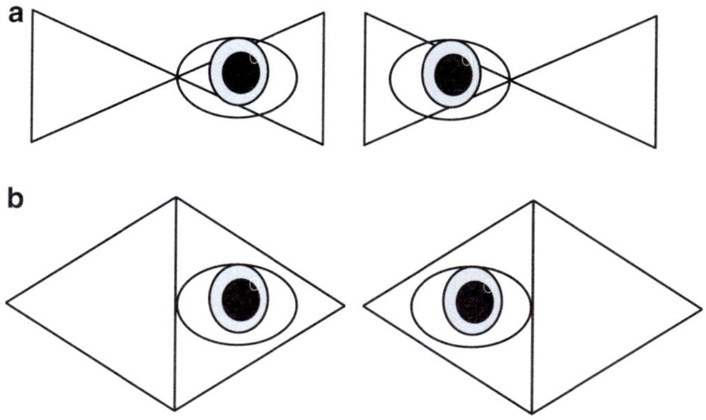

Fig. 2 Beneficial prismatic effects of myopic and hyperopic glasses. In Panel a, a myopic patient with exophoria may enjoy a base-in advantage when converging, especially for reading. In Panel b, a hyperopic patient with esophoria may enjoy a base-out advantage when converging, especially for reading

Finally, we have left *corneal thickness* for last because it deserves a slightly longer and separate discussion. Under this topic, several important concepts include:

1. While optical pachymetry (obtained by topography and Scheimpflug tomography) is helpful for thickness measurements in various parts of the cornea, ultrasonic pachymetry is much more accurate and necessary for the candidacy examination. Thus, the decision for LRS is based on *ultrasonic pachymetry* measurements.
2. Since LRS involves the removal of corneal tissue, it is imperative to ensure that we are not leaving behind a "thin" cornea that may be prone to ectasia (or even perforation with minimal trauma). Historically, the *Munnerlyn formula* has been used to estimate the ablation depth for

[11] A potentially useful mnemonic for remembering this: st**ee**p corneas cause bu**tt**onhole flaps (two e's = two t's).

[12] A patient with existing phoria compensated with glasses may be unhappy after surgery because the beneficial effects of glasses (base-in/base-out effects and/or decreased needs for convergence) may be lost after LRS.

[13] This can happen after cataract surgery as well, as discussed in Chap. 29, Postoperative Optics

myopic corrections.[14] While this formula remains useful, most surgeons use a rule of thumb of approximately 14–15 microns of tissue removed for every 1D of myopic ablation. For example, if we had a patient with a preoperative refractive error −4D sphere, we can use Munnerlyn's formula to calculate that approximately 56.33 microns of corneal tissue will be removed. Similarly, we can "shortcut" the math by multiplying the refractive error by 14 and getting 56 microns.

3. The "*Residual Stromal Bed (RSB)*" is a key measurement for LRS. Recall that with PRK, the epithelium (approximately 50 microns) is removed prior to laser ablation of corneal tissue. With LASIK, a flap (thickness range 90–140 microns) consisting of epithelium, Bowman's layer, and some anterior stroma is lifted prior to laser ablation of corneal tissue. The RSB is considered the amount of corneal tissue that is neither ablated nor part of the flap. *The absolute lowest amount of RSB is 250 microns*, though many refractive surgeons ideally prefer an RSB > 300 microns.
4. The *Percent Thickness Altered (PTA)* is a relatively new measurement that measures the relationship between the flap thickness and ablation depth compared to the preoperative corneal thickness.[15] The PTA is calculated as the sum of the flap thickness (FT) and ablation depth (AD) divided by the preoperative corneal thickness (CCT): PTA = (FT + AD)/CCT. If the PTA is *greater than 40%*, there is an *increased risk of ectasia* even with normal preoperative topography. Most refractive surgeons use PTA as an additional criterion in determining LASIK candidacy rather than a solitary exclusion criterion. Other surgeons may consider a high PTA to be an indication for PRK over LASIK, assuming all other measurements are normal.
5. Custom-based ablations remove slightly more tissue than standard ablations. The full amount varies per laser and the target treatment. The computer-based calculations done by a given laser platform will usually give the exact number of microns to be removed for the proposed treatment. Usually, this is not significantly more than what is calculated by the Munnerlyn or 1D:15-micron rule but may be important for higher treatments.
6. Advanced point: even if you reduce an ablation for higher myopes (for example, 10% reduction for −10.0D myope), the amount of tissue ablated (approximately 140–150 microns) is still the same, not 90% of 140–150 microns. Please consult a refractive surgery text for the finer details on this point.

When considering LRS in presbyopic and pre-presbyopic patients, they should be counseled that they may need reading glasses immediately (or shortly) after LRS if they opt for distance vision only. Therefore, it is necessary to have a preoperative discussion regarding potential *monovision treatment* to allow for some near and intermediate vision after LRS. With this strategy, the dominant eye is corrected for plano while the nondominant eye is left slightly myopic (range: −1.5 to −2D myopia). Remember that some loss of binocularity will result with monovision, so the following additional considerations are necessary:

1. Eye dominance: during the preoperative exam, we can ascertain eye dominance in patients through questions or simple tests. For example, the patient can be asked to make a circle ("OK" sign) with his/her thumb and index finger and look at a distance target; the preferred eye is likely the dominant eye. Additionally, the patient can be asked to make a "diamond sign" using both hands' thumb and index finger to look at a distance target. Other questions include asking a patient which eye they would prefer to sight through a telescope, aim a gun (depending on where you practice, this may be very useful clinically) or take a picture through a camera. **Never assume** that the right eye is the dominant eye, even if the patient is right-handed.[16]
2. Monovision contact lens trial: for patients who seek out LRS and have already been wearing monovision contact lenses, surgical planning is easy. We can simply maintain their monovision. However, for those patients who have not previously experienced monovision, a 1–2-week trial with monovision contact lenses can be an invaluable "test-drive" experience for that patient to determine whether or not he/she likes the monovision. Recall that patients with high demands for binocular vision, type A personalities, and extensive periods of near-vision activities may be poor candidates for monovision LRS to begin with, so a simple monovision contact lens trial can clinch the surgical decision. If a patient undergoes a monovision contact lens trial and is somewhat lukewarm about how much he/she liked it, one option is to perform monovision LRS with the idea that the non-dominant eye can be "touched up" for emmetropia in the future if the patient truly does not acclimate to the monovision.

[14] The Munnerlyn formula: $t = S^2 * D/3$, where t = thickness of the tissue ablated (in microns); S = diameter of the optical zone (in millimeters); and D = dioptric correction. The spherical equivalent can be used for D for cases with significant astigmatism.

[15] Santhiago MR, Smadja D, Gomes BF, Mello GR, Monteiro ML, Wilson SE, Randleman JB. Association between the percent tissue altered and post-laser in situ keratomileusis ectasia in eyes with normal preoperative topography. Am J Ophthalmol. 2014 Jul;158(1):87–95.e1.

[16] Lawsuits have occurred wherein a right-handed patient underwent monovision LRS with the right eye assumed to have been the dominant eye (when in reality the left eye was the dominant eye) without preoperative confirmation using the tests and questions mentioned in the text. A monovision contact lens trial is extremely helpful in these cases.

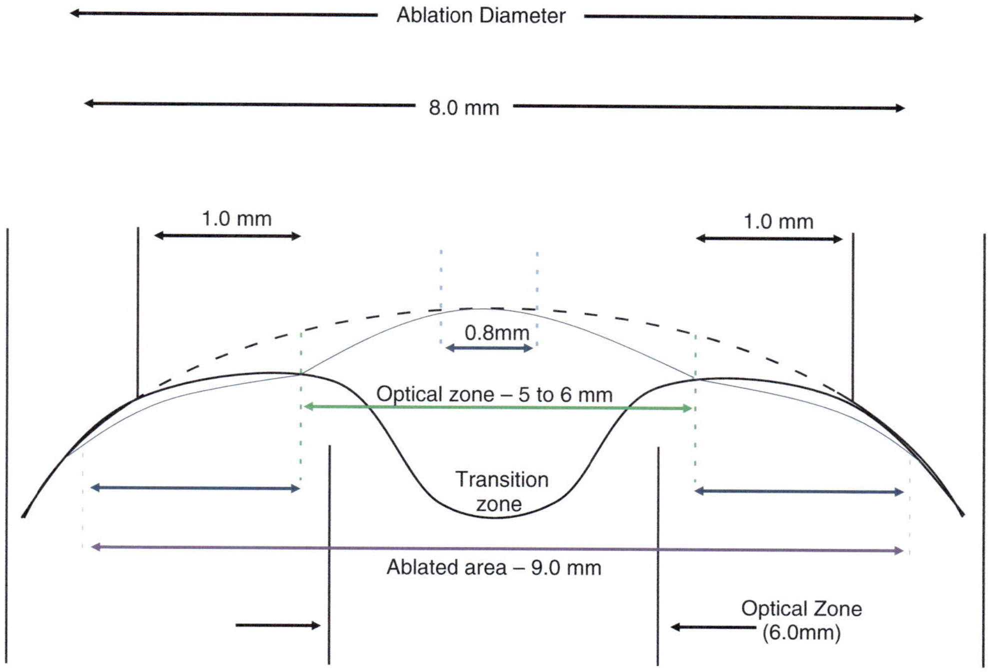

Fig. 3 Representative treatment profile algorithm for a blend zone with variable spot size treatment. Notice that additional treatment is done for the peripheral cornea to reduce potential postoperative HOAs

Conventional Versus Custom Treatments

As discussed in Chap. 14, Physical Optics, recall that all LRS procedures involve *photoablation*, wherein laser energy is used to break covalent bonds (carbon-carbon and carbon-nitrogen) to vaporize collagen polymer chains into individual atoms. The target tissue undergoes sublimation (conversion from solid to gas). Photoablation lasers are considered "cold" lasers since minimal heat/force is generated during the tissue destruction process.

In the early days of LRS (the early 2000s), *conventional treatments* (also known as standard or traditional treatments) were used for all patients. Again, as a simplification, conventional treatments were primarily based on the subjective refraction without a measurement (or consideration) of optical aberrations, especially HOAs. We have the benefit of hindsight, but at that time, it was not known how much impact HOAs had on post LRS outcomes. While conventional treatments objectively treated the refractive error, they treated a small central zone of the cornea (approximately 6–6.5 mm) and created a mostly postoperative oblate corneal shape. This in turn increased HOAs and decreased subjective post-LRS vision, especially in patients with large pupils.[17]

A few other (advanced) points regarding standard treatments, which also apply to custom treatments (discussed in the next section), include:

- Myopic treatments are typically done at lower rates (~6 Hz) than hyperopic treatments (~10 Hz). However, surgeons can choose how slow or how fast to perform the ablation, depending on their preferred practice patterns and/or surgical results (range 1.5–10 Hz)
- Comparatively, the treatment dimensions for hyperopia are larger than the dimensions for myopia. In order to produce a *steeper central cornea* with hyperopic ablations, the bulk of the treatment is directed in a ring-shaped pattern to the peripheral cornea.
- Astigmatism is corrected by focusing the laser treatment to *steepen the flatter axis*, which may seem counterintuitive at first glance.

In contrast, *custom LRS treatments* use wavefront refraction and aberrometry measurements to design an individualized treatment profile for each patient. The most significant feature of custom LRS treatments is the additional treatment done to the peripheral cornea. For example, if a custom LRS treatment is done (using a blend zone) for a patient with 6.00D myopia, then different portions of the cornea will be treated with varying amounts of treatment. Within the central 6 mm optical zone, the laser will treat the full −6D. A blend zone will be additionally treated outside this central zone: −5.00D will be treated at 6.5 mm and −1.00D at 8 mm (Fig. 3). Basically, a gradual slope will be created from the optical zone to the extreme peripheral untreated cornea.

One type of custom LRS treatment is *wavefront guided treatments (WFG)*. In WFG treatments, information from the wavefront map guides the laser to customize the treatment pattern so that irregularities can be corrected, leading to a reduced incidence of glare, haloes, contrast sensitivity, and difficulty with night vision. One potential limitation of WFG is potentially dynamic (or inaccurate) measurements that

[17] These are the patients that end up going on nationally syndicated talk shows hosted by quack doctors to bad mouth LASIK.

vary depending on age, patient accommodation, and pupil diameter. The VISX Star S4 laser (Johnson & Johnson Vision, Santa Ana, CA, USA) is an example of a commonly used WFG laser platform.

Another type of custom LRS treatment is *wavefront optimized (WFO) treatments*, which seek to correct potentially reduced treatments on the peripheral cornea. While the full physics discussion is beyond the scope of this text, we can simplify this concept by realizing that because laser energy directed to the central cornea comes in from a different direction than laser energy directed to the peripheral cornea, there is some unwanted reduction of treatment effect to the peripheral cornea. In turn, this may worsen HOAs, especially SA. With WFO, more energy is directed to the peripheral cornea (transition zone) to compensate for this loss. WFO utilizes preoperative measurements and the attempted correction, compares it to a normative database of patients, and then selects an ablation pattern to minimize optical aberrations (especially HOAs) after surgery. The WaveLight Allegretto Wave Eye-Q Laser (Alcon Laboratories, Fort Worth, TX, USA) is an example of a commonly used WFO laser platform.

Both WFG and WFO are two different philosophical treatment algorithms that seek to improve patients' objective and subjective vision after LRS. WFG primarily seeks to *reduce pre-existing HOAs*, while WFO seeks to *minimize the induction of new (post-LRS) HOAs*. While debate among refractive surgeons may be as intense as the debate between Apple ® and Android ® users about which one is better, suffice it to say that both WFG and WFO produce comparable postsurgical visual outcomes. Most refractive surgeons currently employ either WFG or WGO treatments for most LRS patients.

A few other (advanced) points regarding conventional and custom treatments are as follows:

- As mentioned previously, custom laser treatments remove slightly more corneal tissue than conventional laser treatments. This additional tissue removed is negligible for most patients but may have additional considerations for higher refractive errors.
- While upper limits of treatment vary depending on a given laser's capabilities, conventional LRS can treat slightly higher amounts of myopia as compared to custom LRS. The amount of hyperopia that can be treated is about the same for both custom and conventional treatments.
- For patients with mixed astigmatism (defined as a patient with refractive error with more cylinder than sphere, such as −2.00 + 4.50 × 90), conventional LRS treatments may allow for higher amounts of treatment than custom treatments.
- Depending on a surgeon's practice, custom treatments may incur additional financial costs to the patient compared to conventional treatments.

More recently (FDA approval 2016), *topography-guided ablation treatments (TGA)* have been introduced as a third type of LRS. This technology seeks to improve outcomes of custom LRS and treat corneas that previously may have been considered poor candidates for other types of LRS. In other words, by adding corneal topography measurements (such as areas of elevation and irregularity), TGA may effectively treat irregular corneas (aka "funny looking corneas") to minimize postoperative aberrations. TGA treatments may be especially useful for treating post-LRS complications, such as decentered ablations and irregular astigmatism. The superiority of TGA in routine cases remains to be seen at the time of this writing.

Selected Psychosocial Considerations

Refractive surgeons usually also have to moonlight as psychiatrists: when considering an LRS candidate, while the previously mentioned ophthalmic considerations are essential, there are additional psychosocial considerations that can benefit both the surgeon and the patient:

1. Reasonable postoperative visual expectations: As stated previously, the primary goal of LRS is to provide patients with the same type of vision achieved with glasses and contact lenses. LRS does not enhance or increase a patient's preoperative vision potential. If a patient can only achieve 20/30 in a given eye due to amblyopia, for example, the patient should be counseled that he/she may never achieve 20/20 vision; thus, surgery should be cautiously considered only after extensive preoperative discussion in such patients. If a patient demands unattainable vision through LRS, it's probably best to punt the patient to the local LASIK factory and avoid yourself the headache.[18]
2. Understanding the healing process and appropriate time to achieve the desired vision: Patients should be counseled that despite the advances in LRS, it is still a surgical procedure, and sufficient healing time (especially with PRK) must be given to achieve the desired result. If a patient demands instantaneous vision improvement through LRS or does not want to allow for the natural healing process to occur, it's again probably best to punt the patient to someone else and avoid yourself the headache.

[18]One would then hope that the referral provider would have the knowledge and wherewithal to tell the patient he/she is not a good LRS candidate.

3. Visual acuity does not equal visual function: Many LRS candidates may psychologically feel they have to read a certain line on the eye chart (20/20, 20/15, or even 20/10) to feel they had "successful" surgery. It is necessary to discuss the difference(s) between measured visual acuity and practical visual function. For example, a patient who can see 20/10 may overaccommodate to achieve good distance vision and may suffer from reduced near vision.
4. The ideal LRS patient should have an easy-going nature, reasonable expectations, willingness to follow surgeon instructions, and understand that glasses/contact lenses may still be needed in the near or distant future. After seeing others' misleading advertisements guaranteeing perfect vision, some patients may come in and expect you to provide the same guarantees and outcomes. Any candidate who does not meet these criteria should be punted to… well, you get the theme here.

Postoperative Optics Issues After Excimer Laser Surgery

Every patient after LRS will sing your praises, refer 20 friends and family members to see you for surgery, give you a large briefcase of cash, and commission a statue in your honor. Of course, nothing in the previous sentence is true.

With modern technology and current techniques, LRS is generally a well-tolerated surgical procedure with excellent results. However, as with any surgery, complications may occur and may be encountered by ophthalmologists who do not routinely perform LRS. While we will focus on the optics-relevant postoperative issues after LRS, we would be remiss not to mention that the most common (and usually, thankfully, transient) adverse effect of LASIK is **dry eye syndrome**. As LASIK involves the creation of an anterior flap, corneal nerves may be damaged during flap formation, leading to or exacerbating dry eye syndrome. PRK only ablates the superficial nerve fibers and leaves the deeper nerves intact—therefore, after re-epithelialization, there are significantly fewer dry eye issues with this procedure. The effects of dry eye syndrome on refractive error and vision quality should be evident by now.[19]

We will discuss a few potential postoperative ophthalmic optics issues after LRS below. Please review the discussions on *higher order aberrations* in Chap. 14.[20] Post-LRS corneal ectasia also merits further reading of appropriate texts, especially in the current era of increased awareness and corneal cross-linking.

[19]Please consult other refractive surgery resources for detailed discussion of post-operative dry eye syndrome, as well as other postoperative issues such as striae, flap dislocation, and diffuse lamellar keratitis (DLK; aka "Sands of Sahara")

[20]You were warned previously that you would not be able to escape knowing the higher-order aberrations.

Regression Versus Progression

This is a favorite discussion point as many surgeons (wrongly) interchangeably use these terms when discussing post-LRS refractive misses.

It may be helpful to start with a dictionary definition of each term. *Regression* is a return to a *former* or less developed state. *Progression* is a movement towards a more *advanced* state, especially gradually or in stages. Regarding LRS, both regression and progression may occur, though both are more frequently seen with myopic LRS.

Regression may occur in the *early weeks after myopic LRS* due to asymmetrical epithelial hyperplasia; basically, the eye tries to revert to its original curvature by filling in part of the ablated areas with epithelium. For example, a patient who was −4.00D prior to LRS might be 20/20 (plano) at post-op 1 week, but after 2–3 weeks, may be 20/25 with −0.75D refractive error. If such regression occurs, prolonging or *increasing topical steroids* (+/− topical cyclosporine) may help to reverse the regression. Increasing steroids is the same strategy used to treat early under-correction, and indeed there is likely overlap between regression and under-correction (see the following section). Even in normal postoperative corneas, long-term regression without significant clinical refractive shift may occur (approximately 0.06D of regression may occur per year).

Patients with proven regression of refractive error may need additional LRS treatment if medical therapy and observation fail to improve the symptoms.

Progression usually refers to a significant refractive shift that *occurs years after LRS*. For example, a patient who undergoes LRS at age 19 may have additional myopia 10 years later. In this case, it is unlikely that the laser treatment has "regressed" significantly; it is more likely that myopia progression is the more significant factor here. These patients may need a "touch-up" procedure years later to treat this progression. Therefore, younger LRS patients should be counseled about this potential late-term problem. Additionally, patients who underwent LRS 10–15 years ago, especially during the early days of LRS, may present later in life with myopia due to progression.

As an advanced topic, some surgeons intentionally overtreat young myopes to cause postoperative hyperopia (ranging from 0.50 to 0.75D hyperopia). The idea here is that these patients can comfortably accommodate a bit (which they may have been doing before LRS as well) to neutralize the hyperopia; having this hyperopic "buffer" may allow the patient to have some progression of their myopia with aging and "grow" into emmetropia. Think of this as similar to your parents buying clothes 1–2 sizes bigger when you were younger. Similarly, some surgeons may welcome late progression in myopes >40 years old because this progression may help with presbyopia symptoms (which may not be a bad thing!).

Under-Correction Versus Over-Correction

As a follow-up to the previous topic, a refractive "miss" may occur for various reasons, leading to (early) postoperative under-correction or over-correction. Higher preoperative refractive errors are more likely to be associated with under-/over-corrections. As with many postoperative problems, both of these issues may resolve themselves especially if the magnitude of unintended refractive error is relatively small (up to 0.75D).

Under-correction occurs much more frequently with higher degrees of myopia and hyperopia, especially with smaller optical zones of treatment (<6.0 mm diameter). If seen early in the postoperative period, one option is to *increase steroids* to decrease epithelial hyperplasia and reverse under-correction.[21] This treatment is the same strategy for early regression if you have been paying attention. Indeed, there may be some overlap between early regression and under-correction, but that's a bit of a chicken-egg argument as well.

Over-correction of more than 1.0D at 1 year after LRS occurs much less frequently, and it may also happen more frequently with PRK procedures than LASIK. Younger myopes might not notice over-correction because they may be able to accommodate (generate plus power) to neutralize the unintended hyperopia. If over-correction becomes problematic, intentionally stopping steroids may cause some exuberant healing and reduce the over-correction. Topical NSAIDs may also help.[22]

For persistent under/over-correction, additional laser treatment may be necessary. It is far easier to treat under-correction than over-correction; think of getting a haircut at the barber: it is far easier for the barber to cut more hair (treat the under-correction) than "add" hair (treat the over-correction). One advantage of LASIK compared to PRK is that since refractive stability occurs earlier, this allows for earlier enhancements (within 3 months). For PRK, one should wait >3–6 months to stabilize the refraction and minimize haze risk. When performing a retreatment for LASIK, one can either lift the flap for additional ablation or perform PRK ("PRK over the top") and avoid flap lift.

[21] A mnemonic to remember this: "ISTU" = increase steroids, treat under-correction.

[22] A mnemonic to remember this: "NSAIDS may help NEGATE the correction".

Haze

Any disruptive injury requiring corneal epithelium regrowth can activate fibroblasts and an inflammatory cascade. In PRK, the corneal epithelium is mechanically or chemically removed prior to laser ablation; successful surgery requires regrowth of healthy corneal epithelium. Aberrant tissue growth during this re-epithelialization process can cause corneal opacity and scar formation (haze). Patients at risk for haze formation include higher refractive errors (>−6D), keloid formers, younger age, darker irises, and increased UV light exposure after surgery.

Haze appears in the subepithelial layers, ranging from a lacy, reticular opacity to dense scar-like fibrosis. Haze can present several weeks after PRK, peaking at 1–3 months, and then regressing or disappearing over 6–12 months. Patients with poor epithelial healing history or tendency (e.g., EBMD, diabetes, recurrent corneal erosion syndrome, etc.) may be at increased risk for developing visually significant, non-clearing haze. Why should you care about haze for clinical and exam purposes? Haze can cause *regression* of the refractive correction and astigmatism (including irregular astigmatism).

In terms of prevention, mitomycin-c (MMC; concentration 0.02–0.04%, treatment time range: 12–120 seconds) has been effectively used to decrease the incidence and severity of haze after PRK. Many refractive surgeons advise patients after PRK to use UV light protective sunglasses (3–12 months after surgery) and/or oral vitamin C to further decrease the risk of haze. Persistent, visually debilitating haze may require phototherapeutic keratectomy (PTK) and/or mechanical scraping (with additional MMC) for removal.

Central Island

A central island can be considered as a focal area of untreated corneal tissue within the intended treated zone. Basically, think of this as an area that has been "missed" by the laser. It is defined as an elevation of at least 1D measuring more than 1 mm compared to the surrounding treatment area (Fig. 4). Central islands were more frequently seen with older broad-beam lasers. They may resolve independently (within 6–12 months) but may require additional treatment (PTK or TGA) to remove and improve refractive error.

Central islands can cause unexpected myopia or hyperopia, astigmatism (including irregular), and higher order aberrations.

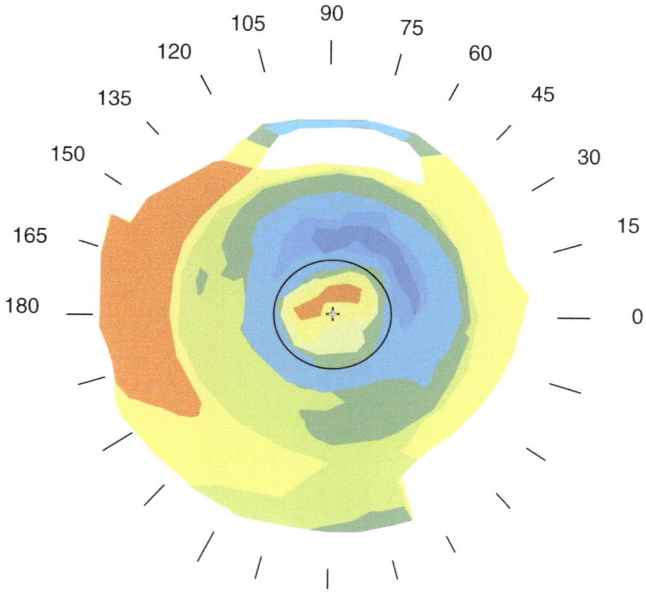

Fig. 4 Central island after LRS. Notice the focal area of elevated cornea (orange) within the treatment zone (blue-green)

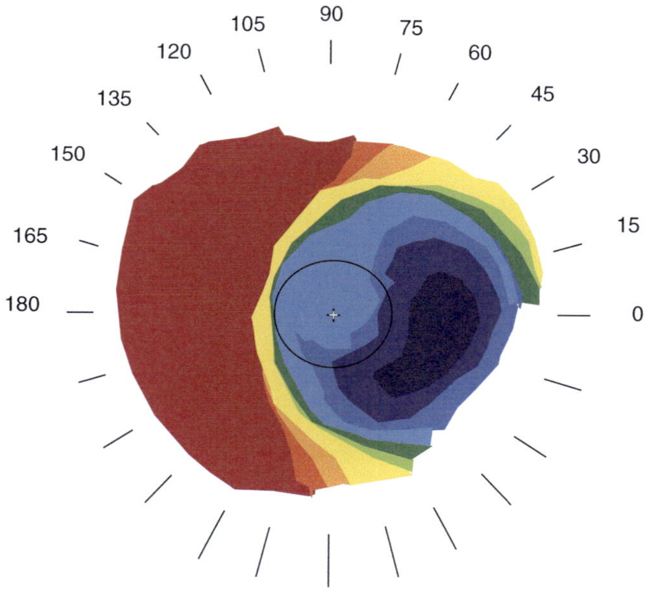

Fig. 5 Decentered ablation. Notice the displacement of the treatment zone (blue-green) with a large crescent-shaped area of untreated cornea (red)

Decentered Ablation

As a summary of our previous discussions on the three important axes,[23] we can understand the importance of centering the ablation such that the patient looks through the treated area. The differences between the visual axis, optical axis, and pupillary axis are negligible for most patients. For LRS, we can introduce the concept of the "line of sight": because of the non-centered optics of the eye, the line of sight isn't necessarily equivalent to the visual and/or optical axes. Therefore, the ideal ablation should be centered on the area of the cornea that overlies the line of sight (i.e., the entrance pupil).

A decentered ablation may appear on topography as a "shift" of the central treatment area to a peripheral sector of the cornea with a larger area of untreated cornea (Fig. 5). Decentration was more frequently seen with older lasers that lacked the ability for real-time eye-tracking. In the early days of LRS, patient fixation on the operating microscope was crucial for proper centration; if the patient's eye drifted during the procedure (or the surgeon did not position the patient's head at the beginning) and the surgeon did not readjust, the ablation would instead be centered on a peripheral area of the cornea—obviously, this is not a good thing. Precise centration on the visual axis, rather than relying on the pupillary axis, is much more critical for hyperopic than myopic treatments, as these eyes may have a significant angle kappa.

Decentration up to 0.5 mm may be asymptomatic and observed. However, decentration of ≥1.0 mm is usually symptomatic. A decentered ablation may cause objective refractive errors (myopia, hyperopia, and astigmatism) and subjective glare, haloes, and other HOAs. Patients with larger pupils may experience more symptoms with even smaller amounts of decentration. RGPCL use or TGA treatment may be necessary for persistent issues with decentration.

Other Types of Refractive Surgery

While LRS is a significant component of Refractive Surgery, there are several additional procedures that we can briefly discuss.

Historical Procedures

While the history of refractive surgery includes many procedures, ranging from ingenious to downright scary, we will focus our discussion on two historical procedures that may still be encountered in patients who present for routine eye care with a remote history of refractive surgery: radial keratotomy (RK) and hexagonal keratotomy (HexK).

Radial Keratotomy (RK)[24]

RK was a procedure introduced in the late 1970s as a procedure to treat myopia by making near-full thickness

[23] See Chap. 26, Preoperative Optics for Cataract Surgery.

[24] See also the discussion on RK in Chap. 26, Preoperative Optics

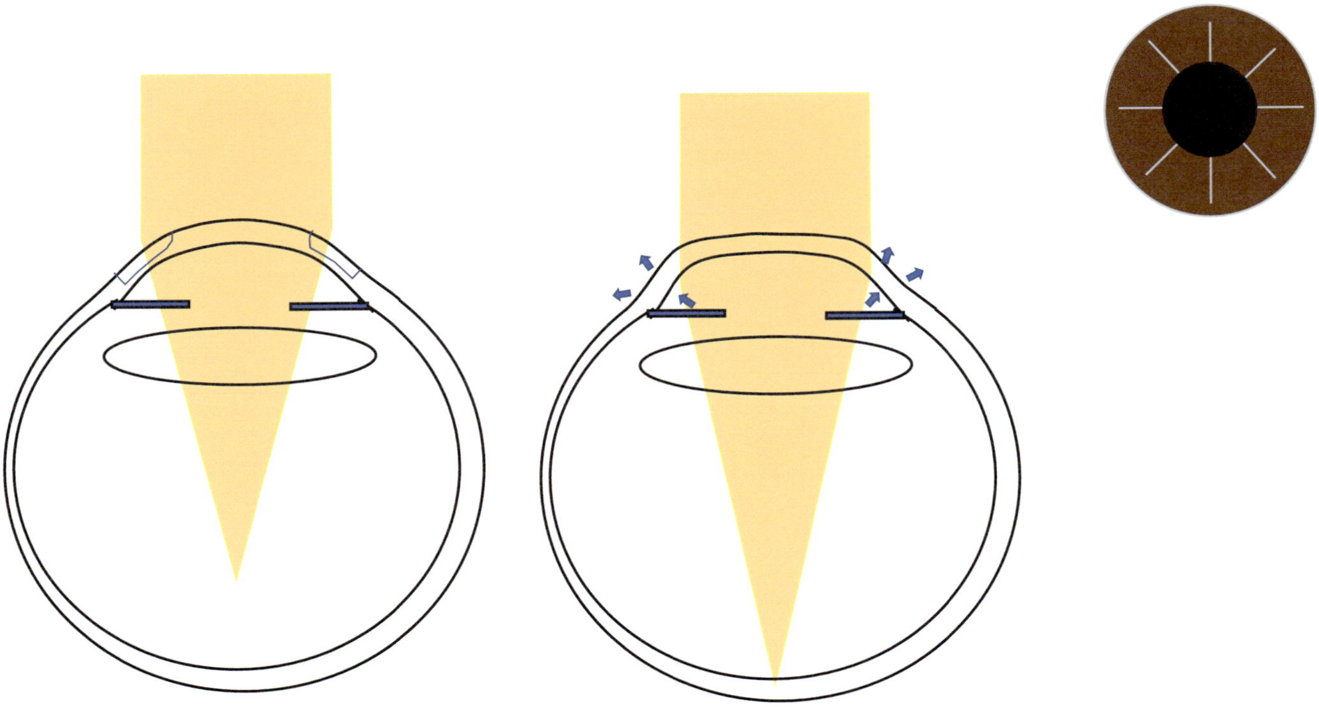

Fig. 6 Radial keratotomy (RK) was an incisional procedure utilizing near-full-thickness radial incisions from the peripheral to central cornea. The resultant corneal flattening would treat the myopic refractive error

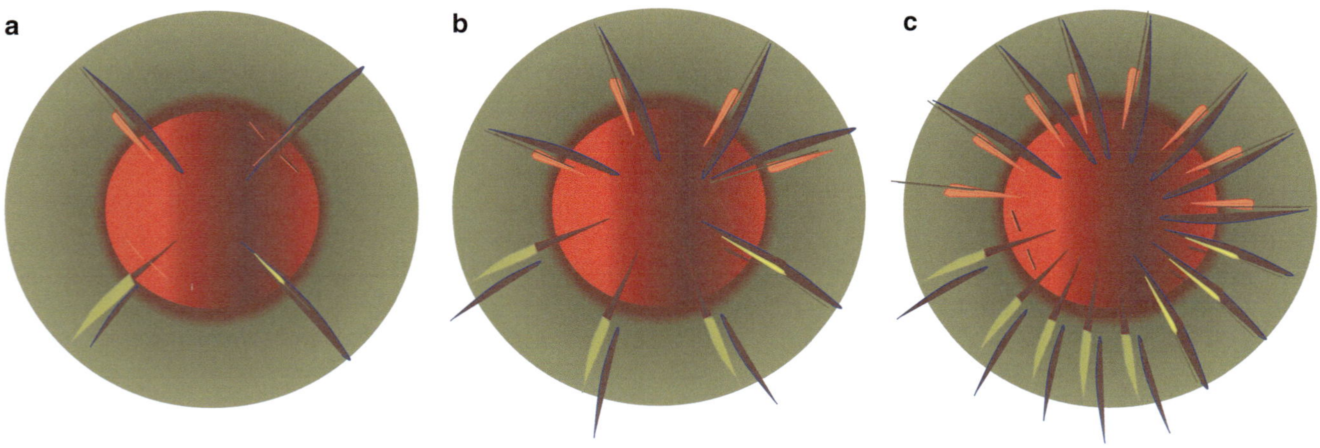

Fig. 7 Radial keratotomy (RK) was an incisional procedure utilizing near-full-thickness radial incisions to cause corneal flattening and secondary treatment of myopia. An increasing number of cuts (4, 8, 16, or more) could be made to treat higher amounts of myopia. Panel A also shows a T-cut (modified astigmatic keratotomy) used to treat astigmatism. Panels b and c show 8 and 16 cut RK, respectively

(approximately 90% corneal thickness) radial incisions to weaken the cornea's mechanical strength and cause corneal flattening (Fig. 6).

An increasing number of incisions, ranging from 4–16 cuts (or even more cuts, making you wonder what the surgeon was thinking at the time), could treat increasing amounts of myopia. RK was primarily used to treat up to 4D of myopia, though surgeons certainly pushed the boundaries in those days (Fig. 7).[25]

Fun fact: excimer lasers were first invented to create more accurate and reproducible RK incisions rather than perform ablations!

of Cataract Surgery.

[25] We've made this joke before, but wow, the 1980s were really an interesting time.

While many RK clinical studies were done, the **PERK Study** (1982–1983) is a landmark study that merits a brief discussion.[26] This study evaluated the safety and efficacy of RK for treatment of −2.00 to −8.75D of myopia. The 10-year results showed that 53% of patients achieved ≥20/20 vision—pretty good! However, the biggest drawback of the procedure was the unpredictability and instability of the treatment effect. For example, a hyperopic shift (≥1D) was seen in 43% of the study patients—not pretty good!

As RK could only treat spherical myopia, for patients with astigmatism, additional transverse incisions ("T-cuts" or modified astigmatic keratotomy (AK) incisions) were placed as seen in Fig. 7, Panel A.

Other complications included diurnal fluctuation of vision, glare, corneal scarring, higher order aberrations and irregular astigmatism. In modern times, this is an abandoned, obsolete procedure. However, you should know about RK for exams and clinical practice, as many of these post-RK patients may now present for cataract surgery. See Chap. 26, Preoperative Optics for Cataract Surgery, for additional information on preoperative assessment and cataract surgery planning.

[26]Waring GO 3rd, Lynn MJ, McDonnell PJ. Results of the prospective evaluation of radial keratotomy (PERK) study 10 years after surgery. *Arch Ophthalmol*. 1994;112(10):1298–1308.

Hexagonal Keratotomy (HexK)

Hexagonal keratotomy (HexK) was a procedure wherein a series of paracentral incisions were made in a hexagonal pattern to induce central corneal steepening and secondary treatment of hyperopia (Fig. 8a). Fittingly enough, HexK was sometimes used to treat sequential hyperopia caused by PRK (Fig. 8b), with varying levels of success.

HexK was abandoned due to many problems and complications, such as glare, photophobia, corneal ectasia, fluctuating vision, and diplopia/polyopia. Again, these post-HexK patients may now present for cataract surgery with skewed corneal measurements making IOL calculations challenging.

Current Incisional Corneal Procedures

Corneal incisional procedures are mainly used in the current era of refractive surgery to reduce corneal (keratometric) astigmatism. These can be performed manually (with a guarded steel or diamond blade) or with the assistance of a femtosecond laser (FSL). They can be combined with cataract surgery or performed outside of cataract surgery to correct naturally occurring and postsurgical astigmatism.

As previously discussed, when treating astigmatism with incisional procedures, the main idea is to "flatten" the steeper meridian of the cornea while "steepening" the flatter meridian 90-degrees away to create a more uniform cornea with reduced corneal astigmatism. This concept of "*coupling*"

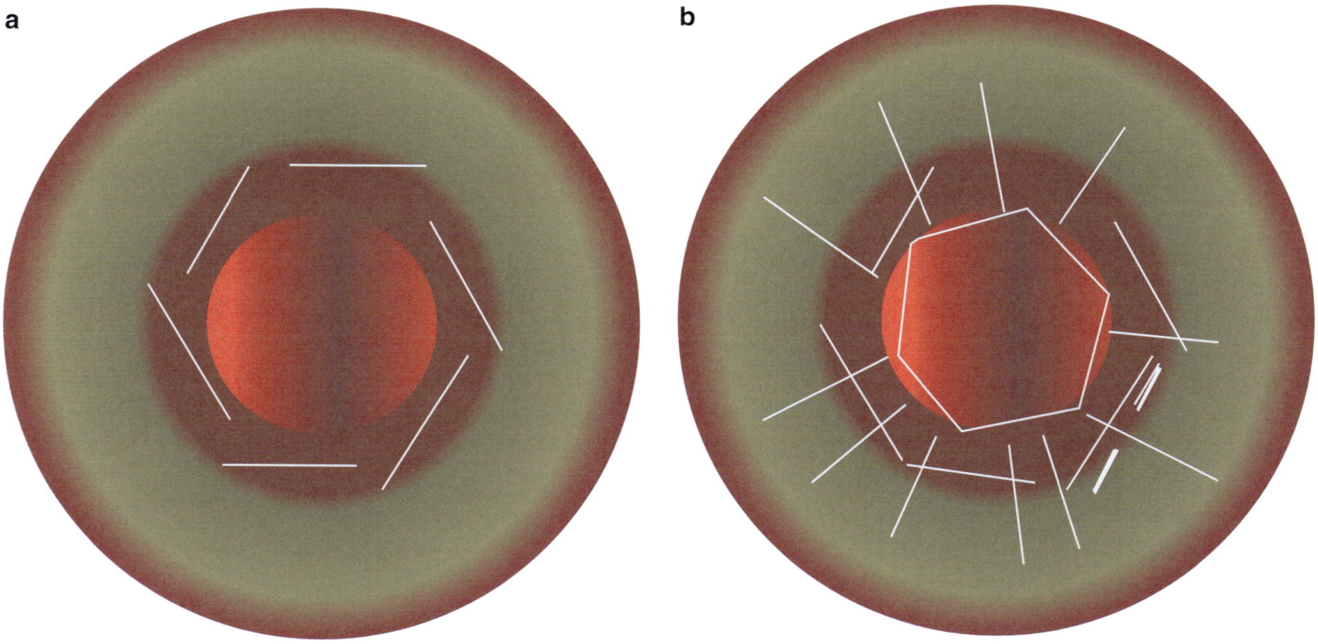

Fig. 8 Hexagonal keratotomy (HexK). Panel a shows 6 paracentral cuts in a hexagonal pattern to cause central corneal steepening. Panel b shows HexK performed after sequential hyperopia from RK (with T-cuts)

states that flattening in one meridian will cause steepening in the meridian 90-degrees away; the amount of coupling depends on how close the incision is placed in relation to the corneal center. A *coupling ratio* of >1.0 (meaning more flattening occurs in the incisional meridian as compared to steepening occurring in the meridian 90-degrees away) is seen with procedures closer to the corneal center, such as astigmatic keratotomy (AK). A coupling ratio closer to 1.0 is seen with procedures closer to the corneal limbus, such as limbal relaxing incisions LRIs.

Both of these procedures may cause under-correction or over-correction of astigmatism, as well as corneal scarring and irregular astigmatism (corneal ectasia). Corneal perforation may occur as a rare complication.

Astigmatic Keratotomy (AK)

Astigmatic keratotomy (AK) procedures refer to tangential incisions made in the mid-peripheral cornea. By definition, AKs are closer to the corneal center than LRIs and thus incur higher risks. We can further divide AKs into manual and FSL-assisted AKs (FSL-AKs).

Manual AKs refer to incisions made with a guarded blade (steel or diamond) at approximately 95% depth in the corneal mid-peripheral zone. A variety of nomograms have been proposed regarding the length, location, and number of AKs to correct higher amounts of astigmatism. Historically, AKs were often (and still) used to treat high amounts of corneal astigmatism after PKP. Manual AKs usually cause a coupling ratio > 1.0.

FSL-AKs have recently been introduced as an alternative method to correct lower amounts of corneal astigmatism (as compared to manual AKs), primarily at the time of cataract surgery. As previously discussed in Chap. 26, Preoperative Optics for Cataract Surgery, this is a highly controversial topic as no large data sets have been published at the time of this writing to demonstrate superiority of this approach.

Limbal Relaxing Incisions (LRIs)

Please see Chap. 26, Preoperative Optics for Cataract Surgery, for a review of limbal relaxing incisions (LRIs) in conjunction with cataract surgery. Outside of this setting, LRIs may be used to treat corneal astigmatism, including post-cataract surgery astigmatism.

A guarded blade (550–600 μm depth) is used to create a partial thickness (approximately 80–90%) circumferential (aka "circum-limbal") incision(s) in the peripheral cornea to cause corneal flattening in the steep meridian and reduction of corneal (keratometric) astigmatism. LRIs can be performed in the office or operating room setting. They produce less astigmatism correction than AKs, but are generally much safer; low-cost to perform; and carry a lower risk of glare, perforation, and irregular astigmatism than AKs. The most significant disadvantage of LRIs is the inevitable regression (up to 50% or more of the intended correction) that occurs over time. LRIs are especially effective for reducing ≤1.5D keratometric astigmatism.

Intrastromal Corneal Ring Segments (ICRS)

While various intrastromal corneal ring segments (ICRS) devices are available in other countries, INTACS (CorneaGen, Seattle, WA, USA) corneal ring segments are the only device available in the USA at the time of this writing. Historically, ICRS were developed around the same time as LRS (the early 2000s) to treat low amounts of myopia by displacing corneal lamellar bundles and shortening corneal arc length. Semi-circle PMMA ring segments are placed in the mid-peripheral corneal stroma (at approximately 70–80% depth) in a lamellar channel created mechanically or with an FSL. More corneal flattening can occur by using thicker and asymmetric segments. For example, a commonly used ICRS strategy for keratoconus involves placing a thicker segment (450 microns) in the inferior cornea and a thinner segment (210 microns) in the superior cornea. Several nomograms and treatment strategies are utilized by surgeons performing ICRS implantation.

While INTACS were initially developed to treat low amounts of myopia, the success of LRS quickly led many refractive surgeons to abandon ICRS in favor of LASIK and PRK, similar to BlueRay ® winning the competition against HD-DVD ®. INTACS fell out of favor but then were repurposed when surgeons began to use them to reduce astigmatism in keratoconus and corneal ectasias. It seemed that INTACS now had a second life! However, while INTACS reduced astigmatism in ectatic corneas, they did not slow disease progression. Thus, keratoconus patients who received INTACS experienced a return (or even increase) of their preexisting astigmatism. Some refractive surgeons again abandoned INTACS because what was the point of a surgical procedure if the potential benefits could not be sustained?

With FDA approval of corneal cross-linking (CXL) in 2016, INTACS have now made their second comeback. Corneal surgeons now use INTACS for patients with mild-moderate keratoconus with CXL to "flatten and freeze" an ectatic cornea. Thus, INTACS can be placed to reverse corneal steepening, and CXL can be used to halt disease progression. Several strategies have been proposed, including combining INTACS with CXL as a single procedure or staging the two procedures by several months. Some surgeons prefer CXL followed by INTACS, while others prefer the opposite when staging. Finally, INTACS can also facilitate contact lens fitting as a result of corneal flattening.

Complications with all ICRS procedures include inadvertent corneal perforation, infection, and extrusion of the ring segment. Other problems include reduced corneal sensitivity, induction of additional astigmatism, and night vision problems (glare, haloes, and HOAs). ICRS does not stop disease

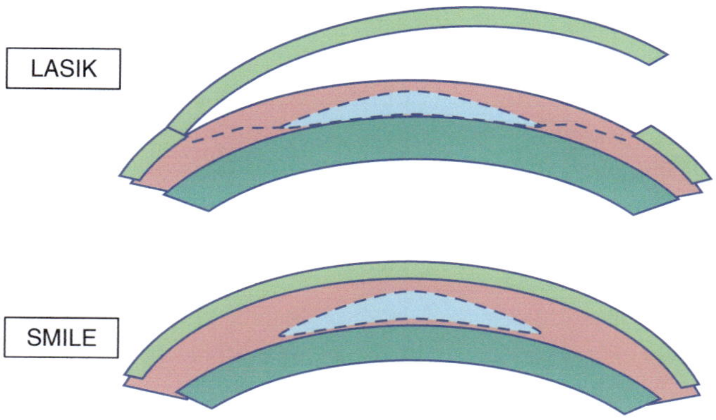

Fig. 9 Comparison of LASIK and Small Incision Lenticule Extraction (SMILE). In LASIK, a flap (blue dotted line) composed of epithelium (~50 μm) and stroma (~50–80 μm) is created prior to the ablation (light blue area). SMILE involves using an FSL to create a stromal lenticule (light blue area) that can be removed via a side-cut incision. The anterior surface of the cornea is not violated with this technique

progression, so if CXL is not done, the disease process may continue, especially in younger patients.

Small Incision Lenticule Extraction (SMILE)

Small Incision Lenticule Extraction (SMILE) is the latest procedure to join the refractive surgery party, achieving excellent postoperative results similar to other LRS procedures.[27] Inclusion and exclusion criteria are similar to LASIK and PRK. Currently, SMILE can treat up to −10D myopia and up to 3D astigmatism.

In this procedure, an FSL is used to create a stromal lenticule that is then extracted through a small side cut incision (Fig. 9). After removing the lenticule, corneal flattening and the desired refractive change occur. No excimer laser ablation is performed, so you can "smile" because the anterior surface of the central cornea is not violated.

Advantages of SMILE compared to LASIK and PRK include preservation of the anterior corneal surface which decreases the risk of dry eye syndrome, induces less biomechanical stress to the cornea, and possibly reduces the severity of induced aberrations. Other benefits include less patient pain and less refractive regression than LASIK and PRK. Furthermore, because the anterior corneal surface is maintained, PRK or LASIK treatment for further reduction of refractive error is still possible.

The main disadvantages of SMILE include potential problems with FSL technology, limited range of treatment for myopic astigmatism, and unknown long-term results compared to LRS. There is significant interest among refractive surgeons about the future of SMILE.

Surgical Treatment of Presbyopia

While we have thus far focused on treating myopia, hyperopia, and astigmatism, several surgical techniques and devices may be considered for the treatment of pure presbyopia in select patient populations.

As an extension of LRS, monovision LASIK or PRK can be used in this patient population in the presence of other refractive errors. Similarly, as an extension of cataract surgery, monovision IOLs or advanced technology IOLs (ATIOLs) for presbyopia can also be offered.

For pure presbyopia, several additional procedures can be offered. These procedures haven't really gained widespread popularity either due to lack of sustained effect and/or postoperative complications.

Presbyopic LASIK (Multifocal Laser Ablation)

Presbyopic LASIK involves combining myopic LASIK with modified laser treatment to create a steep central area in the cornea—essentially creating a "bifocal" cornea. Since then, additional modifications of this "PresbyLASIK" procedure have been used. For example, in peripheral presbyLASIK, the central cornea is treated for distance vision, whereas the peripheral cornea is treated to induce negative spherical aberration and secondarily increase the depth of field for near vision. In central presbyLASIK, a central hyperpositive area is created for near vision, and the peripheral cornea is treated for distance vision.

As with many refractive surgery procedures, PresbyLASIK hasn't achieved widespread popularity due to problems such as decreased contrast sensitivity and some compromise of visual acuity at all distances.[28]

Conductive Keratoplasty (CK)

Conductive keratoplasty (CK) is another one of those procedures where, with the benefit of hindsight, one wonders if this was ever a good idea. CK is a radiofrequency-based collagen shrinking procedure performed in the peripheral cornea in a ring pattern to treat 0.75–3D of hyperopia. A series of 8–32 spots can be placed in a concentric pattern to induce peripheral tightening (flattening) and secondary steeping of the central cornea to correct hyperopia and improve near vision. CK may be performed in an office setting in one or both eyes in a modified monovision ("blended vision") approach.

[27] Zhang Y, Shen Q, Jia Y, et al. Clinical Outcomes of SMILE and FS-LASIK Used to Treat Myopia: A Meta-analysis. J Refract Surg. 2016 Apr;32(4):256–65.

[28] Alio JL, Chaubard JJ, Caliz A, et al. Correction of presbyopia by technovision central multifocal LASIK (presbyLASIK). J Refract Surg 2006; 22(5): 453–460.

Unfortunately, CK had many side effects, including non-clearing corneal edema, irregular astigmatism, and corneal scarring. Clinical evidence suggests that CK has transient effects; significant regression of refractive effect may occur within 4–8 weeks of treatment.[29] At present, some surgeons are utilizing CK in conjunction with CXL in keratoconus patients.

Corneal Inlays

A variety of corneal inlay devices have been introduced (and then subsequently withdrawn from the market) in recent years to treat presbyopia. These devices involve creating a corneal flap (similar to LASIK) and placing a pinhole-style biocompatible polymer inlay designed to increase the depth of field to improve near and intermediate visual acuity without affecting distance vision.[30] Inlays may be combined with LRS. Thus far, results from these surgical devices have not been significantly convincing for widespread adoption.

Phakic IOLs

While not as popular in the USA, phakic IOLs (pIOLs) are commonly used as a primary refractive surgery technique in other countries. Currently, the Visian ICL (Staar Surgical, Monrovia, CA, USA) is the only pIOL available in the USA. Whereas previously, pIOLs could only treat myopic refractive errors, a toric pIOL was recently approved by the FDA in August 2018.

While older pIOLs were placed in the anterior chamber or affixed to the iris, current pIOLs are placed behind the iris and directly in front of the crystalline lens (in the sulcus space). Like cataract surgery, a pIOL requires a corneal incision and is usually performed in the operating room.

Advantages of pIOLs include the following:

- Ability to correct −3.00 to −20.0D myopia with up to 4D of cylinder
- Reversible procedure with no change to the cornea, including maintenance of anterior corneal surface integrity.
- Lower incidence of glare, haloes, and HOAs
- Lower incidence of dry eye syndrome
- Better contrast sensitivity compared to LRS procedures
- Similar patient satisfaction to LRS procedures
- Because the cornea is not altered, IOL calculations for pIOL patients at the time of cataract surgery can be performed as per routine (see below)

Disadvantages of pIOLs include the following:

- Additional cost due to use of an operating room (approximately 2–3× the cost of LRS) that is not covered by medical insurance
- Potential surgical complications for any incisional procedure, such as infection, bleeding, etc.
- Potential damage to iris, anterior chamber angle, and corneal endothelium.
- Pupillary block and angle closure glaucoma. pIOLs require placement of at least 2 (generous) peripheral iridotomies to reduce the risk of this complication.
- Secondary induction of cataract (ASC cataract) due to mechanical damage to the anterior crystalline lens.

As an advanced topic, for extremely high myopic refractive errors (more than -20D myopia), patients may benefit from a staged procedure of pIOL followed by LRS for residual refractive error.

While not all ophthalmologists may place pIOLs, these patients may later present for cataract surgery. Some additional optics-related considerations for these patients include:

- Preoperative biometry considerations: no additional adjustments are needed on modern optical biometry devices to measure the eye and calculate the needed IOL power. You don't have to adjust for the phakic IOL as you would have to adjust for a patient with a previous history of PRK or LASIK. A presbyopia-correcting ATIOL can be considered as the corneal HOAs are similar to a non-refractive surgery patient population.
- Intraoperative considerations: at the time of cataract surgery, the pIOL has to be carefully removed prior to initiating the capsulorhexis, so a surgeon experienced with pIOLs may be better suited for performing cataract surgery in these patients.

Refractive Lens Exchange (RLE)

Refractive Lens Exchange (RLE), also known as clear lens exchange, can be considered "early" cataract surgery wherein a non-cataractous crystalline lens is removed and replaced with a presbyopia-correcting ATIOL. A lengthy discussion of RLE is beyond the scope of this text as this is a controversial topic even among ophthalmologists. RLE may be a potential surgical option for patients with refractive errors, especially presbyopia, who are unsuitable for LRS or other refractive surgical options.

For example, a potential RLE candidate may be a hyperopic patient with presbyopia who has developed contact lens intolerance. RLE may be offered with the placement of monofocal IOLs for monovision or presbyopia-correcting ATIOLs.

While high myopes may be thought of as another good candidate population, in the presence of a formed vitreous,

[29] Rojas MC, Manche EE. Comparison of videokeratographic functional optical zones in conductive keratoplasty and laser in situ keratomileusis for hyperopia. J Refract Surg 2003; 19(3): 333–337.

[30] See the discussions regarding Diffraction and Depth of Field in Chap. 14, Physical Optics and Advanced Optical Principles.

there is a very high risk of retinal detachment even with successful surgery. Please consult other texts and resources for more information. We have included it here for the sake of completeness and for readers to have a cursory awareness of this procedure for exam purposes.

Practice Questions

The following scenarios presented as practice questions will hopefully connect some of the themes, procedures, and strategies discussed thus far in this chapter.

Scenario #1

A 25-year-old male presents to you to discuss surgical options to correct his myopia.

Visual acuity, sc:	OD : HM OS : HM
Manifest Rx:	OD : − 23.50 + 2.00 × 85 (20/15)
	OS : − 24.00 + 2.25 × 95 (20/15)
Topography:	OD : 44.00 × 46.00 @ 85
	OS : 44.00 × 46.25 @ 95
	No ectasia or inferior steepening in both eyes
Pachymetry:	OD : 540 OS : 550

Exam, including DFE: unremarkable OU

What potential surgical options, if any, exist for this patient?

Scenario #2

A 36-year-old patient presents to your office after moving into town a few months ago. She reports that she had LASIK in both eyes approximately 18 years ago at a provider elsewhere. Prior to surgery, she was −8.50D sphere in both eyes. She reports difficulty with glare and halos, especially at night time. She states that she was told that her LASIK might wear off after then years, and she may need a "touch up" procedure. She is very eager to proceed with a LASIK enhancement and has an unmarked envelope full of $100 bills that she casually places on the countertop.

Visual acuity, sc:	OD : 20/20 OS : 20/25 + 1
Visual acuity, cc:	OD : 20/15 OS : 20/15
Manifest Rx:	OD : − 0.50 + 0.25 × 90 (20/15)
	OS : − 0.50 sphere (20/15)
Pupils:	Light : 4.5mm OU Dark : 8.5mm OU
Exam, including DFE:	Unremarkable in both eyes. Well-healed LASIK flaps OU.

Topography: consistent with post-myopic ablation with central flattening changes; no abnormalities or ectatic changes.

What potential surgical options, if any, exist for this patient?

Scenario #3

A 22-year-old patient recently underwent uncomplicated LASIK with you 2 weeks ago. Prior to surgery, she was −7.50D sphere OD and −8.00D sphere OS with 20/20 vision in her glasses. The patient reports that the vision has been intermittently blurry since her surgery, especially at a bdistance, and progressively worsens throughout the day. She is a computer analyst and spends approximately 10 hours a day in front of the computer and other handheld electronic devices. She is highly concerned about an under-correction and wishes to schedule a touch-up enhancement procedure as soon as possible.

Visual acuity, sc (today):	OD : 20/25 OS : 20/30
Manifest Rx (today)	OD : − 2.00 sphere (20/15)
	OS : − 2.25 sphere (20/15)
Exam, including DFE:	Unremarkable OU. Well-healed LASIK flaps OU.
Cycloplegic Rx (today)	OD : plano (20/15) OS : − 0.25 + 0.25 × 80 (20/15)

What potential options, including nonsurgical and surgical, exist for this patient at this time?

Scenario #4

A 60-year-old patient is highly motivated to have refractive surgery to improve his vision as you successfully performed LASIK on his 30-year-old son 6 months ago. He does not currently wear glasses or contact lenses for distance, though occasionally uses some reading glasses for long periods of near work. He works as an accountant and is an avid golfer during the weekends, and he reports some glare while driving at night.

Visual acuity, sc:	OD : 20/25 + , J12 near OS : 20/100 distance, J2 near
Manifest Rx:	OD : − 0.25 + 0.50 × 180 (20/20)
	OS : − 1.75 (20/20)
Cycloplegic Rx:	similar to manifest
Topography:	Unremarkable OU. No evidence of ectasia.
Pupils:	Light : 4 mm OU Dark : 7 mm OU
Exam, including DFE:	Unremarkable OU

What should be discussed and offered to this patient?

Answers

1. There is no single surgical procedure currently available that will correct his entire refractive error. A *staged approach* for myopia correction can be discussed. Given that the patient is beyond the approved limits for LRS, PRK/LASIK is not possible as a primary procedure. However, a cycloplegic refraction and dilated fundus exam should be performed nonetheless prior to any surgical decision in any patient with this amount of myopia due to the high incidence of peripheral retinal pathology in this patient population. RLE would incur arguably unacceptable risks (e.g., retinal detachment) in a young myope, including loss of accommodation postoperatively. Therefore, one potential option is to *first place a toric pIOL* to correct approximately 20D of myopia (recall that pIOLs can correct −3 to −20D myopia, with up to 4D of cylinder) with full correction of the 2D and 2.25D of refractive astigmatism, respectively in each eye, which corresponds to the keratometric astigmatism. After allowing sufficient time for healing and stabilizing the refraction, PRK or LASIK can be performed for the residual refractive error. It is important to inform the patient that temporary glasses may be needed for the residual refractive error while the eyes heal from the pIOL surgery.
2. This vignette is a typical example of a post-LRS patient (who likely received a standard ablation based on LASIK history 18 years ago) with visual decline due to subjective rather than objective issues. The manifest refractive shows a minimal refractive error that is unlikely to cause her primary issues of glare and halos. In other words, her problems are not due to regression or progression of myopia. The more likely explanation for her subjective complaints is due to HOAs, especially spherical aberration, based on the history and the scotopic pupil size.Problems with HOAs are more likely with *higher amounts of laser ablations* and *smaller optical zones* used in the days of standard (conventional) LRS. Recall that in standard LRS, the peripheral cornea is essentially left untouched. During the daytime, her pupil is 4.5 mm and therefore smaller than the likely optical zone (6–6.5 mm), so only the incoming light refracted by the treated central cornea reaches the fovea and a relatively clear (stigmatic) image is formed. However, in low-light conditions, the pupil dilates considerably larger than the optical zone; therefore, incoming light will pass through the treated central cornea and the peripheral ring of untreated cornea to cause a myopic defocus secondary to spherical aberration, which the patient perceives as glare and halos at night-time.As an aside, the Stiles-Crawford effect may also help negate unwanted peripheral light rays during bright-light conditions. The Stiles-Crawford effect states that the light entering the eye near the edge of the entrance pupil produces a lower photoreceptor response than light of equal intensity entering near the center of the pupil. In other words, the brain gives more "preference" to photoreceptors that receive central light rays in photopic conditions, but when more peripheral photoreceptors are activated in mesopic conditions, the brain can't help but notice the peripheral, defocused light rays.Back to our patient: treatment and reassurance would be the best option at this time. The mild myopia may also help the patient delay the need for reading glasses for a few years. Additional LRS to treat the minimal myopic refractive error may help the objective vision but is unlikely to help her main complaints of glare and halos at night time. A mild pupillary constrictor (for example, dilute brimonidine) may be offered for the reduction of symptoms at night time. Glasses and/or contact lenses are also reasonable options. As a final (advanced) point, topography-guided ablation (TGA) could be offered if the topography showed abnormalities.
3. This scenario is a classic example of postoperative LRS refractive error seen in the early postoperative period. The main causes of postoperative LRS refractive error include the following 6 potential reasons:
   - Development of corneal ectasia
   - Development of cataract
   - Progression of myopia
   - Regression of corrective effect
   - Deliberate or unintentional under-correction
   - Spasm of accommodation

   It is unlikely that the patient developed corneal ectasia or a cataract within 2 weeks of LASIK. Similarly, it is unlikely that progression or regression of myopia occurred within such a short time. We should definitely check the LASIK op-notes to ensure that there was no deliberate or unintentional under-correction. However, looking at today's manifest refraction, we notice that she requires a lot of myopic correction for minimal refractive error; this disappears with the cycloplegic refraction. We also notice that she is a young myope who spends a considerable amount of time focusing at close due to her job requirements. Therefore, it is most likely that *spasm of accommodation* is the culprit in this situation.In this case, getting a cycloplegic refraction is the key to solving the puzzle. Initially, reassurance is the mainstay of treatment, along with education regarding methods to break accommodation such as frequent breaks and focusing at distance objects during work hours. For persistent symptoms, a short course of cycloplegia may be offered. Eventually, she should break out of her accommodation so it is *crucial* that we *do not enhance* this patient at this time.

4. Answer:This patient has *naturally occurring monovision*. Despite his enthusiasm for LRS based on his son's excellent outcome, he may not be the best candidate for LRS because he likely functions well without any refractive correction. We may be tempted to correct the left eye, but he would lose his near vision that may hinder his job as an accountant, even if his vision was 20/15 in the left eye. The right eye spherical equivalent is basically plano.Additionally, he is starting to have some glare and has relatively large (especially for a male) scotopic pupils. LRS may further worsen these subjective symptoms.The safest option at this time is to offer him "night-time driving" glasses with anti-glare reflective coating that corrects distance vision in both eyes. Currently, he does not have a visually significant cataract but might be on his way to developing one in a few years. If the patient is highly motivated and additional exam considerations (such as normal axial length, presence of posterior vitreous separation, etc.) are normal, then RLE with presbyopia-correcting ATIOLs may be offered. For exams, conservative options should always be discussed prior to surgical treatments.

Recommended Additional Reading

The following is a recommended, but not comprehensive, list of additional resources for learning more about refractive surgery:

1. Feder RS, Rapuano CJ (eds). The LASIK handbook: a case-based approach. Philadelphia: Lipincott, Williams, & Wilkins; 2007.
2. Azar D, Gatinel D, Ghanem R, Taneri S (eds). Refractive surgery, 3rd edn. Elsevier; 2019.
3. Randleman JB. Refractive surgery: an interactive case-based approach. Slack Incorporated; 2014.
4. Sinjab MM. Corneal topography in clinical practice (Pentacam System): basics & clinical interpretation. Jaypee Brothers Medical Publishers; 2012.

References, Suggested Reading, and Online Sources

Modern Optics Textbooks

1. American Academy of Ophthalmology. Basic and clinical science course, section 3: clinical optics, 2020-2021. San Francisco: American Academy of Ophthalmology; 2021.
2. Babbetts RB. Bennett and Rabbett's clinical visual optics. 4th ed. Philadelphia: Elsevier; 2007.
3. Bennett ES, Henry VA. Clinical manual of contact lenses. 5th ed. Philadelphia: Lipincott, Williams & Wilkins; 2019.
4. Brooks CW, Boorish IM. System for ophthalmic dispensing. 3rd ed. Oxford, UK: Butterworth-Heienemann; 2006.
5. Corboy JM. The retinoscopy book: an introductory manual for eye care professionals. Thorofare: Slack Incorporated; 2003.
6. Dowaliby M. Practical aspects of ophthalmic optics. 4th ed. Oxford, UK: Butterworth-Heinemann; 2000.
7. Elkington AR, Frank HJ, Greaney MJ. Clinical optics. 3rd ed. Hoboken: Wiley-Blackwell; 1999.
8. Hunter DG. Last-minute optics: a concise review of optics, refraction, and contact lenses. 2nd ed. Thorofare: Slack Incorporated; 2010.
9. Kaschke M, Donnerhacke KH, Rill MS. Optical devices in ophthalmology and optometry: technology, design principles and clinical applications. 1st ed. Weinheim: Wiley-VCH; 2014.
10. Katz M. Introduction to geometrical optics. 1st ed. Hackensack: World Scientific Publishing Company; 2002.
11. Keating MP. Geometric, physical, and visual optics. 2nd ed. Oxford, UK: Butterworth-Heinemann; 2001.
12. Shukla AV. Clinical optics primer for ophthalmic medical personnel: a guide to Laws, formulae, calculations, and clinical applications. 1st ed. Thorofare: Slack Incorporated; 2009.

Modern Ophthalmology Textbooks with Optics Sections

Chern KC, Saidel MA. Review questions in ophthalmology. 3rd ed. Philadelphia: Lipincott, Williams & Wilkins; 2018.

Chern KC, Saidel MA. Ophthalmology review manual. 2nd ed. Philadelphia: Lipincott, Williams & Wilkins; 2011.

Friedmann NJ, Kaiser PK, Trattler WB. Review of ophthalmology. 3rd ed. Philadelphia: Elsevier Saunders; 2017.

Luviano DM. Ophthalmology oral board review. 1st ed. Philadelphia: Lipincott, Williams & Wilkins; 2018.

Pemberton JD, Daniels A, Fay A. Ophthalmology clinical vignettes Oral exam study guide II. Little Rock: Crimson House Publishing; 2015.

Tamesis R. Ophthalmology board review: pearls of wisdom. 2nd ed. New York: McGraw-Hill; 2005.

Classic Optics Textbooks

Benjamin WJ. Borish's clinical refraction. 2nd ed. Waltham: Butterworth-Heinemann; 2006.

Campbell CJ. Physiological optics. New York: HarperCollins; 1974.

Duke-Elder S, Abrams D. System of ophthalmology – ophthalmic optics and refraction, vol. 5. Maryland Heights: CV Mosby Company; 1970.

Fry GA. Geometrical optics. Boston: Chilton Book Company; 1969.

Garcia GE. Handbook of refraction. 4th ed. New York: Little, Brown and Company; 1989.

Guyton DL, West CE, Miller JM, Wisnicki HJ. Ophthalmic optics and clinical refraction. Baltimore: Prism Press; 1999.

Henson DB. Optometric instrumentation. Oxford, UK: Butterworth-Heinemann; 1983.

MacInnis BJ. Ophthalmology board review of optics & refraction. Maryland Heights: Mosby, Inc; 1994.

Michaels DD. Basic refraction techniques. New York: Raven Press; 1988.

Milder B, Rubin ML. The fine art of prescribing glasses without making a spectacle of yourself. 3rd ed. Gainesville: Triad Publishing Company; 2004.

Rubin ML. Optics for clinicians. 2nd ed. Gainesville: Triad Publishing Company; 1974.

Reinecke RD, Herm RJ. Refraction: a programmed text. Norwalk: Appleton-Century-Crofts; 1976.

Online Resources: Texts and Lectures

American Academy of Ophthalmology OKAP and Board Review, sections on "Basic Optics", "Lens/Cataract" and "Refractive Surgery". https://www.aao.org/okap-study-presentations.

Ophthalmology Oral Board Review Course. Recorded lectures for written exams and oral exams for optics. www.osler.org/ophthalmology.

Online Resources: Question Banks

Basic and Clinical Science Course Self-Assessment Program. https://store.aao.org/basic-and-clinical-science-course-self-assessment-program.html.

Ophthalmology Question Bank. www.Ophthoquestions.com.

K. M. Riaz et al. (eds.), *Optics for the New Millennium*, https://doi.org/10.1007/978-3-030-95251-8

Index

K. M. Riaz et al. (eds.), *Optics for the New Millennium*, https://doi.org/10.1007/978-3-030-95251-8

C

D

E

F

O

P

MIX
Papier aus verantwortungsvollen Quellen
Paper from responsible sources
FSC® C105338

If you have any concerns about our products,
you can contact us on
ProductSafety@springernature.com

In case Publisher is established outside the EU,
the EU authorized representative is:
Springer Nature Customer Service Center GmbH
Europaplatz 3, 69115 Heidelberg, Germany

Printed by Libri Plureos GmbH
in Hamburg, Germany